Mechanisms of Vascular Disease
A Textbook for Vascular Surgeons

This textbook provides an up-to-date account of the mechanisms and pathophysiology of vascular disease, and the current treatment options open to vascular surgeons. As the scientific basis of vascular disease advances rapidly, it is critical that clinicians have access to relevant information written specifically for vascular surgeons. This account reviews the impact of these scientific advances on established and emerging treatment options. Experts from Australia, North America and Europe have contributed to basic topics such as atherosclerosis, restenosis, thrombosis and haemostasis, ischaemia-reperfusion injury, sepsis, vascular haemodynamics and wound healing. More applied topics such as pain syndromes in vascular surgery and the diabetic foot are also covered in this textbook. This will be a core text for all vascular surgical trainees and vascular surgeons, and specially appropriate for advanced trainees and consultants wishing to refresh their knowledge base.

ROBERT FITRIDGE is Associate Professor of Surgery at the University of Adelaide and Head of Vascular Surgery at the Queen Elizabeth Hospital, Woodville, Australia.

MATTHEW THOMPSON is Professor of Vascular Surgery at St George's Hospital Medical School, London, UK.

Mechanisms of Vascular Disease

A Textbook for Vascular Surgeons

Robert Fitridge
The Queen Elizabeth Hospital, Woodville, Australia
Matthew Thompson
St George's Hospital Medical School, London, UK

CAMBRIDGE
UNIVERSITY PRESS

MI

CAMBRIDGE UNIVERSITY PRESS
Cambridge, New York, Melbourne, Madrid, Cape Town, Singapore, São Paulo

Cambridge University Press
The Edinburgh Building, Cambridge CB2 8RU, UK

Published in the United States of America by Cambridge University Press, New York

www.cambridge.org
Information on this title: www.cambridge.org/9780521860635

First published 2007

Printed in the United Kingdom at the University Press, Cambridge

A catalogue record for this publication is available from the British Library

ISBN-13 978-0-521-86063-5 hardback

10/15/07

Contents

Contributors

Donald J. Adam
University Department of Vascular Surgery
Birmingham Heartlands Hospital
Bordesley Green East
Birmingham
UK

Tahir Ali
Academic Department of Surgery
St Thomas' Hospital
London
UK

Philip J. Barter
Heart Research Institute
Camperdown
New South Wales
Australia

Jill J. F. Belch
Division of Medicine
The Institute of Cardiovascular Research (TICR)
Ninewells Hospital and Medical School
Dundee
Scotland, UK

John Bingley
Department of Surgery
University of Queensland
Royal Brisbane Hospital
Queensland
Australia

Matthew Bown
Department of Surgery
University of Leicester
Leicester
UK

Andrew W. Bradbury
University Department of Vascular Surgery
Birmingham Heartlands Hospital
Bordesley Green East
Birmingham
UK

Nicholas P. J. Brindle
Department of Surgery and Cardiovascular Sciences
University of Leicester
Leicester
UK

Kevin Burnand
Academic Department of Surgery
St Thomas' Hospital
London
UK

Gordon Campbell
Department of Surgery
University of Queensland
Royal Brisbane Hospital
Queensland
Australia

Julie Campbell
Department of Surgery
University of Queensland
Royal Brisbane Hospital
Queensland
Australia

Philip Chan
Division of Clinical Sciences
University of Sheffield
Northern General Hospital
Sheffield
UK

Gloria A. Chin
Department of Surgery
University of Florida
Gainesville, FL
USA

Alexander W. Clowes
Department of Surgery
University of Washington
Seattle, WA
USA

Douglas Coghlan
Department of Haematology
Flinders Medical Centre
Bedford Park
South Australia
Australia

Prue A. Cowled
Department of Surgery
University of Adelaide
Queen Elizabeth Hospital
Woodville
South Australia
Australia

Helen C. S. Daly
MRF Building
Royal Perth Hospital
Perth
Western Australia
Australia

Robert F. Diegelmann
Department of Biochemistry
Medical College of Virginia
Richmond, VA
USA

John Evans
Department of Surgery
Leicester Royal Infirmary
Leicester
UK
and
Department of Vascular Surgery
St George's Hospital
London
UK

Robert A. Fitridge
Department of Surgery
University of Adelaide
Queen Elizabeth Hospital
Woodville
South Australia
Australia

John Fletcher
Westmead Hospital
Westmead
New South Wales
Australia

Gail Gillespie
MRF Building
Royal Perth Hospital
Perth
Western Australia
Australia

George Hamilton
University Department of Vascular Surgery
Royal Free Hospital
London
UK

Natalie J. Hayes
Department of Surgery
University of Leicester
Leicester
UK

Paul D. Hayes
Department of Surgery
University of Leicester
Leicester
UK

Patrick C. H. Hsieh
Department of Surgery
University of Washington
Seattle
WA
USA

Richard D. Kenagy
Department of Surgery
University of Washington
Seattle, WA
USA

Michael Lawrence-Brown
Centre for Health Services Research
School of Population Health
University of Western Australia
Nedlands
Western Australia
Australia

Peter E. Laws
Department of Surgery
University of Adelaide
Queen Elizabeth Hospital
Woodville
South Australia
Australia

Kurt Liffman
CSIRO Manufacturing and Infrastructure Technology and School of Mathematical Sciences
Monash University
Melbourne
Australia

Vidya Limaye
Department of Rheumatology,
Queen Elizabeth Hospital
Woodville
South Australia
Australia

Ian M. Loftus
Department of Vascular Surgery
St George's Hospital
London
UK

Lyle Moldawer
Department of Surgery
University of Florida
Gainesville, FL
USA

Mark J. McCarthy
Department of Surgery and Cardiovascular Sciences
University of Leicester
Leicester
UK

Kevin J. Molloy
Department of Vascular Surgery
St George's Hospital
London
UK

Stephen J. Nicholls
Department of Cardiovascular Medicine
Cleveland Clinic
Cleveland, OH, USA

Dean Patterson
Department of Vascular Medicine
University of Dundee
Scotland
UK

Janet T. Powell
University Hospitals Coventry and Warwickshire NHS Trust
Clifford Bridge Road
Coventry
UK

Denise M. Roach
Department of Surgery
University of Adelaide
Queen Elizabeth Hospital
Woodville
South Australia
Australia

Rachel C. Sam
University Department of Vascular Surgery
Birmingham Heartlands Hospital
Bordesley Green East
Birmingham
UK

Robert Sayers
Department of Cardiovascular Sciences
Leicester Royal Infirmary
Leicester
UK

Stephan A. Schug
MRF Building
Royal Perth Hospital
Perth
Western Australia
Australia

Gregory S. Schultz
Department of Obstetrics and Gynecology
University of Florida
Gainesville, FL
USA

James Semmens
Centre for Health Services Research
School of Population Health
University of Western Australia
Nedlands
Western Australia
Australia

Stanley H. Silverman
University Department of Vascular Surgery
Birmingham Heartlands Hospital
Bordesley Green East
Birmingham
UK

J. Ian Spark
Department of Vascular Surgery
St James University Hospital
Leeds
UK

Michael Stacey
University Department of Surgery
Fremantle Hospital
Fremantle
Western Australia
Australia

Kathryn J. D. Stannard
MRF Building
Royal Perth Hospital
Perth
Western Australia
Australia

Matthew M. Thompson
St George's Hospital Medical School
London
UK

Mathew Vadas
Department of Rheumatology
Queen Elizabeth Hospital
Woodville
South Australia
Australia

Mauro Vicaretti
Westmead Hospital
Westmead
New South Wales
Australia

Stella Vig
Department of Vascular Surgery
St George's Hospital
London
UK

Philip Walker
Department of Surgery
University of Queensland
Royal Brisbane Hospital
Queensland
Australia

Qingbo Xu
Department of Cardiological Sciences
St George's Hospital Medical School
London
UK

1 • The vascular endothelium: structure and function

VIDYA LIMAYE AND MATHEW VADAS

INTRODUCTION

The endothelium provides a cellular lining to all blood vessels in the circulatory system, and forms a structural barrier between the vascular space and the tissues. This cellular layer is no longer viewed as an inert structure, but rather has been recognized to be a dynamic organ, important in several house-keeping functions in health and disease. In adults, the endothelium weighs approximately 1 kg, comprises 1.6×10^{13} cells and has a surface area between 1–7 m^2 [1]. The endothelial cell (EC) is between 25–50 μm in length, 10–15 μm in width and up to 5 μm in depth. Each EC comes into contact with numerous smooth muscle cells and vice versa.

The location of the endothelium at the interface between the blood and vessel wall endows upon it an obligatory role in vasoregulation, the provision of an anti-thrombotic surface facilitating laminar blood flow, and selective permeability to haematopoietic cells and nutrients. These activities are most evident in the microcirculation where the endothelial cell surface area : blood volume ratio is maximal.

Nutrients and macromolecules may flow out of the bloodstream through intercellular spaces between ECs. These intercellular spaces are the result of cellular contraction and have been implicated in local oedema formation. Alternatively, nutrients may be actively transported by transcytosis through the cells themselves.

The endothelium is responsible for regulating the growth of the surrounding connective tissue. In its basal unactivated state, it prevents the proliferation of smooth muscle by the secretion of transforming growth factor-β (TGFβ) and by the surface expression of haparan-like molecules. When activated, however, cytokine/growth factor production by the deranged endothelium results in unchecked smooth muscle proliferation. Enhanced secretion of platelet-derived growth factor (PDGF) along with insulin-like growth factor (IGF) and basic fibroblast growth factor (bFGF) by the dysfunctional endothelium has mitogenic effects on smooth muscle cells, and plays a role in atherosclerotic plaque formation.

Endothelial activation may result from diverse insults such as disordered local cytokine production, viral infection, free radical formation or oxidation of lipids. Perturbations in endothelial function have been implicated in several diseases including atherosclerosis, cancer metastasis, inflammatory diseases and hypertension. Indeed anti-endothelial antibodies have been detected in diabetes mellitus, Raynaud's disease, scleroderma, Kawasaki's disease, vasculitides and in transplant rejection.

ANGIOGENESIS

Angiogenesis is the development of new blood vessels/capillaries from pre-existing vessels (as opposed to vasculogenesis which is the *de novo* formation of vessels important in embryogenesis) and is an essential process in normal growth. In the healthy adult, however, angiogenesis occurs only in select phases of the female reproductive cycle and as a protective mechanism in wound healing/tissue repair. Angiogenesis has been implicated as a key process in pathological conditions such as the proliferative phase of diabetic retinopathy, neovascularization of tumours and in inflammatory diseases such as rheumatoid arthritis. There has been considerable interest in the inhibition of angiogenesis as a therapeutic strategy and hence much research has focused on the underlying mechanisms regulating angiogenesis.

Recent evidence suggests that angiogenic ECs not only arise from contiguous ECs, but may also be derived from bone marrow derived EC precursors. These precursor cells are identified by characteristic cell surface antigen expression and have been demonstrated in the peripheral blood [2]. Bone marrow derived EC precursors have been shown to home to sites of angiogenesis and to be active participants in neovascularization in animal models of limb ischaemia [3; 4].

Angiogenesis involves the degradation of extracellular matrix (ECM) by EC, migration to the perivascular space, proliferation and formation of tubes to line the patent vessels, in association with pericytes. Survival of ECs is dependent on contact with like cells (cell-cell contact), as well as cell-matrix attachments.

Endothelial cell extracellular matrix attachments: the role of integrins

Attachments between the EC and surrounding ECM are mediated by the integrin group of cell surface adhesion receptors. Integrins provide adhesive and signalling functions between ECs and the ECM, and this interaction is critical in maintaining EC polarity and alignment along the vasculature. Integrins are heterodimeric proteins, comprising two non-covalently bound subunits, α and β. There are 18 α and 8 β subunits, which associate in various combinations to provide 24 different heterodimers [5]. The integrins present on ECs include β1, β3, β4, α1, α2, α3, α5, α6, αvβ3 and αvβ5.

Endothelial cell migration

The role of integrins

Migration of ECs involves the development of cell polarity and a leading edge (focal adhesion). The integrins link the cell with the ECM at the focal adhesion and then link with the actin cytoskeleton. This interaction stimulates cell contraction, thus allowing cell movement on adhesive contacts. The focal adhesion is of critical importance and is a site where regulatory proteins are identified. Focal adhesion kinase (FAK) is a cytoplasmic non-receptor tyrosine kinase which becomes phosphorylated on at least seven tyrosine residues when binding its ligands [6]. The FAK mediates its actions through various adaptor proteins and can ultimately activate cell movement via phosphatidyl-inositol-3-kinase (PI3) and Rac-1 (a G-protein).

Eventually integrin inactivation destroys the adhesive complex and allows detachment of the cell in its new location. Migratory deficits have been found in cells lacking FAK and reintroduction of FAK has been shown to restore migratory capacity in ECs [7].

Migration of ECs through the ECM is facilitated by matrix metalloproteinase (MMP) induced degradation of the ECM. Integrins play a role in the regulation of MMP activity. In ECs, α v β 3 not only stimulates MMP-2 production, but interacts with it, to activate the newly synthesized enzyme further [9]. This interaction is critical in EC migration, and indeed, inhibition of MMP-2/α vβ 3 binding has been shown to suppress angiogenesis [10].

The integrin αvβ3 is recognized as a key player in angiogenesis and is highly expressed on growing vessels. However, αvβ3 is barely detectable on quiescent endothelium [11; 12]. It can bind vitronectin, fibronectin, von Willebrand factor, fibrinogen and peptides containing the arginine-glycine-aspartate (RGD) motif. Which ligand binds αvβ3 in angiogenic states has not been established and although vitronectin is the ligand with greatest affinity for αvβ3, it is thought unlikely to be this. The integrin αvβ3 promotes extracellar signal-regulated kinase (ERK) activation and thus stimulates EC proliferation [13], and simultaneously inhibits p53 activity [14]. It promotes cell survival by activating NF-κ B [15]. By inducing cell motility [16] and facilitating ECM degradation (by interaction with MMP-2) [17], αvβ3 is critically important in angiogenesis. Furthermore, αvβ3 ligation promotes its association with vascular endothelial growth factor receptor-2 (VEGF-R2), thus augmenting VEGF-R2 signalling [18].

The use of a monoclonal antibody to αvβ3 (LM609) showed angiogenesis was inhibited in the chorioallantoic membrane assay for angiogenesis [12], thus further establishing the importance of this integrin in angiogenesis. The monoclonal antibody disrupted angiogenesis by promoting apoptosis, suggesting that in the absence of αvβ3 ligation by an endogenous ligand, protective signals are lost, with resultant EC apoptosis [19]. Consistent with this is the observation that disruption of αvβ3 ligation in ECs results in p53 expression in proliferating ECs [14].

The β1 integrins, expressed on both quiescent and growing blood vessels, are involved in cell adhesion and migration, and therefore are also important in angiogenesis. The α5β1 integrin is particularly important – α 5 negative teratocarcinomas have demonstrated reduced neovascularization and delayed tube formation *in vitro* [20]. Although α5β1 ligation enhances angiogenesis, this effect is thought to be secondary to regulation of α vβ 3 [21].

The role of sphingosine-1-phosphate

The bioactive sphingolipid metabolite sphingosine-1-phosphate (S1P), generated by the phosphorylation of membrane associated sphingosine by sphingosine kinase, is involved in cell proliferation and survival, suppression of apoptosis, migration, and angiogenesis. It is a specific ligand for a family of G protein coupled receptors (GPCR), of which five members have been identified (endothelial differentiation gene EDG-1, 3, 5, 6, 8) [22; 23]. The EDG receptors are ubiquitously expressed and most is known about EDG-1, which has been implicated in migration of ECs [24; 25; 26] and smooth muscle cells [27; 28]

The metabolite S1P interacts with PDGF (a factor known to promote cell motility) to enhance cell migration. The receptor for PDGF is physically associated with EDG-1 [29] and indeed migration of cells towards PDGF is dependent on EDG-1 [30].

Cell motility is further regulated by the *Rho* family of small GTPases – Rac, Rho, Cdc42. Binding of S1P to EDG-1 stimulates Rac activity, with cortical actin fibre formation [25; 31], whereas EDG-3 is involved in stress fibre formation [32].

Cell-cell contacts

Endothelial cells must form cell-cell contacts in order to form capillary like networks, and cell-cell adhesion is mediated by cell surface receptors, including vascular endothelial cadherin (VE cadherin) and platelet endothelial cell adhesion molecule-1 (PECAM-1).

Platelet endothelial cell adhesion molecule-1 (PECAM-1)

Platelet endothelial cell adhesion molecule-1 (CD31) is a 130 kDa member of the immunoglobulin superfamily and is normally highly expressed on the vasculature [33]. Heterophilic ligands for PECAM-1 include $\alpha v\beta 3$ [34], glycosaminoglycans [35] and CD38 [36]. It can also form homophilic interactions with itself on adjacent cells via domains 1–2 [37]. It has been proposed that PECAM-1 acts like a docking molecule, which allows other proteins (including integrins) to provide further strength to vascular structures.

Vascular endothelial cadherin (VE cadherin)

Cadherins are transmembrane proteins which form homophilic interactions in a calcium dependent fashion [38]. They provide weak adhesive cell-cell forces, further stabilized by the catenins, which are intracellular proteins linking the cadherin cell surface molecule to the actin cytoskeleton. Vascular endothelial cadherin is abundantly expressed at cell junctions, thus it is thought to be involved in angiogenesis.

E selectin

E selectin is a cell surface adhesion molecule which is primarily involved in leucocyte adhesion to the activated endothelium and is also thought to play a role in angiogenesis. There are normally negligible levels of E selectin on quiescent endothelium; however, it has been detected in non-inflammatory angiogenic tissues such as human placenta [39]. Antibodies to E selectin have been found to inhibit tube formation *in vitro* [40], and conversely, the addition of exogenous E selectin stimulates angiogenesis in the rat cornea [41].

Regulation of angiogenesis: a balance of angiostatic versus proangiogenic factors

Vascular remodelling reflects a balance between angiogenic versus angiostatic factors. Proangiogenic factors include growth factors such as PDGF, epidermal growth factor (EGF), insulin-like growth factor-1 (IGF-1), vascular endothelial growth factor (VEGF), and cytokines such as tumour necrosis factor α (TNFα) and interleukin-2.

Vascular endothelial growth factor is involved not only in angiogenesis but also in vasculogenesis [42]. It interacts with specific tyrosine kinase receptors, receptor 1 (VEGF-RI/flt1) and receptor 2 (VEGF-RII/flk), stimulating receptor autophosphorylation, and EC replication and migration. Mice deficient in VEGF have impaired angiogenesis and vasculogenesis, and die by day 9 of gestation [43].

Also important in vasculogenesis is another family of receptor tyrosine kinases, Tie 1 and Tie 2. Angiopoietin-1 is a specific ligand for Tie 2. Angiopoietin-1/Tie 2 ligation has no effects on tube formation and does not have mitogenic effects on ECs. Instead, angiopoietin-1 regulates the assembly of other components of the vessel wall including smooth muscle cells [42; 44]. Receptor–ligand interaction results in growth factor secretion, which in turn, stimulates the differentiation of surrounding mesenchymal cells into smooth muscle cells. Indeed, Tie 2 mutations in two human families resulted in venous malformations with the absence of smooth muscle cells in the vasculature. Angiopoietin-2 is a naturally occurring antagonist of angiopoietin-1 [45]. The identification of this negative regulator of the Tie 2 system indicates the need for extremely tight control of angiogenesis.

In this highly regulated fashion, therefore, VEGF is involved in the early assembly of the vascular tree and subsequent vessel maturation/stabilization is mediated by angiopoietin-1.

Chemokines are small secreted molecules with both chemoattractant and cytokine activity, which play a role in the regulation of leucocyte trafficking. Chemokines containing the ELR motif (Glu-Leu-Arg) are angiogenic (e.g. interleukin-8), whereas those lacking this critical motif are angiostatic (e.g. platelet factor-4). Angiostatic activity has been demonstrated in fragments of larger proteins, which themselves are not angiostatic [46], e.g. thrombospondin, fragments of fibronectin and prolactin. Angiostatin, a fragment of plasminogen, also inhibits angiogenesis [47] and is thought to be secreted by tumours. It has a long circulating half life and acts to control/inhibit the development of distant metastasis.

VASOREGULATION/ENDOTHELIAL REACTIVITY

Endothelial cells regulate vascular flow and basal vasomotor tone (hence blood pressure) by the highly controlled release of vasodilators (nitric oxide and the prostacyclin, PGI_2) and vasoconstrictors (endothelins and platelet activating factor). Nitric oxide and endothelins are the main regulators of basal vascular tone, and it is only when vascular function/haemodynamics are perturbed that prostaglandin I_2 (PGI_2) and platelet activating factor (PAF) come into play.

Nitric oxide

Nitric oxide (NO) is generated in ECs by the oxidation of L-arginine to L-citrulline by a family of enzymes, NO synthases (NOS) [48]. The endothelial NOS (eNOS) isoform is constitutively active, but is further induced by receptor dependent agonists such as thrombin, adenosine 5′-diphosphate, bradykinin and substance P [49]. Shear stress also stimulates eNOS activity, by virtue of a shear response consensus sequence GAGACC in the eNOS gene promoter [50].

Nitric oxide has pleiotropic effects on the vasculature. It causes vascular smooth muscle relaxation by binding to guanyl cyclase, hence maintaining basal vasomotor tone. It also plays a critical role in the inhibition of thrombosis by inhibiting platelet adhesion, activation and agonist-induced secretion, and in fact, it promotes platelet desegregation [51]. This is thought to be partly through a cyclic guanosine monophosphate (cGMP) dependent mechanism. By suppressing agonist-induced rise in intracellular calcium in platelets, it prevents the conformational change in glycoprotein IIb-IIIa [51; 52]. Nitric oxide also impairs phosphatidyl inositol 3-kinase (PI3-kinase) which normally facilitates conformational changes in glycoprotein IIb-IIIa. These two mechanisms act together to effectively prevent the binding of fibrinogen [53].

Endothelial cell-derived NO has effects beyond that on the vasculature. Nitric oxide inhibits leucocyte/EC adhesion [54; 55], and inhibits injury induced neointimal proliferation by inhibiting the proliferation [56] and migration [57] of smooth muscle cells.

Endothelins

The endothelins (ETs) are a family of 21 amino acid peptides, of which there are three members (ET-1, ET-2, ET-3). They are produced by diverse cell types, and serve to regulate vasomotor tone, cellular proliferation and hormone production. Endothelial cells produce only ET-1, which is also synthesized by vascular smooth muscle cells. Production of ET-1 is induced by hypoxia, ischaemia and shear stress, which induce the transcription of ET-1 mRNA, with prompt secretion of ET-1 within minutes. The kinetics of ET-1 synthesis allow sophisticated regulation of basal vascular tone, as the half life of ET-1 protein and mRNA is 4–7 minutes and 15–20 minutes, respectively [58]. The majority of plasma ET-1 (90%) is cleared by the lung during first passage [59]. The majority (up to 75%) of ET-1 secretion is towards the abluminal side of the EC and thus it acts in a paracrine manner by binding to specific receptors on smooth muscle cells, to cause vasoconstriction [60]. The endothelin ET-2 is produced in the kidney and intestine, while ET-3 has been detected in the brain, gastrointestinal tract, lung and kidney [61].

Synthesis of endothelins

The gene encoding ET-1 is on chromosome 6 [62]. The promoter contains regulatory sites for stimuli such as shear stress, thrombin, hypoxia, growth factors, catecholamines and angiotensin II, which act to induce transcription of ET-1 mRNA. Negative feedback is provided by ET-3, prostacyclin and atrial natriuretic hormone, which inhibit transcription. These factors not only regulate transcription, but can also provide negative feedback at a translational level [63; 64].

Each endothelin is synthesized as a larger precursor, preproendothelin-1 (203 amino acids), which is degraded to the prohormone Big endothelin-1 (39 amino acids). Big endothelin-1 is secreted by ECs into the plasma and has approximately 1% of the potency of ET-1. Endothelin converting enzyme cleaves Big endothelin-1 to generate ET-1 [65].

Production of ET-1 is influenced by other vasoactive substances, vascular stress and numerous hormones (angiotensin II, vasopressin, thrombin, TGFβ, IGF-1, EGF, bFGF), and high and low density lipoproteins. In fact, it is thought that it may be the endothelins which exert the vasoconstriction which is seen in response to some of these stimuli. Conversely, NO and prostacyclin act to inhibit ET-1 production, and this has been shown to be mediated by production of cGMP [66; 67].

Endothelin receptors

There are two endothelin receptors (Type A and B), to which all three endothelins may bind. Type A receptors present on vascular smooth muscle and cardiac myocytes preferentially bind ET-1 with high affinity [68] and are thought responsible for the majority of ET-1 induced vasoconstriction. Ligand binding activates phospholipase C, with the subsequent formation of inositol 1,4,5 triphosphate and diacylglycerol, and a resultant increase in intracellular calcium and vasoconstriction [69]. The rise in intracellular calcium along with diacylglycerol activates protein kinase C, thus accounting for the mitogenic effects of ET-1 [70]. Disassociation of ET-1 from its receptor is outlived by the vasoconstrictive effect, due to the persisting elevated intracellular calcium concentration [71]. Importantly, NO acts to restore the intracellular calcium concentration, thus limiting the duration of the vasoconstrictive response [72]. In atherosclerosis, the protective effects of NO are abolished and thus the unopposed actions of ET-1 result in greatly heightened vasoconstriction [73]. After acute myocardial infarction, in which there is catecholamine induced reduction in the threshold for ventricular arrhythmias, the interaction of ET-1 with the Type A receptor is also important as a protective response and serves to suppress electrical excitability.

Type B receptors are mainly present on ECs [74], but are also detected on smooth muscle cells. Type B receptors are linked to G proteins, which may inhibit cyclic adenosine monophosphate (cAMP), but otherwise their effects are similar to Type A receptors, with phospholipase C activation. They bind ET-1 and ET-3 with similar affinity. The interaction of ET-3 with the Type B receptor is important in the development of cells from neural crest origin. In the absence of ET-3 or in the setting of Type B receptor dysfunction, ganglionic neurons in the intestine fail to develop [75]. Indeed, an inactivating mutation of the Type B receptor has been shown to be associated with a hereditary form of Hirschsprung's disease [76].

Expression of both endothelin receptors is under tight control and their expression often parallels that of the endothelins. Hypoxia induces ET Type A receptor expression and circulating ETs in an attempt to maintain local tissue perfusion.

Effects on the vasculature

The endothelin ET-1 is the most potent known endogenous vasoconstrictor and on a molar basis is 100 times more potent than noradrenaline [77]. Binding to Type A receptors mediates the majority of the vasoconstrictive effect [68; 78], and activation of Type B receptors in the coronary circulation and on other vascular smooth muscle, contributes to a lesser degree [79]. Catecholamines and noradrenaline act in concert with ET-1, each potentiating each other's effects.

Endothelins in disease

There is now convincing evidence that endothelins are involved in various pathological states. Plasma ET-1 levels are normal in essential hypertension but are raised in women with pre-eclampsia [1]. Elevated plasma concentrations of ETs are found in congestive cardiac failure and have prognostic value in this setting [80]. They are also shown to cause bronchoconstriction *in vivo*, an effect which may play a role in the development of pulmonary hypertension. Endothelins have been implicated in vascular diseases of the kidney and cyclosporin induced nephrotoxicity. Plasma ET levels are elevated after ischaemic cerebral infarction [81] and in patients with vasospasm occurring in the context of subarachnoid hemorrhage [82]. An endothelial receptor antagonist, bosentan is now available for the treatment of pulmonary hypertension.

Prostacyclin (PGI_2)

The prostacyclin PGI_2 is an eicosanoid which is not synthesized under resting conditions, but rather its production is induced by disturbances in endothelial function or vascular haemodynamics. It is released from ECs [83] and acts in a paracrine manner. It binds to a specific receptor on platelets and vascular smooth muscle cells to limit vasoconstriction and influence platelet deposition [84].

Platelet activating factor (PAF)

Platelet activating factor is a phospholipid which remains bound to the EC surface and acts in a juxtacrine fashion by binding to its receptor present on leucocytes. It is not constitutively produced and thus not a regulator of basal vasomotor tone. When infused intravenously it has variable effects on vascular dynamics ranging from vasodilatation to vasoconstriction, depending on the dose administered and the vascular bed involved. Its most important effect is in recruiting leucocytes to the EC surface, and its effects on vascular tone are indirect and exerted through the generation of other eicosanoids and leukotrienes [85].

ENDOTHELIUM IN INFLAMMATION

The endothelium plays a critical function in regulating the trafficking of leucocytes from the intravascular space to extravascular sites of inflammation. The mechanisms underlying leucocyte transmigration have been the focus of much attention and the role of adhesion molecules in this process is now well established. The main families of adhesion proteins involved in this process are the selectins, integrins, immunoglobulin supergene family and variants of the CD44 family.

The initial step in leucocyte transmigration is the arrest of leucocytes and random contact with the ECs. This step is mediated by the selectins, which allow the tethering and rolling of the leucocyte on the EC surface [86]. Increasing adhesion occurs with activation of the leucocyte integrins, leucocyte function-associated antigen-1 (LFA-1) and very late antigen-4 (VLA-4). The leucocytes then flatten and migrate along the endothelium, a process known as diapedesis. Extravasation occurs by the migration through EC junctions and subsequent attachment/migration on extracellular matrix components (fibronectin and collagen).

A normal quiescent endothelium does not bind leucocytes – it is only the activated endothelium, in response to cytokines including IL-1, TNFα and lipopolysaccharide, which expresses adhesion molecules and thus can bind leucocytes. Indeed inhibitors of IL-1 (anakinra, an IL-1 receptor antagonist) and TNFα (infliximab, a chimeric monoclonal antibody to TNFα, or etanercept, a Fc- receptor fusion protein) have shown profound therapeutic benefit in inflammatory conditions such as rheumatoid arthritis.

Selectins

All three members of the selectin family (E-selectin L-selectin and P-selectin) are characterized by a C-terminal lectin like domain which binds complex carbohydrates and all are involved in leucocyte recruitment to sites of inflammation. E-selectin (CD62) is a 115 kD antigen which is absent in normal tissues, but is found on the endothelium of post-capillary venules in inflammatory conditions, e.g. rheumatoid arthritis, and the skin in scleroderma. It is induced on ECs after IL-1 or TNFα stimulation. Expression of E-selectin depends on *de novo* protein synthesis, and expression at the cell surface peaks between four and six hours post stimulation. Expression is only transient and levels return to basal levels after 24 hours. It has a C type lectin binding domain, an epidermal growth factor (EGF)-like domain and six complement regulatory protein regions. E-selectin binds a surface glycoprotein, sialyl-Le^x or sialy-Le^y on neutrophils, monocytes and selected subpopulations of lymphocytes.

L-selectin is constitutively expressed on leucocytes and functions in leucocyte recirculation to the lymph nodes, and hence is known as the 'peripheral node homing receptor'. It is also important in leucocyte recruitment to inflammatory sites.

P-selectin (ELAM-1) is stored in the Weibel-Palade bodies (secretory granules) of ECs and platelets. Upon endothelial activation, it undergoes rapid translocation to the cell surface, where it binds cell surface mucin on neutrophils and monocytes.

Integrins

Integrins relevant to leucocyte recruitment are $\beta 1$ (VLA family) and the β 2 integrins. The β 1 integrins α 5β 1 and α 6β 1 mediate binding to the extracellular matrix (fibronectin and laminin, respectively), whereas α 4β 1 principally binds cell surface VCAM-1. The β 2 integrins are present only on leucocytes and their activity depends on conformational changes that occur on leucocyte activation. The β 2 integrins, LFA-1 and Mac-1, both bind intercellular adhesion molecules (ICAMs). The presence of chemokines in the vicinity of the activated endothelium, in conjunction with engagement of selectins, results in leucocyte activation. When activated, the β 2 integrins on leucocytes that are slowly rolling along the endothelium bind ICAM-1 and ICAM-2 on the EC surface. It is this integrin – immunoglobulin superfamily interaction which mediates firm adhesion and is essential for extravasation to occur.

Immunoglobulin gene superfamily

The immunoglobulin gene superfamily comprises numerous cell surface molecules including T cell receptors (CD4, CD8, CD3 and major histocompatibility complex (MHC) class I and II) and adhesion molecules (ICAM-1, ICAM-2, ICAM-3 and VCAM-1). Of the numerous immunoglobulin gene superfamily members, ICAM-1 and VCAM-1 are most relevant to leucocyte transmigration. The adhesion molecule ICAM-1 is constitutively expressed but is further induced by the cytokines IL-1, TNFα and PAF. It is highly expressed on the activated endothelium and is particularly important in mediating the firm adhesion of neutrophils on ECs by acting as a ligand for leucocyte β 2 integrins, and in transendothelial migration by binding LFA-1 and Mac-1 on neutrophils. It has also been implicated in eosinophil migration into the lung in experimental models of allergen induced asthma. Administration of IL-1 or TNFαcauses a gradual rise in ICAM-1 expression, peaking at 24 hours, with continued upregulation for 24–72 hours. This relatively delayed expression pattern is again consistent with its role in the later rather than the initial stages of neutrophil transmigration.

There are two isoforms of VCAM-1 containing six or seven extracellular immunoglobulin like domains and it is the isoform containing seven domains which is expressed on the vascular endothelium. Stimuli for the induction of VCAM include IL-1, TNFα and lipopolysaccharide. Maximum up-regulation takes several hours. The isoform VCAM-1 is a ligand for α 4β 1 (VLA-4) and leucocyte α 4β 7 integrin.

CD44 family

CD44 is the principal receptor that binds hyaluronate, and lymphocytes may use CD44 to form adhesions while rolling on EC surfaces exposing hyaluronate.

The endothelium in cell-mediated immunity

Another function of ECs is in antigen presentation to specific T cells in peripheral tissues. This is important in cell-mediated immunity. Both class I and class II MHC are constitutively expressed by microvascular ECs, but can be induced further by cytokines such as interferon gamma. Endothelial cells can activate only memory T cells [87], in contrast to classical antigen presenting cells which can induce both naïve and memory T cells. In fact, ECs have been described to induce clonal anergy (the prevention of naïve T cells from responding to stimulation) [88].

COAGULATION

The quiescent endothelium possesses anticoagulant activity, and indeed, a pivotal function of the endothelium is to provide an anti-thrombotic surface which inhibits the coagulation cascade. One of the major strategies used by ECs to maintain anticoagulant activity is to prevent activation of thrombin which, if activated, stimulates coagulation by causing platelet activation and the activation of several coagulation factors. Endothelial cells express haparan sulphate which along with glycosaminoglycans in the ECM, stimulates antithrombin-III [89]. They express tissue factor pathway inhibitor (TFPI), which prevents thrombin formation [90], and express thrombomodulin [91]. Thrombin–thrombomodulin interaction activates protein C, which has strong anticoagulant activity. Endothelial cells in fact synthesize protein S, a cofactor for activated protein C. Hence in the healthy endothelium, the balance is towards anticoagulant factors. Endothelial damage, however, results in the endothelium acquiring procoagulant activity in its own right.

The procoagulant activity of the deranged endothelium

An activated endothelium may promote coagulation. Bacterial endotoxin, inflammatory cytokines (e.g. IL-1) and glycosylated proteins may activate the endothelium and promote procoagulant activity. The critical change which occurs on the ECs in the transformation from an endothelial surface with anticoagulant phenotype, to one with procoagulant effects, is the expression of tissue factor (TF). Tissue factor is not detected on the normal endothelium [92]. *In vitro*, agonists capable of inducing TF include thrombin, endotoxin, cytokines, hypoxia, shear stress and oxidized lipoproteins [93]. Tissue factor stimulates the activation of factor IX and factor X, and stimulates prothrombinase activity, with subsequent fibrin formation [94]. The thrombin receptor (protease activated receptor-1, PAR-1) is an EC surface coagulation protein binding site. Binding of thrombin to its receptor causes alterations in the EC surface expression of PAI-1, TF, NO, PAF, ET and PGI_2 [95], and also induces EC permeability by disrupting tight junctions [96]. Tissue factor expression is induced after vascular injury [97] and it has been found in association with ECs in atherosclerotic plaques [98; 99].

Two additional thrombin receptors have been identified – PAR-2 and PAR-3. Some ECs express both PAR-1 and PAR-2, however, PAR-3 has not been identified on ECs.

Endothelial cells and fibrinolysis

Plasminogen activators include tissue plasminogen activator (tPA), urokinase-type plasminogen activator (uPA) and kallikrein. Tissue plasminogen activator is synthesized by ECs and is released as a single chain zymogen, which undergoes proteolytic cleavage to form a two-chain structure, tPA. Stimuli for the formation of tPA include exercise, venous occlusion, vasodilation, thrombin and cytokines. In the plasma, tPA binds the inhibitor, plasminogen activator inhibitor-1 (PAI-1). In healthy states, PAI-1 is in excess, and hence tPA fails to activate plasminogen.

Plasminogen activator inhibitor-1 circulates in much higher concentration than tPA in normal conditions with more than 90% of the total blood PAI-1 being contained within platelets. However, the endothelium and liver are thought to be the main sources of plasma PAI-1. Indeed it is the plasma form of PAI-1 which is mainly active, as opposed to the platelet form which is essentially latent. Synthesis of PAI-1 is stimulated by thrombin, cytokines, lipoprotein a and oxidized low density lipoprotein [100].

Urokinase-type plasminogen activator is not constitutively expressed, but rather it is found in sites of wound repair or angiogenesis [101].

Thrombin–thrombomodulin interactions result in activation of the protein thrombin activatable fibrinolysis inhibitor (TAFI) [102]. This results in a loss of plasmin and tPA binding sites on fibrin, with impaired fibrinolysis. Thus ECs cells reduce the rate of intravascular fibrinolysis through the cell surface expression of thrombomodulin.

CONCLUSIONS

Advances in the understanding of endothelial function/physiology have been the basis for many therapeutic strategies. Many pharmacological interventions have been targeted to the endothelium with the intent of restoring it to its quiescent state. It is foreseeable that expanding the understanding of endothelial function further will lead to targeted therapies to a myriad of diseases, including cancer, cardiovascular disease and inflammatory conditions.

REFERENCES

1. H. G. Augustin, D. H. Kozian & R. C. Johnson, Differentiation of endothelial cells: analysis of the constitutive and activated endothelial cell phenotypes. *Bioassays*, **16**(12) (1994), 901–6.
2. T. Asahara, T. Murohara, A. Sullivan *et al.*, Isolation of putative progenitor endothelial cells for angiogenesis. *Science*, **275** (1997), 964–7.
3. C. Kalka, H. Masuda, T. Takahashi *et al.*, Transplantation of *ex vivo* expanded endothelial progenitor cells for therapeutic neovascularization. *Proceedings of the National Academy of Sciences of the USA*, **97**(7) (2000), 3422–7.
4. T. Murohara, H. Ikeda, J. Duan *et al.*, Transplanted cord blood-derived endothelial precursor cells augment postnatal neovascularization. *Journal of Clinical Investigation*, **105**(11) (2000), 1527–36.
5. R. O. Hynes Cell adhesion: old and new questions. *Trends in Cell Biology*, **9**(12) (1999), M33–7.
6. C. K. Miranti & J. S. Brugge, Sensing the environment: a historical perspective on integrin signal transduction. *Nature Cell Biology*, **4**(4) (2000), E83–90.
7. D. J. Sieg, C. R. Hauck, D. Ilic *et al.*, FAK integrates growth-factor and integrin signals to promote cell

migration. *Nature Cell Biology*, **2**(5) (2000), 249–56.

8. R. A. Klinghoffer, C. Sachsenmaier, J. A. Cooper & P. Soriano, Src family kinases are required for integrin but not PDGFR signal transduction. *EMBO Journal*, **18**(9) (1999), 2459–71.
9. S. Silletti, T. Kessler, J. Goldberg, D. L. Boger & D. A. Cheresh, Disruption of matrix metalloproteinase 2 binding to integrin alpha vbeta 3 by an organic molecule inhibits angiogenesis and tumor growth *in vivo*. *Proceedings of the National Academy of Sciences of the USA*, **98**(1) (2001), 119–24.
10. D. L. Boger, J. Goldberg, S. Silletti, T. Kessler & D. A. Cheresh, Identification of a novel class of small-molecule antiangiogenic agents through the screening of combinatorial libraries which function by inhibiting the binding and localization of proteinase MMP2 to integrin alpha (V)beta (3). *Journal of the American Chemical Society*, **123**(7) (2001), 1280–8.
11. L. Bello, M. Francolini, P. Marthyn *et al.*, Alpha (v)beta 3 and alpha (v)beta 5 integrin expression in glioma periphery. *Neurosurgery*, **49**(2) (2001), 380–9.
12. P. C. Brooks, R. A. Clark & D. A. Cheresh, Requirement of vascular integrin alpha vbeta 3 for angiogenesis. *Science*, **264**(1994), 569–71.
13. B. P. Eliceiri, R. Klemke, S. Stromblad & D. A. Cheresh, Integrin alpha vbeta 3 requirement for sustained mitogen-activated protein kinase activity during angiogenesis. *Journal of Cell Biology*, **140**(5) (1998), 1255–63.
14. S. Stromblad, J. C. Becker, M. Yebra, P. C. Brooks & D. H. Cheresh, Suppression of p53 activity and p21WAF1/ CIP1 expression by vascular cell integrin alpha Vbeta 3 during angiogenesis. *Journal of Clinical Investigation*, **98**(2) (1996), 426–33.
15. M. Scatena, M. Almeida, M. L. Chaisson *et al.*, NF-kappaB mediates alpha vbeta 3 integrin-induced endothelial cell survival. *Journal of Cell Biology*, **141**(4) (1998), 1083–93.
16. D. I. Leavesley, M. A. Schwartz, M. Rosenfeld & D. A., Cheresh, Integrin beta 1- and beta 3-mediated endothelial cell migration is triggered through distinct signaling mechanisms. *Journal of Cell Biology*, **121**(1) (1993), 163–70.
17. P. C. Brooks, S. Stromblad, L. C. Sanders *et al.*, Localization of matrix metalloproteinase MMP-2 to the surface of invasive cells by interaction with integrin alpha vbeta 3. *Cell*, **85**(5) (1996), 683–93.
18. R. Soldi, S. Mitola, M. Strasly *et al.*, Role of alpha vbeta 3 integrin in the activation of vascular endothelial growth factor receptor-2. *EMBO Journal*, **18**(4) (1999), 882–92.
19. P. C. Brooks, A. M. Montgomery, M. Rosenfeld *et al.*, Integrin alpha vbeta 3 antagonists promote tumor regression by inducing apoptosis of angiogenic blood vessels. *Cell*, **79**(7) (1994), 1157–64.
20. D. Taverna & R. O. Hynes, Reduced blood vessel formation and tumor growth in alpha 5-integrin-negative teratocarcinomas and embryoid bodies. *Cancer Research*, **61**(13) (2001), 5255–61.
21. S. Kim, K. Bell, S. A. Mousa & J. A. Varner, Regulation of angiogenesis *in vivo* by ligation of integrin alpha 5beta 1 with the central cell-binding domain of fibronectin. *American Journal of Pathology*, **156**(4) (2000), 1345–62.
22. S. Pyne & N. J. Pyne, Sphingosine 1-phosphate signalling in mammalian cells. *Biochemical Journal*, **349**(Pt 2) (2000), 385–402.
23. S. Spiegel & S. Milstien, Functions of a new family of sphingosine-1-phosphate receptors. *Biochimica et Biophysica Acta*, **1484**(2–3) (2000), 107–16.
24. D. English, Z. Welch, A. T. Kovala *et al.*, Sphingosine 1-phosphate released from platelets during clotting accounts for the potent endothelial cell chemotactic activity of blood serum and provides a novel link between hemostasis and angiogenesis. *FASEB Journal*, **14**(14) (2000), 2255–65.
25. M. J. Lee, S. Thangada, K. P. Claffey *et al.*, Vascular endothelial cell adherens junction assembly and morphogenesis induced by sphingosine-1-phosphate. *Cell*, **99**(3) (1999), 301–12.
26. F. Wang, J. R. Van Brocklyn, J. P. Hobson *et al.*, Sphingosine 1-phosphate stimulates cell migration through a G(i)-coupled cell surface receptor. Potential involvement in angiogenesis. *Journal of Biological Chemistry*, **274**(50) (199), 35343–350.
27. G. Boguslawski, J. R. Grogg, Z. Welch *et al.*, Migration of vascular smooth muscle cells induced by sphingosine 1-phosphate and related lipids: potential role in the angiogenic response. *Experimental Cell Research*, **274**(2) (2000), 264–74.
28. J. P. Hobson, H. M. Rosenfeldt, L. S. Barak *et al.*, Role of the sphingosine-1-phosphate receptor EDG-1 in PDGF-induced cell motility. *Science*, **291**(2001), 1800–3.

29. F. Alderton, S. Rakhit, K. C. Kong *et al.*, Tethering of the platelet-derived growth factor beta receptor to G-protein-coupled receptors. A novel platform for integrative signaling by these receptor classes in mammalian cells. *Journal of Biological Chemistry*, **276**(30) (2001), 28578–85.
30. H. M. Rosenfeldt, J. P. Hobson, M. Maceyka *et al.*, EDG-1 links the PDGF receptor to Src and focal adhesion kinase activation leading to lamellipodia formation and cell migration. *FASEB Journal*, **15**(14) (2001), 2649–59.
31. Y. Liu, R. Wada, T. Yamashita *et al.*, EDG-1, the G protein-coupled receptor for sphingosine-1-phosphate, is essential for vascular maturation. *Journal of Clinical Investigation*, **106**(8) (2000), 951–61.
32. H. Okamoto, N. Takuwa, T. Yokomizo *et al.*, Inhibitory regulation of Rac activation, membrane ruffling, and cell migration by the G protein-coupled sphingosine-1-phosphate receptor EDG5 but not EDG1 or EDG3. *Molecular Cell Biology*, **20**(24) (2001), 9247–61.
33. P. J. Newman, M. C. Berndt, J. Gorski *et al.*, PECAM-1 (CD31) cloning and relation to adhesion molecules of the immunoglobulin gene superfamily. *Science*, **247** (1990), 1219–22.
34. L. Piali, P. Hammel, C. Uherek *et al.*, CD31/PECAM-1 is a ligand for alpha vbeta 3 integrin involved in adhesion of leukocytes to endothelium. *Journal of Cell Biology*, **130**(2) (1995), 451–60.
35. W. A. Muller, M. E. Berman, P. J. Newman, H. M. DeLisser & S. M. Albelda, A heterophilic adhesion mechanism for platelet/endothelial cell adhesion molecule 1 (CD31). *Journal of Experimental Medicine*, **175**(5) (1992), 1401–4.
36. A. L. Horenstein, H. Stockinger, B. A. Imhof & F. Malavasi, CD38 binding to human myeloid cells is mediated by mouse and human CD31. *Biochemical Journal*, **330**(Pt 3) (1998), 1129–35.
37. J. P. Newton, C. D. Buckley, E. Y. Jones & D. L. Simmons, Residues on both faces of the first immunoglobulin fold contribute to homophilic binding sites of PECAM-1/CD31. *Journal of Biological Chemistry*, **272**(33) (1997), 20555–63.
38. E. Dejana, Endothelial adherens junctions: implications in the control of vascular permeability and angiogenesis. *Journal of Clinical Investigation*, **98**(9) (1996), 1949–53.
39. B. M. Kraling, M. J. Razon, L. M. Boon *et al.*, E-selectin is present in proliferating endothelial cells in human hemangiomas. *American Journal of Pathology*, **148**(4) (1996), 1181–91.
40. M. Nguyen, N. A. Strubel & J. Bischoff, A role for sialyl Lewis-X/A glycoconjugates in capillary morphogenesis. *Nature*, (1993), 267–9.
41. A. E. Koch, M. M. Halloran, C. J. Haskell, M. R. Shah & P. J. Polverini, Angiogenesis mediated by soluble forms of E-selectin and vascular cell adhesion molecule-1. *Nature* **376** (1995), 517–19.
42. J. Folkman & P. A. D'Amore, Blood vessel formation: what is its molecular basis? *Cell*, **87**(7) (1996), 1153–5.
43. N. Ferrara, K. Carver-Moore, H. Chen *et al.*, Heterozygous embryonic lethality induced by targeted inactivation of the VEGF gene. *Nature*, **380** (1996), 439–42.
44. S. Davis, T. H. Aldrich, P. F. Jones *et al.*, Isolation of angiopoietin-1, a ligand for the Tie 2 receptor, by secretion-trap expression cloning. *Cell*, **87**(7) (1996), 1161–9.
45. P. C. Maisonpierre, C. Suri, P. F. Jones *et al.*, Angiopoietin-2, a natural antagonist for Tie 2 that disrupts *in vivo* angiogenesis. *Science*, **277**(5322) (1997), 55–60.
46. D. Hanahan & J. Folkman, Patterns and emerging mechanisms of the angiogenic switch during tumorigenesis. *Cell*, **86**(3) (1996), 353–64.
47. M. S. O'Reilly, L. Holmgren, Y. Shing *et al.*, Angiostatin: a novel angiogenesis inhibitor that mediates the suppression of metastases by a Lewis lung carcinoma. *Cell*, **79**(2) (1994), 315–28.
48. J. S. Stamler, D. J. Singel & J. Loscalzo, Biochemistry of nitric oxide and its redox-activated forms. *Science*, **258** (1992), 1898–902.
49. J. N. Topper, J. Cai, D. Falb & M. A. Gimbrone, Jr, Identification of vascular endothelial genes differentially responsive to fluid mechanical stimuli: cyclooxygenase-2, manganese superoxide dismutase, and endothelial cell nitric oxide synthase are selectively up-regulated by steady laminar shear stress. *Proceedings of the National Academy of Sciences of the USA*, **93**(19) (1996), 10417–22.
50. R. C. Venema, K. Nishida, R. W. Alexander, D. G. Harrison & T. J. Murphy, Organization of the bovine gene encoding the endothelial nitric oxide synthase. *Biochimica et Biophysica Acta*, **1218**(3) (1994), 413–20.
51. M. E. Mendelsohn, S. O'Neill, D. George & J. Loscalzo, Inhibition of fibrinogen binding to human platelets by

S-nitroso-N-acetylcysteine. *Journal of Biological Chemistry*, **265**(31) (1990), 19028–34.

52. A. D. Michelson, S. E. Benoit, M. I. Furman, *et al.*, Effects of nitric oxide/EDRF on platelet surface glycoproteins. *American Journal of Physiology*, **270**(5) (1996), H1640–8.
53. A. Pigazzi, S. Heydrick, F. Folli *et al.*, Nitric oxide inhibits thrombin receptor-activating peptide-induced phosphoinositide 3-kinase activity in human platelets. *Journal of Biological Chemistry*, **274**(20) (1999), 14368–75.
54. R. De Caterina, P. Libby, H. B. Peng *et al.*, Nitric oxide decreases cytokine-induced endothelial activation. Nitric oxide selectively reduces endothelial expression of adhesion molecules and proinflammatory cytokines. *Journal of Clinical Investigation*, **96**(1) (1995), 60–8.
55. P. Kubes, M. Suzuki & D. N. Granger, Nitric oxide: an endogenous modulator of leukocyte adhesion. *Proceedings of the National Academy of Sciences of the USA*, **88** AB(11) (1991), 4651–5.
56. U. C. Garg & A. Hassid, Nitric oxide-generating vasodilators and 8-bromo-cyclic guanosine monophosphate inhibit mitogenesis and proliferation of cultured rat vascular smooth muscle cells. *Journal of Clinical Investigation*, **83**(5) (1989), 1774–7.
57. D. S. Marks, J. A. Vita, J. D. Folts *et al.*, Inhibition of neointimal proliferation in rabbits after vascular injury by a single treatment with a protein adduct of nitric oxide. *Journal of Clinical Investigation*, **96**(6) (1995), 2630–8.
58. A. Inoue, M. Yanagisawa, Y. Takuwa *et al.*, The human preproendothelin-1 gene. Complete nucleotide sequence and regulation of expression. *Journal of Biological Chemistry*, **264**(25) (1989), 14954–9.
59. G. de Nucci, R. Thomas, P. D'Orleans-Juste *et al.*, Pressor effects of circulating endothelin are limited by its removal in the pulmonary circulation and by the release of prostacyclin and endothelium-derived relaxing factor. *Proceedings of the National Academy of Sciences of the USA*, **85**(24) (1988), 9797–800.
60. S. Yoshimoto, Y. Ishizaki, T. Sasaki & S. Murota, Effect of carbon dioxide and oxygen on endothelin production by cultured porcine cerebral endothelial cells. *Stroke*, **22**(3) (1991), 378–83.
61. O. Shinmi, S. Kimura, T. Sawamura *et al.*, Endothelin-3 is a novel neuropeptide: isolation and sequence determination of endothelin-1 and endothelin-3 in porcine brain. *Biochemical and Biophysical Research Communications*, **164**(1) (1989), 587–93.
62. M. E. Lee, K. D. Bloch, J. A. Clifford & T. Quertermous, Functional analysis of the endothelin-1 gene promoter. Evidence for an endothelial cell-specific cis-acting sequence. *Journal of Biological Chemistry*, **265**(18) (1990), 10446–50.
63. R. M. Hu, E. R. Levin, A. Pedram & H. J. Frank, Atrial natriuretic peptide inhibits the production and secretion of endothelin from cultured endothelial cells. Mediation through the C receptor. *Journal of Biological Chemistry*, **267**(24) (1992), 17384–9.
64. R. M. Hu, M. Y. Chuang, B. Prins *et al.*, High density lipoproteins stimulate the production and secretion of endothelin-1 from cultured bovine aortic endothelial cells. *Journal of Clinical Investigation*, **93**(3) (1994), 1056–62.
65. D. Xu, N. Emoto, A. Giaid *et al.*, ECE-1: a membrane-bound metalloprotease that catalyzes the proteolytic activation of Big endothelin-1. *Cell*, **78**(3) (1994), 473–85.
66. C. Boulanger & T. F. Luscher, Release of endothelin from the porcine aorta. Inhibition by endothelium-derived nitric oxide. *Journal of Clinical Investigation*, **85**(2) (1990), 587–90.
67. B. A. Prins, R. M. Hu, B. Nazario *et al.*, Prostaglandin E2 and prostacyclin inhibit the production and secretion of endothelin from cultured endothelial cells. *Journal of Biological Chemistry*, **269**(16) (1994), 11938–44.
68. H. Arai, S. Hori, I. Aramori, H. Ohkubo & S. Nakanishi, Cloning and expression of a cDNA encoding an endothelin receptor. *Nature*, **348** (1990), 730–2.
69. M. S. Simonson & M. J. Dunn, Cellular signaling by peptides of the endothelin gene family. *FASEB Journal* **4**(12) (1990), 2989–3000.
70. M. S. Simonson & W. H. Herman, Protein kinase C and protein tyrosine kinase activity contribute to mitogenic signaling by endothelin-1. Cross-talk between G protein-coupled receptors and pp60c-src. *Journal of Biological Chemistry*, **268**(13) (1993), 9347–57.
71. J. G. Clarke, N. Benjamin, S. W. Larkin *et al.*, Endothelin is a potent long-lasting vasoconstrictor in men. *American Journal of Physiology*, **257**(6) (1989), H2033–5.
72. M. S. Goligorsky, H. Tsukahara, H. Magazine *et al.*, Termination of endothelin signaling: role of nitric oxide. *Journal of Cell Physiology*, **158**(3) (1994), 485–94.

73. J. A. Lopez, M. L. Armstrong, D. J. Piegors & D. D. Heistad, Vascular responses to endothelin-1 in atherosclerotic primates. *Arteriosclerosis* **10**(6) (1990), 1113–18.
74. T. Sakurai, M. Yanagisawa, Y. Takuwa *et al.*, Cloning of a cDNA encoding a non-isopeptide-selective subtype of the endothelin receptor. *Nature*, **348** (1990), 732–5.
75. A. G. Baynash, K. Hosoda, A. Giaid *et al.*, Interaction of endothelin-3 with endothelin-B receptor is essential for development of epidermal melanocytes and enteric neurons. *Cell*, **79**(7) (1994), 1277–85.
76. E. G. Puffenberger, K. Hosoda, S. S. Washington *et al.*, A missense mutation of the endothelin-B receptor gene in multigenic Hirschsprung's disease. *Cell*, **79**(7) (1994), 1257–66.
77. E. R. Levin, Endothelins. *New England Journal of Medicine*, **333**(6) (1995), 356–63.
78. K. A. Hickey, G. Rubanyi, R. J. Paul & R. F. Highsmith, Characterization of a coronary vasoconstrictor produced by cultured endothelial cells. *American Journal of Physiology*, **248**(5) (1985), C550–6.
79. B. Seo, B. S. Oemar, R. Siebenmann, L. von Segesser & T. F. Luscher, Both ETA and ETB receptors mediate contraction to endothelin-1 in human blood vessels. *Circulation*, **89**(3) (1994), 1203–8.
80. C. M. Wei, A. Lerman, R. J. Rodeheffer *et al.*, Endothelin in human congestive heart failure. *Circulation*, **89**(4) (1994), 1580–6.
81. I. Ziv, G. Fleminger, R. Djaldetti *et al.*, Increased plasma endothelin-1 in acute ischemic stroke. *Stroke*, **23**(7) (1992), 1014–16.
82. R. Suzuki, H. Masaoka, Y. Hirata *et al.*, The role of endothelin-1 in the origin of cerebral vasospasm in patients with aneurysmal subarachnoid hemorrhage. *Journal of Neurosurgery*, **77**(1) (1992), 96–100.
83. B. B. Weksler, A. J. Marcus & E. A. Jaffe, Synthesis of prostaglandin I2 (prostacyclin) by cultured human and bovine endothelial cells. *Proceedings of the National Academy of Sciences of the USA*, **74**(9) (1977), 3922–6.
84. R. A. Coleman, W. L. Smith & S. Narumiya, International Union of Pharmacology classification of prostanoid receptors: properties, distribution, and structure of the receptors and their subtypes. *Pharmacology Review*, **46**(2) (1994), 205–29.
85. T. A. Imaizumi, D. M. Stafforini, Y. Yamada *et al.*, Platelet-activating factor: a mediator for clinicians. *Journal of Internal Medicine*, **238**(1) (1995), 5–20.
86. R. P. McEver, K. L. Moore & R. D. Cummings, Leukocyte trafficking mediated by selectin-carbohydrate interactions. *Journal of Biological Chemistry*, **270**(19) (1995), 11025–8.
87. A. G. Murray, P. Libby & J. S. Pober, Human vascular smooth muscle cells poorly co-stimulate and actively inhibit allogeneic CD4+ T cell proliferation *in vitro*. *Journal of Immunology*, **154**(1) (1995), 151–61.
88. F. M. Marelli-Berg, R. E. Hargreaves, P. Carmichael *et al.*, Major histocompatibility complex class II-expressing endothelial cells induce allospecific nonresponsiveness in naive T cells. *Journal of Experimental Medicine*, **183**(4) (1996), 1603–12.
89. J. A. Marcum, R. D. Rosenberg, Anticoagulantly active heparin-like molecules from vascular tissue. *Biochemistry*, **23**(8) (1984), 1730–7.
90. G. J. Broze, Jr., Tissue factor pathway inhibitor. *Thrombosis and Haemostasis*, **74**(1) (1995), 90–3.
91. C. T. Esmon & K. Fukudome, Cellular regulation of the protein C pathway. *Seminars in Cell Biology*, **6**(5) (1995), 259–68.
92. T. A. Drake, J. H. Morrissey & T. S. Edgington, Selective cellular expression of tissue factor in human tissues. Implications for disorders of hemostasis and thrombosis. *American Journal of Pathology*, **134**(5) (1989), 1087–97.
93. Y. Nemerson, Tissue factor: then and now. *Thrombosis and Haemostasis*, **74** (1995), 180
94. D. Stern, P. Nawroth, D. Handley & W. Kisiel, An endothelial cell-dependent pathway of coagulation. *Proceedings of the National Academy of Sciences of the USA*, (1985), 2523–7.
95. C. Kanthou, Cellular effects of thrombin and their signalling *Cellular Pharmacology*, **2** 293.
96. J. G. N. Garcia, Vascular endothelial cell activation and permeability responses to thrombin. *Blood Coagulation and Fibrinolysis*, **6** (1995), 609.
97. J. D. Marmur, M. Rossikhina, A. Guha *et al.*, Tissue factor is rapidly induced in arterial smooth muscle after balloon injury. *Journal of Clinical Investigation*, **91**(5) (1993), 2253–9.
98. S. V. Thiruvikraman, A. Guha, J. Roboz *et al.*, *In situ* localization of tissue factor in human atherosclerotic plaques by binding of digoxigenin-labeled factors VIIa and X. *Laboratory Investigation*, **75**(4) (1996), 451–61.
99. K. Hatakeyama, Y. Asada, K. Marutsuka *et al.*, Localization and activity of tissue factor in human

aortic atherosclerotic lesions. *Atherosclerosis*, **133**(2) (1997), 213–9.

100. D. J. Luskutoff, *Progress in Haemostasis and Thrombosis*, (Philadelphia: Saunders, 1989).

101. J. Wojta, R. L. Hoover & T. O. Daniel, Vascular origin determines plasminogen activator expression in human endothelial cells. Renal endothelial cells produce large amounts of single chain urokinase type plasminogen activator. *Journal of Biological Chemistry*, **264**(5) (1989), 2846–52.

102. L. Bajzar, J. Morser & M. Nesheim, TAFI, or plasma procarboxypeptidase B, couples the coagulation and fibrinolytic cascades through the thrombin-thrombomodulin complex. *Journal of Biological Chemistry*, (1996), 16603–8.

2 • Vascular smooth muscle cells: structure and function

PHILIP CHAN

What is a smooth muscle cell ? This deceptively simple question continues to elude a straight answer; perhaps, as I hope to argue in this chapter, because it may contain assumptions that cannot be upheld in the age of modern biology.

Arguably, if an artery or vein is stripped of adventitia and its luminal surface scraped free of endothelium, the substantial remnant is a fairly pure mass of vascular smooth muscle. The smooth muscle cell and its associated extracellular matrix is the major structural component of the vessel wall in both arteries and veins. There are far fewer smooth muscle cells in the lymphatics, and none in the lymphatic capillaries and precollector vessels. There are negligible amounts of other cell types in the arterial and venous media, only the small number of endothelial cells and adventitial fibroblasts accompany the vasa vasorum and innervating nerves. This was known to be true in the 1950s and 1960s and has not changed today, so contemporary references to vascular fibroblasts and scarring are poorly informed.

The difficulties in defining a vascular smooth muscle cell (VSMC) reflect the difficulties in defining any cell type so as to be both comprehensive and exclusive at the same time [1]. This concept may be outdated as we come to accept gradations of cell type and cell type plasticity, even in adults. Specific difficulties centre on the questions of how vascular smooth muscle is distinguished from other tissues of mesenchymal origin in the body and what precursors can contribute to the vascular smooth muscle mass in pathological conditions of human vessels.

STRUCTURE

Vascular smooth muscle cells exist in the media of arteries and veins, bounded by the internal and external elastic laminae. Classically, the outer media is described as circular and the inner as longitudinal, reflecting the orientation of the cells. There are occasional VSMCs in the normal intima; there are many more intimal VSMCs in pathological circumstances. Normally there are no VSMCs in the adventitia, which is thought to be mostly fibroblasts and fat cells, as well as containing the vasa vasorum and nerves.

The primary functions of the VSMC in the vessel wall are structural and contractile. The bulk of the vessel wall is composed of VSMCs. It serves as an elastic reservoir of energy from the pulse wave and it can regulate local blood flow in response to nervous or humoral stimuli. The structure of the vessel wall VSMC subserves contraction and is dominated by actin/myosin filaments. The actual arrangement of VSMC contractile apparatus is not as clear as that determined for skeletal muscle.

Expression of the alpha-1 isoform of actin and the smooth muscle isoform of myosin heavy chain has been regarded as a definitive identification of the VSMC. However, this concept is rather old-fashioned and certainly blurred at the edges; for example, alpha actin expression is down-regulated during the cell cycle, so an actin-negative cell can still be a vascular smooth muscle cell. Other protein markers are also significantly associated with vascular smooth muscle (Table 2.1), but no single protein can be regarded as being a canonical definition of the cell type.

A structural definition of the VSMC is further blurred by the existence of a spectrum of myofibroblasts. Myofibroblasts are intermediate in structure between classical smooth muscle and their mesenchymal relative, the fibroblast. They can express protein markers that are characteristic of both types and represent a spectrum of intermediate forms. *In vivo*, myofibroblasts are prominent in contracting granulation tissue of wounds in virtually all tissues except neural. They represent tissue fibroblasts which proliferate, migrate and undergo smooth muscle type differentiation, chiefly by synthesis of contractile microfilaments [2; 3]. If an established VSMC proliferates and migrates, for example, in cell

Table 2.1. *Vascular smooth muscle cell markers*

Alpha smooth muscle actin
Myosin heavy chain (smooth muscle)
Smoothelin
Smooth muscle specific isoforms of
Alpha tropomyosin
Calponin
Caldesmon
Calvasculin
Myosin regulatory light chain 2
SM22
CHIP28
Vinculin/meta-vinculin

Table 2.2. *Vascular smooth muscle contractile agonists*

Acetylcholine
Alpha adrenergic agonists
Angiotensin 2
ATP
Bradykinin
Endothelin
Lipoproteins
Serotonin (via 5HT-2 receptor)
Thrombin
Thromboxane
Vasopressin

culture from an explant (see below), it undergoes relative loss of contractile microfilaments, and may end up indistinguishable from a fibroblast-derived myofibroblast, having arrived there from the other end of the spectrum. Arguably, every VSMC in culture can be regarded as a type of myofibroblast.

Vascular smooth muscle derives from diverse embryological origins. From avian embryology models, it appears that head and neck vessels, and part of the aorta derive from the neural crest; local mesoderm is recruited by angioblasts to form VSMCs in other parts of the body. There are considerable differences in expression of cytoskeletal proteins, at least in avian embryos between these two cell lineages; whether this persists into adult life and whether this pattern is strictly conserved in mammals is an open question [4]. Recruitment and organization of smooth muscle cells into new circulations is discussed in the following section on angiogenesis and arteriogenesis.

CONTRACTILE FUNCTION

What does the VSMC do? Simply put, there is a primary function within the vessel wall and a secondary, reparative function relevant to disease.

The primary function of vascular smooth muscle is to maintain tone in the vessel wall and to serve as the principal structural component of the vessel. The physiology of vascular smooth muscle contraction and its regulation are outside the scope of this chapter. In very simple terms, phosphorylation of myosin light chain is the critical biochemical event in the initiation of contraction; ordinarily dependent on elevation of intracellular calcium, as in other muscle cells.

Intracellular calcium elevation involves mobilization of calcium stores from the sarcoplasmic reticulum. Different types of calcium channels are responsible for this and for entry of calcium from the extracellular space into the cell.

Contractile signal transduction is effected through several pathways. A key role is assigned to protein kinase C and its activators, membrane phospholipids. Agonists producing smooth muscle contraction are many and varied, and include many classes of compounds, some of which are listed in Table 2.2.

The chief vasorelaxant agent in nature is NO, nitric oxide. It is the mechanism by which endothelium chiefly regulates vessel tone in the intact vessel. There is a default tendency to vasoconstriction in vascular smooth muscle within the vessel wall, which is regulated by endothelial production of NO (endothelium-dependent relaxation). Nitric oxide is the product of metabolism of L-arginine by two types of NO synthase enzymes, the inducible (iNOS), and the constitutive (eNOS in endothelium) types.

The main pathologies of vascular smooth muscle contractile function are vasoconstriction and hypertension. Vasoconstrictive diseases generally present with peripheral Raynaud's phenomenon. Vasodilators such as thymoxamine (an alpha adrenergic antagonist) have been shown to have some effect, as have prostanoid infusion. Graft vasoconstriction during surgical bypass tends not to respond to adrenergic antagonists; more rational treatment centres on promoting NO function, and direct high dose nitrate administration may be effective.

Hypertension is a multisystem, multifaceted disease and is certainly not as simple as a disease of primary vasoconstriction. Undeniably, however, there is increased vascular tone in hypertension. Direct vasodilator agents (prazosin, doxazosin) are sometimes effective treatments.

VASCULAR SMOOTH MUSCLE PROLIFERATION

Vascular smooth muscle has a response to injury function within the vessel, which involves proliferation. The mechanisms of proliferation have been elicited by animal models of vascular injury, chiefly the rat carotid balloon injury model.

From the studies led by Alex Clowes, Michael Reidy, Steve Schwartz and the late Russell Ross in Seattle, the events of vascular healing after injury are currently quite well described [5; 6].

There are three waves of response to vascular injury in the rat carotid artery. The balloon injury causes complete loss of endothelium and extensive death and damage of medial VSMCs. The first response is a wave of medial VSMC replication and occurs around 24 hours after injury. Most of this response is stimulated by the release of basic fibroblast growth factor (bFGF) by dead and damaged VSMCs.

Migration of medial VSMCs across the internal elastic lamina into the intima constitutes the second wave. This occurs around three days post injury and continues for an unknown length of time. Many molecules can mediate or influence this second wave, particularly including platelet-derived growth factor (PDGF), previously regarded as a pre-eminent smooth muscle cell mitogen, as well as angiotensin II and transforming growth factor-β (TGFβ).

Intimal smooth muscle cells replicate and secrete matrix weeks to months after the injury, forming the third wave of the response. This is not under the control of bFGF or PDGF. The factors that control continued proliferation over such a long period after the initial damage stimulus are not known [6; 7].

Vascular smooth muscle proliferation is of great interest in human pathology. The two chief pathologies of human arteries, atherosclerosis and vascular restenosis after intervention, both involve an important component of VSMC proliferation.

The Ross model of human atherosclerosis visualizes this ubiquitous disease as a response to vascular injury; not just physical injury, but also more subtle injuries inflicted by biochemical imbalances, particularly involving lipids, and by flow changes producing haemodynamic disturbances [6]. The three waves of response are not classically expressed in these situations; the role of lipid-laden macrophage foam cells in the arterial wall is now stressed. However, there is still smooth muscle replication in the diseased intima, which can stabilize the developing plaque by forming a 'fibrous cap' between the lipid lesion and the lumen [7].

Vascular smooth muscle cell proliferation plays a much more central role in restenosis after vascular intervention, be it surgery, angioplasty or stenting. A neointimal response to injury is seen in which VSMC hyperplasia creates a new thickened intima. In around 30% of cases, this will lead to significant luminal stenosis after the intervention (which, of course, was performed to relieve a luminal stenosis). Histologically, the neointimal lesion is vascular smooth muscle and associated extracellular matrix; the matrix accounting for 75% of the lesion volume.

It has been unclear to what extent VSMC proliferation contributes to the lesion. Pickering *et al.* found very high rates of VSMC proliferative markers, while O'Brien *et al.* found very low proliferative indexes in human restenosis samples. Different techniques were used in these studies, and there may have been a fixation artefact; one study used methanol and the other formalin for their samples [8; 9].

There are striking similarities and some important differences in restenosis after different procedures and in different parts of the circulation. The rates of restenosis are surprisingly similar in all vessels at 20%–40%, be it carotid, coronary or femoro-popliteal, after any kind of intervention. However, endovascular techniques of stent and angioplasty occur in the diseased artery, on a background of established, stenotic atheroma. Vein graft bypass excludes this tissue and the stenotic process occurs *de novo* on a background of relatively healthy vein wall. It is indeed surprising that cytological and histological differences are minimal; if the background is masked out the restenotic tissue is identical in all situations, be it stent, angioplasty or vein graft. The cellular picture, that of VSMC proliferation, neointimal formation and matrix secretion, are indistinguishable. Presumably the biological modulators are also similar.

At first, antiproliferative treatments with various drugs, all tested in the rat carotid injury model and found to be effective against VSMC proliferation, were unsuccessful in the prevention of human restenosis. This led to a de-emphasis of the role of VSMC proliferation in this condition and concentration on a set of alternative factors, such as constrictive recoil after vascular stretching with the angioplasty balloon or a less well understood, longer-term process termed remodelling. Remodelling is a set of processes that tends to increase the lumen size despite thickening of the intima by outward expansion of the vessel wall, first described in relation to the atherosclerotic plaque. These processes may include smooth muscle apoptosis, extracellular matrix synthesis, metabolism and breakdown. Little is understood about how these processes are co-ordinated in response to vascular wall thickening. Attribution of the pathology of restenosis to defective remodelling is, in effect, the same as attribution to defective, but unknown factors. This is not an especially creative or revealing line of thought.

Recently, overtly antiproliferative strategies using localized radioactivity (brachytherapy, by incorporation of isotope into stent material) and cell cycle inhibitor drugs, also bound to stents, have begun to show quite dramatic effects of neointimal formation. It is therefore likely that the restenosis process, at least in the scenario of stent restenosis, is chiefly mediated by VSMC proliferation.

Proliferation of VSMCs occurs under the influence of a number of growth factors. Platelet-derived growth factor was the first to be implicated; however, it appears that PDGF is not directly mitogenic to VSMC, but can act as a co-mitogen. There is no single growth factor that is responsible for VSMC proliferation *in vivo*. Therapeutic attempts at targeting single growth factors to inhibit proliferation are therefore misled, and no such effort has been successful. In the real situation of vascular injury, there is extensive cellular disruption, activation of platelets and inflammatory cells as well as the response of the vessel wall itself. These activated multiple pathways are all stimulatory to VMSC proliferation. Even if a therapy could knock out one pathway, there are many others that are left active. Antiproliferative therapies that have met with a measure of success target the VSMC response, generally to a component regulating cell cycle progression, with local specificity conferred by incorporation into a stent.

HOW ARE VSMCS STUDIED?

Vascular smooth muscle cells are conventionally studied within the intact vessel wall, as isolated cells or as cultured cells, in cell or organ culture.

Vessel wall rings have been used in physiological studies of contraction for over a century. In an appropriate electrolyte medium, freshly isolated rings of arteries and veins can exhibit contractile responses to a variety of agonist molecules. The myograph is a miniaturized convenient extension of this design. A segment of vessel is placed between two fixed transducer points and isometric contraction is induced, this produces strain which is quantified by the apparatus (see, for example, http://www.dmt.dk).

Vascular smooth muscle cell proliferation can be studied in the intact vessel by using metabolic labels. In experimental animals, labelled nucleotides (BrdU) can be administered at the time of a vascular injury intervention and the labelling index gives a measure of proliferative activity in the studied vessel segment. In histological preparations of human material, cell proliferation markers, such as PCNA or Ki67 can be studied. These markers are associated with cells that have recently undergone mitosis.

Vascular smooth muscle cells isolated from vessels by a combination of enzymatic and mechanical methods have also been used to study the physiology of individual cells. Generally, contractile functions have been examined in one of two ways; labelling with fura-2 dye produces an intracellular colour change when intracellular calcium is released at the initiation of contraction; or more directly, patch-clamp methods have recorded electric potentials from the cell membrane directly associated with ion channel opening during contraction.

Vascular smooth muscle cell culture is well established in many centres. It is not a difficult procedure, as VSMCs proliferate in standard cell culture media and fetal calf serum, and adhere well to tissue culture plastics. Vascular smooth muscle cells can be cultured from explants of vessel wall tissue or from enzyme digest preparations. Generally, VSMC cultures are used to study proliferation, as this can be easily quantified in cell culture by simple cell counting. The VSMC cultures can be passaged on; adult human VSMC cultures will usually propagate to the fifth or sixth culture passages with preserved and consistent function.

Finally, organ culture of VSMCs places the dissected wall of a vessel into tissue culture conditions. Histological analysis of VSMC proliferation is made, using BrdU labelling, usually after two weeks. Viability of the organ culture becomes impaired after this time period.

All methods of VSMC study have to be adapted to the research question. Exposure to enzyme digestion has significant effects on the cell membrane and may alter its electrophysiology. Explant cultures represent a selected set of VSMCs which are advantaged in adhesion to culture plastic and grow rapidly in reponse to serum stimulus. Organ cultures cannot be reliably studied beyond two weeks. These and many other related considerations have to be made before selecting the most suitable method.

ARE THERE DIFFERENT SUBTYPES OF VSMCS?

On one level, it would be very surprising if there were not different types of VSMCs. There are clearly different types of skin on the palm and sole compared with the face, and still a different type in specialized regions such as the nipple and scrotum. As VSMCs are present in arteries and veins, with as wide a distribution throughout the body and as much variation in function as skin, it would indeed be surprising if there were no local or functional variants. It has been proposed that there are different types of fibroblasts, dependent on their locality and immediate function; e.g. fibrogenesis, tissue skeleton or barrier, intercellular communication system, contractile machinery, endocrine activity and vitamin A storage. There is considerable consistency in the expression of characteristic proteins to subserve these individual functions, even in the absence of visible morphological differences [10].

There is one clearly acknowledged specialist variant of the VSMC, the mesangial cell of the renal glomerulus. However, there may also be different types of VSMC within vessel walls. Pharmacological phenotypes are recognized. The differential effect of various types of adrenergic agonists on vessel constriction was initially studied on vessel rings in organ baths; leading to description of alpha and beta receptors. Vascular smooth muscle rings from coronary and splanchnic circulations have different responses to adrenergic stimulation, due to different receptor populations.

Vascular smooth muscle cells have been proposed as two phenotypes by Julie and Gordon Campbell, synthetic and contractile. These phenotypes reflect the two functions of the VSMC; the Campbells assigned typical morphologies to these types and produced them in culture. The contractile VSMC is typically spindle shaped, with abundant actin and myosin fibres; the synthetic phenotype is broader, with a greater amount of cytoplasm. This was expressed quantitatively as the volume fraction of myofibrils in the cell, which was greater in contractile than synthetic type cells. It was proposed that the phenotype changes from contractile to synthetic states and back regulated proliferation of VSMC within the vessel wall after injury. There was also explicit recognition of a spectrum of intermediate phenotypes [11].

A further phenotype of VSMCs has been proposed as a major component of the vascular response to injury. Vascular smooth muscle cells cultured from the intimal hyperplastic lesion after carotid balloon injury in rats has a similar morphology to cells from infant rats; being polygonal and growing in monolayers in culture, somewhat like an epithelial or endothelial cell line. This pup-intimal (PI) phenotype is stable in culture and characterized by growth in soft agar, and expression of PDGF-B [12].

One interpretation of the PI phenotype is that it represents a specific, fetal-like subset of VSMCs within the vessel wall. While other cells are terminally differentiated, to serve their vascular wall functions, PI cells might exist as fetal 'rests' activated by injury to form a neointima. The difficulty with this concept is that the PI phenotype is defined in culture and not *in situ* in the vessel wall. Human neointimal cultures do not consistently yield this cell phenotype. There is something clearly different about cultured intimal cells compared with cultured medial cells. Whether this difference existed before the vascular injury, or whether it represents a differentiation phenomenon in response to that injury, remains unknown.

Nevertheless, it is an attractive concept that proliferative phenotypes of VSMCs exist in the vessel wall; as we know that major arterial pathologies are based on abnormal VSMC proliferation, this concept provides a theoretical basis for these diseases, in the form of an abnormal phenotype.

In support of this concept, Murry *et al.* studied clonality in the VSMC populations of coronary atherosclerotic plaques. Using laser micro-dissection of plaques, they demonstrated that 'patches' of VSMCs exist within plaques; all VSMCs within the plaques expressed genetic markers indicating that they originated from a single, or very few founder cells. The size of the plaques could extend up to 2 mm. This evidence of clonal proliferation (not necessarily the same as a clonal selection process) in vascular disease supports the concept that there is something abnormal about VSMCs that participate in the disease process [13].

Our group have over many years defined an abnormal VMSC phenotype, characterized by its relative resistance to growth inhibition by heparin, which is associated with human vein graft 'restenosis'. This phenotype does not have a characteristic morphology like the PI cell, but has reproducible resistance to heparin which is heritable in culture [14]. We have been able to produce clonal cultures with different heparin responses and characterize these cultures by gene expression profile, using cDNA microarrays.

All phenotypes of vascular smooth muscle described have been identified in culture. There does not seem to be any explanation of why tissue culture should produce a variety of phenotypes artefactually while no such diversity exists in the intact vessel. Nevertheless, there is little direct proof for the existence of diverse VSMC phenotypes *in situ*.

There has been intense speculation as to whether the proliferating VSMCs in intimal lesions after vascular injury derive from VSMC lineages at all.

From angioplasty experiments, it has been theorized that the intimal VSMC is derived from adventitial origin. Certainly, in the rat balloon injury model, proliferation in the adventitia outside the vessel is seen after injury and before intimal proliferation [15]. Labelling of adventitial fibroblasts in experimental models indicate that these cells may form the intimal layer after vascular injury [3]. However, labelling of the adventitia is non-selective, and can be incorporated into any cell that is actively synthesizing DNA at the time of labelling, not just the adventitial cell. Subsequent appearance of the labelled cell in the intima is not a conclusive proof that the cell has migrated from adventitia to intima. Undoubtedly in models such as pig coronary angioplasty, the radial splitting injury found in the medial layer facilitates the transit of cells from adventitia to intima and there is some evidence to support a connection between increased intimal proliferation with deeper medial injury.

Alternatively, another school of thought has theorized that the intimal VSMC is derived from blood-borne precursors. This idea originates from the disparity between the rather quiescent arterial wall and the rapid, intense activity in the intima after injury. Vascular injury models have been set up in bone-marrow transplanted animals, who therefore have different cells making up the vessel wall to haematogenous cell lines. The transplanted, bone-marrow derived cells express a marker, either male cells marked by a Y chromosome in a female recipient, or a reporter gene transfection. Analysis of the intimal response to vascular injury indicates that the cells involved may derive from the transplanted, haematogenous precursors, rather than the recipient vessel wall. Again, there may be an element of confusion here; the intima undoubtedly contains inflammatory cells as well as smooth muscle, especially at early time points, and labelling of the neointima after vascular injury is never completely positive for donor cells or recipient [16; 17]. Heterogeneity of the intimal tissue confounds the picture. There may also be local stem cells within tissues that contribute to VSMCs in newly forming or renewing vessels (see below).

ANGIOGENESIS AND ARTERIOGENESIS

Smooth muscle cells participate in the formation of arteries, in development and in neovascular responses. Formation of new blood vessels is initiated by endothelial tube assembly (angiogenesis); which is then shortly invested with smooth muscle (arteriogenesis). The origin of this smooth muscle is discussed above; in the adult animal it develops from locally derived cells, either from the vessel wall or adventitial cells. The term pericyte is often used, but it is deliberately imprecise and does not define either origin or stage of differentiation. Eventually these investing cells differentiate along clear VSMC lines [18].

The mechanisms involved are interesting and complex. Mouse knock-out models have provided a number of clues to the molecular mechanisms involved. Smooth muscle cell recruitment to stabilize new vessels may be mediated by angiopoietin-1 and ephrin B2 and B4. In adult animals, there may be a contribution from locally resident stem cells, for example, in skeletal muscle, which may differentiate into VSMCs. These considerations, combined with the heterogeneity of established VSMC types are examples of adult cell type plasticity, and further confound attempts to define what is, and what is not, a VSMC.

The process of arteriogenesis is the conversion of thin walled capillary vessels into small arteries capable of carrying flow. This process is important in the formation of collateral circulations around vascular occlusions and can be thought of as the major therapeutic goal in biological vascular research. The biological processes are thought to recapitulate the arteriogenesis phase of new blood vessel formation, with different stimulating factors.

When a vessel is occluded, blood is channelled into surrounding pre-existing capillary networks. There is increased fluid flow through these channels, resulting in increased hydrostatic pressure, wall tension, shear stress and other haemodynamic factors. In response, endothelial cells are thought to express monocyte chemokines and monocyte adhesion molecules, thus attracting, holding and activating monocytes. These monocytes destroy the existing vessel wall, and allow new smooth muscle recruitment and vessel enlargement, in response to further growth factor stimulus from the endothelium, chiefly involving bFGF, PDGF-BB and TGFβ1. The important role of monocytes/macrophages is evidenced by increased collateral growth after macrophage stimulation in a hindlimb ischaemia model [19].

SUMMARY

The VSMC is the major structural component of the blood vessel. It therefore plays a significant role in most diseases and adaptations to disease of blood vessels. Restenosis and vein graft stenosis can be regarded as a primary disease of vascular smooth muscle.

Suggested further reading; S. M. Schwartz & R. P. Mecham ed., *The Vascular Smooth Muscle Cell*. San Diego: Academic Press, 1995.

REFERENCES

1. S. M. Schwartz, Definition of a cell type. *Circulation Research*, **84** (1999), 1234–5.
2. G. Gabbiani, G. B. Ryan & G. Majno, Presence of modified fibroblasts in granulation tissue and their possible role in wound contraction. *Experientia*, **27** (1971), 549–50.
3. A. Zalewski & Y. Shi, Vascular myofibroblasts. *Arteriosclerosis, Thrombosis and Vascular Biology*, **17** (1997), 417–22.
4. P. F. Gadson, Jr., C. Rossignol, J. McCoy & T. H. Rosenquist, Expression of elastin, smooth muscle alpha-actin, and c-jun as a function of the embryonic lineage of vascular smooth muscle cells. *In vitro Cellular and Developmental Biology*, **29A** (1993), 773–81.
5. A. W. Clowes, M. M. Clowes & M. A. Reidy, Kinetics of cellular proliferation after arterial injury, III. *Laboratory Investigation*, **54** (1986), 295–303.
6. R. Ross, The pathogenesis of atherosclerosis, *Nature*, **362** (1993), 801–9.
7. V. J. Dzau, R. C. Braun-Dullaeus & D. C. Sedding, Vascular proliferation and atherosclerosis: new perspectives and therapeutic strategies. *Nature Medicine*, **8** (2002), 1249–56.
8. J. G. Pickering, L. Weir, J. Jekanowski, M. A. Kearney & J. M. Isner, Proliferative activity in peripheral and coronary atherosclerotic plaque among patients undergoing percutaneous revascularisation. *Journal of Clinical Investigation*, **91** (1993), 1469–80.
9. E. R. O'Brien, C. E. Alpers, D. K. Stewart, *et al.* Proliferation in primary and restenotic coronary atherectomy tissue: implications for antiproliferative therapy. *Circulation Research*, **73** (1993), 223–31.
10. T. Komuro, Re-evaluation of fibroblasts and fibroblast-like cells. *Anatomy and Embryology*, **182** (1990), 103–12.
11. G. R. Campbell & J. H. Campbell, The phenotypes of smooth muscle expressed in human atheroma. *Annals of the New York Academy of Sciences*, **598** (1990), 143–58.
12. M. W. Majesky, C. M. Giachelli, M. A. Reidy & S. M. Schwartz, Rat carotid neointimal smooth muscle cells reexpress a developmentally regulated mRNA phenotype during repair of artery injury. *Circulation Research*, **71** (1992), 759–68.
13. C. E. Murry, C. T. Gipaya, T. Bartosek *et al.*, Monoclonality of smooth muscle cells in human atherosclerosis. *American Journal of Pathology*, **151** (1997), 697–705.
14. P. Chan, M. Patel, L. Betteridge *et al.*, Abnormal growth regulation of vascular smooth muscle cells by

heparin in patients with restenosis. *Lancet*, **341** (1993), 341–2.

15. N. A. Scott, G. D. Cipolla, C. E. Ross *et al.*, Identification of a potential role for the adventitia in lesion formation after balloon overstretch injury of porcine coronary arteries. *Circulation*, **93** (1996), 2178–87.
16. C. L. Han, G. R. Campbell & J. H. Campbell, Circulating bone marrow cells can contribute to neointimal formation. *Journal of Vascular Research*, **38** (2001), 113–19.
17. K. Shimizu, S. Sugiyama, M. Aikawa *et al.*, Host bone-marrow cells are a source of donor intimal smooth-muscle-like cells in murine aortic transplant arteriopathy. *Nature Medicine*, **7** (2001), 738–41.
18. P. Carmeliet, Mechanisms of angiogenesis and arteriogenesis. *Nature Medicine*, **6** (2000), 389–95.
19. M. Arras, W. D. Ito, D. Scholz *et al.*, Monocyte activation in angiogenesis and collateral growth in the rabbit hindlimb. *Journal of Clinical Investigation*, **101**(1) (1998), 40–50.

3 • Vascular haemodynamics

MICHAEL LAWRENCE-BROWN, KURT LIFFMAN
AND JAMES SEMMENS

INTRODUCTION

Vascular interventions have developed rapidly since the first aortic replacement with dacron by Dubois in 1952. Understanding vascular haemodynamics and the biological response to implanted materials is essential for vascular surgeons and scientists developing new interventional technologies [1; 2].

This chapter will summarize and discuss the following laws, equations and phenomena in order to give a basic understanding of the haemodynamic principles of the conduits and fluids with which we work:

Laplace's law of wall tension
Newtonian fluid
Shear thinning fluid
Poiseuille flow
Bernoulli's equation
Young's modulus and pulsatile flow
Mass conservation
Reynolds' number: laminar and turbulent flow
Shear stress and pressure
Forces on a single tube graft system

For those who understand electrical circuit theory, there is much similarity with haemodynamics. Understanding the physiology and physics of blood flow is aided by the use of that recognition. When considering fluid dynamics instead of:

$$V = IR \tag{1}$$

where V is the voltage, I is the current and R is the electrical resistance. This formula maybe substituted by:

$$P = QR \tag{1}$$

with P the pressure, Q the volume flow rate and R the flow resistance.

Resistors in series and parallel govern the degrees of ischaemia, and the behaviour of blood flow and contribution of collaterals, and hence the degree of limb ischaemia.

LAPLACE'S LAW OF WALL TENSION

Laplace's law relates the tension in an arterial or venous wall with the pressure that the elastic tube can apply to material inside the tube. To assist in understanding this law we consider Figure 3.1. In this figure, w represents the thickness of the arterial wall, r is the inner radius of the artery or vein, P is the inward pressure force due to the elastic nature of the artery and T is the tensional stress within the vessel wall, where the tensional stress points in a direction that is tangential to the vessel wall. The formula for Laplace's law is given by equation 2:

$$P = \frac{w}{r}T \tag{2}$$

where it is usually assumed that the wall thickness, w is small relative to r. This law tells us that the inward pressure that is exerted by the vessel wall on the blood is directly proportional to the tensional stress in the wall and inversely proportional to the radius of the wall. Thus the smaller the vessel the larger the pressure it can apply on the blood.

One consequence of this behaviour is that, to a certain extent, an artery acts like a long cylindrical party balloon. When one attempts to blow up such a balloon, it is quite difficult to do at the first blow, however, once the balloon reaches a particular radius, it usually becomes much easier to expand the balloon. That is you require less pressure to increase the size of the balloon. This phenomenon is known as instability. If this happens to an artery, then we are dealing with an aneurysm and the relatively constant blood pressure will keep on increasing the size of the aneurysm.

The radius of the artery at which this instability occurs is difficult to compute accurately, but some fairly general arguments suggest that r_c is the critical radius

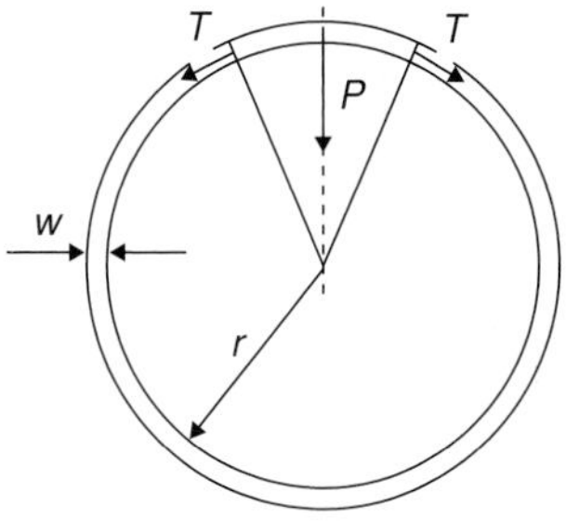

Fig. 3.1. Cross section of an artery showing the various physical components that make up Laplace's law.

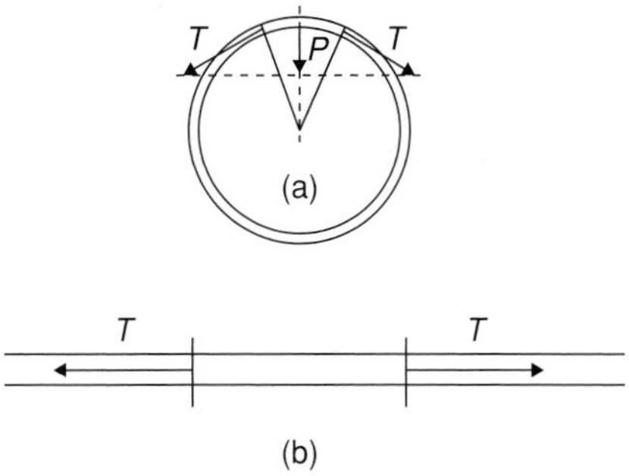

Fig. 3.2. Cross section of (a) a small artery and (b) a very large artery. Each shows the stress distribution within the artery.

for the onset of the instability and r_0 is the initial radius of the artery, as shown in equation 3:

$$r_c \sim 2r_0 \tag{3}$$

The median diameter of the aorta is 23 mm and an aortic rupture is very rare when less than 50 mm in diameter, which is consistent with recent clinical data [3; 4]. How arterial wall instability arises is illustrated in Figure 3.2, where in Figure 3.2 (a) we show the stress structure within a small artery. Here the tensile stresses have a component in the radial direction, where the letter T labels this component. In Figure 3.2 (b) the aneurysm/balloon has become very large, such that over a small segment of the wall the artery has hardly any curvature. This is an extreme case, but it does show that there is now no radial component to the tensile stresses. In such a case, the aneurysm can expand freely for just about any internal arterial pressure. The performance of endoluminal grafts (ELGs) was found to be different to open repair with a sewn replacement of the artery because of unsuspected influences, as mentioned above, that relate to sustained physical forces [1]. The openly sewn prosthesis binds the wall of the artery to the prosthesis with a transmural suture. The artery may expand above or below the prosthesis. However, at the point of attachment the artery wall is held to the fixed diameter by the through wall suture for as long as the suture holds. Endoluminal grafts to date do not bind the adventitia to the prosthesis – they merely attach. The ELG must continue to act to bridge the gap between the normal artery above and below until, if ever, the aneurysm's cavity shrinks right down. In open surgery, the suture is binding and the tissues around supportive. The diameters of the grafts used for the same aortic abdominal aneurysm (AAA) differ markedly between the open and ELG methods. The common diameters used for tube replacement surgically of infrarenal AAA are 18 or 20 mm. The commonest diameter for an ELG is 26 or 28 mm, and 30+ mm is not that uncommon. Why is there such a discrepancy when the surgeon judges the diameter to be a suitable fit? This discrepancy is due to the different types of attachment of an open graft and an ELG. With the former, there are sutures through the graft and the full thickness of the aortic wall. This means that the aortic diameter at that point is permanently fixed to the diameter of the graft in its pressurized state. The diameter of a crimped vascular graft is, by definition, the minimum internal distance between the crimps in the non-pressurized state. It is increased by approximately 10% when pressurized. With the ELG, a residual radial force is required for seal and the attachment may or may not be enhanced by latching barbs. The oversize allowance must accommodate elasticity and compliance while maintaining the seal between pulsations for the whole of the length of the sealing zone.

With an ELG the device must bridge a gap for an indeterminate time before the body reabsorbs the contents of the aneurysm and encases the graft in foreign body fibrous tissue support. Therefore the long term function and durability demands are` different and more demanding [1]. Understanding the forces involved is basic to the design and use of new technology, and an understanding of the weaknesses that lead to aneurysmal disease provides a challenge [1; 5].

A mistaken clinical impression is that the forces on a thoracic ELG should be greater than those on an abdominal ELG is a good example. The flow and diameter of the thoracic aorta are greater, and the haemodynamic forces potentially much larger. However, because the diameter of the graft changes little, if at all, the downward displacement force in the thoracic ELG is small as the resistance in the graft is low – except on the curve. The resistance of any graft that extends into the iliac vessels is much greater because of the significant change in diameter and high resistance, with the graft acting like a windsock or sea anchor [5]. An aorto-uni-iliac device affords greater resistance than a bifurcated graft, and detachment at the neck and migration are common problems due to high displacement forces. In contrast with the thoracic aorta there is little drag because there is little or no change in diameter and the force applied to the graft is on the curve – centrifugal forces apply. Since every action has an equal and opposite reaction (Newton's third law), one must ask where is the reaction. The reaction is to pull the graft out from the top and the bottom almost equally. When ELGs were first used in the thorax, unexpected upward migration of the distal end emerged as the problem, especially when there was a significant curve on the graft. For the same reason, this 'lift out' may also be seen from the iliacs when the graft fixation is weak because of ectasia and/or a short length of attachment.

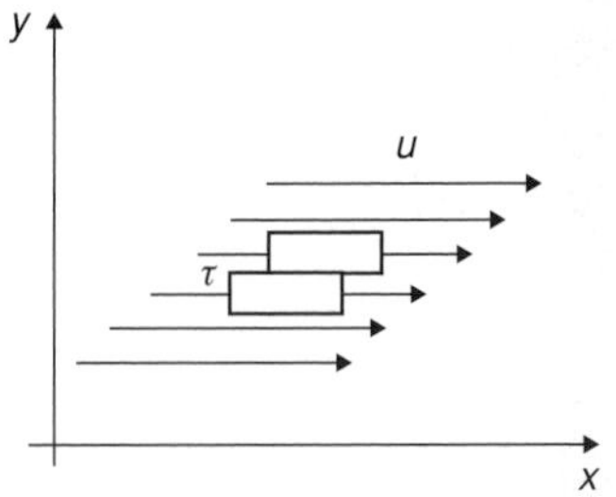

Fig. 3.3. Elements of fluid slide past each other and generate a frictional shear stress τ.

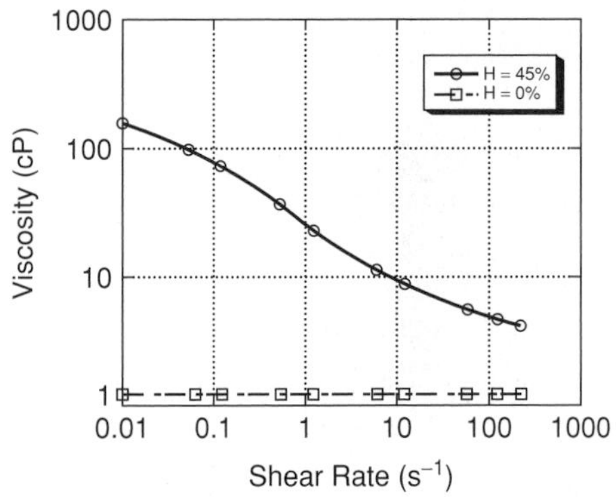

Fig. 3.4. Blood viscosity as a function of shear rate for 0% and 45% haematocrit (H) [6].

NEWTONIAN FLUID

When we wish to describe the behaviour of a fluid it is necessary to know something about the frictional properties of the fluid. Consider the schematic depiction of a fluid shown in Figure 3.3. In this figure, fluid is flowing from left to right along the x direction. For purposes of illustration, we assume that the speed of the fluid, u, is increasing with increasing height (i.e. increasing y). This means that elements of fluid are sliding past each other and so generate some frictional stress τ. In a Newtonian fluid, the frictional stress is proportional to the rate at which the speed changes as a function of distance, where μ is the viscosity (see equation 4). To a reasonable approximation, one can assume that blood is a Newtonian fluid, at least for flow along the major arteries.

$$\tau = \mu \frac{du}{dy} \qquad (4)$$

SHEAR THINNING FLUID

A shear thinning fluid is a fluid that changes from 'thick' to 'thin' when force is applied to the fluid. Examples of such fluids are shampoos and paints. This behaviour usually occurs because at rest a shear thinning fluid typically has a tangled molecular structure, which makes the fluid relatively viscous. When force is applied, the molecules become ordered, the fluid viscosity decreases and the fluid begins to flow more easily. In Figure 3.4 we show the experimentally determined shear thinning behaviour of blood, where the haematocrit value for the blood is 45%. These data show that for high shear rates, which may occur in the large arteries of the body, the viscosity of blood is about four times that of water (where the viscosity of water is approximately 1 centipoise (cP)). However, for lower shear rates, the viscosity of blood can be over 100 times that of water. This change in viscosity is mostly due to the collective behaviour of red blood cells. At low shear rates, red blood cells form aggregates where they stack one upon another, somewhat like a cylindrical pile of coins. These 'stacks' of red blood cells are known as 'rouleaux' (Figure 3.5). When the shear rate increases, these aggregates of blood cells are broken down and the blood

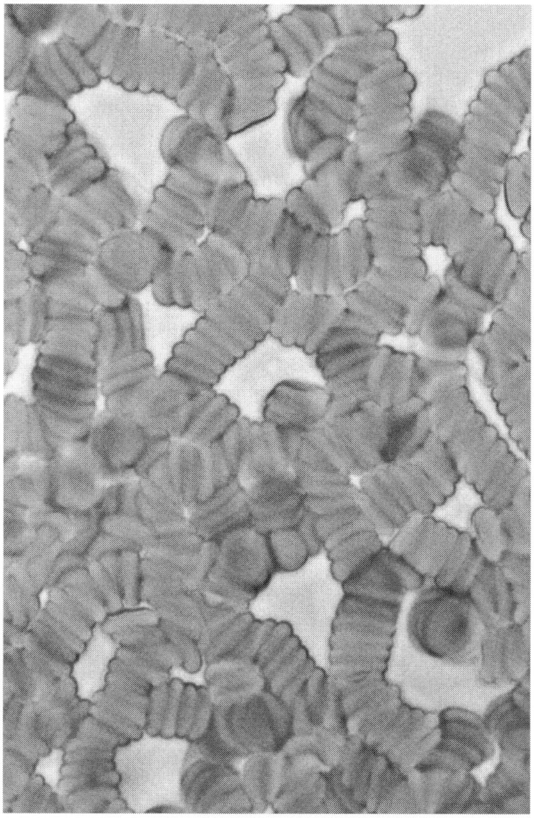

Fig. 3.5. Rouleaux blood cell network (see colour plate section).

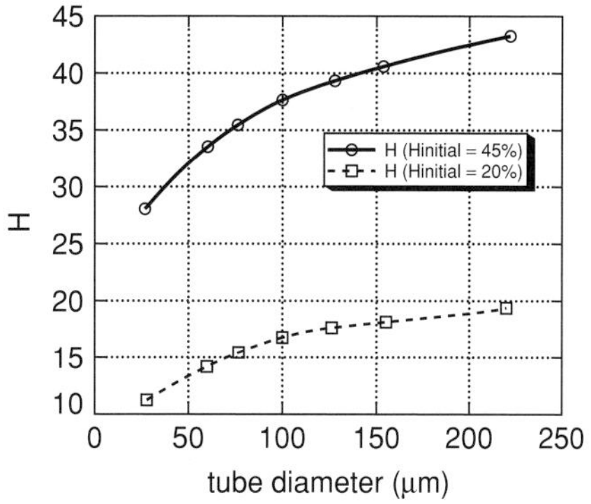

Fig. 3.6. Haematocrit (H) as a function of tube diameter. The initial haematocrit value for each line is shown in the inset box [7].

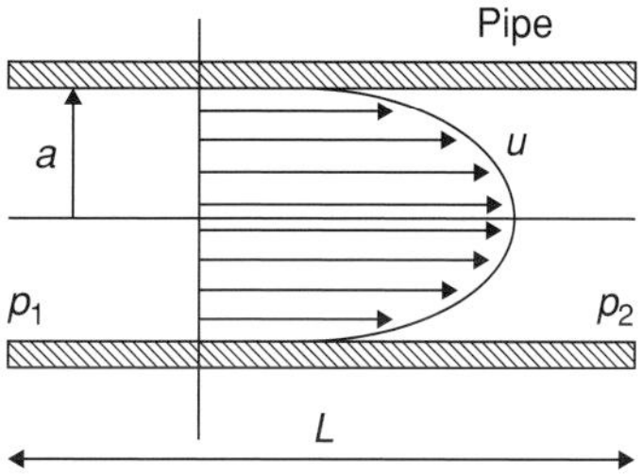

Fig. 3.7. Parabolic velocity profile for fully developed Poiseuille flow.

viscosity decreases. For high shear rates, the blood cells tend to become elongated and line up with the flow of the liquid. This also tends to decrease the viscosity of the blood. Given that the viscosity of blood increases with decreasing shear, one would think that the viscosity of blood within the body should increase as blood travels from the arteries through the arterioles and into the capillaries. This is because the shear rate and velocity of the blood decreases as the blood travels from the arteries through to the capillaries. The viscosity of blood, however, may be approximately constant throughout much of the body. This effect arises due to separate physical flow phenomena.

First, the viscosity of blood is dependent on the haematocrit. If the haematocrit decreases then the blood viscosity decreases. For example, in Figure 3.4 we show the viscosity of blood as a function of shear rate for 45% and 0% haematocrit. For the 0% haematocrit line the viscosity of the blood is constant and has a value of approximately 1.6 cP.

Second, the haematocrit level is dependent on the diameter of the blood vessel. As the blood vessel decreases in diameter, the haematocrit level also decreases (Figure 3.6). This effect occurs because the blood cells tend to move away from the vessel walls and travel to where the flow velocity is at a maximum. This behaviour is known as the Fahraeus effect and it has been shown to occur in tubes with a diameter as small as 29 μm. Given that a blood cell has a diameter of around 8 μm it is possible that the Fahraeus effect may occur in tubes with diameters less than 29 μm. The combination of these two effects implies that the viscosity of blood is approximately constant throughout the body.

POISEUILLE FLOW

Suppose that you have a Newtonian fluid flowing, in a steady, non-pulsatile manner, down a cylindrical, non-elastic pipe of length L and radius a. If the pipe is long enough, the flow will develop a parabolic velocity profile, which is generally called a Poiseuille flow profile (Figure 3.7). The flow takes its name from Jean Louis Poiseuille, a physician with training in physics and mathematics, who first described the flow structure in 1846. The volumetric flow rate (q) for Poiseuille flow, i.e. the volume of fluid flowing along the tube per unit time is given in equation 5:

$$q = \frac{(p_1 - p_2)\pi a^4}{8\mu L} \qquad (5)$$

where $p_1 - p_2$ is the pressure difference between the two ends of the tube and μ is the viscosity of the fluid.

The physics of the flow is nicely described by this equation. That is, flow is driven by the pressure gradient in the tube or, conversely, when there is flow in a tube then you must have a pressure gradient to drive the flow.

Prostheses are subject to the intermittent forces of pulsation and flow. The large elastic vessels are capacitors and provide on-flow in diastole, and the muscular peripheral vessels maintain pressure by altering resistance mediated via physiological feed back. Current prostheses are not able to do this and have to withstand the forces.

Note also the parameter of length. Flow is therefore also related to length. Patency, such as in femoropopliteal synthetic conduits, maybe as much, if not more, related to the length of the conduit as it is to angulation across the bend points, depending on the haematological factors depositing the thrombus. This may also partly explain better patency in shorter bypass grafts.

BERNOULLI'S EQUATION

Johann Bernoulli (1667–1748) was a professor in Basel and taught physics, anatomy and physiology. His understanding lies at the heart of vascular physics and relates pressure to motion and energy. For a fluid that has no viscosity, one can write:

$$p + \rho\frac{u^2}{2} + \rho g y = \text{constant of the flow} \qquad (6)$$

where p is the pressure, ρ the mass density of the liquid, u the speed of the fluid, g the gravitational acceleration and y the height. In other words, the Bernoulli equation states that the pressure plus the kinetic energy per unit volume, $\rho\frac{u^2}{2}$, plus the potential energy per unit volume, $\rho g y$, is a constant at any point along the blood vessel. So for a constant height, an increase in flow speed implies a decrease in pressure, while for constant flow speed, an increase in height implies a decrease in pressure.

It should be understood that equation 6 is an approximation, as it ignores the loss of energy due to shearing friction between the flowing blood and the walls of the artery. Even so, it does provide us with an intuitive understanding of the physics of the arterial/venous system. For example, suppose we wish to measure the blood pressure of a person. Typically one places a sleeve or an external cuff around the upper arm. The upper arm is chosen because it is at approximately the same level as the heart and so the pressure will not be affected by any difference in height. To measure the systolic pressure, the cuff pressure is increased until all blood flow ceases. From equation 6 we know that this 'cut-off' pressure is the maximum pressure in the artery. The pressure in the external cuff is then decreased until the flow is a maximum. We then know that the pressure will be a minimum and this is the diastolic pressure in the artery.

In practice, the arterial system has two sources of potential energy to drive the blood forward. The first is blood pressure and this is transformed into kinetic energy of flow during the period between systole and diastole, and the second is stored energy in the wall of the artery – its capacitance. Consider what might happen when the kinetic energy meets a resistive obstacle – some energy is dissipated as heat, as with circuit theory, and some is stored for use in diastole for onward flow in the period of heart filling by the elasticity of the great vessels acting as a capacitor. However, some energy is used up as a water hammer. The repetitive alterations in forward pressure and resistive back pressure with pulsatile flow in a physiologically responding, pressurized system sets up the potential for the water hammer. The injury and healing cycle effect of these water hammers on atherogenesis and aneurysm behaviour at stress points has yet to be fully determined.

YOUNG'S MODULUS AND PULSATILE FLOW

Blood flows through the arteries in a pulsatile fashion. Arteries are semi-elastic tubes, and the arteries expand and contract as the pulse of blood flows along the artery. The speed, c, at which blood flows along an artery is determined by the speed that a pulse of fluid can travel along an elastic tube. This speed is given, approximately,

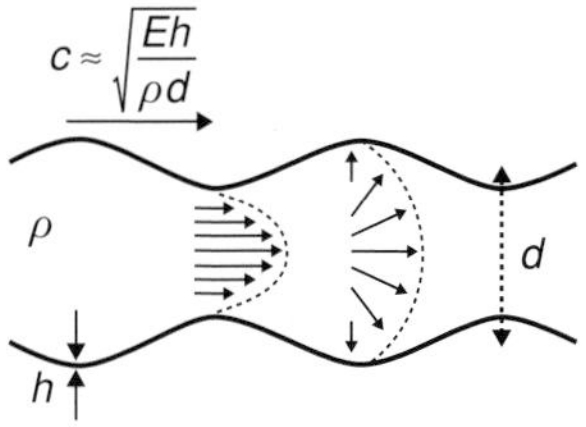

Fig. 3.8. An exaggerated, schematic view of blood flow in an artery.

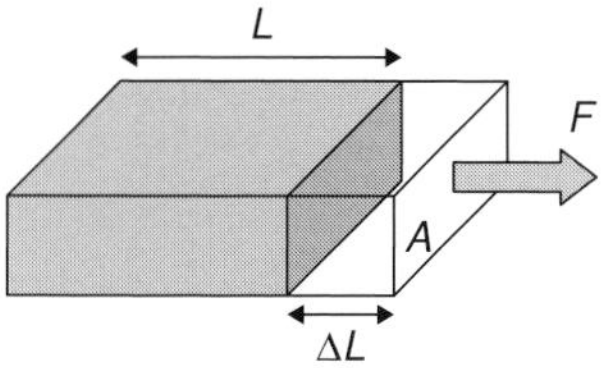

Fig. 3.9. A block of material with a length, L, and side area A is subject to a force F. The applied force stretches the block a distance ΔL.

by the Moen-Korteweg formula:

$$c \approx \sqrt{\frac{Eh}{\rho d}} \tag{7}$$

where E is Young's modulus for the wall of the artery, h is the thickness of the artery, d is the inner diameter of the artery and ρ is the density of blood. A schematic depiction of how a pulsatile wave propagates along an artery is given in Figure 3.8. As can be seen from equation 7, the speed at which blood travels along an artery is partially dependent on the Young's modulus of the arterial wall. To illustrate the definition of Young's modulus it is useful to consider Figure 3.9, where a block of material is being stretched due to an applied surface on one end of the block. The block has a natural length denoted by L; when a force F is applied to one side of the block then the length of the block increases by ΔL. This change in length is known as a *strain*, ε, and it is defined by equation 8:

$$\varepsilon = \frac{\Delta L}{L} \tag{8}$$

The *stress* that the force applies to the block of material has the definition

$$\sigma = \frac{F}{A} \tag{9}$$

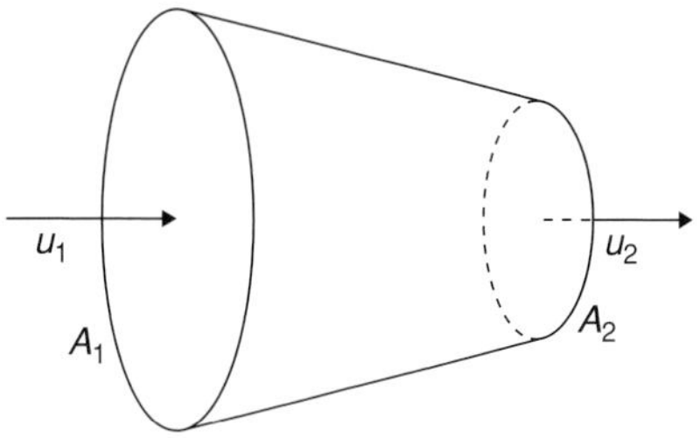

Fig. 3.10. A change in the diameter of an artery leads to a change in the blood flow speed.

Young's modulus is defined as the stress over the strain, i.e.

$$E = \frac{\sigma}{\varepsilon} \tag{10}$$

Thomas Young (1773–1829) was a medical physician who made significant contributions to fields of physics (through his experiments which demonstrated the wave-like nature of light), linguistics (via his identification of the Rosetta stone), medicine (with his studies of blood flow) and structural mechanics (e.g. Young's modulus). He was well aware of the elastic nature of the arteries, but, somewhat ironically, does not appear to have used Young's modulus to describe their properties.

One consequence of aging is increasing stiffness in the arteries. This means that the Young's modulus increases and this, as a consequence of equation 7, increases the speed of pulsatile flow within the arterial system.

MASS CONSERVATION

In Figure 3.10 we view a schematic depiction of an artery that is changing in shape as one travels along the artery. The blood flows in at one end with a speed u_1. The area at the inlet of the artery is given by A_1. In its simplest form, the mass conservation equation provides us with the relationship between the quantities at the proximal and distal ends of the artery:

$$u_1 A_1 = u_2 A_2 \tag{11}$$

here u_2 and A_2 are the outlet flow speed and diameter, respectively. In plain English, equation 11 is another way of saying 'what goes in must come out'.

We can see from equation 11 that if an artery becomes narrower, i.e. A_2 becomes smaller, then the flow speed, u_2, increases. This occurs because the mass flow is conserved and so if the tube becomes narrower then the flow rate has to increase.

REYNOLDS' NUMBER

The Reynolds' number is a dimensionless number, which provides an indication of how blood is flowing in an artery. The Reynolds' number is given by:

$$Re = \frac{UD\rho}{\mu} \quad (12)$$

where U is the speed of the flow, D is the diameter of the blood vessel, ρ the blood density and μ the blood viscosity. For an artery, the flow tends to change from laminar to turbulent at a Reynolds' number of approximately 2000. This number should be treated as only a representative value, since the transition from laminar to turbulent flow may occur at higher Reynolds' numbers.

To see a representative peak value of Reynolds' number, we consider an abdominal aorta of diameter $D = 2.5$ cm $= 0.025$ m, peak blood flow speed $U = 60$ cm/s $= 0.6$ m/s, blood density $\rho = 1$ gram/cc $= 1000$ kg/m^3 and blood viscosity $\mu = 0.0036$ Pa s. These values give Re ≈ 4200. So, in principle, it is possible for turbulent flow to occur in the aorta during the systolic phase.

Fluid flowing in a laminar fashion is dominated by the viscosity and at a high Reynolds' number by its inertia. A bruit is audible chaotic flow at high velocity with energy transformed to noise – inefficient flow that may be disruptive as in a carotid stenosis – and blood needs to be able to flow fast in order to deliver its load at a cardiac output of up to 30 L/min in an athlete.

Turbulent flow is less efficient relative to laminar flow. This means that more energy or a greater pressure drop is required to drive turbulent flow compared with laminar flow. A quantitative way of measuring this inefficiency is given by the formula for energy or 'head' loss for flow along a pipe:

$$h_L = f\frac{L}{D}\frac{U^2}{2g} \quad (13)$$

where f is the loss coefficient, L the length of the artery or appropriate subsection of an artery and g the acceleration due to gravity. For laminar flow:

$$f_{\text{lam}} = \frac{64}{Re} \quad (14)$$

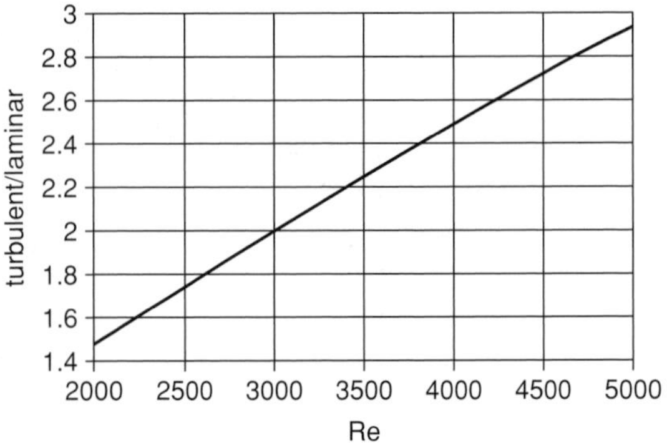

Fig. 3.11. Plot of the ratio of turbulent to laminar energy loss coefficients.

while for turbulent flow:

$$f_{\text{turb}} \sim \frac{0.316}{Re^{1/4}} \quad (15)$$

One can show that $f_{\text{turb}} > f_{\text{lam}}$ when Re > 1200, which implies that turbulence consumes more energy relative to laminar flow. This result is represented schematically in Figure 3.11, where we have plotted the ratio $f_{\text{turb}}/f_{\text{lam}}$ as a function of Re. Here we see that at a Reynolds' number of around 2000, turbulent flow loses 1.5 times more energy relative to laminar flow. As Re approaches 5000, turbulent flow tends to lose three times as much energy as laminar flow. It is interesting to speculate that the particulate nature of blood and plasma composition may act to discourage the formation of turbulent flow. Each red cell, being bi-concave, could change the local interactions between the cells and the blood plasma so that the flow tends to remain laminar. The shape of the red cell then may enhance the efficiency of blood flow, in addition to increasing surface area for oxygen delivery.

SHEAR STRESS AND PRESSURE

All vascular clinicians are familiar with the ultimate shearing force injury of high velocity impact when the mobile arch of the aorta and heart continue to move forward while the descending aorta, held by the intercostals and posterior mediastinum, is held to the vertebral bodies. What of subtle persistent long term shear stresses and the relationship with the greatest risk factor for arterial disease – age? There are known common

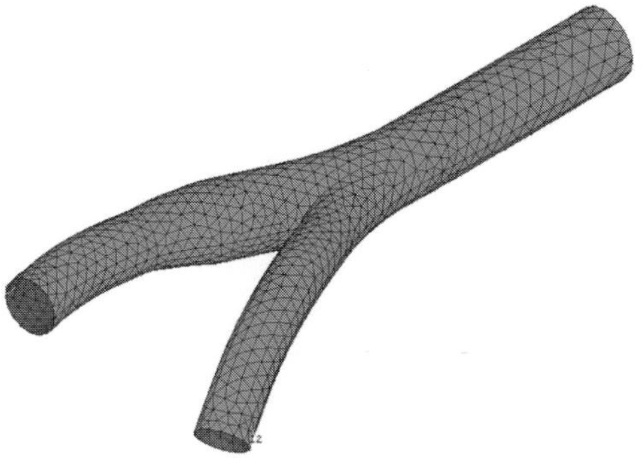

(a) Finite element computational mesh of a carotid bifurcation.

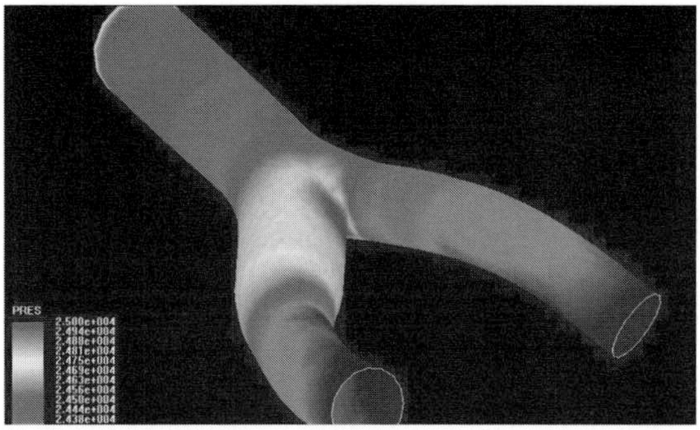

(b) Distribution of wall pressure.

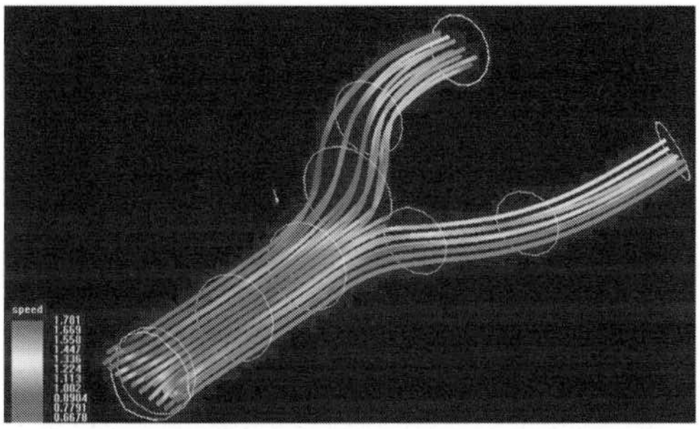

(c) Flow streamlines.

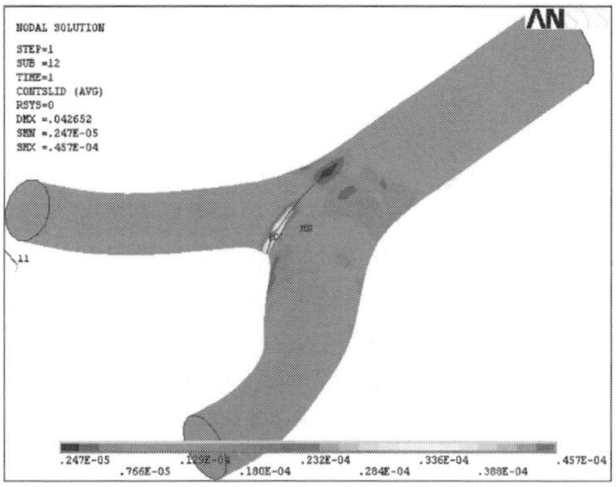

(d) Inter-layer sliding distance.

Fig. 3.12. Finite element stress/strain and computational fluid dynamic model of a carotid bifurcation (see colour plate section).

sites for occlusive atheromatous plaques, e.g. the carotid bifurcation, aortic bifurcation, origins of branches of the aorta and coronary arteries, and shear stress points like the adductor canal.

Atheroma is an arterial lesion. It is only seen in veins subject to long term pulsatile pressure when they are said to be 'arterialized'. Pressure and pulsatility are the forces involved, and the biochemical and biological responses act as the accelerators and decelerators. These are the accelerators to any predisposition that is genetically and age determined.

The clinically known common sites of atheromatous occlusive lesions in the arterial tree – be it cardiac, cerebrovascular, visceral or peripheral are stress focal points that can be predicted mathematically and illustrated with finite element stress/strain analysis. They correspond so much so that the appearance of a typical plaque of a carotid bifurcation lesion imaged with angio-computed tomography (CT) can, to a certain extent, be duplicated by the computational stress area chart of a simulated carotid bifurcation.

In Figure 3.12 (a) we show the computational mesh for a finite element model that computes the stresses and strains on a carotid bifurcation. Simulated blood was allowed to flow through the model at a systolic speed of 1 m/s and an entrance pressure of 180 mm Hg. The subsequent pressure inside the bifurcation is shown in Figure 3.12 (b). Interestingly, it shows that a region of maximum pressure occurs at the bifurcation between the internal and external carotids. This is probably due to ram pressure where the moving fluid rams directly into the arterial wall. Figure 3.12 (c) illustrates some of the flow streamlines, while Figure 3.12 (d) shows the sliding distance between two layers within the arterial wall. In this case, the maximum displacement between the two layers is approximately 40 microns. Shear stress on an arterial wall, τ_w, due to Poiseuille fluid flow is given in equation 16:

$$\tau_w = \frac{4\mu q}{\pi a^3} \quad (16)$$

where a is the radius of the artery and q is the volume flow rate of blood through the artery. From this formula it can be seen that shear stress increases with the increase of blood flow through the artery and tends to increase as the artery becomes smaller in diameter – provided that the volume flow rate and the viscosity are approximately constant.

Shear stress may play a more important role in atherogenesis than flow stress due to the damaging effect of transmural forces. There might be a greater contribution to wall damage from fatigue stress than flow stress and thereby to atherogenesis because of its greater role in the damage and healing response that is lesion generating.

The arterial wall is constructed like a tyre and tube. The outer wall is strong and built to handle pressure. The inner wall is smooth for minimal disruption to laminar flow, but has little strength. The media is the infrastructure between and the layers into which feed the vasa vasorum, via the adventitia. Movement of the adventitia with respect to the intima sets up a shearing moment that is enhanced by pressure and pulse rate increases. Should this shear force be sufficient to tear a penetrating vasa vasorum a subintimal haematoma results and an atheromatous lesion may follow. Separation of the layers and the injury healing cycle progress the lesion. Intraplaque haemorrhage without intimal defect is common. This same shear force may rupture the established plaque. Plaque rupture and intraplaque haemorrhage are recognized causes of cardiac events.

A pressure of 180 mm Hg produces a movement differential of 0.04 mm in the arterial wall at a typical carotid bifurcation stress point, in finite element analysis of a simulated carotid bifurcation. This movement is repeated with every pulse.

Although these results are from very preliminary calculations, they suggest a mechanism for anti-hypertensive agents – such as ace inhibitors and beta blockers that are effective in vascular event reduction – by reducing the forces, especially during activity, and protecting the arterial structural system.

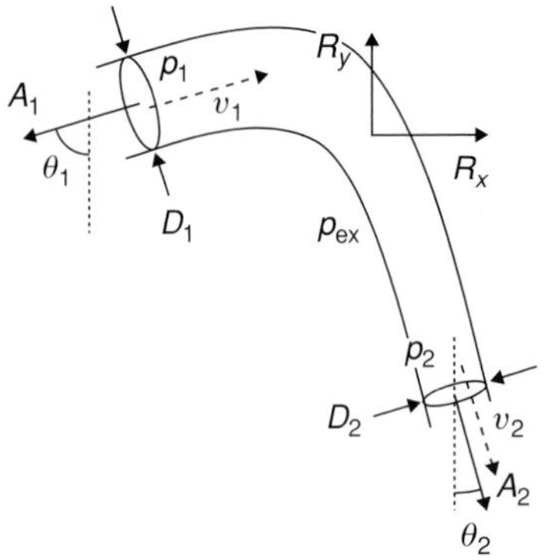

Fig. 3.13. The characteristic velocity, pressure, area and force vectors required to compute the restraining forces on a bent, single-tube graft system.

FORCES ON A SINGLE TUBE GRAFT SYSTEM

An important issue in vascular intervention is the durability of ELGs. Such grafts are often used to protect aneurysms from the effects of arterial pressure. Unfortunately, haemodynamic forces can displace a graft and thereby, possibly, interrupt the seal between the graft and the neck of the aneurysm. it is important, therefore to have an understanding of the possible forces that may be exerted on a graft.

To illustrate the steps used in determining the forces on a graft system, via analytic equations, we consider the steady flow of blood through a bent pipe (Figure 3.13). In this figure, the proximal inlet entrance is labelled 1 and the distal exit 2. D_1, A_1 and D_2, A_2 are the diameters and cross-sectional areas, respectively, of the graft at the points 1 and 2. The vector normals of the cross-sectional areas are, respectively, at angles of θ_1 and θ_2 to the vertical. Similarly p and v refer to the pressures and velocities at these points. R_x and R_y are the x and y components of the restoring force. The external pressure on the graft system is denoted by p_{ex}.

In our analysis, we assume steady-state, i.e. non-pulsatile, flow. We do this for two reasons: first, it gives us a basic idea of how the system is behaving. Second, we are in the process of deriving and testing the appropriate equations for pulsatile flow, so it would be premature to release those results at this stage.

The first equation is the steady-state mass conservation equation (equation 11), which we rewrite in the form:

$$v_1 A_1 = v_2 A_2 \tag{17}$$

One should note that v_1 and v_2 are average flow speeds, where the average is taken over the areas of A_1 and A_2, respectively.

The next analysis tool at our disposal is the momentum conservation equation, which can be expressed in the form:

$$R_x = \begin{array}{l}(p_2 - p_{ex})A_2 \sin\theta_2 - (p_1 - p_{ex})A_1 \sin\theta_1 \\ +\rho v_2^2 A_2 \sin\theta_2 - \rho v_1^2 A_1 \sin\theta_1\end{array} \tag{18}$$

and

$$R_y = \begin{array}{l}-(p_1 - p_{ex})A_1 \cos\theta_1 - (p_2 - p_{ex})A_2 \cos\theta_2 \\ -\rho v_1^2 A_1 \cos\theta_1 - \rho v_2^2 A_2 \cos\theta_2\end{array} \tag{19}$$

where in these formulae, we have ignored the weight of the graft and the weight of blood in the graft. These terms are easily included into the equations, if required.

An interesting point about the above equations is that they compute the force on the graft, but that the length of the graft does not explicitly enter into the equations. Only the pressure and flow of blood through the faces of the graft are explicitly shown. This is because we have assumed steady-state flow. If we had assumed pulsatile flow, then the equations would be the same, except there would be an extra term, which does include the length of the graft. The relative magnitude of this pulsatile term is still under investigation and will not be discussed here.

Energy is the final conserved quantity that we can use in our analysis. The energy conservation equation has the form:

$$\frac{p_1}{\gamma} + \frac{\alpha_1 v_1^2}{2g} + z_1 = \frac{p_2}{\gamma} + \frac{\alpha_2 v_2^2}{2g} + z_2 + h_L \tag{20}$$

where g is the gravitational acceleration, $\gamma = \rho g$ is the weight density of blood, z_1 and z_2 are the vertical heights of the proximal and distal ends of the graft, respectively, and h_L is the 'head loss' in the pipe, i.e. the amount of

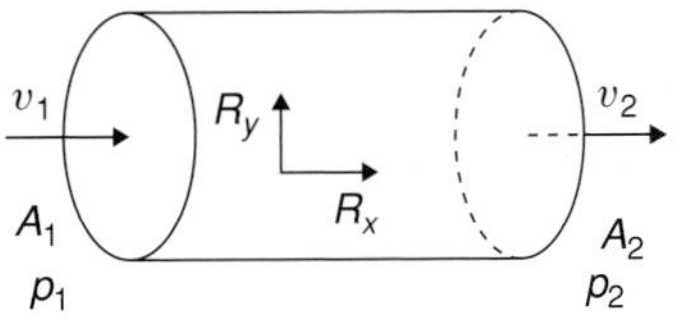

Fig. 3.14. Cylindrical graft.

pressure or energy that is lost due to frictional viscous effects as the fluid travels through the pipe. Head loss is usually given by the equation:

$$h_L = K_L \frac{v_2^2}{2g} \tag{21}$$

where K_L is a constant, the value of which is usually dependent on the shape, length and diameter of the pipe. The coefficients α_1 and α_2 are kinetic energy correction factors that have different values depending on the type of flow. For example, for uniform flow $\alpha = 1$, turbulent flow has $\alpha \approx 1$ and laminar flow gives $\alpha = 2$.

By combining equations 17, 20 and 21 one obtains:

$$p_2 = p_1 + \frac{\gamma v_1^2}{2g}\left(\alpha_1 - (\alpha_2 + K_L)\left(\frac{A_1}{A_2}\right)^2\right) + \gamma(z_1 - z_2) \tag{22}$$

So, by using equations 22 and 17 we can express p_2 and v_2 in terms of quantities at the entrance of the graft. This then allows us to compute the restraining forces on the graft system by then using equations 18 and 19.

Case 1 – the cylindrical graft

For this case, see Figure 3.14, the inlet and the outlet areas are the same, so, as given by equation 17, the inlet and outlet flow speeds are also equal. The angles θ_1 and θ_2 are equal and have a value of 90°. The inlet and outlet pressures are not equal due to the frictional, shear interaction between the blood and the graft (i.e. the head loss as given by equation 21). This frictional interaction causes the outlet pressure, p_2, to be less than the inlet pressure, p_1. This is called a pressure drop.

From all of this information, one can write down the restraint forces on the graft. So, from equations 18 and 19:

$$R_y = 0 \tag{23}$$

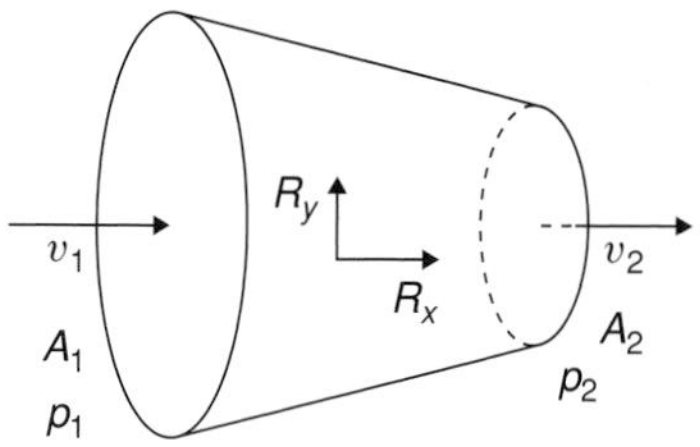

Fig. 3.15. An endoluminal graft in the shape of a windsock.

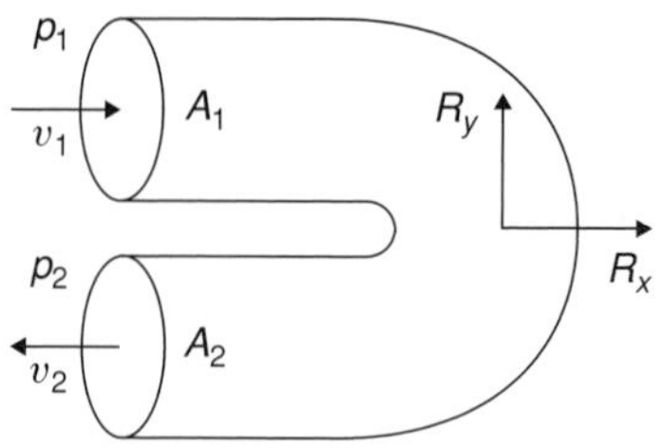

Fig. 3.16. Curved graft.

i.e. there are no vertical forces generated by blood flowing through a horizontal graft and:

$$R_x = (p_2 - p_1)A_1 \tag{24}$$

where we have set the external pressure to zero. In this case, the horizontal force on the graft is quite small, because p_1 will only be a little larger than p_2. One can conclude from this analysis that straight, cylindrical grafts only feel a relatively small drag force in the direction of the flow.

Case 2 – the windsock graft

Suppose now we consider a graft in the shape of a windsock, such as in Figure 3.15.

For this case, the inlet area is now larger than the outlet area, so, as given by equation 17, the outlet flow speed is greater than the inlet flow speed as:

$$v_2 = \left(\frac{A_1}{A_2}\right) v_1 \tag{25}$$

As in the previous case, the angles θ_1 and θ_2 are equal and have a value of 90°, and the inlet and outlet pressures are not equal due to the frictional, shear interaction between the blood and the graft.

The restraint forces on the graft are from equations 18 and 19:

$$R_x = p_2 A_2 - p_1 A_1 + \rho v_2^2 A_2 - \rho v_1^2 A_1, \tag{26}$$

and

$$R_y = 0 \tag{27}$$

When you put the appropriate numbers into equation 26, it is found that the dominant term in this equation is the $p_1 A_1$ term. Many ELGs have this 'windsock' shape, an exit, distal area that is smaller than the proximal, inlet area. This shape has a much larger drag force than for a cylindrical graft.

Case 3 – the curved graft

From Figure 3.16, the inlet and outlet areas are the same, so, as given by equation 17, the inlet and outlet flow speeds are also equal. Due to the symmetry of the situation, the vertical restraint force is zero. The horizontal restraint force is given by:

$$R_x = -p_2 A_2 - p_1 A_1 - \rho v_2^2 A_2 - \rho v_1^2 A_1. \tag{28}$$

So, now both the pressure and velocity components add together to produce a greater total force on the graft. This result suggests that a curved graft may be subject to greater forces than a windsock shaped graft.

CONCLUSION

Understanding the physics of the vascular system in health and disease will influence vascular management. This is a rich field for further research. Further clues to atherogenesis may lie in the differences of the fluid dynamics and physical forces applied to the arterial systems, in particular the pressure patterns.

REFERENCES

1. M. M. D. Lawrence-Brown, J. B. Semmens, D. E. Hartley *et al.*, How is durability related to patient selection and graft design with endoluminal grafting for abdominal aortic aneurysm? In *Durability of Vascular and Endovascular Surgery*, ed. R. M. Greenhalgh & W. B. Saunders. (London: Saunders Company Ltd, 1999), pp. 375–85.
2. P. L. Harris, J. Buth, C. Mialhe, H. O. Myhre & L. Norgren, The need for clinical trials of endovascular

abdominal aortic aneurysm stent-graft repair: the EUROSTAR project. *Journal of Endovascular Surgery*, **4** (1997), 72–7.

3. The UK Small Aneurysm Trial Participants. Mortality results for randomized controlled trial of early elective surgery or ultrasonographic surveillance for small abdominal aortic aneurysms. *Lancet*, **352** (1998), 1649–55.
4. M. M. D. Lawrence-Brown, P. E. Norman, K. Jamrozik, *et al.*, Initial results of the western Australian ultrasound screening project for aneurysm of the abdominal aorta: relevance for endoluminal treatment of aneurysm disease. *Cardiovascular Surgery*, **9** (2001), 234–40.
5. K. Liffman, M. M. D. Lawrence-Brown, J. B. Semmens *et al.*, Analytical modelling and numerical simulation of forces in an endoluminal graft. *Journal of Endovascular Therapy*, **8** (2001), 358–71.
6. S. Chien, S. Usami, R. J. Dellenbeck & M. Gregersen, Shear dependent deformation of erythrocytes in rheology of human blood. *American Journal of Physiology*, **219** (1970), 136–42.
7. J. H. Barbee & G. R. Cokelet, The Fahraeus effect. *Microvascular Research*, **3** (1971), 6–16.

4 • Haemostasis – a clinician's perspective

DOUGLAS COGHLAN AND DONALD J. ADAM

NORMAL HAEMOSTASIS

Under normal conditions, blood circulates through the intact vasculature without appreciable thrombus formation or haemorrhage. Normal haemostasis acts to minimize haemorrhage, maintain vascular integrity, maximize perfusion, and facilitate healing and repair.

Vascular injury leads to temporary vasoconstriction and increased tissue tension due to blood loss into adjacent tissues. Subsequent formation of a platelet-fibrin plug at the site of vessel injury restores the integrity of circulation. Inhibition of thrombus formation in intact areas ensures that this occurs with minimal interruption to blood flow. The end result is healing of the vascular injury, removal of the blood clot and restoration of function. Normal haemostasis is a dynamic balance between fibrin formation and resolution, and is dependent on interactions between endothelium, platelets, coagulation and fibrinolysis.

EVOLUTION OF OUR UNDERSTANDING OF HAEMOSTASIS

In 1892, Schmitt described the process of clot formation by thrombin-mediated clotting of fibrinogen. In 1905, Morowitz demonstrated that tissue extracts could induce clotting in plasma and that this formed the basis for an 'extrinsic' pathway of coagulation. The first test of the coagulation pathway exploiting this finding was described by Quick in 1935. This is now formalized as the prothrombin time (PT) assay. Macerated tissue and calcium are added to citrate-anticoagulated plasma and the time to clot formation is determined. The macerated tissue contains a source of tissue factor (TF) and phospholipids. The variability in the nature of these thromboplastins gave rise to variability in the PT and derived prothrombin ratio (PTR). The development of the international normalized ratio (INR) has addressed this problem. Deficiencies of factors VII, V, X, prothrombin or fibrinogen may result in the prolongation of the PT. The PT will also be prolonged in the presence of an inhibitor and so this test is commonly used to monitor the anticoagulant effect of warfarin.

The extrinsic pathway of coagulation was therefore described on the basis that something needed to be added to plasma to initiate clot formation. Langdell and colleagues investigated the spontaneous clotting of recalcified citrated plasma and developed the partial thromboplastin time (PTT). As activation of coagulation occurred with exposure of plasma to surfaces such as glass and did not require the addition of compounds extrinsic to the plasma, this was referred to as the 'intrinsic' pathway of coagulation. The presently formulated activated partial thromboplastin time (aPTT) test is sensitive to deficiencies in factors XII, XI, IX and VIII as well as those in the common pathway (see below). Inhibitors may prolong the aPTT which is used to monitor unfractionated heparin activity.

The models were brought together by McFarlane (Cascade model) and Davie and Ratnoff (Waterfall model) in 1964 [1; 2]. These models emphasized the extrinsic and intrinsic coagulation pathways coming together at the activation of factor X with a final common pathway of thrombin activation and fibrin formation. Work done in the late 1970s and the 1980s emphasized the links between these artificially defined pathways. Various inhibitors were identified and the discovery of thrombomodulin (TM) allowed the integration of the procoagulant and anticoagulant pathways. The cascade model was then elaborated as initial amplification of a procoagulant stimulus leading to thrombin formation. Thrombin cleaves fibrinogen to fibrin and also activates factors V and VIII augmenting its own production. The binding of thrombin to TM leads to an alteration of its target with resultant activation of protein C which is an anticoagulant enzyme responsible for the inactivation of factors V and VIII. Thus thrombin is not only the major procoagulant enzyme but also the major anticoagulant enzyme. The cascades were now cast as positive feedback loops augmenting the activation of coagulation and negative feedback loops switching it off.

LIMITATIONS OF THE CASCADE MODEL

The cascade model describes clot formation *in vitro*, and allows an understanding of the laboratory monitoring of anticoagulation therapy and the diagnosis of coagulation disorders.

However, this arbitrary model is inadequate for the study of clot formation *in vivo*. For example, patients who have hereditary factor XII deficiency or deficiency in prekallikrein or high molecular weight kininogen have a markedly prolonged aPTT but no bleeding diathesis. These proteins are not, therefore, required to maintain haemostasis *in vivo*.

The cascade model gives no insight into the initiation of *in vivo* coagulation as macerated tissues and synthetic surfaces are not applicable *in vivo*. Tissue factor is a normal constituent of the surface of non-vascular cells and stimulated monocytes and endothelial cells (ECs). The central role of TF in the initiation of blood coagulation became clear during the 1980s and is *the* central component of any present model of haemostasis. The TF-factor VIIa complex activates not only factor X but also factor IX thus interconnecting the arbitrarily defined intrinsic and extrinsic pathways.

The cascade model further inhibits our understanding of haemostasis because it precludes questions concerning the roles of platelets and ECs both of which are critical to the development of the thrombus.

At a deeper level the model is circular – if the only tests are plasma clot based and the model is described by these tests then it will adequately predict the results of the tests. It will not, however, provide any information outside the model. Blood and plasma clot *in vitro* when only approximately 5% of prothrombin is converted to thrombin. Thus a clot based end point ignores the vast bulk of thrombin formation. An example of this is the common point mutation involving the prothrombin gene which gives rise to an increased level of prothrombin in the plasma but normal PT. Thus one of the common prothrombotic states is completely unrecognized by standard tests. Another example is massive blood transfusion which can lead to marked impairment of haemostasis with normal PT and aPTT. Replacement of clotting factors can normalize the tests without fully correcting the haemostatic defect.

COMPONENTS OF THE COAGULATION PATHWAY

Introduction

A zymogen is an inactive precursor protein which by proteolytic cleavage gains enzymatic function. This may be catalysed by other enzymes. An active form is generally indicated by a lower case 'a'. A protein domain is a sequence of amino acids (referred to as residues) which may confer a function. Often the sequence will resemble that from another protein and this may give insight into structure and function. For example, TF has a domain structure similar to a type 2 cytokine receptor suggesting that it may have a signalling function. Conformation refers to the three dimensional structure of the protein.

When a protein is synthesized from the amino to the carboxy terminus, the initial process of protein synthesis is referred to as translation (mRNA is *translated* into protein in the ribosome). Leader or signal sequences may direct the protein to cellular organelles where further modification such as carboxylation may occur. These sequences are subsequently cleaved from the mature protein. The DNA sequences of the genes for the coagulation proteins are known and the control of their expression is an area of intensive study. As a generalization, exons ('coding' regions) are the genetic sequences which are expressed in mRNA and subsequently in protein. Within the gene there are 'non-coding' regions referred to as introns.

To facilitate understanding of the pathway it is worthwhile grouping the various components by structure and function:

(1) Vitamin K-dependent zymogens – factors II, VII, IX, X and protein C
(2) Co-factors and transport molecules – factors V, VIII, protein S and von Willebrand factor (vWF)
(3) Factor XI and the 'contact factors'
(4) Cell associated co-factors – tissue factor (TF) and thrombomodulin (TM)
(5) Fibrinogen
(6) Factor XIII and thrombin-activatable fibrinolysis inhibitor (TAFI)

(7) Plasma coagulation protease inhibitors – antithrombin (AT)-III and tissue factor pathway inhibitor (TFPI)
(8) Platelets
(9) Endothelial cells

The vitamin K-dependent zymogens (factors II, VII, IX, X and protein C)

These proteins are all synthesized in the liver. A serine residue is present in the active site of the enzymes and thus they are described as serine proteases. These enzymes bind to phospholipid surfaces and this greatly increases their activity. The presence of specific receptors on cell surfaces may further enhance activity. Calcium is necessary for this binding and seems to induce conformational change so that the protein is anchored to the membrane.

The specific functions of all of these enzymes in the coagulation pathway seem to relate to surface loop domains which confer specificity to binding and co-factor interaction. Tissue factor is the co-factor for factor VIIa; factor VIIIa is the co-factor for factor IXa; factor Va for factor Xa; and activated protein C (aPC) is the co-factor protein S. Although thrombin does not have a co-factor, its activity is altered by binding to TM.

Co-factors have binding sites for their specific enzyme and its substrate. If we think of these as molecules interacting we can visualize how this might enhance activity by bringing these molecules into close physical proximity. The binding of the co-factor to its enzyme can also enhance activity by generating conformational change. The binding of a procoagulant enzyme to its co-factor and to an appropriate surface may enhance its activity more than one-million-fold. These assemblies are referred to as complexes named for their substrate. Factor VIIa-TF complex is referred to as the extrinsic tenase complex, factor IXa-VIIIa complex as the intrinsic tenase complex and the factor Xa-Va complex as the prothrombinase complex.

Prothrombin (factor II) is cleaved in two places by the Xa-Va complex and this gives rise to thrombin and a detectable fragment (prothrombin fragment, PF1+2). Assays of PF1+2 allow measurement of thrombin activation *in vitro*. Thrombin cleaves fibrinogen to yield fibrin monomers which polymerize to form a fibrin clot. It also activates factors V, VIII and XI providing for increased thrombin formation by positive feedback. Thrombin is the principal activator of platelets. Thrombin has anticoagulant properties at low concentrations by increasing the activation of protein C. At high concentrations, thrombin has a procoagulant and antifibrinolytic effect by overcoming the effect of aPC and activating TAFI. The major inhibitor of thrombin in plasma is AT-III. There are several polymorphisms of the prothrombin gene. One occurring at position 20210 (G-A) in a non-coding region increases the level of the circulating protein and is associated with an increased risk of venous thrombo-embolism.

Factor VII binds to TF and is activated. This active complex is the major physiological activator of both factors X and IX. It is inhibited by AT-III in the presence of heparin but the major inactivator is TFPI.

Factor IX is activated by TF-factor VIIa complex or by factor XIa. In the presence of factor VIIIa and a phospholipid surface, this complex is a very efficient activator of factor X. Activated platelets not only provide a negatively charged phospholipid surface but seem to have specific receptors which enhance complex formation and substrate binding. AT-III inhibits factor IXa.

Factor X can be auto-catalytically cleaved (beta Xa) but the major activation is by the intrinsic or extrinsic tenase complexes. In association with factor Va and a phospholipid surface (preferentially the activated platelet membrane), it is the physiological activator of thrombin (the prothrombinase complex). Factor Xa can activate factors VII, VIII and V. Factor Xa can be inhibited by AT-III or TFPI.

Protein C is activated by thrombin when it is bound to TM. Activated protein C in association with protein S inactivates factors Va and VIIIa. Reduced levels of protein C or the production of a mutant protein with defective function gives rise to an increased risk of venous thrombo-embolism. Activated protein C is inhibited by protein C inhibitor.

Co-factors and transport molecules (factors V, VIII, protein S and von Willebrand factor)

Factor V is activated by cleavage by thrombin and also factor Xa. Inactivation is by aPC at two sites (Arg 306 and Arg 506). The Arg 506 site is abolished by a mutation to glutamine, referred to as factor V Leiden. This is the most common cause of aPC resistance and the most commonly identified genetic thrombophilia. In addition to circulating free factor V there are substantial stores in platelet alpha granules some of which may be in a partially activated form.

Factor VIII is synthesized in the liver and circulates in a non-covalent complex with vWF. Factor VIII is activated by cleavage at three sites by thrombin or factor Xa. Activation is accompanied by release from vWF. Activated factor VIII is unstable and spontaneously loses activity. Proteolytic inactivation occurs by aPC and also thrombin.

Protein S does not contain a catalytic domain and is a co-factor for aPC in the inactivation of factors Va and VIIIa. It competes with factor Xa for bindng to factor Va and therefore has some intrinsic anticoagulant activity.

Von Willebrand factor is synthesized by ECs and megakaryocytes. It is the carrier molecule for factor VIII and mediates platelet adhesion to the subendothelium which is essential for the formation of occlusive platelet thrombi at sites of arterial injury. Von Willebrand factor derived from ECs accounts for 40% of total platelet adhesion, with the remaining 60% provided by plasma vWF.

Factor XI and the 'contact factors'

Factor XI is a zymogen and circulates in complex with high molecular weight kininogen (HMWK). Its catalytic domain is that of a serine protease and within its other domains there are sites for binding to HMWK, prothrombin, platelets, factor IX, thrombin and factor XIIa. The most likely mechanism of activation *in vivo* is by thrombin on the surface of activated platelets. In the laboratory, factor XIIa activates it in the aPTT test. Thrombin can activate it in the fluid phase and on charged surfaces. Deficiency of factor XI gives rise to a haemorrhagic tendency. Although factor XIa does not require a co-factor to activate factor IX, this reaction is calcium dependent. There are several circulating protease inhibitors of factor XIa and binding to platelets may partially protect it from degradation. The significance of factor XII, prekallikrein and HMWK to coagulation *in vivo* is uncertain. Their principal physiological roles appear to be in the inflammatory response.

Cell associated co-factors (tissue factor and thrombomodulin)

Tissue factor is an integral membrane protein. It is the receptor and co-factor for factors VII and VIIa. Tissue factor is expressed on many extravascular cells constitutively including vascular adventitia, microglia and stromal cells. It is not normally expressed on cells which are in contact with flowing blood. Tissue factor is expressed when ECs or monocytes are exposed to bacterial components such as lipopolysaccharide or inflammatory cytokines. When an injury exposes extravascular tissues, blood comes into contact with TF and coagulation is initiated. Factor VIIa represents 1%–2% of circulating factor VII and this binds to the exposed TF. Factor VII competes for this binding and acts as a negative regulator. The TF-VIIa complex becomes an efficient activator of factors X and IX. Although the complex does not need phospholipid its presence enhances activity by improving substrate localization. A major inhibitor of the complex is TFPI but AT-III may also play a role.

Thrombomodulin is the cellular co-factor for thrombin. It is a transmembrane protein which is constitutively expressed on vascular ECs. It can bind thrombin and protein C. When thrombin binds to TM it undergoes conformational change and profoundly alters its substrate. It no longer activates platelets, factors V and VIII or cleaves fibrinogen, but it becomes an efficient activator of protein C and TAFI.

Fibrinogen

This large molecule is found in plasma and the alpha granules of platelets. It supports the initial platelet plug and is cross-linked to generate the solid haemostatic clot. The plasma half life of fibrinogen is 3–5 days and only a small proportion is consumed in the formation of clots. Fibrinogen is also an acute phase reactant produced by the liver.

Fibrinogen is activated when thrombin binds and releases two fibrinopeptides A and B. This exposes binding sites in the E domain which bind complementary sites in the D domain. Fibrinogen monomers are linked at the E domain by disulphide bonds into dimers which are the dominant circulating form. This gives rise to the formation of fibrin protofibrils which are able to bind together to give rise to thick fibres. Protofibrils can bind to generate a three dimensional meshwork. Lateral growth is enhanced by calcium binding. As polymerization occurs other molecules bind. Adhesive molecules including fibronectin, thrombospondin and vWF are added at this time, as are elements of the fibrinolytic system. Fibrin also has specific binding sites for platelets. These elements influence further generation of fibrin, its cross-linking and ultimately its rate of breakdown. Cross-linking is achieved by factor XIIIa and degradation occurs by fibrinolysis. Fibrinolysis mediated by plasmin leads to a progressive proteolytic breakdown with D-dimer only generated by the breakdown of cross-linked fibrin.

Factor XIII and thrombin-activatable fibrinolysis inhibitor

This is a glycoprotein which is activated by thrombin when calcium is present. It is found in plasma, platelets, monocytes and macrophages and circulates in association with fibrinogen. Plasma factor XIII is activated by thrombin and cross-links the alpha and gamma chains of fibrin. It also cross-links α-2 antiplasmin to fibrin reducing the efficacy of plasmin-initiated fibrinolysis and thus stabilizing the fibrin plug. Thrombin-activatable fibrinolysis inhibitor is not strictly a procoagulant enzyme. It is activated by thrombin bound to TM. Carboxy terminal lysine residues on fibrin are exposed when plasmin begins to lyse fibrin. Activated TAFI reduces fibrinolysis by removing these residues from fibrin and their loss as binding sites greatly reduces the efficiency of plasmin.

There is a hypothesis that the high levels of thrombin required to activate TAFI are generated by factor XI-augmented thrombin activation. Clinically, factor XI deficiency gives rise to bleeding after initial fibrin clot formation and the clot is more readily lysed. The haemorrhagic diathesis is corrected when TAFI is added to a factor XI deficient model.

Plasma coagulation protease inhibitors (antithrombin-III and tissue factor pathway inhibitor)

In addition to Protein S and C, the best characterized inhibitors are TFPI and AT-III.

Tissue factor pathway inhibitor binds to and inhibits factor Xa. Only after this binding is it able to bind to and inhibit the TF-factor VIIa complex. Tissue factor pathway inhibitor is thus the major inhibitor of the TF pathway. It is also a significant inhibitor of factor Xa although quantitatively less important than AT. Tissue factor pathway inhibitor is synthesized in ECs and circulates in association with lipoproteins. Heparin releases TFPI from EC glycosaminoglycans.

Antithrombin-III is a serine protease inhibitor (serpin). This is a class of proteins which bind to their substrates (serine proteases) in a 1:1 fashion and inhibit their action. The serpin-serine protease complex is degraded by liver mediated endocytosis. The major targets are factors IIa, Xa and IXa. Antithrombin-III binds to thrombin to form the thrombin-antithrombin (TAT) complex. Antithrombin-III deficiency is a cause of a significant thrombophilia.

Heparins are glycosaminoglycans of varying molecular weight. They greatly augment AT-III activity and are able to bind both AT-III and its protease substrate. This binding brings the reactants into physical proximity and may also cause conformational change. Unfractionated heparins greatly facilitate binding of thrombin to AT-III. Lower molecular weight heparins may have relatively more effect on the binding and inactivation of factor Xa.

ENDOTHELIAL CELLS AND COAGULATION

The vascular endothelium forms the physical interface between blood and the underlying tissues, allows exchange and active transport of substances across the vessel wall, and has an important role in the regulation of haemostasis and the maintenance of vascular tone. Injured endothelium initiates thrombus formation by exposing the subendothelial surface to platelets and coagulation factors. Healthy intact endothelium provides an anticoagulant environment. It is negatively charged and forms a physical barrier which prevents the interaction between platelets and clotting factors, and subendothelial TF and collagen. Healthy ECs also contain an endogenous heparin-like factor called haparan sulphate which acts to increase the rate of thrombin inactivation by AT. Thrombin also binds to TM expressed on the surface of ECs and the resultant thrombin-TM complex activates protein C which, together with the endothelial product protein S, inactivates coagulation factors Va and VIIIa, and the tenase and prothrombinase complexes. Endothelial cells are the main site of synthesis of TFPI and express tissue plasminogen activator (tPA), which activates fibrinolysis and ensures that coagulation is confined to areas of vessel injury.

As discussed in chapter 1 EC activation involves a change in function and morphology, and consists of: change in phenotype from anticoagulant to procoagulant; loss of vascular integrity; cytokine production; expression of leucocyte adhesion molecules; and up-regulation of human leucocyte antigen molecules. Endothelial cell activation is induced by a wide range of agents including ischaemia, endotoxaemia and cytokines. *In vitro*, these cytokines induce TF expression by ECs (and leucocytes) and up-regulate the release of vWF into plasma resulting in a procoagulant state. The procoagulant effects of EC activation consist of: increased plasminogen activator inhibitor (PAI) release which inhibits fibrinolysis; increased PAF expression; diminished platelet anti-aggregatory effects due to reduced prostacyclin expression; vasodilation secondary to increased nitric oxide (NO) production; increased TF expression; and shedding of haparan sulphate.

FIBRINOLYSIS

Fibrinolysis is a physiological consequence of fibrin deposition. At the same time as thrombin generation and fibrin deposition are taking place, the fibrinolytic system is secondarily activated in order to limit clot formation to the site of vessel wall injury and recanalize blood vessels after repair has taken place.

Tissue plasminogen activator is the principal endogenous activator of plasminogen (Figure 4.1) and is rapidly released from vascular endothelial and smooth muscle cells in response to thrombin, endotoxins, cytokines and ischaemia. Plasminogen is concentrated into the forming clot and tPA binds to the fibrin surface to form the tPA/plasminogen/fibrin complex. Tissue plasminogen activator activates plasminogen to the enzyme plasmin. Plasmin activity is maximal in the clot where it is protected from the circulating plasmin inhibitor, α-2 antiplasmin. Plasmin causes lysis of fibrin, fibrinogen and a cross-linked fibrin clot to produce split products including fibrin degradation products (FDPs) and a D-dimer which further stimulate plasmin formation. Plasmin acts specifically in areas of excessive fibrin deposition as tPA is a poor plasminogen activator in the absence of fibrin.

The availability and activity of tPA is dependent not only on its release from the endothelium, but also on neutralization by its inhibitors, α-2 antiplas-

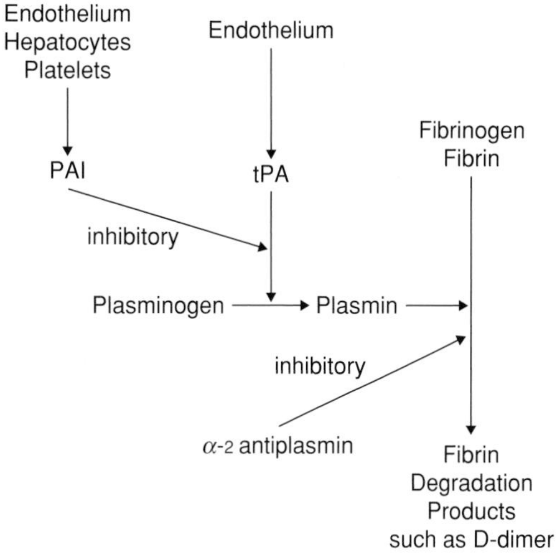

Fig. 4.1. Fibrinolytic system.

min and PAIs, and first-pass PAI-independent hepatic clearance. Plasminogen activator inhibitor is the principal fast-acting inhibitor of tPA and is synthesized by vascular endothelial and smooth muscle cells as well as hepatocytes, and is found in the alpha granules of platelets and normal plasma. Plasminogen activator inhibitor rapidly complexes with tPA to reduce its activity in plasma, prevent excessive plasmin formation and thus localize fibrinolysis to fibrin deposits. The binding of PAI to clot-bound tPA is much slower. High concentrations of thrombin activate TAFI which acts on partially degraded fibrin to prevent formation of the tPA/plasminogen/fibrin complex and thus limit plasmin formation. Plasminogen activator inhibitor's short half life, its inactivation by aPC and thrombin, and the diffusion of tPA into a fibrin clot, all favour fibrinolysis.

THE PRESENT MODEL OF HAEMOSTASIS

The present model of haemostasis was proposed in 1990, elaborated subsequently and is summarized in Figure 4.2.

Injury to the blood vessel wall leads to the exposure of subendothelial collagen, and exposure and release of TF. Tissue factor forms a complex with coagulation factor VII which leads to the activation of factor VII itself. The TF-factor VIIa complex is the physiological

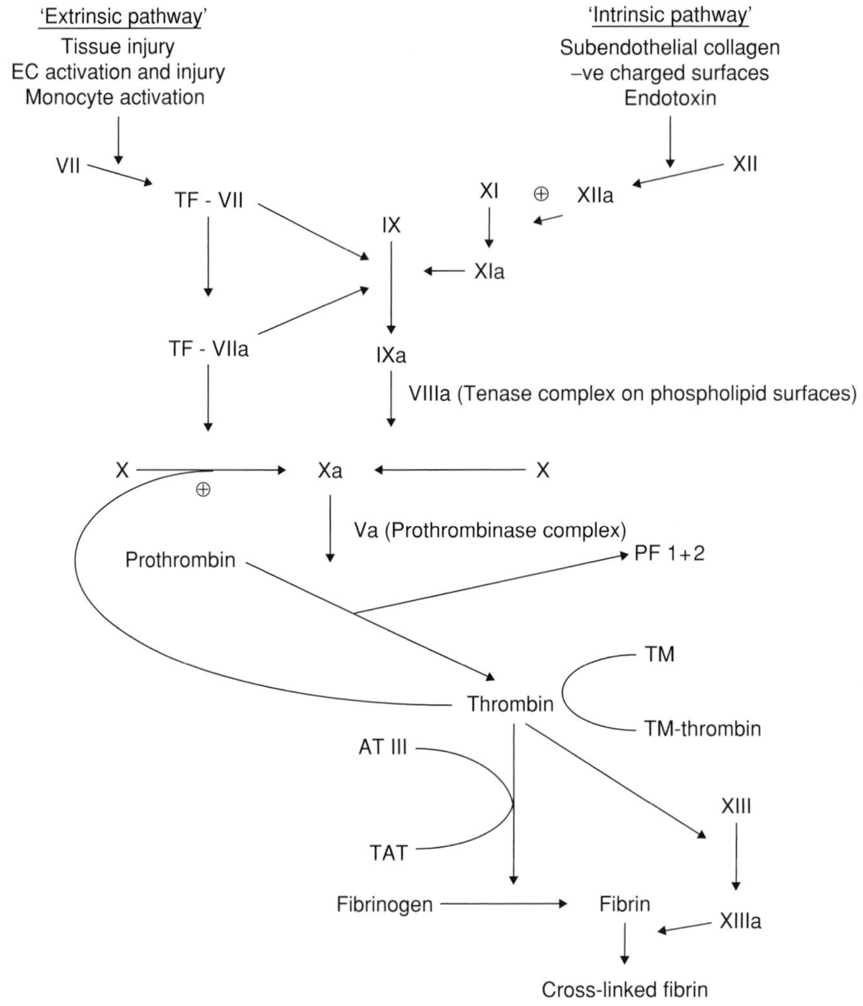

Fig. 4.2. Coagulation cascade. Major activation of factor X is by thrombin. Activation by the 'instrinsic' pathway is probably irrelevant *in vivo*.

initiator of haemostasis. It activates factor X directly and indirectly via activation of factor IX. Factors IXa and Xa act in a positive feedback pathway to increase activation of factor VII.

Factor IXa is able to bind to the activated platelet surface and is not inhibited efficiently by AT-III. Once bound to the activated platelet surface, it becomes the major activator of factor X. This requires calcium ions and is increased almost 1000 times in the presence of factor VIIIa and negatively charged phospholipid. The combination of factor IXa, vWF, factor VIIIa, calcium and phospholipid constitutes the tenase complex on activated platelets.

Factor Xa is a weak but sufficient activator of factor V. Factor Xa converts prothrombin to thrombin which, through another positive feedback pathway, activates factor V. Factor Xa, factor Va and calcium bind to phospholipid to form the prothrombinase complex on activated platelets. This increases the conversion of prothrombin to thrombin at over 300 000 times the rate of factor Xa alone. Thrombin augments its own production by positive feedback involving activation of factors V, VIII and XI. Once produced, thrombin cleaves fibrinopeptides A and B from fibrinogen in platelets and plasma, converting it into a fibrin monomer. The fibrin monomer polymerizes to form strands and thrombin activates factor XIII which, in the presence of calcium, stimulates the formation of a dense open mesh of insoluble cross-linked fibrin. This binds platelets via glycoprotein IIb-IIIa to form the platelet-fibrin plug and allows plasmin to enter the clot to initiate fibrinolysis. The cross-linked fibrin in association with aggregated platelets seals the site of injury.

Small amounts of activated procoagulants are rapidly inhibited and only when a stimulus of injury is adequate does coagulation take place. Tissue factor pathway inhibitor binds and inhibits factor Xa. This, in turn, rapidly inhibits the TF-factor VIIa complex. This negative feedback pathway inhibits activation of factor X unless there is massive expression and release of TF. Thrombin generation adjacent to normal intact endothelium is inactivated by a number of ATs, the most important of which is AT-III. Thrombin binds to AT-III, which is concentrated by intact endothelium, and splits it to form the inactive TAT complex. Thrombomodulin is expressed on the surface of the endothelium and binds thrombin. The thrombin-TM complex inhibits fibrin formation and platelet activation, and activates protein C which inactivates factors Va and VIIIa and decreases thrombin generation. Protein C activity is increased ten times in the presence of protein S. Coagulation is localized to areas of tissue injury because damaged endothelium is incapable of neutralizing thrombin, whereas adjacent intact endothelium continues to express agents such as AT-III, TM and protein C. This model begins to integrate the known effects of tissue injury and incorporates the effects of activation of platelets in boosting coagulation. The effect of blood flow and intact endothelium in localizing clot formation is also understandable.

THE FUTURE

This is not the final model of coagulation. We still tend to analyse coagulation as a series of chemical reactions and platelet activity as separate activities. New techniques are allowing experiments that are integrating these dynamic systems. We are now able to analyse platelet activities such as activation, calcium fluxes and adhesion in real time in individual platelets. As these results inform our models there will be further insights. The effects of other blood cells such as monocytes is also being actively explored. Integration of haemostasis into other aspects of host defence such as inflammation and wound healing is now an area of intense study. The relationship between coagulation and malignancy is also being actively investigated.

SUGGESTED READING

The present model of haemostasis is presented in any standard book of haematology.

1. E. Beutler, M. A. Lichtman, B. S. Coller, T. J. Kipps & U. Seligsohn, *Williams Hematology*, 6th edn (McGraw-Hill, 2001).
2. R. W. Colman, J. Hirsh, V. J. Marder, A. W. Cloews, & J. N. George, *Haemostasis and Thrombosis: Basic Principles and Clinical Practice*, 4th edn (Philadelphia: Lippincott Williams and Wilkins, 2001).

HISTORICAL REFERENCES

1. R. G. MacFarlane, An enzyme cascade in the blood clotting mechanism, and its function as a biological amplifier. *Nature*, **202** (1964), 498.
2. E. W. Davie & O. D. Ratnoff, Waterfall sequence for intrinsic blood clotting. *Science*, **145** (1964), 1310.

5 • Hypercoagulability and vascular disease

STELLA VIG

INTRODUCTION

Hypercoagulability has a profound effect on the vascular tree with thromboses in the cerebrovascular, cardiovascular and peripheral vascular systems. The association between venous thromboses and hypercoagulability has now been firmly established. The association between arterial disease, arterial thromboses and hypercoagulability is now becoming accepted.

COAGULATION CASCADE

Thrombus forms at the end point of the coagulation cascade, a complex interaction of enzymes, co-factors and platelets as shown in Figure 5.1. Classically the clotting cascade has been depicted with an intrinsic and extrinsic pathway as the initial step in activation. These are now thought to occur almost simultaneously rather than in isolation.

Collagen and tissue factor released at the endothelial level initiate the coagulation pathways. Both pathways converge at factor X, which converts prothrombin to thrombin using factor V as a co-factor. Thrombin activates factors VIII and V further increasing thrombin formation. Thrombin proteolytically converts soluble fibrinogen to insoluble fibrin. This activates factor XIII and allows the formation of cross-links and stabilization of the clot. Protein C is a potent inhibitor of thrombus formation and protein S is a co-factor for protein C. Other inhibitors of thrombin generation are antithrombin-III and tissue factor pathway inhibitor. The fibrinolytic system converts plasminogen to plasmin, which digests the fibrin clot.

A fine balance exists between this clotting cascade and regulators of fibrinolysis. Co-factors, which inhibit and potentiate thrombus generation, may be deficient or have abnormal function thereby causing increased clotting or lysis. Hypercoagulability is an umbrella term that incorporates these thrombophilia defects and those as yet unidentified causes, which promote clotting. Identifiable defects are defined as thrombophilia defects and may be classified into two sub-groups: inherited and acquired. One problem with this classification is that disorders such as protein C and S may have both a congenital and acquired form.

Schafer described three categories of patients with thromboses [1]:

1. Those where there is a definite identifiable defect
2. Those where the mechanism of thrombosis remains unclear
3. Those who are 'thrombosis prone' where individuals may have recurrent thromboses but have no recognizable predisposing factor

These last two categories are also loosely termed 'prothrombotic states'. Hypercoagulability therefore must include all three of the above categories. Factors currently known to predispose to hypercoagulability are shown in Table 5.1.

INDIVIDUAL FACTORS

Inherited thrombophilia defects

Antithrombin-III deficiency

Antithrombin-III is a vitamin K dependent, irreversible inhibitor of clotting factors, especially factors XIIa, XIa, Xa and thrombin. Deficiency of this factor decreases inhibition of these clotting factors and leads to hypercoagulability. Antithrombin-III deficiency is inherited as an autosomal dominant trait. The prevalence in the general population is 0.05%–3.1% [2; 3]. There are two types of inherited antithrombin-III deficiency. The first is due to decreased formation of the normal inhibitor. The second is due to normal formation of an inhibitor with decreased biological function due to a mutation, substitution or gene deletion.

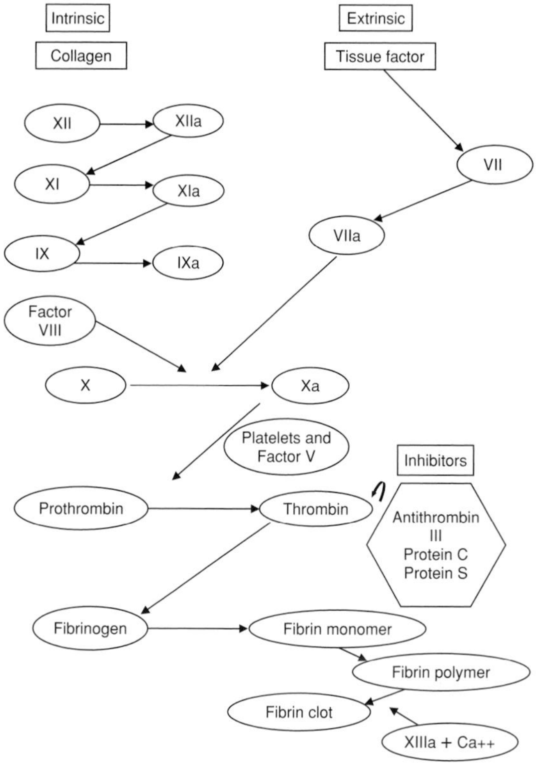

Fig. 5.1. Clotting cascade.

Protein C deficiency

Protein C is a vitamin K dependent membrane bound inhibitor of the clotting cascade. Protein C is activated by thrombin bound to thrombomodulin. Once activated this complex requires protein S to inactivate factors Va and VIIIa and inhibit generation of thrombin and factor Xa. Protein C has an autosomal dominant inheritance. Homozygous protein C deficiency may present at birth with purpura fulminans. This is characterized by skin vessel thrombosis and disseminated intravascular coagulation that can be lethal. The heterozygous form occurs in up to 1 in 200 of the general population [2].

Recently there has been investigation of the pathophysiology of disseminated intravascular coagulation in sepsis [4]. There appears to be a down regulation of protein C and it is suggested that treatments designed to overcome any functional defect maybe of benefit.

Factor V Leiden

A single point mutation in the gene for factor V (factor V Leiden) leads to resistance to activated protein C

Table 5.1. *Factors known to contribute to hypercoagulability*

Inherited hypercoagulability	Acquired hypercoagulability
Antithrombin-III deficiency	Lupus anticoagulant/ antiphospholipid syndrome
Protein C deficiency	Malignancy
Activated protein C resistance	Drugs
Protein S deficiency	Myeloproliferative syndrome
Decreased fibrinolysis	Nephrotic syndrome
Dysfibrinogenaemia	Inflammatory bowel disease
Homocystinaemia	Behçet's syndrome

(APCR) [5]. The prevalence may be as high as 5% in the general population [6]. If warfarin is administered to patients with APCR in the absence of heparin, the protein C levels fall more rapidly than other vitamin K dependent coagulation factors. This renders them acutely and severely protein C deficient and may lead to skin necrosis [7].

Protein Z is a vitamin K dependent protein. The first cases of protein Z deficiency were described in patients suffering from a bleeding tendency from an otherwise unknown origin [8]. However, patients with both the factor V Leiden mutation and low protein Z levels show earlier onset and higher frequency of thromboembolic events than do patients presenting with factor V Leiden mutation and normal protein Z levels. Protein Z enhances the inhibition of factor Xa by protein Z dependent protease inhibitor (ZPI) and therefore reduction in protein Z levels would induce a prothrombotic tendency due to lowered co-factor activity for ZPI [9].

Protein S deficiency

This is a vitamin K dependent inactivator of factors Va and VIIIa and acts as a co-factor for protein C. Some 60% circulates as a protein bound form but only the unbound form has co-factor function. Protein S deficiency is inherited as an autosomal dominant trait. Again, the homozygous state is associated with potentially lethal neonatal purpura fulminans. Protein S has also been associated with warfarin induced skin necrosis but far less commonly than protein C. The prevalence in the general population is 0.7% [10].

Prothrombin mutation

Prothrombin is the precursor of thrombin. The common genetic variant involves a GA20210 mutation in the prothrombin gene. This mutation is present in 1% of healthy controls and 4%–18% of patients with a documented family history of venous thrombophilia [11]. The mutation is associated with elevated prothrombin levels [12].

Fibrinogen

Fibrinogen is converted to fibrin by thrombin and in excess may lead to hyperviscosity. In dysfibrinogenaemia the fibrinogen molecule is functionally defective due to a structural abnormality that is inherited as an autosomal dominant trait. The clinical manifestations of this condition can range from excessive bleeding to thrombotic events and are dependent on the specific mutation. Increased plasma levels of fibrinogen were associated with peripheral arterial occlusive disease (PAOD) in one epidemiological study [13], while several studies, including Framingham, have now established the role of high fibrinogen levels as a thrombotic risk [14; 15].

Abnormalities of fibrinolysis

Abnormalities of fibrinolysis include hypoplasminogenaemia, dysplasminogenaemia, abnormal tissue plasminogen activator release and elevated plasminogen activator inhibitor. These disorders lead to a condition in which the thrombus lyses slowly, therefore allowing propagation of a clot that would otherwise have been removed by an intact fibrinolytic system. Decreased fibrinolytic activity is found in patients with atherosclerosis and diabetes. These abnormalities are often only diagnosed at the time of an acute thrombosis such as a deep venous thrombosis, pulmonary embolus or acute myocardial infarction.

Acquired thrombophilia defects

The antiphospholipid syndrome and lupus anticoagulant

The antiphospholipid syndrome occurs due to the presence of immunoglobulins directed at negatively charged phospholipids such as cardiolipin (anticardiolipin antibody) and the lupus anticoagulant. The lupus anticoagulant is interestingly named as it has no inherent anticoagulant property but interferes with phospholipid dependent coagulation tests. Antiphospholipid antibodies may be present secondary to systemic lupus erythematosus (SLE), malignancy and after administration of drugs such as phenothiazines. The actual mechanism of action of these autoantibodies is not known but it is hypothesized that they may inhibit prostacycline production and protein C activation.

Drugs

Hypercoagulability can be induced following the administration of chemotherapeutic agents such as bleomycin, cyclophosphamide, methotrexate, vinca alkaloids, mitomycin and vinblastine. The oral contraceptive pill (OCP) also increases the risk of venous thrombosis. High dose oestrogen preparations may increase the risk by 2–4 times. The risk reduces with low dose oestrogen OCPs and even further with progesterone only pills.

Heparin can induce a thrombocytopenia (heparin induced thrombocytopenia (HITS)) in 5%–10% of cases that can be classified into two types [16]. Type 1 is characterized by a mild thrombocytopenia, type 2 is a more serious immune response with antibodies specific for complexes consisting of heparin and platelet factor 4 (PF4), a heparin-binding protein found in platelet alpha granules [17]. It is not fully understood why this should induce hypercoagulability but it is suggested that immunological endothelial damage and intravascular platelet aggregation may contribute to thrombus formation. This usually occurs 6 to 14 days after heparin treatment and there is a 10% risk of developing thrombo-embolic arterial or venous events [18].

Malignancy

The myeloproliferative disorders such as polycythaemia rubra vera and essential thrombocythaemia are associated with hypercoagulability due to increased blood viscosity. Mucin secreting adenocarcinomas such as pancreatic, lung, gastric, prostatic and cholangiocarcinomas have been also been associated with a prothrombotic state even if not clinically manifest (Trousseau's syndrome). The incidence of cancer in patients with a deep venous thrombosis without an identifiable risk factor is reported to be as high as 10% [19]. Tumour cells are able to interact with the coagulation and fibrinolytic cascade,

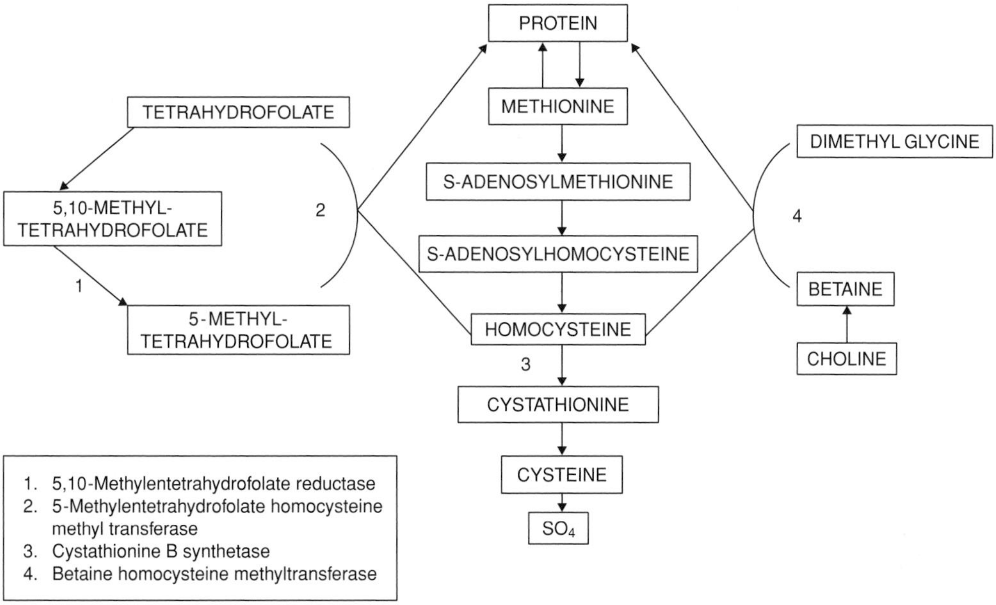

Fig. 5.2. Homocysteine metabolism.

directly activating plasmin and thrombin and therefore thrombus formation [20].

Miscellaneous

Pregnancy, nephrotic syndrome, inflammatory bowel disease, pre-eclampsia, liver disease, malnutrition and autoimmune diseases such as Behçet's can increase the risk of hypercoagulability.

It is interesting to note that although the prevalence of thrombophilia defects in the normal population maybe as high as 11%, most individuals do not have clinical thrombotic complications [21]. It is likely that clinically apparent hypercoagulable states result from multigene interaction and that thromboses are precipitated by an insult in a patient with an inherited predisposition to thrombosis [22].

HOMOCYSTEINE

Homocysteine is associated with thrombosis although the actual mechanism is unclear. Homocysteine may down-regulate thrombomodulin function, inhibit tissue plasminogen activation and decrease endothelial protein C activation and the activity of antithrombin-III [23; 24; 25]. Homocysteine may also increase factor VIIIC and von Willebrand factor leading to hypercoagulability and thrombus formation [26]. The auto-oxidation of homocysteine leads to the release of potent reactive oxidative species such as superoxide and hydrogen peroxide, which may lead to vascular damage [27]. The lipid peroxidation may cause direct endothelial damage initiating the coagulation cascade, the proliferation of smooth muscle cells and atherogenesis [28].

Homocysteine is formed by the conversion of methionine, which is abundant in animal protein (Figure 5.2). In plasma, homocysteine is present in several forms:

(1) 1% circulates as a free thiol
(2) 70%–80% is bound to plasma proteins such as albumin
(3) 20%–30% occurs as a dimer or in association with cysteine [29]

Total plasma homocysteine (or serum) (tHcy) refers to the pool of all these forms.

Congenital deficiencies of any of the enzymes involved in the homocysteine pathway may result in hyperhomocysteinaemia. Homozygous cystathionine synthase deficiency (autosomal recessive) may present with premature atherosclerosis, venous thrombosis, lens dislocation, osteoporosis and mild mental retardation [30; 31; 32; 33]. The heterozygous form is more common (1 in 150) and is associated with normal levels of tHcy. The most common cause of a moderately elevated homocysteine is the point mutation (C-677T) in the gene coding for MTHFR resulting in a thermolabile form of methylene tetrahydrofolate reductase (MTHFR C-677T) that has reduced enzymatic activity [34; 35]. The TT genotype is found in about 10% of the normal population and is associated with a raised homocysteine especially in the presence of suboptimal folate intake [36]. Heterozygosity due to the MTHFR mutation does not appear to be clinically significant.

Homocysteine levels are inversely correlated to folate, vitamin B_{12} and to a lesser extent vitamin B_6, and nutritional deficiencies of these co-factors are associated with elevations in homocysteine [37; 38]. Renal impairment is also associated with increased levels due to reduced homocysteine excretion by the kidney [39; 40; 41]. Levels are also increased with drugs that interfere with folate such as methotrexate, phenytoin, carbamazepine and thiazide diuretics. Cigarette smoking interferes with the synthesis of vitamin B_6 thereby reducing levels [42]. This could therefore lead to hyperhomocysteinaemia and may suggest one possible mechanism by which cigarette smoking could promote atherogenesis and atherothrombosis.

PREVALENCE AND RISK OF THROMBOPHILIA DEFECTS AND VENOUS DISEASE

One study detailed the current consensus amongst vascular surgeons in Great Britain and Ireland regarding the investigation and management of patients with suspected or proven deep vein thrombosis (DVT). Despite the association between DVT and thrombophilia only 14% of consultants would request a thrombophilia screen [43].

The prevalence of thrombophilia defects in patients with venous thromboses may be up to 12% but they do not appear to be equally associated with the development of a venous thrombosis [44]. Data suggest that a protein S or C deficiency is more likely to be associated with the development of a DVT [45]. Factor V Leiden has also been suggested as a strong risk factor in venous thrombosis (odds ratio of 3.6) present in 26.5% of patients [44; 46]. The prevalence of the prothrombin mutation was 3.1% [44]. The prevalence of thrombophilia defects is similar in patients with DVTs or pulmonary emboli.

Although it has now been well established that thrombophilia defects may be associated with venous thromboses, the data regarding association with recurrent DVTs are less clear [47]. The incidence of a recurrent venous thrombosis appears lowest after a surgical related venous thrombosis (0%) and highest after unprecipitated venous thrombosis (19.4%) ($p < 0.001$) [48]. Recurrence rates were not related to the presence of laboratory evidence of heritable thrombophilia (hazard ratio 1.50 (95% CI 0.82–2.77); $p = 0.187$).

Deep venous thrombosis is a major risk factor for chronic venous ulceration. The prevalence of thrombophilia defects in this group was 41% [49]. This rate was two to 30 times higher than the rate in the general population but was similar to that reported for patients with previous DVT. The presence of a thrombophilia defect does not appear to relate to the pattern of reflux or severity of the disease [50].

PREVALENCE AND RISK OF HOMOCYSTEINE AND VENOUS DISEASE

The data regarding the association of elevated homocysteine levels, genetic variants and venous thrombosis are conflicting. The prevalence of hyperhomocysteinaemia in patients with venous thromboses is 18%–34% compared to 5% in the control group and maybe more prevalent than other identifiable thrombophilia defects [44; 51]. Plasma homocysteine levels were significantly higher in patients with a venous thrombosis and carried a four- to nine-fold increase in risk for DVT, irrespective of clinical predisposition, as well as other thrombophilic risks surveyed [52]. One meta-analysis reported that the odds ratio for venous thromboses was 2.5 (95% CI 1.8–3.5) for a fasting plasma homocysteine concentration above the 95th percentile whilst another suggested that the odds ratio for a 5 μmol/l increase in serum homocysteine was 1.60 for DVT with or without pulmonary embolism [53; 54].

Patients with unprovoked venous thromboses, recurrent venous disease or a first episode at a late age were more likely to have an elevated homocysteine compared with those with a single episode associated with another causative risk factor [55]. Mild hyperhomocysteinemia therefore appears to be associated with venous thrombosis but a causal relationship has not yet been established. The VITRO (VItamins and ThROmbosis) trial was the first multicentre, randomized, double-blind and placebo-controlled study to evaluate the effect of homocysteine-lowering therapy by means of 5 mg folic acid, 0.4 mg vitamin B_{12} and 50 mg vitamin B_6. The study was a secondary prevention trial in 600 patients who suffered from a first episode of idiopathic DVT, pulmonary embolism (PE) or both. The results of this trial have not been reported yet [56]. Hyperhomocysteinaemia has also been associated with a four-fold increased risk of cerebral vein thrombosis [57].

The prevalence of the MTHFR mutation was 13.7% in patients with venous disease and although an important cause of mild hyperhomocysteinaemia, it did not seem to be a risk factor for venous thrombosis [58; 59]. The Longitudinal Investigation of Thromboembolism Etiology (LITE) study reported that although hyperhomocysteinaemia was associated with venous thromboses, carriers of the MTHFR C-677T polymorphism were not at higher risk for venous thrombosis than those with normal genotype [60]. The homocysteine polymorphisms may not be associated with an increased risk of venous thromboses but the data conflict with some suggesting that the MTHFR mutation was a significant variable in both venous ($p = 0.03$) and arterial thrombosis ($p = 0.004$) [44; 61]. The MTHFR gene may become a risk factor for venous thromboses when combined with a known thrombophilia defect although, again, the data are conflicting [62; 63; 64]. The odds ratio for recurrent venous thrombosis was 1.8 (95% CI 1.1–3.0) for fasting hyperhomocysteinaemia, 5.1 (95% CI 3.0–8.6) for factor V Leiden and 1.8 (95% CI 0.7–4.2) for prothrombin G20210A. A combined hyperhomocysteinemia and factor V Leiden yielded an odds ratio of 11.6 (95% CI 3.2–42.5). The individual relative risk for MTHFR mutation was 1.5 but the combined risk for MTHFR and factor V Leiden was 18.7 (95% CI 3.3–108) [65].

A recent meta-analysis concluded that it is unlikely that the suggested relationship between hyperhomocysteinaemia and venous thrombo-embolism is mediated by the MTHFR gene defect. This meta-analysis did not recommend routine testing for the MTHFR C-677T polymorphism in venous thrombosis [66].

PREVALENCE AND RISK OF THROMBOPHILIA DEFECTS AND ARTERIAL DISEASE

Data regarding the prevalence of thrombophilia defects in large population based studies are lacking. The few studies recording the prevalence of thrombophilia defects in patients with vascular disease are based in different cohorts and use individualized thrombophilia screens, and are therefore difficult to compare.

There was a higher prevalence of thrombophilia defects in patients with vascular disease compared with the general population increasing from 25% in stable claudicants to 40% in those requiring revascularization [21]. Some 30% of patients with symptomatic peripheral vascular disease presenting at an early age will have an identifiable thrombophilia defect [67; 68; 69; 70]. The data from studies of the more typical patients presenting with peripheral vascular disease also suggest that the prevalence of thrombophilia in this group is also 20% to 30% [21; 71; 72; 73; 74; 75; 76; 77]. These studies are summarized in Table 5.2.

The most commonly identified thrombophilia defect was the antiphospholipid syndrome, present in one series in one-third of the vascular population. Protein C and S deficiencies are present in almost 20%, double the prevalence of the antithrombin-III deficiency and APCR. The prothrombin mutation is the least common thrombophilia defect detected.

Although the data are limited it appears that the prevalence of thrombophilia defects was more common in patients with symptomatic peripheral vascular disease compared with aortic or carotid disease. The prevalence of APCR was 14%–16% in symptomatic PAOD, compared to 12%–14% in aneurysmal disease, 9% in venous disease and 5%–9% in carotid disease [76; 78]. In comparison another study suggested that the prevalence of antithrombin-III deficiency was similar in carotid, aneurysmal and peripheral arterial disease at 13%–18% [72]. It also appears that thrombophilia defects are associated with increased progression of distal lower limb arterial disease compared to suprapopliteal disease [79].

The literature reviewed so far suggests that almost 30% of patients who present with PAOD may have a thrombophilia defect. The data support the suggestion that thrombophilia defects are associated with the progression of distal peripheral vascular disease and are more prevalent in those patients who require intervention.

Thrombophilia defects may be associated with increased coronary artery and cerebrovascular thrombotic disease, but again the data are conflicting. Some studies show that the antiphospholipid syndrome was associated with thrombotic events in coronary and cerebrovascular disease [80; 81; 82; 83]. Another comparison

Table 5.2. *Prevalence of thrombophilia defects in vascular patients*

Patients			Thrombophilia screen							
Study	Age	Number	Overall %	Anti-phospholipid syndrome	Low protein C	Low protein S	Low anti-thrombin	APCR (factor V Leiden)	Platelet function	Prothrombin mutation
A. Peripheral vascular disease										
Eldrup-Jorgensen *et al.* 1989 [68]	23–50	20	30%	15%	15%	20%	NT*	NT*	47%	NT*
Aronsen *et al.* 1989 [69]	<45	37	<30%	NT*	0%	8%	2.7%	NT*	NT*	NT*
Valentine *et al.* 1996 [67]	<45	50	15%	26%	13.3%	0%	2%	NT*	NT*	NT*
Levy *et al.* 1996 [70]	<45	51	<30%	19.6%	15.6%	7.8%	9.8%	NT*	NT*	NT*
Ray *et al.* 1997 [89]	Mean 67	60	35%	15%	5%	18.5%	1.7%	NT*	NT*	NT*
Lee *et al.* 1996 [71]		262	32%	32%	NT*	NT*	NT*	NT*	NT*	NT*
Evans *et al.* 1999 [77]	Median 65	116	21%	13%	1.7%	1.7%	0.8%	2.6%	NT*	NT*
Vig *et al.* (unpublished) 2002	Mean 71	150	27%	4%	4%	11%	<1%	7%	NT*	4%
B. Mixed Vascular Pathology										
Flinn *et al.* 1984 [72]	Mean 69		16.4%	NT*	NT*	NT*	16.4%	NT*	NT*	NT*
Donaldson *et al.* 1990 [73]	Mean 65	158	9.5%	3.2%	2.5%	0.6%	1.2%	NT*	2.5%	NT*
Taylor *et al.* 1994 [75]	Mean 64	234	27%	26%	0.4%	1.2%	0.4%	NT*	NT*	NT*
Ouriel *et al.* 1996 [76]		173	11.6%	NT*	NT*	NT*	NT*	11.6%	NT*	NT*
Sampram *et al.* 2001 [78]		775	12%	NT*	NT*	NT*	NT*	12%	NT*	NT*

of the coagulation status of patients with coronary artery disease awaiting surgery reported no difference in coagulation status compared with controls [84]. Heterozygous factor V Leiden mutation may be found in 8% of patients diagnosed with an acute myocardial infarction but there is no evidence in the literature of causality [85]. Studies associating the prothrombin mutation and factor V Leiden with myocardial infarction have yielded conflicting results possibly due to complicated gene–gene interactions or small sample sizes. A study using simultaneous analysis of multiple gene variants in a large sample size from a genetically isolated population in Newfoundland reported that the prevalence of the prothrombin mutation was 3.2% in myocardial infarction patients and almost six-fold higher in patients younger than 51 years diagnosed with a myocardial infarction. The prevalence of factor V Leiden was four-fold greater in young patients than in patients older than 50 years. This study suggested that the prothrombin mutation is a risk factor for myocardial infarction especially for early onset cardiac ischaemia and that factor V Leiden may predispose patients to early-onset myocardial infarctions [86].

The prevalence of thrombophilia was between 2.4%–27% in patients with ischaemic strokes [44]. Protein S deficiency was the most common disorder, followed by protein C deficiency and again these were more prevalent in the younger age group. Factor V Leiden may be present in up to 11% and the prothrombin mutation in 2% [44]. Antithrombin did not appear to be associated with ischaemic stroke in a later study [87].

THROMBOPHILIA AND FAILURE OF INTERVENTION IN PERIPHERAL VASCULAR DISEASE

Thrombophilia defects (especially protein C deficiency) have been strongly associated with acute ischaemia ($p < 0.01$), prior vascular intervention ($p < 0.01$) and major amputation ($p < 0.01$). It was also suggested that hypercoagulability played an important role in early ischaemia and poor results reported for lower extremity vascular procedures in patients with premature atherosclerosis. These patients were almost six times more likely to develop complications than controls [88].

An antithrombin-III deficiency was associated with a 30-day revascularization failure rate three times higher than controls [72]. The presence of APCR was also associated with early graft occlusion and again appeared to increase the risk of failure following infrainguinal revascularization by a factor of three [76]. It was also noted that patients who were positive and occluded were so secondary to thrombosis whereas patients who were APCR negative often had a demonstrable anatomical lesion explaining the occlusion.

The risk of occlusion increases within a study, dependent on how comprehensive a thrombophilia screen is undertaken. A positive thrombophilia screen may be associated with almost a thirteen-fold increase in failure rate after infrainguinal revascularisation [73]. Ray *et al.* reported a 92% failure rate after revascularization in patients with an identifiable thrombophilia defect compared to only 2% in the 'normal' cohort at 30 days [89]. At a one year follow-up the difference was not as dramatic with 65% occluding in the thrombophilic group compared with 18% in the 'normal' cohort, suggesting that the risk of thrombotic failure was highest within the first 30 days. Nearly 40% of patients in this study who had undergone a previous revascularization had evidence of a thrombophilia defect compared to 27% of those with no thrombophilia defect [89]. Taylor *et al.* also reported that patients with evidence of antiphospholipid syndrome were twice as likely to have had a previous failed lower limb vascular procedure and six times more likely to have had an occlusive cause for failure than those without [75].

An isolated thrombophilia defect appears to confer a three-fold increase of failure following lower limb revascularization. The larger the number of thrombophilia defects detected the higher the risk of thrombotic occlusion. The data are not available to determine whether a particular thrombophilia defect was more aggressive in causing failure or whether the presence of multiple thrombophilia defects in an individual also caused a higher risk.

PREVALENCE AND RISK OF HYPERHOMOCYSTEINAEMIA IN ARTERIAL DISEASE

The prevalence of hyperhomocysteinaemia in patients developing premature PAOD was 19%–30% [32; 90; 91; 92]. The prevalence in symptomatic patients was 13%–47% and up to 60% in the general vascular population compared to 1%–5% in the general population

[93; 94; 95; 96]. Hyperhomocysteinaemia maybe also be present in 16% of patients with an ischaemic stroke [44]. The prevalence of the MTHFR mutation is lower at 10.6%. Several studies have now confirmed that hyperhomocysteinaemia may be an independent risk factor for cardiovascular morbidity and mortality [97; 98; 99]. A meta-analysis of 27 studies concluded that the odds ratio for fatal or non-fatal events in coronary artery disease was 1.6 and 1.8 in men and women, respectively. The odds ratio increased to 2.5 for the cerebral circulation and 6.8 for symptomatic PAOD. Therefore hyperhomocysteinaemia may be a stronger risk factor for PAOD than for coronary artery disease.

The meta-analysis also suggested that hyperhomocysteinaemia may account for 10% of the population risk for coronary artery disease. If this can be expanded to patients with PAOD then it may be the most important haematologically detected risk factor for PAOD [100]. There was in fact a graded relationship for homocysteine and vascular risk in a similar way to cholesterol. A 5 μmol/l increase of homocysteine produced an increase in vascular risk by one-third. This was of the same magnitude as a 0.5 mmol/l increase in plasma cholesterol. The odds ratios for a 5 μmol/l increase in serum homocysteine were 1.42 for ischaemic heart disease and 1.65 for stroke [53]. More recent studies continue to show that homocysteine is an independent risk factor for atherosclerotic disease. The European Concerted Action Project showed that a 5 μmol/l increase in homocysteine was associated with a relative risk of atherosclerotic vascular disease of 1.35 in men and 1.42 in women [101]. Another study showed that homocysteine levels of 12 μmol/l carried an increased risk of vascular risk independent of other factors [102].

The MTHFR mutation was previously shown to be associated with an increased risk for coronary heart disease [103; 104] but a recent meta-analysis has failed to confirm this [105]. There are also conflicting data regarding the causal association with peripheral arterial disease [106].

HOMOCYSTEINE AND FAILURE OF INTERVENTION IN PERIPHERAL VASCULAR DISEASE

There are very few data on the association of hyperhomocysteinaemia and failure of angioplasty or lower limb bypass grafts in the literature. A comparison of patients undergoing coronary artery bypass grafting suggested that there was no significant difference in levels of homocysteine or lipoprotein (a) between patients with an occluded graft and those with a patent graft at a one year follow-up [107].

Young age, diabetes and hyperhomocysteinaemia were reported as independent risk factors for the failure of vascular procedures, with a further study clearly demonstrating an association of hyperhomocysteinaemia with vein graft stenosis following femorodistal vein bypass [94; 108]. This association was also supported as plasma homocysteine levels were significantly elevated in patients with vein graft stenosis following infrainguinal vein grafts [109]. These studies contrast with the report by Caldwell *et al.*, which showed that whilst hyperhomocysteinaemia was more common in patients with peripheral vascular disease, it was not associated with neointimal hyperplasia detected after infrainguinal venous grafts [99]. The Dutch BOA (Bypass Oral anticoagulants or Aspirin) study also investigated the influence of hyperhomocysteinaemia on graft patency after infrainguinal bypass surgery and found no significant differences between serum levels of homocysteine in patients with and without graft occlusion [110].

THE PREVALENCE AND RISK OF HYPERFIBRINOGENAEMIA IN VASCULAR DISEASE

The largest cross sectional epidemiological study has shown that fibrinogen levels are higher in women compared with men and also elevated in black men. Fibrinogen levels also increased with age, smoking, weight, diabetes, low density lipoprotein and lipoprotein (a) [111]. Framingham data confirmed that there was a dose dependent increase of fibrinogen with smoking, an effect that was reversible on cessation [112; 113]. Hyperfibrinogenaemia may also be present in half of the patients with peripheral arterial disease [114].

In the Scottish Heart Health study [115], the odds ratios for intermittent claudication in men with plasma fibrinogen levels in the middle and high thirds of the fibrinogen distribution were 2.33 and 2.73, respectively, compared with those individuals with levels in the lower third. This association remained significant after adjusting for other variables. Plasma fibrinogen increases with age and cigarette smoking but when corrected for these factors it still emerged as a risk factor for claudication on multivariate analysis [116; 117]. Patients with elevated fibrinogen levels in the range of 10.2–12.2 mol/l and above 12.2 mol/l had a significantly increased adjusted risk for all-cause mortality (hazard ratios (HR) 1.87 and 1.90, $p = 0.025$ and $p = 0.020$, respectively) compared to patients in the lowest quartile (fibrinogen below 8.61/4 mol per l). This study concluded that elevated fibrinogen levels in high-risk patients with PAOD indicate an increased risk for poor outcome, particularly for fatal cardiovascular complications [118].

Fibrinogen is part of the acute phase reaction and will become raised subsequent to any episode of ischaemia. It could therefore be argued that it is merely a marker for ischaemic disease. However, there is a massive body of indirect evidence to suggest that a raised plasma fibrinogen is a true causal risk factor for a range of cardiovascular diseases. The ultimate proof, that is a proven decrease in the progression of PAOD with normalizing or lowering plasma fibrinogen, is still lacking. It is also thought that hyperfibrinogenaemia may hinder blood flow by its rheological effect, i.e. rheological claudication [119].

Hyperfibrinogenaemia was associated with restenosis following angioplasty and surgical revascularization [120; 121; 122]. The relative risk for developing a restenosis within six months following an angioplasty with a fibrinogen >2.8g/l was 2.8 (95% CI 1.30–6.02) [123]. The mean fibrinogen levels were significantly higher in patients with stenosed femoro-distal vein bypass grafts compared to the non-stenosed group [106]. Longitudinal data suggests that a high fibrinogen level was also a significant predictor for reocclusion of femoro-popliteal vein bypass grafts [122].

SCREENING

The data presented suggest that one-third of patients with peripheral vascular disease have a thrombophilia defect, one-third have hyperhomocysteinaemia and half may have hyperfibrinogenaemia. All three risk factors increase the likelihood of failure of either radiological or surgical intervention. However, wide scale screening for hypercoagulable states is not advocated at present [124].

The Transatlantic Inter-Society Consensus document recommends that 'a hypercoagulable profile should be obtained in individuals with a personal or family history of thrombotic events, early onset of disease (onset <45 years), or the absence of any of the usual risk factors for PAOD, including a family history of atherosclerotic complications' [125]. This document also suggests that plasma homocysteine levels should be obtained on any patient who presents with claudication who does not have any of the usual risk factors that are associated with peripheral arterial disease. The British Committee for Standards in Haematology (BCSH) has also issued recommendations for thrombophilia screening. The groups include patients who present with a venous thrombosis before the age of 40 or arterial thrombosis before the age of 30 years. They also recommend screening for patients with unexplained, recurrent or unusual venous thromboses, and of patients with a family history of thrombophilia or venous thrombosis [126]. Most patients with symptomatic peripheral vascular disease would fall outside these recommendations. A recent review of thrombophilia defects in vascular disease recommended that all vascular patients undergoing intervention should be screened, as a positive screen appeared to confer a poorer prognosis following intervention [127].

The arguments against screening are becoming less robust. Historically thrombophilia screens were difficult to perform, costly and results became available after a time delay. The thrombophilia assays are now largely automated, and are therefore more readily available and have become less expensive.

Homocysteine assays have also been difficult to perform. Most laboratories recommend that subjects be fasted, whilst some suggest methionine loading. Methionine loading is thought to stress the homocysteine pathway and therefore be a more sensitive test. The procedure involves baseline testing followed by an oral methionine load. Homocysteine levels are then repeated between two and eight hours post ingestion. Although methionine loaded homocysteine assays may increase the diagnosis of hyperhomocysteinaemia by 55%, they are cumbersome to carry out and are not well tolerated by the patient [128]. As red blood cells also metabolize homocysteine, homocysteine levels will increase when separation of red cells from plasma is delayed. The absolute increase in homocysteine is independent of the initial plasma concentration and the rate of increase is 0.5 μmol/l per hour during the first 24 hours at 22°C [129]. Blood samples therefore either need to be centrifuged within one hour of removal or placed on ice until the plasma is separated. The homocysteine assays have now become more simplified and screening is now possible.

Patients with vascular disease could therefore undergo a hypercoagulabilty screen that would comprise of:

(1) Full blood count (polycythaemia, thrombocytosis)
(2) Fibrinogen, erythrocyte sedimentation rate
(3) Test for lupus anticoagulant
(4) Activated protein C resistance
(5) Antithrombin-III assay
(6) Protein C assay
(7) Free protein S assay
(8) Factor V Leiden and prothrombin gene mutation by PCR.
(9) Homocysteine assay

It is recommended that patients should undergo testing prior to any intervention as hypercoagulability may manifest *de novo* in post-operative patients. By the third post-operative day, 55% of patients may have a thrombophilia abnormality, normally a low protein C or S. At a six-month follow-up these tests appeared to have returned to baseline levels. This may be secondary to the artificial surfaces providing thrombogenic potential and activating the coagulation system creating a transient hypercoagulable state [130].

THERAPEUTIC OPTIONS

Hypercoagulability is often diagnosed retrospectively following a failed primary procedure. It has therefore been very difficult to carry out prospective clinical trials to evaluate best medical practice and so there is little published work on the management of patients with a positive hypercoagulability screen. In addition, many pharmaceutical agents used to modulate graft patency have only been evaluated in cardiac surgery.

Lindblad *et al.* surveyed the use of prophylaxis against graft occlusion worldwide [131]. Although prophylaxis is common, the actual drug therapy used is widely variable. Aspirin (ASA) is used most commonly but the use of oral anticoagulants is more prevalent in Europe. In contrast, ASA/dipyridamole (DIP) is the favoured combination in South America. A survey of the Vascular Surgical Society of Great Britain and Ireland (VSSGBI) concluded that almost all surgeons used some form of antiplatelet prophylaxis [132].

The following review highlights those drugs that are used or potentially may be of benefit in patients with hypercoagulability. Figure 5.3 schematically demonstrates the sites of action of these drugs.

HEPARIN

Unfractionated heparin (UFH) potentiates the anticoagulant activity of factors IX, X, XI, XII and antithrombin-III. It suppresses platelet function and inhibits neointimal hyperplasia in animal models following vascular injury [133]. Low molecular weight (LMWT) heparin causes an anti-thrombin dependent inhibition of factor Xa. It has a longer half life than UFH and maybe administered once or twice daily subcutaneously. It is safer than UFH as it has a lower potential for bleeding [134].

There are only a few published trials of heparin in peripheral vascular disease. An Italian study prospectively randomized patients with Leriche-Fontaine IIb peripheral arterial occlusive disease (stable claudicants) to heparin or ticlodipine for three months [135]. The claudication distance appeared to improve by 50% and 30%, respectively. A prospectively randomized trial of daily LMWT heparin or aspirin/dipyridamole for three months in patients undergoing vascular reconstruction reported that patency was significantly higher in the heparin group [136]. Analysis by indication for surgery indicated that there was a significant benefit for those undergoing salvage surgery in both groups. The difference in patency was not significant for those undergoing surgery for claudication. Interestingly, although the treatment period was only three months, the benefit from heparin appeared to continue for one year. A comparison of perioperative intravenous heparin versus LMWT heparin for infrainguinal polytetrafluoroethylene (PTFE) grafts reported no increase in graft failure before discharge in patients treated with LMWT heparin. The use of LMWT heparin reduced the in hospital stay before full coagulation. However, there was a non-significant higher haemorrhagic complication rate in those patients treated with IVH [137].

A randomized multicentre trial compared heparin-bonded dacron (HBD) with PTFE in below-knee popliteal or tibioperoneal trunk bypass grafts. Each patient was given aspirin (300 mg) before surgery, and this was continued unless the patient had an intolerance to aspirin. Patency at 1, 2 and 3 years for HBD was 70%, 63% and 55% compared with 56%, 46% and 42%, respectively, for PTFE ($P = 0.044$). Heparin-bonded

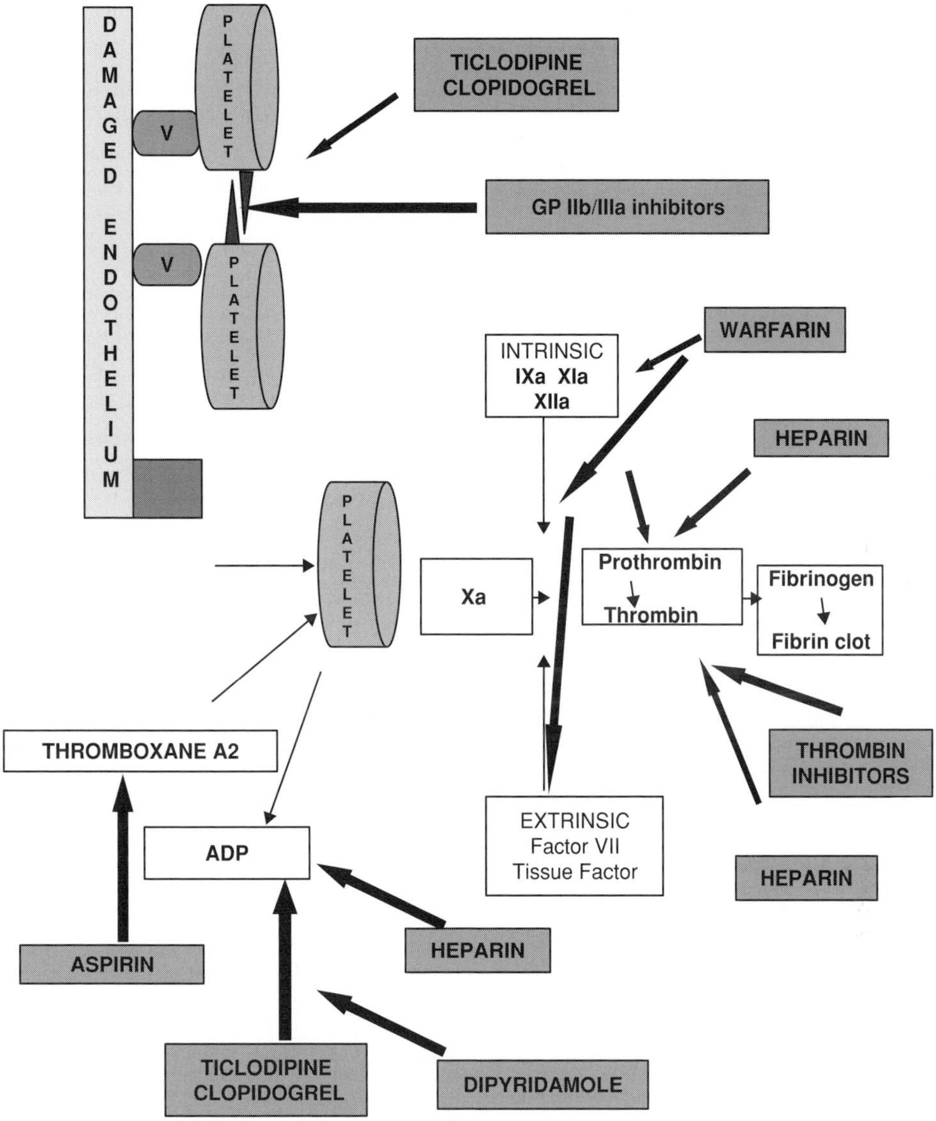

Fig. 5.3. VWF = von Willebrand factor; TF = Tissue factor; GP IIa/IIIb = Glycoprotein receptors.

dacron therefore achieved better patency compared with PTFE bypass grafts, which carried a higher risk of subsequent amputation [138].

Another study randomized patients undergoing peripheral angioplasty with evidence of dissection to seven-day post-PTA intravenous treatment with either full heparinization or nadroparin calcium followed by adjunctive oral aspirin for six months. When angioplasty was performed in the superficial femoral artery the degree of restenosis was significantly lower ($p < 0.01$) among patients receiving nadroparin calcium compared to those given heparin [139].

Reviparin sodium is as effective as UFH in preventing deep vein thrombosis (DVT) in moderate risk surgery (general and abdominal) and significantly reduced DVT in patients with brace immobilization of the legs [132]. A prospective, randomized, double-blind trial was performed with a parallel group comparison of four-dose regimen of reviparin sodium, in patients undergoing major arterial reconstructive surgery. Patients randomized into the two lower dose groups, experienced a relatively high incidence of restenosis, whereas patients receiving the highest dose of reviparin, experienced an unacceptably high rate of bleeding events (all bleeds, 43%; major bleeding, 14.3%). Thus, the optimal dose of reviparin sodium to be administered in patients undergoing major arterial reconstructive surgery is half the therapeutic dose: 5950 to 6300 anti Xa IU (75–85 anti Xa IU/kg body weight per day). Patients included in this group had no major bleeding events (95% confidence interval, 0% to 6.6%) and a significant improvement of the ankle-brachial systolic pressure index. The efficacy and safety of this dosage regimen in comparison to the standard of care needs to be further substantiated in larger trials [140].

The usage of LMWT heparins is difficult in the long term as they require an intravenous or subcutaneous mode of administration. An interesting development is the potential development of an orally absorbable heparin. A phase II study in patients undergoing total hip replacement indicated that oral heparin was as effective and safe as UFH given subcutaneously. A phase III clinical trial comparing two doses of SNAC heparin given orally with LMWT heparin by subcutaneous injection for the prevention of venous thromboembolism in patients undergoing total hip replacement is currently underway [141].

WARFARIN

Warfarin is a vitamin K antagonist, which competitively inhibits the activity of vitamin K dependant clotting factors (II, VII, IX and X). The effect of warfarin on an individual's coagulation is variable and therefore requires regular monitoring. Overall, the annual risk of bleeding on warfarin treatment is approximately 6%, with major and fatal bleeding events estimated to be 2% and 0.8%, respectively [142].

Kretschmer *et al.*, a leading advocate of warfarin, reported a prospective randomized series of patients with autologous vein bypasses followed for ten years [143; 144; 145]. Graft patency and survival was improved in those treated with warfarin compared with controls. However, the control group did not receive any antiplatelet medication. Some 10% of patients had to discontinue warfarin due to haemorrhage. The risk of death from warfarin was calculated at 0.3% per patient per year in this study.

The effect of warfarin and heparin versus heparin alone on lower limb graft patency, salvage and patient survival has also been studied prospectively [146]. There was no statistically significant difference between the two groups. However, 5% of patients had a serious haemorrhage on warfarin and 15% of patients discontinued treatment due to bleeding, drug interactions or inability to manage the anticoagulation therapy. Other studies suggest that ASA/DIP is superior to warfarin in the patency of distal autologous vein grafts and prosthetic above knee grafts [147; 148]. A decision as to the overall benefit of extended anticoagulation once a thrombophilia defect is identified in the individual patient requires assessment of the risk of recurrence in the absence of treatment, versus the bleeding risk associated with prolonged anticoagulation [149].

ANTIPLATELET AGENTS

Aspirin and dipyridamole

Aspirin (ASA) inhibits platelet aggregation by irreversibly affecting platelet cyclo-oxygenase and blocking the production of thromboxane A2. Dipyridamole (DIP) appears to inhibit platelet phosphodiesterase. Both inhibit platelet adherence to the vascular endothelium, platelet aggregation and development of fibrointimal hyperplasia [150].

Aspirin reduces non-fatal myocardial infarctions and non-fatal strokes by one-third and deaths from all vascular causes by one-sixth [151]. The absolute risk reduction of having a serious vascular event was 36 (SE 5) per 1000 treated for two years amongst patients with previous myocardial infarction; 38 (5) per 1000 patients treated for one month among patients with acute myocardial infarction; and 36 (6) per 1000 treated for two years among those with previous stroke or transient ischaemic attack. The absolute risk reduction of having a serious vascular event was less amongst those with acute stroke: 9 (3) per 1000 treated for three weeks and 22 (3) per 1000 treated for two years among other high risk patients (with separately significant results for those with stable angina, peripheral arterial disease and atrial fibrillation).

A further meta-analysis of patients with peripheral vascular disease reported that the number suffering a non-fatal myocardial infarction, non-fatal stroke or vascular death was 6.5% in the antiplatelet group compared with 8.1% in the placebo group (odds ratio 0.78; 95% CI 0.63–0.96), favouring antiplatelet treatment [152]. This meta-analysis also suggested that the data in five trials of ASA against another antiplatelet agent showed that 8.4% in the ASA group suffered a vascular event compared with 6.6% in the second antiplatelet group (odds ratio 0.76; 95% CI 0.64–0.91; $P < 0.01$). These data therefore favour ticlopidine/clopidigrel/ASA + DIP against ASA alone.

However, a recent Cochrane systematic review looking specifically at the role of DIP suggested that DIP had no clear effect on vascular death (RR 1.02; 95% CI 0.90–1.17) compared with the control [153]. Dipyridamole appeared to reduce the risk of vascular events (RR 0.90; 95% CI 0.83–0.98), but this effect was only statistically significant due to a single large trial in patients presenting with cerebral ischaemia (6602 patients). There was no clear difference in vascular death (RR 1.03; 95% CI 0.87–1.22) when DIP plus ASA was compared with ASA alone. This review therefore concluded that for patients presenting with arterial disease there was no evidence that DIP, in the presence or absence of another antiplatelet drug (chiefly ASA) reduced the risk of vascular death, though it may reduce the risk of further vascular events [154].

Both ASA and DIP delay radiological progression of established atherosclerotic disease and ASA also decreases the scintigraphically detectable uptake of platelets at sites of vascular injury, e.g. angioplasty sites [155].

Aspirin however has the potentially serious adverse effect of gastrointestinal bleeding. There is a theoretical risk that ASA may potentiate bleeding from peptic ulceration at a time of stress in patients undergoing vascular surgery [156]. Some surgeons are therefore wary of prescribing ASA pre-operatively. However, antiplatelet therapy started pre-operatively does appear to have a greater effect in improving graft patency than if it is started post-operatively [157; 158; 159]. This has also been the experience in coronary vein bypass grafting where treatment initiated after the second post-operative day had no effect on graft patency [160; 161]. Kester demonstrated improved early patency rates in femoro-popliteal dacron grafts if treated with ASA/DIP compared with placebo [162].

Another study examined the effect of a six-week course of ASA/DIP in bypass grafts. The controls did not receive any antiplatelet medication and ASA was started post-operatively in the treated group. There was no significant improvement in patency rates of infrainguinal vein grafts. However, patency of prosthetic bypass grafts was improved from 53% to 85% in the treated group, which was equivalent to autologous vein graft patency at one year in this study. It is interesting to note that the majority of grafts failed within the first month and that this may therefore be due to undiagnosed hypercoagulability in these patients [163]. A retrospective study of 200 autologous vein grafts, compared six-month treatment with warfarin versus ASA/DIP, versus no medication. Patency rates were twice as high for the ASA/DIP group compared to warfarin treated and controls at ten year follow-up. In addition, the limb salvage rate in the ASA/DIP group was 100% compared to 85% in the warfarin treated group. However, this can in part be explained by the fact that those patients with poor outflow and deemed to be at a higher risk of graft failure are often placed on warfarin [146].

Aspirin in combination with warfarin improved patency in distal reconstructions with poor run off but did not improve patency in more proximal reconstructions [145]. A large multicentre trial by McCollum *et al.* showed no difference in patency of autologous vein femoro-popliteal bypasses at a long term follow-up between placebo and ASA/DIP. However, there was a significant reduction in the risk of myocardial infarctions and strokes in these patients [164]. There was also no improvement in patency rates in autologous vein, PTFE or composite grafts over 13 months when ASA was compared to the placebo [165]. A meta-analysis of ten trials of infrainguinal bypass surgery and two of percutaneous angioplasty suggested that antiplatelet therapy might be of benefit but that the results did not reach statistical significance [147].

Aspirin maybe an effective anti-thrombotic agent for many patients but some patients develop thrombotic events despite treatment. These patients may exhibit aspirin resistance, which has been reported with cardiovascular, cerebrovascular and peripheral vascular disease. The true significance of the problem remains unknown, as there are differences in the definition of resistance, variations in detection methods and lack of controlled trials. Multiple mechanisms for resistance have been proposed, including increased reactivity to platelet aggregating factors, genetic polymorphisms and alternative pathways for thromboxane synthesis [166]. If diagnosed these patients might benefit from alternative or combined antiplatelet therapy.

A Cochrane systematic review examined the evidence for antiplatelet agents after revascularization [167]. The review concluded that the administration of a variety of platelet-inhibitors resulted in improved venous and artificial graft patency compared to no treatment. The analysis indicated that patients with a prosthetic graft were more likely to benefit from administration of platelet-inhibitors than those with a venous graft. Antiplatelet therapy with ASA appeared to have a slight beneficial effect on the patency of peripheral bypasses, but seemed to have an inferior effect on venous graft patency compared with artificial grafts. The effect of ASA on cardiovascular outcomes and survival was mild and not statistically significant. It was thought that this might be due to the fact that the majority of patients receiving a peripheral graft had severe critical ischaemia with high cardiovascular mortality rates of 20% per year. A further meta-analysis suggested that compared with non-active controls, ASA with DIP improved patency (odds ratio 0.69; 95% CI 0.53–0.90) and mortality (odds ratio; 0.80; 95% CI 0.57–1.14) [168].

Glycoprotein IIb/IIIa platelet receptor inhibitors

Platelet glycoprotein (GP) IIb/IIIa receptors are the final common pathway to platelet aggregation and thrombus formation. Coller developed an inhibitor to these receptors using a recombinant murine/human chimeric antibody Fab fragment, ReoPro (abciximab, c7E3) [169]. This exhibited both a high affinity and absolute specificity for the GP IIb/IIIa receptor and inhibited platelet aggregation. In coronary artery disease, the administration of ReoPro at the time of angioplasty or atherectomy has been shown to be highly effective in reducing acute ischaemic events by 35% when compared with placebo [170]. During a six-month follow-up, it was found that further ischaemic events were reduced by 26%. In discussing these findings, it was postulated that ReoPro might in fact cause 'passivation' of the vessel wall [171]. This occurs when the wall develops a platelet non-reactive surface reducing the risk of thrombus formation and intimal hyperplasia. However, ReoPro can be immunogenic and cause thrombocytopenia. Initially there was a significant risk of major adverse bleeding events if administered during cardiac catheterization with standard dose heparin, which was minimized when low dose heparin regimens were used subsequently.

Synthetic inhibitors of platelet GP IIb/IIIa receptors have been developed such as eptifibatide (integrilin). In the IMPACT study, patients undergoing coronary angioplasty and administration of integrilin had lower rates of myocardial infarction, unplanned coronary revascularization and mortality [172]. This benefit has been confirmed in the enhanced suppression of the platelet IIb/IIIa receptor with integrilin therapy (ESPRIT) trial [173]. Lamifiban and tirofiban are non-peptide GP IIb/IIIa inhibitors and have longer half lives. These have yet to show a beneficial effect in cardiac revascularization and infarction. Oral preparations such as xemlofiban are under development. Trials are needed to evaluate their role in peripheral vascular surgery.

A novel use for GP IIb/IIIa platelet receptor inhibitors was investigated in conjunction with peripheral arterial thrombolysis. Two studies have suggested that the addition of abciximab or tirofiban significantly shortened the duration of lysis without an increase in major bleeding events [174; 175].

Ticlodipine and clopidigrel

Ticlodipine and clopidigrel inhibit platelet aggregation by specifically antagonizing the ADP-dependant activation of platelet GP IIb/IIIa receptors. They both appear to have a beneficial effect in the prevention of strokes and myocardial infarctions. Ticlodipine reduces the relative risk of all vascular deaths by 33% compared with 25% with ASA but can cause profuse diarrhoea and severe bone marrow depression (0.85%) [176; 177]. The CAPRIE multicentre study involving 19 185 patients investigated the role of ASA and clopidigrel in vascular disease [178]. Long term administration (three years) of clopidigrel to patients with atherosclerotic vascular disease was more effective than ASA in reducing the combined risk of ischaemic stroke, myocardial infarction or vascular death. The safety profile of 75 mg of clopidigrel in this study was similar to medium dose ASA and without the severe side effects of ticlodipine.

Blanchard *et al.* reported results from EMATAP, a double blind placebo controlled trial of ticlodipine in patients with intermittent claudication [179]. There was a reduction in the number of sudden deaths, myocardial infarctions and need for vascular surgery. A further study reported an improvement in claudication distance by 30% on a three-month regimen of ticlodipine in patients with Leriche-Fontaine IIb peripheral arterial occlusive disease [180]. There has been little human work on the role of ticlodipine in vascular reconstruction but it has been suggested that ticlopidine may improve patency (odds ratio 0.53; 95% CI 0.33–0.85) and reduce the risk of amputation (odds ratio 0.29; 95% CI 0.08–1.01) [171]. In animal models, ticlodipine increases patency of microvascular grafts and PTFE grafts possibly by inhibiting intimal hyperplasia [181]. In humans, ticlodipine inhibited platelet deposition in prosthetic aorto-femoral grafts and may therefore have a role in increasing the early patency rate [182]. However, in this series blood loss and transfusion requirements were higher in the ticlodipine group compared with the placebo group. A Japanese study compared ticlodipine or placebo in supra and infrainguinal reconstructions and found no improvement in late patency rates [183]. This negative result may be because half of the patients underwent suprainguinal reconstructions, which have very good long term patency rates. However, the sub-group of patients undergoing salvage surgery appeared to benefit. The role of clopidigrel clearly needs to be evaluated in a multicentre randomized, controlled trial in patients undergoing vascular reconstruction. This is especially so as it has been established that it has a greater benefit than ASA in reducing mortality from vascular causes and has a safety profile similar to ASA.

Cilostazol, naftidrofuryl and pentoxifylline

Cilostazol is a specific inhibitor of phosphodiesterase 3 and activator of lipoprotein lipase. It is suggested that this drug increases pain-free and absolute walking distances in claudicants [184]. However, cilostazol does cause minor side effects including headache, diarrhoea, loose stools and flatulence. Naftidrofuryl is a serotonin (5-HT2) receptor antagonist and antiplatelet drug, and may also be beneficial for claudicants.

Pentoxifylline has been shown to reduce red cell rigidity, fibrinogen concentration and blood viscosity. A large double-blind, multicentre trial showed an improvement in claudication by 45% compared to 23% in the placebo group at a six-month follow-up [185]. Many trials have been carried out subsequently with conflicting results. A critical review of these trials concluded that the actual improvement in walking distance attributable to pentoxifylline is often unpredictable, may not be clinically significant in comparison to the placebo and does not justify the added expense. However, it was felt that there was a role in severe claudicants, who did not respond to or could not engage in exercise therapy, and for whom even a small improvement would allow a great improvement in lifestyle [186].

Thrombin inhibitors

Hirudin and hirulog are derived from the leech *Hirudo medicinalis*. Argatroban, efegatran and hirugen are synthetic thrombin inhibitors. These are specific inhibitors of both free and clot bound thrombin. They cannot be reversed with protamine but have a short half life. They have been tested in animal models and have been found to exert an anti-thrombotic effect on prosthetic grafts [187]. Argatroban has been evaluated as an alternative anticoagulant to replace heparin in various clinical studies, especially in patients with coronary artery disease or cerebral vascular disease but data are still not available to reach a consensus decision [188]. However, three trials assessing the role of hirudin and heparin in acute myocardial infarctions were stopped prematurely due to unacceptable rates of major bleeding [189; 190; 191]. Hirulog appears to have a better safety profile. Despite this narrow therapeutic window, these drugs may have a limited role at the time of vascular surgery in preventing thrombus deposition. A randomized, controlled trial of hirudin or hirulog versus heparin in bypass grafting is awaited.

Folic acid

There are now several studies suggesting that homocysteine levels may be reduced by the administration of 0.4 mg folic acid even in non-folate-deficient patients. The addition of vitamins B_{12} and/or B_6, to folic acid supplementation may provide a small further reduction in homocysteine levels in certain groups of patients. Renal impairment, an important cause of hyperhomocysteinaemia, requires significantly higher doses of folic acid (5–40 mg) to achieve maximal therapeutic effect [192]. One study has suggested that lowering homocysteine concentrations by 3 micromol/l would reduce the risk of ischaemic heart disease by 16% (11%–20%), DVT by 25% (8%–38%) and stroke by 24% (15%–33%) [53]. These data are further compounded by the suggestion that vitamin B_6 plus folic acid is protective against a further event in patients with premature atherothrombotic cerebrovascular disease and hyperhomocysteinaemia [193].

OVERVIEW

Patients with peripheral vascular disease present a high-risk group with an overall mortality rate three times higher than the controls [194]. The relative risk of death in claudicants from coronary artery disease is as high as six times that of normal populations.

A further high-risk group may be defined for whom therapy could be optimized. Patients with hypercoagulability present with early atherosclerosis and are more likely to occlude vascular reconstructions. Prevalence studies suggest that this group may compose 40% of patients requiring revascularization. At present, screening for hypercoagulability is only routine when there is a presentation of premature atherosclerosis, an acute thrombosis or recurrent graft failure. However, it would seem sensible to screen patients for thrombophilia in vascular clinics to allow the optimization of medical therapy at the time of intervention. With limited budgets, this is difficult as the tests are expensive. However, the costs of screening must be considered against the costs of graft failure, further revascularization and possible amputation.

It is difficult to define the best possible medical therapy in these patients. There are no published trials of medical therapy in patients with hypercoagulability and peripheral vascular disease. Treatment of asymptomatic hypercoagulable patients is not routinely recommended unless there is a strong family history of thrombosis. However, prophylaxis during surgery or angioplasty is recommended. It must be remembered that these patients also have generalized atherosclerosis and so there can be no justification in withholding antiplatelet therapy as it has been shown to reduce vascular deaths. In addition, the systematic overview of the Antiplatelet Trialists' Collaboration provided unequivocal evidence that antiplatelet therapy reduces the odds of arterial or graft occlusion among patients who have had a range of vascular operations. The choice between the individual drugs remains the surgeon's choice.

Medium dose aspirin remains the most widely tested, most convenient and least expensive antiplatelet treatment. Aspirin has been shown to reduce overall vascular mortality as well as improving graft patency. Evidence suggests that it should be started pre-operatively to gain maximum benefit despite the theoretically increased risk of gastrointestinal bleeding. Aspirin appears to improve the patency of prosthetic distal grafts more significantly than autologous vein grafts.

Heparin is used perioperatively to inhibit thrombus formation at the site of revascularization. Heparin is used widely despite the lack of good published evidence in clinical series. Low molecular weight heparin carries a lower risk of bleeding and reduces the need for intensive monitoring of coagulation therefore decreasing overall treatment costs.

Warfarin is prescribed at present if there is an acute thrombosis or a failed graft requiring revascularization. It is difficult to recommend the use of warfarin routinely in these patients without a large prospectively randomized, controlled trial because of the potentially lethal side effects such as bleeding.

Ticlodipine and clopidigrel have been shown to be more effective than aspirin in reducing overall mortality and could have a substantial role in preventing graft failure due to thrombus. However, there are no robust clinical trials in patients undergoing revascularization. Ticlodipine requires haematological monitoring as it has a 1% risk of inducing an aplastic anaemia and therefore appears less desirable. However, clopidigrel has great potential, as its safety profile appears to be better than ticlodipine and equivalent to medium dose aspirin.

The role of the newer glycoprotein IIb/IIIa platelet receptor inhibitors needs to be carefully evaluated. These drugs could potentially decrease graft failure secondary to thrombus in hypercoagulable patients. Whether a single infusion at the time of surgery would be enough or whether longer treatment with oral agents is required needs to be evaluated with a prospective randomized, controlled trial.

A recent leading article in the *British Medical Journal* advocated the prescription of the polypill [195]. It suggested that a single pill containing 10 mg atorvastatin or 40 mg simvastatin; three anti-hypertensive agents (for example, a thiazide, a beta blocker and an angiotensin converting enzyme inhibitor) each at half standard dose; 0.8 mg folic acid and 75 mg aspirin may be beneficial in reducing cardiovascular and cerebrovascular events. Patients with hypercoagulability might benefit from this to a greater degree but might require a further antithrombotic agent.

By optimizing best medical practice the number of failed grafts may be reduced. If 40% of patients undergoing revascularization exhibit hypercoagulability and around 60% occlude their grafts, then this would account for 24 patients out of 100. Even if only one-third of these patients required re-intervention and possibly amputation the costs are huge. Any pharmaceutical manipulation that could positively influence the outcome of surgery should be evaluated.

REFERENCES

1. A. I. Schafer, The hypercoagulable states. *Annals of Internal Medicine*, **102** (1985), 814–28.
2. B. M. Alving, The hypercoagulable states. *Hospital Practice*, (1993), 109–21.
3. J. G. van der Bom, V. L. Bots, H. H. D. M. van Vliet *et al.*, Antithrombin and atherosclerosis in the Rotterdam study. *Arteriosclerosis, Thrombosis and Vascular Biology*, **16** (1996), 864–7.
4. S. N. Faust, R. S. Heyderman & L. Levin, Coagulation in severe sepsis: a central role for thrombomodulin and activated protein C. *Critical Care Medicine*, **29**(7) (2001), S62–7.
5. J. S. Greengard, X. Sun, X. Xu *et al.*, Activated protein C resistance caused by Arg506Gln mutation in factor Va. *Lancet*, **343** (1994), 1361–2.
6. P. M. Ridker, C. H. Hennekens, K. Lindpainter *et al.*, Mutation in the gene coding for coagulation factor V and the risk of myocardial infarction, stroke and venous thrombosis in apparently healthy men. *New England Journal of Medicine*, **332** (1995), 912–17.
7. P. C. Comp, Coumarin induced skin necrosis. Incidence, mechanisms, management and avoidance. *Drug Safety*, **8** (1993), 128–35.
8. B. Kemkes-Matthes & K. J. Matthes, Protein Z. *Seminars in Thrombosis and Hemostasis*, **27** (2001), 551–6.
9. B. Kemkes-Matthes, M. Nees, G. Kuhnel, A. Matzdorff, & K. J. Matthes, Protein Z influences the prothrombotic phenotype in factor V Leiden patients. *Thrombosis Research*, **106** (2002), 183–5.
10. F. Rodeghiero & A. Tossetto. The VITA project: population based distributions of protein C, antithrombin III, heparin cofactor II and plasminogen – relationship with physiological variables and establishment of reference ranges. *Thrombosis and Haemostasis*, **76** (1996), 226–33.
11. V. R. Arruda, J. M. Annichino-Bizzacchi, M. S. Goncalves & F. F. Costa, Prevalence of the prothrombin gene variant (nt20110A) in venous thrombosis and arterial disease. *Thrombosis and Haemostasis*, **78** (1997), 1430–3.
12. S. R. Poort, F. R. Rosendaal, P. H. Reitsma, & R. M. Bertina, A common genetic variation in the 3′-untranslated region of the prothrombin gene is associated with elevated plasma prothrombin levels and an increase in venous thrombosis. *Blood*, **88** (1996), 3698–703.
13. W. G. Hughson, J. I. Mann & A. Garrod, Intermittent claudication: prevalence and risk factors. *British Medical Journal*, **1** (1978), 1379–81.
14. W. B. Kannel, P. A. Wolf, W. B. Castelli & R. B. D'Agostino, Fibrinogen and risk of cardiovascular disease. The Framingham Study. *Journal of the American Medical Association*, **258** (1987), 1183–6.
15. W. B. Kannel, R. B. D'Agostino & A. J. Belanger, Update on fibrinogen as a cardiovascular risk factor. *Annals of Epidemiology*, **2** (1992), 457–66.
16. T. E. Warkentin & J. G. Kelton, Heparin induced thrombocytopaenia. *Progress in Hemostasis and Thrombosis*, **10** (1991), 1–34.

17. S. H. Lee, C. Y. Liu & G. PaoloVisentin, Heparin-induced thrombocytopenia: molecular pathogenesis. *International Journal of Hematology*, **76** (2002), 346–51.
18. D. J. King, & J. G. Kelton, Heparin associated thrombocytopenia. *Annals of Internal Medicine*, **100** (1984), 535–40.
19. P. Pradoni, A. W. A. Lensing, H. R. Buller *et al.*, Deep vein thrombosis and the incidence of subsequent symptomatic cancer. *New England Journal of Medicine*, **327** (1992), 1128–33.
20. G. J. Caine, P. S. Stonelake, G. Lip & S. T. Kehoe, The hypercoagulable state of malignancy: pathogenesis and current debate. *Neoplasia*, **4** (2002), 465–73.
21. S. A. Ray, M. R. Rowley, A. Loh *et al.*, Hypercoagulable states in patients with leg ischaemia. *British Journal of Surgery*, **81** (1994), 811–14.
22. A. I. Schafer, Hypercoagulable states: molecular genetics to clinical practice. *Lancet*, **344** (1994), 1739–42.
23. G. M. Rodgers & M. T. Conn, Homocysteine, an atherogenic stimulus, reduces protein C activation by arterial and venous endothelial cells. *Blood*, **75** (1990), 895–901.
24. S. R. Lentz & J. E. Sadler, Inhibition of thrombomodulin surface expression and protein C activation by the thrombogenic agent homocysteine. *Journal of Clinical Investigation*, **88** (1991), 1906–14.
25. G. Puerto & S. Coccheri, Lowered antithrombin-III activity and other clotting changes in homocysteinuria. *Blood*, **19S** (1989), 24–8.
26. G. Freyburger, S. Labrouche, G. Sassoust *et al.*, Mild hyperhomocysteinaemia and haemostatic factors in patients with arterial vascular diseases. *Thrombosis and Haemostasis*, **77** (1996), 466–71.
27. G. N. Welch, G. R. Upchurch & J. Loscalzo. Hyperhomocysteinaemia and atherothrombosis. *Annals of the New York Academy of Sciences*, **811** (1997), 48–58.
28. M. F. Bellamy & I. F. W. McDowell, Putatative mechanisms for vascular damage by homocysteine. *Journal of Inherited Metabolic Disease*, **29** (1996), 307–15.
29. P. M. Ueland, Homocysteine species as components of plasma redox thiol status. *Clinical Chemistry*, **41** (1995), 340–2.
30. E. Cacciari & S. Saladari, Clinical and laboratory features of homocysteinuria. *Haemostasis*, **19** (1989), 10–13.
31. S. H. Mudd, F. Skovby, H. L. Levy *et al.*, The natural history of homocysteinuria due to cystathionine beta-synthetase deficiency. *American Journal of Human Genetics*, **37** (1985), 1–31.
32. G. H. Boers, A. G. Smals, F. J. Trijbels *et al.*, Heterozygotes for homocysteinuria in premature peripheral and cerebral occlusive arterial disease. *New England Journal of Medicine*, **313** (1985), 709–15.
33. D. E. L. Wilcken & B. Wilcken, The pathogenesis of coronary artery disease: a possible role for methionine metabolism. *Journal of Clinical Investigation*, **57** (1976), 1079–82.
34. S. S. Kang, J. Zhou, P. W. Wong, J. Kowalisyn & G. Strokosch, Intermediate homocysteinemia: a thermolabile variant of methylentetrahydrofolate reductase. *American Journal of Human Genetics*, **43** (1988), 414–21.
35. A. M. Engbersen, D. G. Franken, G. H. Boers *et al.*, Thermolabile 5,10-methylentetrahydrofolate reductase as a cause of mild hyperhomocysteinaemia. *American Journal of Human Genetics*, **56** (1995), 142–50.
36. P. Frosst, H. J. Blom, R. Milos *et al.*, A candidate genetic risk factor for vascular disease. *Nature Genetics*, **10** (1995), 111–13.
37. J. Selhub, P. F. Jacques, P. W. Wilson, D. Rush & I. H. Rosenberg, Vitamin status and intake as primary determinants of homocysteinemia in an elderly population. *JAMA*, **270** (1993), 2693–8.
38. S. S. Kang, P. W. K. Wong & M. Norusis, Homocysteinemia due to folate deficiency. *Metabolism*, **36** (1987), 458–62.
39. D. E. Wilcken & V. J. Gupta, Sulphur containing amino acids in chronic renal failure withparticular reference to homocysteine and cysteine-homocysteine mixed disulphide. *European Journal of Clinical Investigation*, **9** (1979), 301–7.
40. K. Robinson, A. Gupta, V. Dennis *et al.*, Hyperhomocysteinaemia confers an independent risk of atherosclerosis in end stage renal disease and is closely linked toplasma folate and pyridoxine concentrations. *Circulation*, **94** (1996), 2743–8.
41. A. G. Bostom & L. Lathrop, Homocysteinemia in end stage renal disease; prevalence, aetiology and potential relationship to arteriosclerotic outcomes. *Kidney International*, **52** (1997), 10–20.
42. W. J. Vermaak, J. B. Ubbink, H. C. Barnard *et al.*, Vitamin B_6 nutrition status and cigarette smoking.

American Journal of Clinical Nutrition, **51** (1990), 1058–61.
43. E. P. Turton, P. A. Coughlin, D. C. Berridge & K. G. Mercer, A survey of deep venous thrombosis management by consultant vascular surgeons in the United Kingdom and Ireland. *European Journal of Vascular and Endovascular Surgery*, **21** (2001), 558–63.
44. M. Gaustadnes, N. Rudiger, J. Moller *et al.*, Thrombophilic predisposition in stroke and venous thromboembolism in Danish patients. *Blood Coagulation and Fibrinolysis*, **10**(5) (1999), 251–9.
45. T. Y. Chen, W. C. Su & C. J. Tsao, Incidence of thrombophilia detected in southern Taiwanese patients with venous thrombosis. *Annals of Hematology*, **82** (2003), 114–17.
46. D. J. Harrington, A. Malefora, V. Schmeleva *et al.*, Genetic variations observed in arterial and venous thromboembolism – relevance for therapy, risk prevention andprognosis. *Clinical Chemistry and Laboratory Medicine*, **41** (2003), 496–500.
47. M. A. Crowther & J. G. Kelton, Congenital thrombophilic states associated with venous thrombosis: a qualitative overview and proposed classification system. *Annals of Internal Medicine*, **138** (2003), 128–34.
48. T. Baglin, R. Luddington, K. Brown & C. Baglin, Incidence of recurrent venous thromboembolism in relation to clinical and thrombophilic risk factors: prospective cohort study. *Lancet*, **16** (2003), 523–6.
49. R. K. Mackenzie, C. A. Ludlam, C. V. Ruckley *et al.*, The prevalence of thrombophilia in patients with chronic venous leg ulceration. *Journal of Vascular Surgery*, **35** (2002), 718–22.
50. A. W. Bradbury, R. K. MacKenzie, P. Burns & C. Fegan, Thrombophilia and chronic venous ulceration. *European Journal of Vascular and Endovascular Surgery*, **24** (2002), 97–104.
51. L. J. Langman, J. G. Ray, J. Evrovski, E. Yeo & D. E. Cole, Hyperhomocyst(e)inemia and the increased risk of venous thromboembolism: more evidence from a case-control study. *Archives of Internal Medicine*, **160** (2000), 961–4.
52. T. S. Hsu, L. A. Hsu, C. J. Chang *et al.*, Importance of hyperhomocysteinemia as a risk factor for venous thromboembolism in a Taiwanese population. A case-control study. *Thrombosis Research*, **102** (2001), 387–95.
53. D. S. Wald, M. Law & J. K. Morris, Homocysteine and cardiovascular disease: evidence oncausality from a meta-analysis. *British Medical Journal*, **325** (2002), 1202.
54. M. den Heijer, F. R. Rosendaal, H. J. Blom, W. B. Gerrits & G. M. Bos, Hyperhomocysteinemia and venous thrombosis: a meta-analysis. *Thrombosis and Haemostasis*, **80** (1998), 874–7.
55. P. Hainaut, C. Jaumotte, D. Verhelst *et al.*, Hyperhomocysteinemia and venous thromboembolism: a risk factor more prevalent in the elderly and in idiopathic cases. *Thrombosis Research*, **10** (2002), 121–5.
56. H. P. Willems, M. den Heijer, G. M. Bos, Homocysteine and venous thrombosis: outline of a vitamin intervention trial. *Seminars in Thrombosis and Hemostasis*, **26** (2000), 297–304.
57. I. Martinelli, T. Battaglioli, P. Pedotti, M. Cattaneo & P. M. Mannucci, Hyperhomocysteinaemia in cerebral vein thrombosis. *Blood*, **102** (2003), 1363–6.
58. M. L. Varela, Y. P. Adamczuk, R. R. Forastiero *et al.*, Major and potential prothrombotic genotypes in a cohort of patients with venous thromboembolism. *Thrombosis Research*, **104** (2001), 317–24.
59. M. den Heijer & M. B. Keijzer, Hyperhomocysteinaemia as a risk factor for venous thrombosis. *Clinical Chemistry and Laboratory Medicine*, **39** (2001), 710–13.
60. A. W. Tsai, M. Cushman, M. Y. Tsai *et al.*, Serum homocysteine, thermolabile variant of methylene tetrahydrofolate reductase (MTHFR), and venous thromboembolism: Longitudinal Investigation of Thromboembolism Etiology (LITE). *American Journal of Hematology*, **72** (2003), 192–200.
61. T. B. Domagala, L. Adamek, E. Nizankowska, M. Sanak & A. Szczeklik, Mutations C677T and A1298C of the 5,10-methylenetetrahydrofolate reductase gene and fasting plasma homocysteine levels are not associated with the increased risk of venous thromboembolic disease. *Blood Coagulation and Fibrinolysis*, **13**(5) (2002), 423–31.
62. C. Rintelen, C. Mannhalter, K. Lechner *et al.*, No evidence for an increased risk of venous thrombosis in patients with factor V Leiden by the homozygous 677 C to T mutation in the methylene tetrahydrofolate reductase gene. *Blood Coagulation and Fibrinolysis*, **10** (1999), 101–5.
63. V. M. Morelli, D. M. Lourenco, V. D'Almeida *et al.*, Hyperhomocysteinaemia increases the risk of venous thrombosis independent of the C677T mutation of the methylene tetrahydrofolate reductase gene in selected

Brazilian patients. *Blood Coagulation and Fibrinolysis*, **13**(3) (2002), 271–5.

64. H. Fujimura, T. Kawasaki, T. Sakata *et al.*, Common C677T polymorphism in the methylenetetrahydrofolate reductase gene increases the risk for deep vein thrombosis in patients with predisposition of thrombophilia. *Thrombosis Research*, **98** (2000), 1–8.
65. M. B. Keijzer, M. den, Heijer, H. J. Blom *et al.*, Interaction between hyperhomocysteinaemia, mutated methylenetetrahydrofolate reductase (MTHFR) and inherited thrombophilic factors inrecurrent venous thrombosis. *Thrombosis and Haemostasis*, **88**(5) (2002), 723–8.
66. J. G. Ray, D. Shmorgun & W. S. Chan, Common C677T polymorphism of the methylenetetrahydrofolate reductase gene and the risk of venous thromboembolism: meta-analysis of 31 studies. *Pathophysiology of Haemostasis and Thrombosis*, **32** (2002), 51–8.
67. R. J. Valentine, H. S. Kaplan, R. Green *et al.*, Lipoprotein (a), homocysteine and hypercoagulable states in young men with premature peripheral atherosclerosis: a prospective controlled analysis. *Journal of Vascular Surgery*, **23** (1996), 53–63.
68. J. Eldrup-Jorgensen, D. P. Flanigan, L. Brace *et al.*, Hypercoagulable states and lower limb ischaemia in young adults. *Journal of Vascular Surgery*, **9** (1989), 334–41.
69. D. C. Aronson, T. Ruys, J. H. van Bockel *et al.*, Aprospective survey of the risk factors in young adults with arterial occlusive disease. *European Journal of Vascular Surgery*, **3** (1989), 227–32.
70. P. J. Levy, M. F. Gonzalez, C. A. Hornung *et al.*, A prospective evaluation of the atherosclerotic risk factors and hypercoagulability in young adults with premature lower extremity disease. *Journal of Vascular Surgery*, **23** (1996), 36–45.
71. R. W. Lee, L. M. Taylor, G. J. Landry *et al.*, Prospective comparison of infrainguinal bypass grafting in patients with and without antiphospholipid antibodies. *Journal of Vascular Surgery*, **24** (1996), 524–33.
72. W. R. Flinn, M. D. McDaniel, J. S. Yao, V. A. Fahey & D. Green, Antithrombin III deficiency as areflection of dynamic protein metabolism in patients undergoing vascular reconstruction. *Journal of Vascular Surgery*, **1** (1984), 888–95.
73. M. C. Donaldson, D. S. Weinberg, M. Belkin, A. D. Whittemore & J. A. Mannick, Screening for hypercoagulable states in vascular surgical practice. *Journal of Vascular Surgery*, **11** (1990), 825–31.
74. J. D. Eason, J. L. Mills & W. C. Beckett, Hypercoagulable states in arterial thromboembolism. *Surgery, Gynecology and Obstetrics*, **174** (1992), 211–15.
75. L. M. Taylor, Jr, R. W. Chitwood, R. L. Dalman *et al.*, Antiphospholipid antibodies in vascular surgery patients: a cross sectional study. *Annals of Surgery*, **220**(4) (1994), 544–51.
76. K. Ouriel, R. M. Green, J. A. DeWeese & C. Cimino, Activated protein C resistance: prevalence and implications in peripheral vascular disease. *Journal of Vascular Surgery*, **23** (1996), 46–57.
77. S. M. Evans, J. Brittenden, D. J. Adam, C. Ludlam, A. W. Bradbury, Vascular Surgical Society of Great Britain and Ireland; prevalence and significance of thrombophilia in patients with intermittent claudication. *British Journal of Surgery*, **86** (1999), 702–3.
78. E. S. K. Sampram & B. Lindblad, The impact of factor V mutation on the risk of occlusion in patients undergoing peripheral vascular reconstructions. *European Journal of Vascular and Endovascular Surgery*, **22** (2001), 134–8.
79. E. Y. Lam, L. M. Taylor, Jr, G. J. Landry, J. M. Porter & G. L. Moneta, Relationship between antiphospholipid antibodies and progression of lower extremity arterial occlusive disease after lower limb bypass operations. *Journal of Vascular Surgery*, **33** (2001), 976–82.
80. K. E. Morton, T. P. Gavaghan, S. A. Krilis *et al.*, Coronary artery bypass graft failure – an autoimmune phenomenon? *Lancet*, **2** (1986), 1353–7.
81. A. Hamsten, R. Norberg, U. Bjorkholm, de Faire & G. Holm, Antibodies to cardiolipin in young survivors of myocardial infarction: an association with recurrent cardiovascular events. *Lancet*, **1** (1986), 113–15.
82. S. J. Kittner & P. B. Gorelick, Antiphospholipid antibodies and stroke: an epidemiological perspective. *Stroke*, **23** (1992), I-19–22.
83. D. C. Hess, Stroke associated with antiphospholipid antibodies. *Stroke*, **23** (1992), I-23–8.
84. P. Gorog, C. D. Ridler, G. M. Rees & I. B. Kovacs, Evidence against hypercoagulability in coronary artery disease. *Thrombosis Research*, **79** (1995), 377–85.
85. M. S. Gowda, M. L. Zucker, J. L. Vacek *et al.*, Incidence of factor V Leiden in patients with acute myocardial infarction. *Journal of Thrombosis and Thrombolysis*, **9** (2000), 43–5.

86. C. Butt, H. Zheng, E. Randell *et al.*, Combined carrier status of prothrombin 20210A and factor XIII-A Leu34 alleles as a strong risk factor for myocardial infarction: evidence of a gene-gene interaction. *Blood*, **101** (2003), 3037–41.
87. W. H. Chen, M. Y. Lan, Y. Y. Chang, S. S. Chen & J. S. Liu, The prevalence of C. protein, S. protein, and antithrombin III deficiency in non-APS/SLE Chinese adults with noncardiac cerebral ischaemia. *Clinical and Applied Thrombosis/Haemostasis*, **9** (2003), 155–62.
88. G. Collins, R. L. Heymann & R. Zajtchuk, Hypercoagulability in patients with peripheral vascular disease. *The American Journal of Surgery*, **130** (1975), 2–6.
89. S. A. Ray, M. R. Rowley, D. H. Bevan, R. S. Taylor & J. A. Dormandy, Hypercoagulable abnormalities and postoperative failure of arterial reconstruction. *European Journal of Vascular and Endovascular Surgery*, **13** (1997), 363–70.
90. M. R. Malinow, P. B. Duell, D. L. Hess *et al.*, Reduction of plasma homocysteine levels by breakfast cereal fortified with folic acid in patients with coronary artery disease. *New England Journal of Medicine*, **338** (1998), 1009–15.
91. R. Clarke, L. Daly, K. Robinson *et al.*, Hyperhomocysteinaemia: an independent risk factor for vascular disease. *New England Journal of Medicine*, **324** (1991), 1149–55.
92. D. C. Aronson, W. Onkenhout, A. M. Raben *et al.*, Impaired homocysteine metabolism: a risk factor in young adults with atherosclerotic arterial occlusive disease of the leg. *British Journal of Surgery*, **81** (1994), 1114–18.
93. M. van de Berg & G. H. J. Boers, Homocysteinuria: what about mild hyperhomocysteinaemia? *Postgraduate Medical Journal*, **72** (1996), 513–18.
94. I. C. Currie, Y. G. Wilson, J. Scott *et al.*, Homocysteine: an independent risk factor for the failure of vascular intervention. *British Journal of Surgery*, **83** (1996), 1238–41.
95. K. S. McCully, Homocysteine and vascular disease. *Nature Medicine*, **2** (1996), 386–9.
96. G. J. Hankey & J. W. Eikelbloom, Homocysteine and vascular disease. *Lancet*, **354** (1999), 407–13.
97. S. S. Kang, P. W. K. Wong & R. Malinow, Hyperhomocysteinaemia as a risk factor for occlusive vascular disease. *Annual Review of Nutrition*, **12** (1992), 279–98.
98. I. Fermo, S. Vigano' D'Angelo, R. Paroni *et al.*, Prevalence of moderate hyperhomocysteinaemia in patients with early onset venous and arterial occlusive disease. *Annals of Internal Medicine*, **123** (1995), 747–53.
99. S. Caldwell, M. McCarthy, S. C. Martin *et al.*, Hyperhomocysteinaemia, peripheral vascular disease and neointimal hyperplasia in elderly patients. *British Journal of Surgery*, **85** (1998), 709.
100. C. J. Boushey, S. A. Beresford, G. S. Omenn & A. G. Motulsky, A quantitative assessment of plasma homocysteine as a risk factor for vascular disease. *JAMA*, **274** (1995), 1049–57.
101. I. M. Graham, L. E. Daly, H. M. Refsum *et al.*, Plasma homocysteine as a risk factor for vascular disease; the European Concerted Action Project. *JAMA*, **277** (1997), 1775–81.
102. K. Robinson, K. Arheart, H. Refsum *et al.*, Low circulating folate and vitamin B_6 concentrations: risk factors for stroke, peripheral vascular disease and coronary heart disease. *Circulation*, **97** (1998), 437–43.
103. P. M. Gallagher, R. Meleady, D. C. Shields *et al.*, Homocysteine and risk of premature coronary heart disease. *Circulation*, **94**(9) (1996), 2154–8.
104. H. Morita, J. Taguchi, H. Kurihara *et al.*, Genetic polymorphism of 5,10-methylenetetrahydrofolate reductase as a risk factor for coronary artery disease. *Circulation*, **95**(8) (1997), 2032–6.
105. L. Brattstrom, D. E. Wilcken, J. Ohrvik & L. Brudin, Common methylenetetrahydrofolate reductase gene mutation leads to hyperhomocysteinaemia but not vascular disease. *Circulation*, **98**(23) (1998), 2520–6.
106. T. G. Deloughery, A. Evans, A. Sadeghi *et al.*, Common mutation in methylenetetrahydrofolate reductase: correlation with homocysteine metabolism and late onset vascular disease. *Circulation*, **94** (1996), 3074–8.
107. J. Eritsland, H. Arnesen, I. Seljeflot *et al.*, Influence of serum lipoprotein (a) and homocysteine levels on graft patency after coronary artery bypass grafting. *American Journal of Cardiology*, **74** (1994), 1099–102.
108. M. Mireskandari, M. Schachter, I. G. Timms *et al.*, Plasma homocysteine is an independent risk factor for vein graft stenosis. *British Journal of Surgery*, **85**(1) (1998), 27.
109. C. Irvine, Y. G. Wilson, I. C. Currie *et al.*, Hyperhomocysteinaemia is a risk factor for vein graft stenosis. *European Journal of Vascular and Endovascular Surgery*, **12**(3) (1996), 304–9.

110. G. J. de Borst, M. J. Tangelder, A. Algra *et al.*, Dutch BOA (Bypass Oral anticoagulants or Aspirin) study group. The influence of hyperhomocysteinaemia on graft patency after infrainguinal bypass surgery in the Dutch BOA study. *Journal of Vascular Surgery*, **36** (2002), 336–40.
111. A. Folsom, Fibrinogen and cardiovascular risk in the atherosclerotic communities (ARIC) study. In *Fibrinogen, a New Cardiovascular Risk Factor*, ed. E. Ernst (Oxford: Blackwell, 1992).
112. W. B. Kannel, R. B. d'Agostino & Belanger. Fibrinogen, cigarette smoking and risk of cardiovascular disease; insights from the Framingham study. *American Heart Journal*, **113** (1987), 1006–10.
113. E. Ernst & A. Matrai, Abstention from chronic cigarette smoking normalises blood rheology. *Atherosclerosis*, **64** (1987), 75–7.
114. S. W. K. Cheng, A. C. W. Ting, H. Lau *et al.*, Epidemiology of atherosclerotic peripheral arterial occlusive disease in Hong Kong. *World Journal of Surgery*, **23** (1999), 202–6.
115. W. C. S. Smith, M. Woodward & H. Tunstall-Pedoe, Intermittent claudication in Scotland. In *Epidemiology of Peripheral Vascular Disease*, ed. F. G. R. Fowkes. (London: Springer-Verlag, 1991) pp. 117–23.
116. T. W. Meade, R. Chakrabarti, A. P. Haines *et al.*, Characteristics affecting fibrinolytic activity and plasma fibrinogen concentration. *British Medical Journal*, i (1979), 153–5.
117. T. W. Meade, J. Imeson & Y. Stirling, Effect of changes in smoking and other characteristics on clotting factors and the risk of ischaemic heart disease. *Lancet*, **2** (1987), 986–8.
118. L. Doweik, T. Maca M. Schillinger *et al.*, Fibrinogen predicts mortality in high risk patients with peripheral artery disease. *European Journal of Vascular and Endovascular Surgery*, **26**(4) (2003), 381–6.
119. J. A. Dormandy, E. Hoare, J. Colley *et al.*, Clinical, haemodynamic, rheological and biochemical findings in 126 patients with intermittent claudication. *British Medical Journal*, **4** (1973), 576–81.
120. K. R. Woodburn, A. Rumley, G. D. Lowe *et al.*, Clinical, biochemical and rheological factors affecting the outcome of infrainguinal bypass grafting. *Journal of Vascular Surgery*, **24** (1996), 639–46.
121. J. D. Hamer, F. Ashton & M. J. Meynell, Factors influencing prognosis in the surgery of peripheral vascular disease: platelet adhesiveness, plasma fibrinogen and fibrinolysis. *British Journal of Surgery*, **60** (1973), 386–9.
122. S. Wiseman, G. Kenchington, R. Dain *et al.*, Influence of smoking and plasma factors on patency of femoropopliteal vein grafts. *British Medical Journal*, **299** (1989), 643–6.
123. M. Tschopl, D. A. Tsakiris, G. A. Marbet *et al.*, Role of haemostatic risk factors for restenosis in peripheral arterial occlusive disease after transluminal angioplasty. *Arteriosclerosis, Thrombosis and Vascular Biology*, **17** (1997), 3208–14.
124. D. G. Hackam, & S. S. Anand, Emerging risk factors for atherosclerotic vascular disease: a critical review of the evidence. *JAMA*, **290**(7) (2003), 932–40.
125. TASC Working Group, Management of peripheral arterial disease. *International Angiology*, **19** (2000), 65–72.
126. British Society for Haematology, Guidelines on the investigation and management of thrombophilia. *Journal of Clinical Pathology*, **43** (1990), 703–10.
127. P. J. Burns, D. A. Mosquera & A. W. Bradbury, Prevalence and significance of thrombophilia in peripheral arterial disease. *European Journal of Vascular and Endovascular Surgery*, **22** (2001), 98–106.
128. R. van der Griend, F. J. Haas, M. Duran *et al.*, Methionine loading is necessary for the detection of hyperhomocysteinaemia. *Journal of Laboratory and Clinical Medicine*, **132** (1998), 67–72.
129. H. Refsum, T. Fiskerstrand, A. B. Guttormsen & P. M. Ueland, Assessment of homocysteine status. *Journal of Inherited Metabolic Disease*, **20** (1997), 286–94.
130. A. I. Scafer, The hypercoagulable states. *Annals of Internal Medicine*, **102** (1985), 814–28.
131. B. Lindblad, T. W. Wakefield, T. J. Stanley *et al.*, Pharmacological prophylaxis against postoperative graft occlusion after peripheral vascular surgery: a world wide survey. *European Journal of Vascular and Endovascular Surgery*, **9**(3) (1995), 267–71.
132. S. Sarin, S. K. Shami, T. R. Cheatle *et al.*, When do vascular surgeons prescribe antiplatelet therapy? Current attitudes. *European Journal of Vascular Surgery*, **7**(1) (1993), 6–13.
133. R. D. Rosenberg, Vascular smooth muscle proliferation: basic investigators and new therapeutic approaches. *Thrombosis and Haemostasis*, **70** (1993), 10–16.
134. H. K. Breddin, Reviparin sodium – a new low molecular weight heparin. *Expert Opinion on Pharmacotherapy*, **3**(2) (2002), 173–82.

135. G. M. Andreozzi, S. S. Signorelli, G. Cacciaguerra, *et al.*, Three month therapy with calcium heparin in comparison with ticlodipine in patients with peripheral arterial occlusive disease at Leriche-Fontaine IIb Class. *Angiology*, (1993), 307–313.
136. R. A. Edmondson, A. T. Cohen, S. K. Das, M. B. Wagner & V. Kakkar, Low molecular weight heparin versus aspirin and dipyridamole after femoropopliteal bypass grafting. *Lancet*, **344** (1994), 914–18.
137. W. D. McMillan, W. J. McCarthy, S. J. Lin, J. S. Matsumura, W. H. Pearce & J. S. T. Yao, Perioperative low molecular weight heparin for infrageniculate bypass. *Journal of Vascular Surgery*, **25**(5) (1997), 796–800.
138. C. Devine, B. Hons & C. McCollum, Heparin-bonded Dacron or polytetrafluoroethylene for femoropopliteal bypass grafting: a multicenter trial. *Journal of Vascular Surgery*, **33**(3) (2001), 533–9.
139. J. Schweizer, A. Muller, L. Forkmann, G. Hellner & W. Kirch, Potential use of a low-molecular-weight heparin to prevent restenosis in patients with extensive wall damage following peripheral angioplasty. *Angiology*, **52**(10) (2001), 659–69.
140. P. Kujath, C. Eckmann & F. Misselwitz, Low-molecular-weight heparin in arterial reconstructive surgery: a double-blind, randomized dose-finding trial. *Clinical and Applied Thrombosis/Haemostasis*, **8**(4) (2002), 337–45.
141. G. F. Pineo, R. D. Hull & V. J. Marder, Orally active heparin and low-molecular-weight heparin. *Current Opinion in Pulmonary Medicine*, **7**(5) (2001), 344–48.
142. A. E. Schusshaim & V. Fuster, Thrombosis, antithrombotic agents and the antithrombotic approach in cardiac disease. *Progress in Cardiovascular Diseases*, **40**(3) (1997), 205–38.
143. G. Kretshmer, E. Wenzl, O. Wagner *et al.*, Influence of anticoagulant treatment in preventing graft occlusion following saphenous vein bypass for femoropopliteal occlusive disease. *British Journal of Surgery*, **73**(9) (1986), 689–92.
144. G. Kretshmer, E. Wenzl, M. Schemper *et al.*, Influence of postoperative anticoagulant treatment on patient survival after femoropopliteal vein bypass surgery. *Lancet*, **1** (1988), 797–9.
145. G. Kretshmer, F. Herbst, M. Prager *et al.*, A decade of oral anticoagulant treatment to maintain autologous vein grafts for femoropopliteal atherosclerosis. *Archives of Surgery*, **127** (1992), 1112–15.
146. B. Arfvidsson, F. Lundgren, C. Drott, T. Schersten & K. Lundholm. Influence of coumarin treatment on patency and limb salvage after peripheral arterial reconstructive surgery. *American Journal of Surgery*, **159** (1990), 556–60.
147. D. Rosenthal, M. J. Mittenthal, D. M. Ruben *et al.*, The effects of aspirin, dipyridamole and warfarin in femorodistal reconstructions: long term results. *American Surgeon*, **58**(9) (1987), 477–81.
148. K. Ala Kulju, P. Ketonen, J. Salo *et al.*, Effect of antiplatelet and anticoagulant therapy on patency of femorotibial bypass grafts. *Journal of Cardiovascular Surgery*, **31** (1990), 651–5.
149. K. A. Bauer, Management of thrombophilia. *Journal of Thrombosis and Haemostasis*, **1**(7) (2003), 1429–34.
150. A. P. Basile, T. T. G. S. Fiala, Yaremchuk & J. W. May, The antithrombotic effects of ticlodipine and aspirin in a microvascular thrombogenic model. *Plastic and Reconstructive Surgery*, **95**(7) (1995), 1258–64.
151. Antiplatelet Trialists' Collaboration, Secondary prevention of vascular disease by prolonged antiplatelet treatment. *British Medical Journal*, **296** (1988), 320–31.
152. P. Robless, D. P. Mikhailidis & G. Stansby, Systematic review of antiplatelet therapy for the prevention of myocardial infarction, stroke or vascular death in patients with peripheral vascular disease. *British Journal of Surgery*, **88**(6) (2001), 787–800.
153. E. L. De Schryver, A. Algra, J. van Gijn, Dipyridamole for preventing stroke and other vascular events in patients with vascular disease. *Cochrane Database Systematic Reviews*, (1) (2003), CD001820.
154. E. L. De Schryver, A. Algra & J. van Gijn, Cochrane review: dipyridamole for preventing major vascular events in patients with vascular disease. *Stroke*, **34**(8) (2003), 2072–80.
155. D. A. Cunningham, B. Kumar, B. A. Siegel *et al.*, Aspirin inhibition of platelet deposition at angioplasty sites: demonstration by platelet scintigraphy. *Radiology*, **151** (1984), 487–90.
156. C. A. C. Clyne, R. F. McCloy & J. H. Baron, Gastric function in peripheral vascular disease. *British Medical Journal*, **1** (1979), 235.
157. M. R. Green, L. R. Roedersheimer & J. A. DeWeese, Effects of aspirin and dipyridamole on expanded polytetrafluroethylene graft patency. *Surgery*, **92**(6) (1982), 1016–26.
158. M. Goldman, C. Hall, J. Dykes, R. J. Hawkes & C. N. McCollum, Does indium platelet deposition predict

patency in prosthetic arterial grafts? *British Journal of Surgery*, **70** (1983), 635–8.

159. T. R. Kohler, J. L. Kaufman, G. Kacoyanis *et al.*, Effect of aspirin and dipyridamole on the patency of lower extremity bypass grafts. *Surgery*, **96** (1984), 462–6.
160. A. W. Clowes, The role of aspirin in enhancing arterial graft patency. *Journal of Vascular Surgery*, **3** (1986), 381–5.
161. B. Stein, V. Fuster, D. H. Israel *et al.*, Platelet inhibitor agents in cardiovascular disease: an update. *Journal of the American College of Cardiology*, **14** (1989), 813–36.
162. R. C. Kester, The thrombogenicity of dacron arterial grafts and its modification by platelet inhibitory drugs. *Annals of the Royal College of Surgeons of England*, **66** (1984), 241–6.
163. C. A. C. Clyne, T. J. Archer, L. K. Atuhaire, A. D. B. Chant & J. H. H. Webster, Random control trial of a short course of aspirin and dipyridamole (perstatin) for femorodistal grafts. *British Journal of Surgery*, **74**(4) (1987), 246–8.
164. C. McCollum, C. Alexander, G. Kenchington, P. J. Franks & R. Greenhalgh, Antiplatelet drugs in femoropopliteal vein bypasses: a multicenter trial. *Journal of Vascular Surgery*, **13** (1991), 150–62.
165. B. Satiani, A prospective randomised trial of aspirin in femoral popliteal and tibial bypass grafts. *Angiology*, **36** (1985), 608–16.
166. P. A. Howard, Aspirin resistance. *Annals of Pharmacotherapy*, **36**(10) (2002), 1620–4.
167. J. Dorffler-Melly, M. M. Koopman & D. J. Adam, Antiplatelet agents for preventing thrombosis after peripheral arterial bypass surgery. *Cochrane Database Systematic Reviews*, (3) (2003), CD000535.
168. B. Girolami, E. Bernardi, M. H. Prins *et al.*, Antiplatelet therapy and other interventions after revascularisation procedures in patients with peripheral arterial disease: a meta-analysis. *European Journal of Vascular and Endovascular Surgery*, **19**(4) (2000), 370–80.
169. B. S. Coller. A new murine monoclonal antibody reports an activation dependent change in the conformation and/or microenvironment of the glycoprotein IIb/IIIa complex. *Journal of Clinical Investigation*, **76** (1985), 101–8.
170. The EPIC Investigators. Use of a monoclonal antibody directed against the platelet glycoprotein IIb/IIIa receptor in high-risk coronary angioplasty. *New England Journal of Medicine*, **330** (1994), 956–61.
171. J. Leftovits, E. F. Plow & E. J. Topol, Platelet glycoprotein IIb/IIIa receptors in cardiovascular medicine. *New England Journal of Medicine*, **332**(4) (1995), 1553–9.
172. The IMPACT 11 Investigators, Effect of competitive platelet glycoprotein IIb/IIIa inhibition with intergilin in reducing complications of percutaneous coronary interventions: results of the randomised clinical trial IMPACT-11. *Lancet*, **349** (1997), 1422–8.
173. J. C. O'Shea & J. E. Tcheng, Eptifibatide: a potent inhibitor of the platelet receptor integrin glycoprotein IIb/IIIa. *Expert Opinion of Pharmacotherapy*, **3**(8) (2002), 1199–210.
174. J. Schweizer, W. Kirch, R. Koch *et al.*, Short- and long-term results of abciximab versus aspirin in conjunction with thrombolysis for patients with peripheral occlusive arterial disease and arterial thrombosis. *Angiology*, **51**(11) (2000), 913–23.
175. J. Schweizer, W. Kirch, R. Koch *et al.*, Use of abciximab and tirofiban in patients with peripheral arterial occlusive disease and arterial thrombosis. *Angiology*, **54**(2) (2003), 155–61.
176. Antiplatelet Trialists' Collaboration. Collaborative overview of randomised trials of antiplatelet therapy. 1. Prevention of death, myocardial infarction and stroke by prolonged antiplatelet therapy in various categories of patients. *British Medical of Journal*, **308** (1994), 81–106.
177. R. B. Haynes, R. S. Sandler, E. B. Larson, J. L. Pater & F. M. Yatsu, A critical appraisal of ticlopidine, a new antiplatelet agent. Effectiveness and clinical indications for prophylaxis of atherosclerotic events. *Archives of Internal Medicine*, **152** (1992), 1376–80.
178. CAPRIE Steering Committee. A randomised, blinded, trial of clopidogrel versus aspirin in patients at risk of ischaemic events (CAPRIE). *Lancet*, **348** (1996), 1329–39.
179. J. Blanchard, L. O. Carreras, M. Kindermans *et al.*, Results of EMATAP: a double-blind placebo-controlled multicentre trial of ticlopidine in patients with peripheral arterial disease. *Nouvelle Revue Francaise D'Hematologie*, **35** (1993), 523–8.
180. G. M. Andreozzi, S. S. Signorelli, G. Cacciaguerra *et al.*, Three-month therapy with calcium-heparin in comparison with ticlopidine in patients with peripheral arterial occlusive disease at Leriche-Fontaine IIb class. *Angiology*, **44**(4) (1993), 307–13.

181. K. J. Hansen, H. R. Howe, T. A. Edgerton *et al.*, Ticlodipine versus aspirin and dipyridamole: influence on platelet deposition and three month patency of polytetrafluroethylene grafts. *Journal of Vascular Surgery*, **4**(2) (1986), 174–8.
182. A. Nevelsteen, L. Mortelmans, A. Van de Cruys, E. Merckx & R. Verghaeghe, Effect of ticlodipine on blood loss, platelet turnover and platelet deposition on prosthetic surfaces in patients undergoing aortofemoral bypass grafting. *Thrombosis Research*, **64**(3) (1991), 633–9.
183. S. Shionoya & T. Sakurai, Influence de la ticlodipine sur les results de la chirurgie arterielle reconstructive peripherique; etude prospective multicentrique de 3 ans. *Sang, Thrombose, Vaiseaux*, **2**(Suppl) (1990), 12–16.
184. S. A. Doggrell, Pharmacotherapy of intermittent claudication. *Expert Opinion on Pharmacotherapy*, **2**(11) (2001), 1725–36.
185. J. Porter, B. Cutler & B. Lee, Pentoxifylline efficacy in the treatment of intermittent claudication: multicenter controlled double blind trial with objective assessment of chronic occlusive arterial disease patients. *American Heart Journal*, **104** (1982), 66–72.
186. K. Radack & R. J. Wyderski, Conservative management of intermittent claudication. *Annals of Internal Medicine*, **113** (1990), 135–146.
187. L. A. Harker, S. R. Hanson & A. B. Kelly, Antithrombotic benefits and hemorrhagic risks of direct thrombin antagonists. *Thrombosis and Haemostasis*, **74**(1) (1995), 464–72.
188. J. L. Chen, Argatroban: a direct thrombin inhibitor for heparin-induced thrombocytopenia and other clinical applications. *Heart Disease*, (3) (2001), 189–198.
189. K. L. Neuhaus, R. von Essen, U. Tebbe *et al.*, Safety observations for the pilot phase of the randomised r-hirudin for improvement of thrombolysis (HIT11) study. *Circulation*, **90** (1994), 1638–42.
190. Global use of strategies to open occluded coronary arteries (GUSTO IIa Investigators). Randomised trial of intravenous heparin versus recombinant hirudin for acute coronary syndromes. *Circulation*, **90** (1996), 1631–7.
191. A. M. Antman (for the TIMI 9A Investigators), Hirudin in acute myocardial infarction: safety report from the thrombolysis and thrombin inhibition in myocardial infarction (TIMI) 9A trial. *Circulation*, **90** (1994), 1624–30.
192. J. O'Donnell & D. J. Perry, Pharmacotherapy of hyperhomocysteinaemia in patients with thrombophilia. *Expert Opinion on Pharmacotherapy*, **3**(11) (2002), 1591–98.
193. E. G. Vermeulen, J. A. Rauwerda, P. Erix *et al.*, Normohomocysteinaemia and vitamin-treated hyperhomocysteinaemia are associated with similar risks of cardiovascular events in patients with premature atherothrombotic cerebrovascular disease. A prospective cohort study. *Netherlands Journal of Medicine*, **56**(4) (2000), 138–46.
194. M. H. Criqui, R. D. Langer, A. Fronek *et al.*, Mortality over a period of 10 years in patients with peripheral arterial disease. *New England Journal of Medicine*, **326** (1992), 381–6.
195. N. J. Wald & M. R. Law, A strategy to reduce cardiovascular disease by more than 80%. *British Medical Journal*, **326** (7404) (2003), 1419.

6 • The role of platelets in vascular disease

PAUL D. HAYES AND NATALIE J. HAYES

INTRODUCTION

Following an injury to the endothelial lining of a blood vessel, platelets are essential for targeting the coagulation cascade to the site of injury, amplifying the inflammatory response and providing the initial plug at the site of the defect in the vessel wall to limit blood loss. Consequently, they are a fundamental component of the haemostatic response to bleeding and injury, and defects in their function can give rise to a number of conditions usually characterized clinically by increased bleeding tendencies and abnormal haemostasis after injury.

However, pathological conditions also exist whereby platelet function is abnormally increased and this can lead to conditions associated with hypercoagulable states. In these cases, inappropriate intravascular platelet activation and aggregation causes occlusion of blood vessels, leading to ischaemia and organ damage.

In this chapter, basic platelet physiology in the normal circulation will be discussed, before a review of the more common disorders of platelet function. The role of platelets in vascular diseases and the use of antiplatelet agents will be considered, and finally the implications of this for vascular surgery will be outlined along with a review of the major clinical trials in this area

PLATELET PHYSIOLOGY

Large cells known as megakaryocytes are the precursors of platelets and are found primarily in the bone marrow, where they constitute around 0.5% of the cells. Mature megakaryocytes are large in size with abundant cytoplasm and numerous granules [1]. A characteristic feature of megakaryocytes is their ability to undergo endomitosis and divide into up to 64 portions, called proplatelets [2]. Megakaryocytopoiesis is regulated by multiple cytokines, most notably thrombopoietin [3], and it is thought that after synthesis, megakaryocytes are shed into the circulation and fragment into platelets in the pulmonary circulation. Another theory has suggested that platelets are shed gradually into the bloodstream from megakaryocytes lying adjacent to the vascular endothelium (Figure 6.1).

Platelets themselves are therefore not cells, but small disc-like subcellular fragments without nuclei that circulate in the blood and are an integral component of haemostasis. Under normal physiological conditions, their resting size and shape means that they are forced close to the endothelial cell wall by normal haemodynamic factors. Adhesion to the endothelium is prevented by high local concentrations of anti-thrombotic factors such as prostacyclin and nitric oxide, which are continuously released by endothelial cells lining the blood vessel.

Platelet activation

In the event of an endothelial injury, the platelets are exposed to the subendothelium which is highly thrombogenic and causes them to become activated extremely quickly. Adherence of the activated platelets to the endothelium at the site of injury is facilitated by von Willebrand factor (vWF). This is normally secreted into the subendothelium by endothelial cells and following an injury to the vessel wall, circulating vWF binds to extracellular collagen exposed by the defect in the endothelium. Platelet adherence to vWF occurs via a specific receptor interaction between glycoproptein receptors on the platelet surface (GpIβ receptors) and vWF bound to subendothelial collagen. Von Willebrand factor is multimeric, i.e. it has numerous binding sites, and this allows receptors on multiple platelets to bind to it, therefore increasing the amount of platelet aggregation arising from a single vWF molecule. The receptors on these activated and adherent platelets subsequently undergo a conformational change themselves that enables them to bind to both vWF and fibrin, which

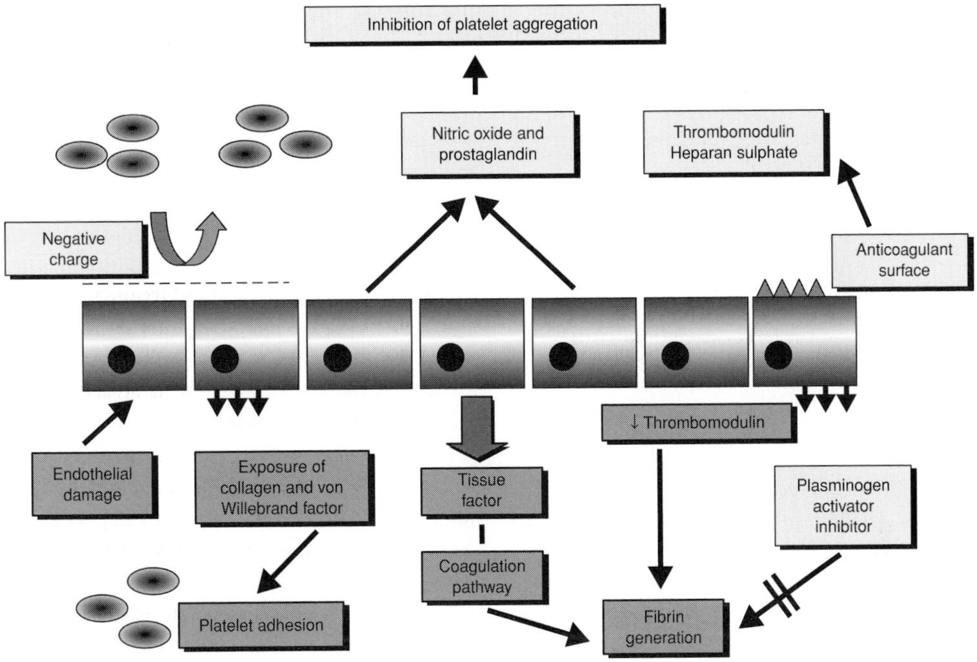

Fig. 6.1. Endothelial haemostatic function. Events shown in green denote anti-thrombotic activity. Those shown in red depict pro-thrombotic response to endothelial injury.

results in irreversible platelet aggregation and adherence to the endothelial defect [4].

Platelet activation is characterized by two important events which allow the platelets to effectively cover the damaged endothelial surface, help to plug bleeding points and assist in the recruitment of other inflammatory cells to the area.

(i) *Structural changes to the platelet shape*
The smooth biconcave disc is replaced by a spherical form, with numerous protruberant frond-like structures, or pseudopodia. These extensions from the platelet surface attach to other platelets, flatten out across the damaged endothelial surface and help to increase the stability of the newly forming plug over the defect.

(ii) *Secretion of pro-inflammatory factors*
Granules stored within the resting non-activated platelet contain numerous chemoattractant and pro-thrombotic factors, including growth factors, coagulation proteins, adhesion molecules, cytokines, angiogenic factors and inflammatory molecules. When the platelet becomes activated, these granules move to the platelet surface and release their contents into the local circulation, thus facilitating the recruitment of further platelets and inflammatory cells to the site of injury.

Three types of platelet granules have been identified to date, and these are referred to as **alpha granules, dense granules** and lysosomes [5]. The majority of platelet granules are of the alpha subtype, with the average platelet containing around 80 alpha granules [6]. They contain platelet-specific molecules that are synthesized exclusively by megakaryocytes, such as platelet factor-4 and beta thromboglobulin. They also contain coagulation factor V, thrombospondin, p-selectin (CD62P) and vWF, which are referred to as platelet selective molecules due to the fact that only a small number of cells besides platelets are able to synthesize them. In addition to these molecules, alpha granules also contain a number of non-platelet specific secretory proteins, including fibrinogen, and these are listed in Table 6.1

In contrast, the average platelet contains only around seven dense granules [7], and these contain important platelet activating molecules such as ADP, serotonin and nucleotides. These molecules are involved

Table 6.1. *Platelet granule contents*

Alpha granule contents	• P-selectin *(selective)* • Factor V *(selective)* • Platelet-derived growth factor (PDGF) *(not specific)* • Beta-thromboglobulin *(specific)* • Platelet factor 4 *(specific)* • VWF *(specific)* • Plasminogen activator inhibitor-1 *(selective)* • Thrombospondin (*not specific)* • Fibrinogen *(selective)* • Factor VIII (*not specific)* • Albumin (*not specific)* • IgG (*not specific)* • Transforming growth factor-β (*not specific)* • Epidermal growth factor (*not specific)* • Insulin-like growth factor (*not specific)* • Fibronectin (*not specific)* • Vascular endothelial growth factor (*not specific)*
Dense granule contents	• ATP • GTP • ADP • GDP • Calcium • Magnesium • Pyrophosphate • Serotonin

in the activation of resting circulating platelets, causing an amplification of the initial platelet response.

Lysosomes are present in the smallest numbers, with the majority of platelets containing only one or two [8]. They contain lysosomal membrane proteins and their exact role in platelet function has yet to be elucidated.

Platelet receptors

The ability of platelets to bind to each other as well as the endothelium is due to the presence of specific surface receptors, which are vital for their aggregatory and adhesive functions, and the expression of which determines the level of activity of the platelet. Because platelets have no nuclei and therefore cannot synthesize proteins according to requirement, additional receptor proteins are stored within granules inside the platelet and transported to its surface membrane when additional 'expression' is required. Despite their small size, platelets express a large range of receptors that include molecules involved in their haemostatic function such as the integrin receptor family and the fibrinogen receptor, as well as receptors for platelet agonists, including ADP, thrombin, collagen and thromboxane A2.

P-selectin is a member of the integrin family of platelet receptors and plays a vital role in platelet aggregation. Following activation of the platelet, it is expressed on the platelet surface in vastly increased numbers and provides an adhesion site for the attachment of a neighbouring platelet. In this way, it enables the formation of a mass of aggregated platelets, which then forms the basis of the platelet rich thrombus at the site of endothelial injury.

Following activation and aggregation, the ability of platelets to bind circulating fibrinogen to their surfaces is imperative for the formation and maintenance of a stable thrombus, and this heralds the final stage in its development. Fibrinogen binding occurs via the GPIIb-GPIIIa fibrinogen receptor and its expression is a reliable indicator of platelet activation. As the platelets are increasingly activated, so the amount of fibrinogen bound to the platelets' fibrinogen receptors also increases.

The actions of these two receptors underlie the major haemostastic functions of the platelet, and abnormalities in the structure or function of either can lead to a clinical syndrome of prolonged bleeding time, non-traumatic mucosal haemorrhage and florid ecchymoses.

PLATELET DISORDERS

Disorders of platelet structure and function can be acquired or congenital, and characteristically present with features of a haemostatic disorder. By this, they can be distinguished from a coagulation disorder primarily by history and examination. Disorders of haemostasis, including abnormalities of platelet function cause a distinct collection of symptoms and signs; petechiae and bruising is common, with epistaxes and menorrhagia

Table 6.2. *Causes of thrombocytopenia*

• *Increased platelet destruction*	Immune thrombocytopenic purpura (ITP) Disseminated intravascular coagulation (DIC) Drug-induced thrombocytopenia Systemic lupus erythematosus (SLE) Human Immunodeficiency virus (HIV) Haemolytic-uraemic syndrome (HUS) Massive blood transfusion
• *Decreased platelet production*	Giant platelet syndromes Hypersplenism and sequestration
• *Haemodilution*	Massive blood transfusion Extracorporeal perfusion

Table 6.3. *Causes of thrombocytosis*

• *Primary*	Essential thrombocythaemia Chronic myeloproliferative disorders, including polycythaemia rubra vera and myelofibrosis Chronic myeloid leukaemia Myelodysplastic syndrome
• *Secondary (reactive)*	Infection Post-chemotherapy Tissue damage, including surgery Chronic inflammation Malignancy Renal disease Haemolytic anaemia Iron deficiency Asplenia

also featuring prominently. Conversely, haemarthroses are rarely seen and intramuscular haematomas are uncommon. This is in direct contrast with coagulation abnormalities, which are characterized by spontaneous bleeds into joints and muscle compartments, but in which bruising and mucosal bleeding are infrequently seen.

Platelet disorders can be due to abnormal numbers of platelets (increased or decreased) or due to abnormal function (reduced function on overactivity). A comprehensive list of the well known disorders is given in Tables 6.2, 6.3 and 6.4, and the more common and clinically relevant platelet disorders are outlined below.

Autoimmune thrombocytopenic purpura (AITP)

This condition is characterized by a thrombocytopenia secondary to immune destruction of platelets, with the platelets becoming coated in antibody and then removed from the circulation by macrophages. It is defined clinically as a thrombocytopenia in the presence of a normal haemoglobin level, white blood cell count and differential, and in the absence of any underlying disease [9]. An acute form of the disease is usually seen in children and often follows a viral infection. The development of autoantibodies to platelets accounts for shortened platelet survival, and patients present with increased bruising and epistaxis, with major haemorrhage occurring extremely infrequently. Remission is usually spontaneous, with steroidal or immunoglobulin therapy required only in cases where the platelet count is $<20 \times 10^9/L$ and there is significant blood loss.

Chronic AITP is usually a disease of adult females and is frequently associated with other autoimmune disorders, including systemic lupus erythematosus (SLE) and thyroid disease, and with generalized immunodeficiency states such as human immunodeficiency virus (HIV) and malignancy. Platelet autoantibodies are usually present and this form of AITP rarely remits spontaneously. Treatment is aimed at reducing platelet autoantibody levels and usually comprises steroid therapy, with a reducing dose once remission has been achieved. Splenectomy can be useful for those patients who fail to respond to steroids, or in whom relapse occurs. Immunosuppressive agents such as azathioprine and cyclosporine are reserved for the small proportion of patients who demonstrate further relapse despite splenectomy.

Thrombotic thrombocytopenic purpura (TTP)

This is an uncommon condition, although its incidence is currently increasing. There is a characteristic

Table 6.4. *Causes of disorders of platelet function*

• *Acquired*	Uraemia	
	Myeloproliferative disorders	Essential thrombocythaemia
		Polycythaemia rubra vera
		Chronic myeloid leukaemia
	Acute leukaemias	
	Extracorporeal perfusion	
	Acquired von Willebrand's disease	
	Acquired storage pool deficiency	
	Antiplatelet antibody production	
	Liver disease	
	Drugs	
• *Inherited*	Platelet adhesion disorders	Von Willebrand's disease
	Agonist receptor deficiency	Collagen
		ADP
		Thromboxane A2
	Signalling pathway deficiencies	Phospholipase
		Cyclooxygenase
		Thromboxane
		Lipooxygenase
		Calcium
	Secretion deficiencies	Storage pool diseases
	Aggregation abnormalities	Glanzmann thrombasthenia
		Congenital afibrinogenaemia

pattern of symptoms and signs, including widespread purpura, pyrexia and fluctuating cerebral disturbance, often coupled with a haemolytic anaemia and red cell fragmentation that can lead to renal failure in severe cases. It is therefore a condition associated with substantial morbidity and not inconsequential mortality, in which unregulated platelet destruction results in a major thrombocytopenia, with disease severity directly related to the extent of microvascular platelet aggregation.

The aetiology of this condition is not fully understood, but it is thought that a genetic abnormality in the protease responsible for the degradation of von Willebrand's factor (vWF) renders it inactive. This allows large numbers of vWF molecules to accumulate, causing damage to the endothelium [10]. Platelet aggregation and adherence to the vessel walls then occurs, resulting in spontaneous vessel thrombosis and large-scale platelet consumption and a relative thrombocytopenia.

It is associated with pregnancy, SLE [11], viral and bacterial infections including HIV [12; 13; 14], and oral contraceptive use, although in many cases no cause is identified. Treatment is aimed at restoring normal levels of vWF by the use of plasma exchange and fresh frozen plasma (FFP) administration to replace the missing vWF protease.

Von Willebrand's disease (vWD)

Although not strictly a disease of platelets per se, this condition adversely affects platelet function and so is often considered in this group of haematological disorders. It arises as a result of mutations of the vWF gene on chromosome 12 and can be categorized into three clinical types. Type 1 is inherited as an autosomal condition and results in only a mild reduction in the amount of functional vWF. Type 2 is also inherited as an autosomal dominant condition and is characterized by the presence of abnormal vWF multimers with defective function. Type 3 is autosomal recessive and patients with this subtype of the disease have virtually no normal circulating vWF.

The clinical effects of types 1 and 2 are often mild, with patients experiencing frequent episodes of epistaxis and menorrhagia, but have no catastrophic bleeding tendencies. In contrast, patients with type 3 disease are prone to more significant bleeding, although this is rarely as severe as that seen in haemophilia sufferers. Characteristic laboratory findings occur, with a prolonged bleeding time but normal prothrombin time, and vWF levels are reduced to as little as 5% of normal values in type 3 disease.

Von Willebrand's factor is also necessary for the stabilization of factor VIII:C in plasma. Consequently, a reduced level of vWF is associated with decreased levels of functional factor VIII:C and this can be measured to assist in the diagnosis of vWD.

Treatment varies according to the severity of the disease and is aimed at increasing the amount of functional circulating factor VIII by the use of desmopressin acetate (DDAVP) or factor VIII concentrates. Von Willebrand's factor concentrates are reserved for bleeding patients, or those undergoing surgery.

Disseminated intravascular coagulation (DIC)

This potentially life-threatening condition is characterized by an inappropriate, spontaneous and sustained intravascular activation of the coagulation cascade. Its causes are numerous but all result in the release of prothrombotic material into the circulation, which results in extensive fibrin production and platelet aggregation within the vasculature. The resultant consumption of platelets and clotting factors leads to an increased bleeding tendency and haemorrhage, paradoxically coupled with widespread vessel thrombosis and tissue infarction. Common causes include malignancy, sepsis, haemolytic transfusion reactions, trauma, burns, amniotic fluid embolism and placental abruption, and the likely source is usually evident from the history and examination.

Clinically, a spectrum of disease exists from no bleeding abnormality to a severely ill patient with haemodynamic compromise and extensive haemorrhage. Bleeding is often from the mucosal membranes, and vessel occlusion by platelet aggregates and fibrin characteristically causes focal infarction in the microvasculature of the skin, kidneys and cerebral tissue.

Prothrombin time, activated partial thromboplastin time and thrombin time are all increased in these patients, and high levels of fibrin degradation products are found, owing to extensive fibrinolytic activity in response to abnormally high levels of fibrin in the circulation. A severe thrombocytopenia is seen as a result of excessive platelet consumption and this contributes to the increased bleeding tendency seen with this condition.

Treatment is targeted towards resolution of the causative pathology and often no further specific measures are required. Supportive therapy is often the mainstay of treatment in DIC, with the restoration and maintenance of normovolaemia and adequate tissue perfusion being paramount. If bleeding is excessive and sustained, platelet concentrates, red cell transfusions, fresh-frozen plasma and cryoprecipitate can be used to correct the consumption coagulopathy.

Thrombocytosis and essential thrombocythaemia

Thrombocytosis is defined as a platelet count greater than $500 \times 10^9/L$ [15; 16]. It may occur as the result of a clonal abnormality of production, referred to as primary thrombocytosis, or may be secondary to an underlying disease process such as infection, malignancy, chronic inflammation or tissue damage. In these cases, it is classified as a secondary or reactive thrombocytosis.

Reactive thrombocytosis is more common than primary thrombocytosis in both adults and children [17; 18] and is thought to be cytokine-mediated, rather than due to clonal proliferation of megakaryocytes [19; 20; 21]. It is thought that a systemic acute phase reaction to the causative disease process leads to an excess of thrombopoietic growth factors that stimulate excessive platelet production. Factors implicated to date include interleukin-1, -4, and -6, and tumour necrosis factor-α [20; 21; 22; 23]. Clinical manifestations of a raised platelet count such as vasomotor disturbances, bleeding and thrombosis, are less common when due to a reactive cause rather than primary thrombocytosis, although the reasons for this remain unclear at present [24; 25; 26; 27; 28; 29]. Consequently, there is rarely a specific indication for the use of antiplatelet therapies in the vast majority of patients with reactive thrombocytosis and the platelet count usually falls to within normal limits upon treatment of the underlying cause [18; 30; 31].

Primary thrombocytosis is due to an abnormal clonal proliferation of megakaryocytes leading to an elevated platelet count and is classified as a myeloproliferative disorder [32; 33]. The commonest cause is referred to as essential thrombocytosis and is defined as a persistent elevation in platelet count which is not reactive nor associated with other myeloproliferative disorders, such as chronic myeloid leukaemia, polycythaemia rubra vera or myelodysplastic syndrome [24]. Patients often present with a persistent and isolated thrombocytosis in the absence of any causative disease. Most patients are completely free of symptoms at diagnosis, although some may complain of atypical chest pain, headaches and visual disturbances suggestive of vasomotor dysfunction [34; 35; 36]. Bleeding and thrombosis occur in around 5% and 20% of patients, respectively, with the most common complication being transformation into acute leukaemia. This occurs in around 5% of patients at ten years from diagnosis [34; 35; 36; 37].

Treatment is aimed at limiting the haemorrhagic and thrombotic complications of the disorder by the use of antiplatelet agents such as aspirin, and platelet-reducing compounds including hydroxyurea depending on the incidence of these events in each patient. In addition to managing these specific sequelae, surveillance for leukaemic transformation is also important in the long term management of this condition.

Defects of platelet adhesion

A vast number of inherited disorders of platelet adhesion have been described, most of which are due to an abnormality of a platelet surface receptor protein. The effect of this is that affected patients have platelets with defective adhesive and aggregatory properties that manifest clinically as an increased bleeding tendency, frequent non-traumatic mucosal bleeds and excessive bruising. Abnormalities of almost all platelet receptors and intracellular metabolic pathways have been described, and most of these are extremely rare. Although consideration of all of these conditions is beyond the scope of this chapter, two of the most clinically relevant and commoner conditions are outlined below.

Bernard–Soulier syndrome is an autosomal recessive disorder that arises from a defect in a family of glycoprotein receptors expressed on the platelet surface. This group of molecules, referred to as the GP I complex is implicated in normal platelet adhesivity and aggregation, and this is evidenced by the fact that patients with this condition have a prolonged bleeding time, and structurally abnormal platelets that are unable to aggregate in response to platelet agonists [38; 39].

Glanzmann thrombasthenia is also an autosomal recessive condition in which there is a mutation of the integrin gene. The integrin molecule, or GP IIb/IIIa receptor is vital for normal platelet–platelet aggregation, and the absence of normal aggregation in response to platelet agonists such as adenosine diphosphate (ADP) and collagen is a characteristic feature of this disease. The classical symptoms of platelet dysfunction are present, with purpura, epistaxis and menorrhagia exhibited by almost all patients with this condition. Bleeding from the gastrointestinal tract and spontaneous haemarthroses are rare [38].

THE ROLE OF PLATELETS IN VASCULAR DISEASE

Arterial thrombosis and atherosclerosis

Platelets in plaque development and thrombus generation

In the course of atherogenesis, lipid enters the vessel wall through damaged endothelial cells to produce a fatty streak [40; 41]. The resulting gaps between endothelial cells also expose the subendothelium to the circulation, or the endothelial cells can detach, leaving an exposed site to which platelets can adhere. In addition, these dysfunctional endothelial cells lose their anti-thrombotic properties and instead become pro-thrombotic with increased adhesiveness for platelets and white blood cells [42]. This creates thrombogenic sites around the fatty streak and promotes platelet aggregation and adherence to the vessel wall. Primarily, this again involves the attachment of vWF to the endothelial defect, and platelet activation then occurs in the same manner as in response to vessel injury by any other means. Von Willebrand factor release is increased in areas of disturbed blood flow and high flow rates, and this would help to explain why platelet aggregation to plaques increases as the plaque grows and affects normal laminar flow in the vessel.

As lipid accumulation progresses and the plaque increases in size, it becomes less stable and more prone to rupture. Significantly more platelet deposition occurs on plaques with high lipid content and this enhances the thrombogenic potential of the plaque. Activated platelets adherent to the plaque attract pro-thrombotic inflammatory cells and more platelets, which in turn are activated and adhere to the growing plaque. [43; 44; 45; 46; 47; 48]. In this way, platelets are directly involved in initiating and maintaining plaque propagation and disease progression.

Ischaemic cerebrovascular disease

Stroke

The disruption of a carotid plaque is a major cause of ischaemic stroke and may cause this in one of two ways; namely, secondary to embolic occlusion from either the plaque or resulting thrombus, or by thrombotic occlusion of the internal carotid artery with a failure of the collateral blood supply to adequately support the metabolic needs of the dependent cerebral tissue.

Currently, the most common cause of stroke is embolic and secondary to the dislodging of platelet microthrombi from the disrupted atheromatous plaque [49; 50]. In this case, this collection of activated and aggregating platelets occludes an end artery causing distal ischaemia, and, in addition, provides a prothrombotic surface for the propagation of a new thrombus at the site of occlusion.

Evidence is emerging to suggest that patients with large ischaemic strokes have platelets with an increased tendency to become activated and aggregate, and that these abnormally sensitive platelets are probably involved in the pathogenesis of this condition [51; 52]. This may explain the diversity in clinical manifestations of carotid atheromatous disease, and why some patients progress from transient ischaemic attack (TIA) to stroke more readily that others.

Peripheral vascular disease

The involvement of platelets in occlusive peripheral arterial disease [53; 54] is suggested by their presence in the causative arterial thrombi, atherosclerotic plaques, and the fact that they are known to be instrumental in the development of restenosis after surgical and percutaneous revascularization procedures [41; 55]. In addition, a number of studies have demonstrated increased levels of circulating resting and activated platelets in patients with peripheral vascular disease when compared with healthy volunteers without vascular pathology [56; 57].

Diabetes mellitus

Vascular disease is the cause of death in the majority of patients with diabetes mellitus and this also accounts for a substantial proportion of the morbidity associated with the disease [58]. In addition to pathology of larger vessels including the coronary and cerebral vessels, diabetic patients also exhibit a characteristic pattern of occlusive vascular disease that has a predilection for the microvasculature of the limbs, digits and retina.

Platelet emboli derived from atherosclerotic lesions cause microvascular occlusion and multiple areas of distal ischaemia, leading to tissue loss and infection. Platelets in these patients also exhibit an increased sensitivity to thrombogenic stimuli, and are therefore prone to inappropriate intravascular activation and aggregation [59]. This is thought to be due to the inherent metabolic disturbances arising as a result of this disease and can be partly reduced by fastidious glycaemic control. This in part explains the dramatic reduction in diabetic complications seen with adequate and sustained metabolic control.

Hypercoagulability secondary to increased platelet responsiveness occurs in both type I and type II diabetic disease, and this would support the assumption that metabolic disturbances underlie the abnormal interactions between platelets and the microvasculature that cause the organ damage seen in both sub-groups of patients [60]. This fact may also explain the observation that diabetic patients often obtain poor results from revascularization procedures such as angioplasty, exhibiting much higher rates of restenosis than those patients with normoglycaemia.

ANTIPLATELET AGENTS AND THEIR USE IN VASCULAR DISEASE

Aspirin

Acetylsalicylic acid, or aspirin, is the synthetic acetic acid ester of salicylic acid and has anti-inflammatory, antipyretic, analgesic, and antiplatelet properties. Since its introduction into the pharmaceutical arena in the late 1890s, it has become one of the most widely used therapeutic agents ever marketed, and its ability to inhibit platelet activity has made it a vital weapon in the armoury against cardiovascular disease and its complications.

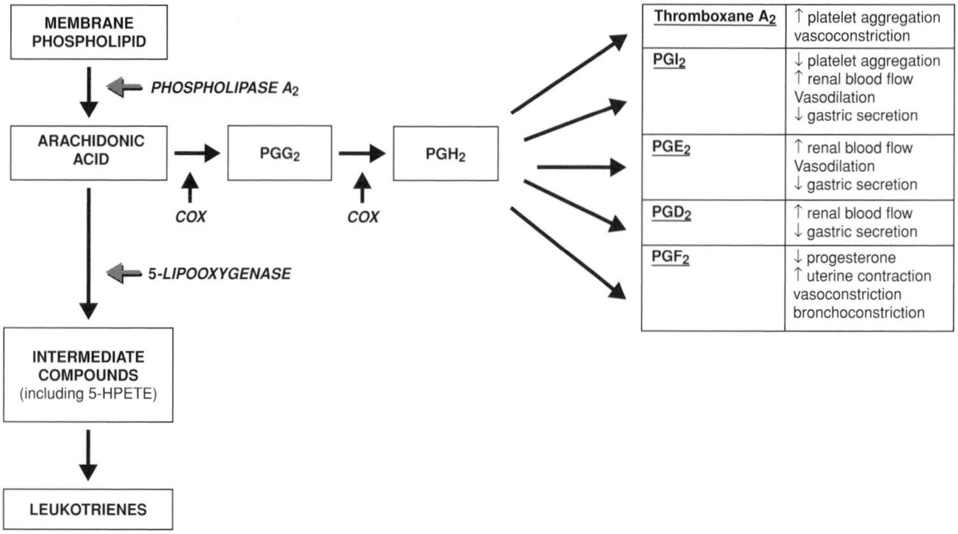

Fig. 6.2. Leukotriene and prostaglandin synthesis via the lipo-oxygenase and cyclo-oxygenase pathways.

Mechanism of action

Aspirin exerts the majority of its pharmaceutical effects by disrupting prostaglandin synthesis. In this pathway, arachidonic acid is synthesized from membrane phospholipids by phospholipase A_2 and can then take one of two metabolic routes. In the lipooxygenase pathway, 12-lipo-oxygenase, converts arachidonic acid to a number of intermediate compounds that are ultimately metabolized to form a family of leukotrienes. In the cyclo-oxygenase pathway (COX), cyclo-oxygenase (also known as prostaglandin H synthase) converts arachidonic acid to prostaglandin G_2, which is then further metabolized to form thromboxane A2 and the prostaglandin family of molecules (I_2, E_2, D_2, $F_{2\alpha}$). These synthetic pathways are illustrated in Figure 6.2.

Two isoforms of the COX enzyme have been identified, namely, COX-1 and COX-2. COX-1 is a constitutive enzyme that is expressed by all cells and facilitates the production of the prostaglandins that are involved in physiological cellular functions. For example, COX-1 mediated prostaglandin synthesis is implicated in gastric mucosal protection, maintenance of normal renal blood flow, and platelet activation and aggregation. In contrast, COX-2 is not a constitutive enzyme, but is produced in response to inflammatory stimuli such as cytokines and growth factors, and facilitates the synthesis of the prostaglandins that mediate the inflammatory response.

Aspirin blocks prostaglandin synthesis by irreversible acetylation of the cyclo-oxygenase enzymes resulting in a conformational alteration that prevents the binding of arachidonic acid and conversion to prostaglandin H_2. This molecule is an essential precursor for prostaglandin synthesis. In this way, aspirin is able to block the actions of both COX isoforms, although its inhibitory effect on COX-1 has been shown to be over 150 times greater than on COX-2.

The antiplatelet activity of aspirin is due to inhibition of the COX-1 isoform, which leads to a reduction in thromboxane A2 production via the cyclo-oxygenase pathyway. Thromboxane A2 is a powerful platelet agonist and aspirin therapy effectively blocks this route of platelet activation. Conversely, inhibition of COX-2 does not prevent platelet thromboxane production, and so results in no antiplatelet action and is therefore of little benefit in the treatment of vascular disease.

Aspirin use in the treatment of cardiovascular disease

The use of aspirin in the treatment of cardiovascular disease is primarily due to its antiplatelet, and anti-thrombotic actions. As previously discussed, platelet activation occurs in response to a number of pro-thrombotic and inflammatory stimuli including exposure to collagen, ADP, fibrinogen and thrombin. This results in a morphological change in the platelet and the release of further inflammatory material including thromboxane A2. which is synthesized by the activated platelet itself. This is in turn a powerful agonist of non-activated circulating platelets and assists in amplifying the overall platelet response. It can be seen from this that by inhibiting the ability of the platelet to produce thromboxane, platelet aggregation can be limited. If the pathogenesis of atherosclerotic disease and its thrombo-embolic sequelae are considered, the potential benefits of antiplatelet activity are clear.

As a result of numerous large-scale, multicentre clinical trials, aspirin now has an established role in both the prevention of cardiovascular disease and in the management of acute thrombotic events. Long term aspirin administration has been proven to decrease the incidence of recurrent myocardial infarction, and its use in the acute setting has been proven by the findings of the Second International Study of Infarct Survival (ISIS-2) trial. This showed that aspirin use in acute myocardial infarction was associated with a reduced mortality at five weeks post-event, and a significantly lower rate of early reinfarction and non-fatal stroke [61]. In addition to this, aspirin use in these settings was not associated with an increased risk of bleeding or haemorrhagic stroke.

Cerebrovascular and carotid artery disease
Early studies of the effect of aspirin use in the prevention of further cerebrovascular events in patients with previous stroke and TIA were not conclusive and yielded conflicting results [62; 63; 64]. However, a review of 145 such studies by the Antiplatelet Trialist Group found that the use of aspirin in patients with a prior episode of stroke or TIA resulted in a highly significant reduction in further non-fatal stroke and a similarly significant reduction in mortality from all causes. There was also a significant decrease in the incidence of all vascular events, including acute myocardial infarction [65]. These findings were applicable to both patients with completed strokes and those patients with previous TIA only. It is likely that by inhibiting platelet activation and aggregation, aspirin is able to limit the extension of thrombi in the cerebral and extracranial vessels and reduce the rate of propagation of embolic material arising from these lesions.

In addition to this, substantial work has been directed at reducing the post-operative thrombo-embolic complications of carotid endarterectomy surgery for the treatment of carotid atherosclerotic disease. Aspirin has been conclusively shown to decrease the incidence of post-operative stroke, acute myocardial infarction and death from vascular causes in patients undergoing this procedure [66].

In light of these findings, aspirin is established as playing a vital role in both secondary prevention of cerebrovascular disease, and in the prevention of postoperative complications following carotid artery surgery. However, in contrast to coronary artery disease, there is no proven indication for the use of aspirin in the primary prevention of cerebral ischaemia at present [65].

Aspirin use after revascularization procedures
Percutaneous revascularization of occluded vessels is associated with a certain degree of vascular endothelial trauma that is largely unavoidable. This inevitably results in local platelet aggregation and activation, which left unchecked, can progress to acute and sub-acute thrombosis of the affected vessel in up to 6% of cases [67]. Aspirin has been used alongside other antiplatelet agents including dipyridamole and clopidogrel to significantly reduce the incidence of this complication [68], although this effect is not as dramatic when aspirin is used alone [69].

Aspirin has also been proven to reduce the rates of thrombosis and restenosis in surgical revascularization procedure [70]. Again, localized vascular injury and endothelial disruption at the anastamotic site predispose the vessel to platelet aggregation and further thrombosis formation. In coronary artery bypass grafting, the use of aspirin has significantly reduced the rate of thrombotic graft occlusion and its use pre-operatively is associated with decreased in-patient mortality rates.

Dipyridamole

Dipyridamole has been available for a number of years, yet only a limited amount of information is known about its mode of action. It was initially marketed as a coronary vasodilator in the 1960s but was also found to inhibit adenosine uptake, which reduced platelet aggregation and inhibition. These findings led to its use as an antithrombotic and antiplatelet agent and a renewed interest in its mechanism of action.

A number of theories have suggested that dipyridamole exerts its effect via a number of actions on the vessel wall as well as the platelet population:

Anti-thrombotic action on vessel walls
Dipyridamole causes increased levels of prostacyclin release by the vessel wall. This directly inhibits platelet aggregation and adhesion to the endothelium and prevents thrombus formation.

Elevation of platelet camp and guanosine monophosphate (GMP) levels
This occurs secondary to inhibition of phosphodiesterases by dipyridamole, which potentiates the vasodilatory effects of nitric oxide on the endothelium and further inhibits platelet activation, aggregation and adhesion.

Inhibition of cellular uptake of adenosine
As previously discussed, by inhibiting adenosine uptake and metabolism, platelet aggregation is further inhibited by dipyridamole.

Inhibition of smooth muscle proliferation
This directly inhibits restenosis of revascularized vessels.

At present, it is not thought that dipyridamole use is superior to aspirin in the primary and secondary prevention of major vascular events. However, the European Stroke Prevention Study-2, demonstrated that combined use of these agents is more effective than aspirin alone in the secondary prevention of cerebrovascular disease. It was noted that co-administration of aspirin and dipyridamole reduced the recurrence of stroke by 37% compared with reductions of 18% and 16%, respectively, when these agents were used alone [71].

Ticlopidine and clopidogrel

Ticlopidine and its more recently developed analogue clopidogrel, are thienopyridine derivatives that are known to inhibit platelet function. Both agents can be administered orally and require post-digestion modification to the active metabolite form. Ticlopidine and clopidogrel both act by inhibiting the binding of ADP to its platelet receptor [11] and this ADP receptor blockade leads to direct inhibition of fibrinogen binding to its GP IIb/IIIa receptor to cause platelet aggregation [72]. Evidence also exists to suggest that ticlopidine can interfere with the platelet–vWF interaction, resulting in a decreased tendency to thrombosis [73].

Two types of ADP receptor exist on the platelet surface, with one exhibiting low affinity and one possessing high affinity for ADP. The low affinity site is G protein coupled and causes the release of intracellular calcium stores when activated. This results in a conformational change and subsequent activation of the glycoprotein GP IIb/IIIa, or fibrinogen receptor. Both ticlopidine and clopidogrel inhibit this site, which leads to a reduction in platelet aggregation and thrombus formation

Both drugs require administration for between three and four days to reach maximal effect, and appear to irreversibly inhibit platelet function over the subsequent seven days.

Three major trials have demonstrated a small but significant benefit in the reduction of vascular events after the administration of ticlodipine and clopidogrel. The largest of these was the CAPRIE study (Clopidogrel versus Aspirin in Patients at Risk of Ischaemic Events) [74], which assigned over 19 000 patients to treatment with either clopidogrel or 325 mg of aspirin. The mean follow-up period was 1.9 years, and an overall relative reduction in major vascular events of 8.7% was revealed. Sub-group analysis demonstrated that clopidogrel conferred no benefit over aspirin in the prevention of either stroke or myocardial infarction. The sole group to benefit from clopidogrel administration were those patients with severe peripheral vascular disease. Two further smaller studies have shown a small reduction in the risk of cerebral ischaemia following ticlopidine administration [43].

Inhibitors of platelet-fibrinogen binding

Following initial platelet activation through its binding to subendothelial vWF, there is a rapid up-regulation in the number of fibrinogen receptors (GP IIb/IIIa) expressed on the platelet surface, to a figure of approximately 50 000 per platelet. Fibrinogen has active sites for platelet binding at both ends of its structure, which enables it to cross-link platelets and therefore form large platelet aggregates as the basis for thrombus formation. This is the final common pathway by which most forms of stimulation cause platelet aggregation.

The active sites within the fibrinogen molecule contain a specific arginine-glycine-aspartic acid sequence, referred to as the RGD sequence. The RGD sequence is also found on other adhesive proteins including vWF, and, therefore, inhibition of binding to this sequence should exert a profound effect upon platelet ability to form a thrombus.

The first group of compounds found to act at this site were peptides retrieved from monoclonal antibodies targeted against the active site and include 7E3 or Reopro [75]. These agents now have a proven role in the prevention of coronary thrombosis and restenosis following angioplasty, although there currently exists little evidence of their role in stroke prevention. However, as coronary angioplasty provides a similar environment to carotid endarterectomy in that there is significant localized damage to the endothelium, it follows that Reopro may also be useful in the prevention of thrombotic complications and restenosis in patients who have undergone carotid endarterectomy.

Dextran polymers

The dextran molecule consists of a long chain of polysaccharide moieties produced by the organism *Leuconstoc mesenteroides*. It was first used in 1944 as a plasma expander and initial reports of its ability to induce a bleeding tendency in patients did not emerge until the 1960s.

Although dextrans have been in use in clinical practice for many years, the mechanism behind their effect on bleeding time and platelet function has yet to be fully established. The infusion of between 500 and 1000 ml of dextran into healthy volunteers and patients undergoing minor surgical procedures is known to induce a significant reduction in platelet aggregating ability in response to collagen, but the effect of dextran on bleeding time is variable. Dextran sulphate binds clotting factor VIII and the loss of this factor from circulating plasma is associated with a decrease in aggregation in response to platelet agonists. Dextran is also known to inhibit the function of platelet factor-3, can reduce plasma concentrations of antithrombin-III in the post-operative period and can cause an increase in thrombus fragility.

Most of the clinical studies using dextran have focused on its ability to reduce the incidence of post-operative deep venous thrombosis (DVT). The first clinical study of this effect reported that the incidence of postoperative DVT was reduced from 21% to 4% in patients who received dextran when compared to those patients who did not. This conclusion has now been reproduced in as many as 28 other studies.

The findings of studies that have investigated the prevention of arterial occlusions by dextrans have been less convincing; a recent clinical study of autogenous infrainguinal grafting in patients with peripheral vascular disease failed to demonstrate any benefit in dextran administration in terms of graft patency in the short term or in the long term [76].

Conversely, a number of studies have demonstrated that small volumes of dextran-40 can reduce the number of post-operative carotid thromboses seen following CEA and indeed a decrease in embolization rates from the endarterectomized vessel can be seen after a peripheral infusion of only 20–30 ml of dextran-40 [77; 78; 79]. However, the exact mechanisms that underlie this dramatic effect have yet to be elucidated and are the subject of ongoing trials.

Cilostazol

Cilostazol was first marketed in Japan for the treatment of symptoms due to ischaemia in chronic arterial occlusive disease, and is now licensed for use in intermittent claudication in Asia and the USA. It exerts an antiplatelet effect by its selective inhibition of the phosphodiesterase (PDE)3 family of intracellular isoenzymes [80], which are important in the regulation of intracellular cyclic adenosine monophosphate (cAMP) and cyclic guanosine monophosphate (cGMP). These molecules act as second messengers in intracellular transduction and assist in the control of numerous cellular functions in many cell populations, including platelets. Inhibition of PDE3 in human platelets increases their cAMP content, causing a reduction in intracellular calcium concentrations. This results in inhibition of platelet aggregation and activation in response to platelet agonists including thrombin, ADP and collagen [80]. By this mechanism, cilostazol can inhibit both primary platelet aggregation, and secondary aggregation induced by platelet-synthesized ADP. In this respect, it differs from aspirin, which inhibits secondary aggregation only.

In addition to its inhibitory effect on platelet aggregation, cilostazol has also been shown to reduce thromboxane production, platelet factor-4 release and platelet-derived growth factor release by inhibiting platelet activation [81]. Evidence also exists to suggest that cilostazol has vasodilatory properties [82] and can inhibit proliferation of vascular smooth muscle cells [83].

Perhaps unsurprisingly, given its antiplatelet and anti-thrombotic activity, cilostazol has been shown to be of use in a number of thrombo-embolic and occlusive vascular scenarios. The Cilostazol Stroke Prevention Study (CSPS) found that the administration of cilostazol post cerebral infarction was associated with significantly lower rates of reinfarction within the first five years [84]. In addition, seven large-scale trials conducted in the USA concluded that cilostazol conferred a significant benefit to patients with chronic lower limb ischaemia and intermittent claudication. When compared with placebo, the absolute claudication distance, or distance walked prior to disabling symptoms was significantly prolonged in patients taking cilostazol [85]. Furthermore, unlike aspirin and ticlodipine, cilostazol has been proven to prevent restenosis following revascularization by percutaneous transluminal coronary angioplasty (PTCA) or stent insertion [83].

CONCLUSIONS

Since platelets adhere to sites of endothelial damage it is unsurprising that platelets can be found adhering to angioplasty and endarterectomy sites, and to vascular grafts inserted into the arterial circulation. Indeed, even the small amount of suture that is exposed to the lumen of an arterial anastomosis acts as a stimulus to platelet adherence [86]. As well as platelets adhering to the endarterectomy zone of a carotid end (CEA) they adhere to the patch angioplasty, regardless of whether the patch is made of autologous vein, dacron or polytetrafluoroethylene (PTFE) [87]. Application of arterial clamps also leads to platelet deposition very shortly after flow restoration [88]. Laboratory analysis of vascular grafts that had subsequently failed demonstrated the presence of a platelet rich thrombus as the cause of the failure in the majority of cases.

It is now clear that platelets play a major role not only in the pathogenesis of thrombo-embolic vascular disease itself, but also in the development of post-procedural complications following surgical and percutaneous revascularization. The ever-expanding body of evidence confirming the beneficial effects of antiplatelet agent use in the management of these problems provides a powerful weapon in the battle against these debilitating and often life-threatening conditions. Advancements in our understanding of platelet physiology coupled with the development of new antiplatelet agents with novel therapeutic targets suggest that this mode of therapy will continue to play an important role in the treatment of a disease process that continues to pose one of the greatest threats to global health in modern times.

REFERENCES

1. M. B. Zucker, E. G. Puszkin, I. Sussman & E. A. Mauss, Inhibition of vWF platelet agglutination by ADP. *Journal of Laboratory and Clinical Medicine*, **116** (1990), 305–14.
2. J. M. Paulus, DNA metabolism and development of organelles in guinea pig megakaryocytes. *Blood*, **35** (1970), 298–311.
3. E. S. Choi, J. C. Nichol, M. M. Hokom, A. C. Hornkohl & P. Hunt, Platelets generated *in vitro* from proplatelet-displaying human megakaryocytes are functional. *Blood*, **15** (1995), 402–13.
4. K. S. Sakariassen, Role of platelet membrane glycoproteins and von Willebrand factor in adhesion of platelets to subendothelium and collagen. *Annals of the New York Academy of Science*, **516** (1987), 52–65.
5. J. L. Costa & D. L. Murphy, Platelet 5-HT uptake and release is stopped rapidly by formaldehyde. *Nature*, **255** (1975), 407–8.
6. J. J. Sixma, J. W. Slot & H. J. Geuze, Immunocytochemical localization of platelet granule proteins. *Methods in Enzymology*, **169** (1989), 301–11.
7. J. L. Costa, T. S. Reese & D. L. Murphy, Serotonin storage in platelets: estimation of storage-packet size. *Science*, **183** (1974), 537–8.
8. M. Menard, K. M. Meyers & D. J. Prieur, Demonstration of secondary lysosomes in bovine megakaryocytes and platelets using acid phosphatase chemistry with cerium as a trapping agent. *Thrombosis and Haemostasis*, **63** (1990), 127–32.
9. J. N. George, S. H. Woolf, E. Raskob, *et al.*, Idiopathic thrombocytopenic purpura: the recommendations of the American Society of Haematology. *Blood*, **88** (1996), 3–40.
10. Y. Asada, A. Sumiyoshi, T. Hayashi, J. Suzumiya & K. Kaketani, Immunochemistry of vascular lesions in thrombotic thrombocytopenic purpura, with special reference to factor VIII related antigen. *Thrombosis Research*, **38** (1985), 469–79.

11. G. Nesher, V. E. Hanna, T. L. Moore, M. Hersh & T. G. Osborn, Thrombotic microangiopathic haemolytic anaemia in systemic lupus erythematosus. *Seminars in Arthritis and Rheumatology*, **24** (1994), 172–5.
12. L. S. Yospur, N. C. Sun, P. Figueroa & Y. Niihara, Concurrent thrombotic thrombocytopenic purpura and immune thrombocytopenic purpura in an HIV-positive patient. *American Journal of Haematology*, **51** (1996), 73–8.
13. A. N. Leaf, L. J. Laubenstein, B. Raphael *et al.*, Thrombotic thrombocytopenic purpura associated with immunodeficiency virus type 1 (HIV-1) infection. *Annals of Internal Medicine*, **109** (1988), 194–7.
14. J. Nair, R. Bellevue, M. Bertoni & H. Dosik, Thrombotic thrombocytopenic purpura in patients with the acquired immunodeficiency syndrome (AIDS)-related complex. *Annals of Internal Medicine*, **109** (1988), 209–12.
15. S. Sacchi, G. Vinci & L. Gugliotta, Diagnosis of essential thrombocythaemia at platelet counts between 400 and 600×10^9/L. *Haematologica*, **85** (2000), 492–5.
16. E. Lengfelder, A. Hochhaus & U. Kronawitter, Should a platelet limit of 600×10^9/L be used as a diagnostic criterion in essential thrombocythaemia? An analysis of the natural course including early stages. *British Journal of Haematology*, **100** (1998), 15–23.
17. M. D. Yohannan, K. E. Higgy, S. A. al-Mashhadani & C. R. Santhosh-Kumar, Thrombocytosis. Aetiological analysis of 663 patients. *Clinical Paediatrics*, **33** (1994), 340–3.
18. H. L. Chen, S. S. Chiou, J. M. Sheen *et al.*, Thrombocytosis in children at one medical centre of souhern Taiwan. *Acta Paediatrica Taiwan*, **40** (1994), 309–13.
19. C. W. Hollen, J. Henthorn, J. Koziol & S. Burstein, Elevated serum interleukin-6 levels in patients with reactive thrombocytosis. *British Journal of Haematology*, **79** (1991), 286–90.
20. I. Haznedaroglu, I. Ertenli & O. I. Ozcebe, Megakaryocyte-related interleukins in reactive thrombocytosis versus autonomous thrombocythaemia. *Acta Haematologica*, **95** (1996), 107–11.
21. K. Dan, S. Gomi & K. Inokuchi, Effects of interleukin-1 and tumor necrosis factor on megakaryocytopoeisis: a mechanism for reactive thrombocytosis. *Acta Haematologica*, **93** (1995), 67–72.
22. A. Ishiguro, T. Ishikita, T. Shimbo, Elevation of serum thrombopoeitin precedes thrombocytosis in Kawasaki disease. *Thrombosis and Haemostasis*, **79** (1998), 1096–100.
23. S. Chuncharunee, N. Archararit, P. Hathirat, U. Udomsubpayakul & V. Atichartakarn, Levels of serum interleukin-6 and tumor necrosis factor in postsplenectomised thalassemic patients. *Journal of the Medical Association of Thailand*, **80** (1997), S86–S91.
24. M. Griesshammer, M. Bangerter, T. Sauer *et al.*, Aetiology and clinical significance of thrombocytosis: analysis of 732 patients with an elevated platelet count. *Journal of Internal Medicine*, **245** (1999), 295–300.
25. M. L. Randi, F. Stocco, C. Rossi, T. Tison & A. Girolami, Thrombosis and haemorrhage in thrombocytosis: evaluation of a large cohort of patients (357 cases). *Journal of Medicine*, **22** (1991), 213–23.
26. D. H. Buss, J. J. Stuart & G. E. Lipscomb, The incidence of thrombotic and haemorrhagic disorders in association with extreme thrombocytosis: an analysis of 129 cases. *American Journal of Haematology*, **20** (1985), 365–72.
27. P. J. van Genderen & J. J. Michiels, Erythromelalgia: a pathognomic microvascular thrombotic complication in essential thrombocythaemia and polycythaemia vera. *Seminars in Thrombosis and Haemostasis*, **23** (1997), 357–63.
28. M. Johnson, T. Gernsheimer & K. Johansen, Essential thrombocytosis: underemphasized cause of large vessel thrombosis. *Journal of Vascular Surgery*, **22** (1995), 443–7.
29. M. Schmuziger, J. T. Christenson, J. Maurice, F. Simonet & V. Velebit, Reactive thrombocytosis after coronary bypass surgery. An important risk factor. *European Journal of Cardiothoracic Surgery*, **9** (1995), 393–7.
30. D. H. Buss, A. W. Cashell, M. L. O'Connor, F. Richards & L. D. Case, Occurrence, aetiology, and clinical significance of extreme thrombocytosis: a study of 280 cases. *American Medical Journal*, **96** (1994), 247–53.
31. W. W. Coon, J. Penner, P. Clagett & N. Eos, Deep venous thrombosis and postsplenectomy thrombo-cytosis. *Archives of Surgery*, **113** (1978), 429–31.
32. A. L. Taksin, J. P. Couedic & I. Dusanter-Fourt, Autonomous megakaryocyte growth in essential thrombocythemia and idiopathic myelofibrosis is not related to a c-mpl mutation or to an autocrine stimulation by Mpl-L. *Blood*, **93** (1999), 125–39.
33. J. Thiele, H. M. Kvasnicka, V. Diehl, R. Fischer & J. J. Michiels, Clinicopathological diagnosis and differential

criteria of thrombocythaemias in various myeloproliferayive disorders by histopathology, histochemistry and immunostaining from bone marrow biopsies. *Leukmia and Lymphoma*, **33** (1999), 207–18.

34. A. Tefferi, R. Fonseca, D. L. Pereira & H. C. Hoagland, A long-term retrospective study of young women with essential thrombocythaemia. *Mayo Clinic Proceedings*, **76** (2001), 22–8.
35. C. Besses, F. Cervantes & A. Pereira, Major vascular complications in essential thrombocythaemia: a study of the predictive factors in a series of 148 patients. *Leukaemia*, **13** (1999), 150–4.
36. P. Fenaux, M. Simon, M. T. Caulier *et al.*, Clinical course of essential thrombocythaemia in 147 cases. *Cancer*, **66** (1990), 549–56.
37. F. Cervantes, D. Tassies, C. Salgado *et al.*, Acute transformation in non-leukaemic chronic myeloproliferative disorders. *Acta Haematologica*, **85** (1991), 124–7.
38. A. T. Nurden & J. N. George, Inherited abnormalities of the platelet membrane: Glanzmann thrombasthenia, Bernard-Soulier syndrome, and other disorders. In *Haemostasis and Thrombosis. Basic Principles and Clinical Practice*, ed. R. W. Colman, J. Hirsh, J. Marder, A. W. Clowes & J. N. George. (Philadelphia: Lippincott, Williams, and Wilkins, 2001), pp. 921–43.
39. J. A. Lopez, R. K. Andrews, V. Afshar-Kharghan & M. C. Berndt, Bernard-Soulier syndrome. *Blood*, **91** (1998), 4397–418.
40. O. Faergeman, The atherosclerotic epidemic: methodology, nosology, and clinical practice. *American Journal of Cardiology*, **88**(Suppl) (2001), 4E–7E.
41. V. Fuster, L. Badimon, J. J. Badimon & J. H. Chesebro, The pathogenesis of coronary artery disease. *New England Journal of Medicine*, **326**(4) (1992), 242–50.
42. V. Fuster, The pathogenesis of coronary artery disease and the acute coronary syndromes. *New England Journal of Medicine*, **326** (2002), 310–18.
43. J. N. Wilcox, Molecular and cellular mechanisms of atherogenesis: studies of human lesions linked with animal modelling. In *Haemostasis and thrombosis*, ed. A. L. Bloom. (London: Churchill Livingstone, 1994), pp. 1139–52.
44. P. A. Merlini, Activated factor VII and increased thrombin activity in acute coronary syndromes. *Circulation*, **90** (1994), 179.
45. S. M. A. Evers, G. L. Engel & A. J. Ament, Cost of stroke in the Netherlands from a social perspective. *Stroke*, **28**(7) (1997), 1375–81.
46. M. Thorngren & B. Westling, Utilization of health care resources after stroke. A population-based study of 258 hospitalized cases followed during the first year. *Acta Neurologica Scandinavia*, **84** (1991), 303–10.
47. P. D. Hayes, A. J. Lloyd, N. J. M. London, P. R. F. Bell & A. R. Naylor, Transcranial ultrasound is a cost effective method of stroke prevention. *European Journal of Vascular and Endovascular Surgery*, **19** (2000), 56–61.
48. C. J. Frijns, L. J. Kappelle, J. van Gijn *et al.*, Soluble adhesion molecules reflect endothelial cell activation in ischaemic stroke and in carotid atherosclerosis. *Stroke*, **28** (1997), 2214–18.
49. J. P. Mohr, L. R. Caplan, J. W. Melski *et al.*, The Harvard Cooperative Stroke Registry: a prospective registry of patients hospitalized with stroke. *Neurology*, **28** (1978), 754–62.
50. R. L. Sacco, P. A. Wolf, W. B. Kannel & P. M. McNamara, Survival and recurrence following stroke: The Framingham Study. *Stroke*, **13** (1982), 290–5.
51. F. van Kooten, G. Ciabattoni & P. J. Koudstaal, Evidence for episodic platelet activation in acute ischaemic stroke. *Stroke*, **25** (1994), 278–81.
52. J. A. Zeller, D. Tschoepe & C. Kessler, Circulating platelets show increased activation in patients with acute cerebral ischaemia. *Thrombosis and Haemostasis*, **81** (1999), 373–7.
53. M. H. Criqui, A. Fronek, E. Barrett-Connor *et al.*, The prevalence of peripheral arterial disease in a defined population. *Circulation*, **71** (1995), 510–15.
54. M. H. Criqui, R. D. Langer, A. Fronek *et al.*, Mortality over a 10-year period in patients with peripheral arterial disease. *New England Journal of Medicine*, **326** (1992), 381–6.
55. A. Turpie, A. C. de Boer & E. Genton, Platelet consumption in cardiovascular disease. *Seminars in Thrombosis and Haemostasis*, **8** (1982), 161–85.
56. F. Zeiger, S. Stephan, D. Hoheisel, C. Pfeiffer & C. Ruehlmann, P-selectin expression, platelet aggregates, and platelet-derived microparticle formation are increased in peripheral arterial disease. *Blood Coagulation and Fibrinolysis*, **11** (2000), 723–8.
57. C. Reininger, J. Graf, A. J. Reininger *et al.*, Increased platelet and coagulatory activity in peripheral atherosclerosis flow mediated platelet function is a

sensitive and specific disease indicator. *International Angiology*, **15** (1996), 335–43.
58. C. Eastman & H. Keen, The impact of cardiovascular disease on people with diabetes: the potential for prevention. *Lancet*, **350**(1) (1997), 129–32.
59. J. A. Colwell, Vascular thrombosis in type II diabetes mellitus. *Diabetes*, **42** (1993), 8–11.
60. A. B. Sobol & C. Watala, The role of platelets in diabetes-related vascular complications. *Diabetes Research in Clinical Practice*, **50** (2000), 1–16.
61. Second International Study of Infarct Survival (ISIS-2) Collaborative Group, Randomised controlled trial of intravenous streptokinase, oral aspirin, both, or neither, among 17,187 cases of suspected acute myocardial infarction: ISIS-2. *Lancet*, **2** (1998), 349–60.
62. P. S. Sorensen, H. Pedersen, J. Marquardsen *et al.*, Acetylsalicylic acid in the prevention of stroke in patients with reversible cerebral ischaemic attacks. A Danish cooperative study. *Stroke* **14** (1983), 15–21.
63. UK-Transient-Ischaemic Attack Study Group, United Kingdom transient ischaemic attack aspirin trial: interim results. *British Medical Journal*, **296** (1988), 316–20.
64. The Swedish Cooperative Study Group, High doses of acetylsalicylic acid after cerebral infarction. A Swedish cooperative study. *Stroke*, **18** (1986), 325–34.
65. Antiplatelet Trialists' Collaboration. Collaborative overview of randomised trials of antiplatelet therapy. *British Medical Journal*, **308** (1994), 81–106.
66. D. W. Taylor, H. J. M. Barnett, R. B. Haynes *et al.*, Low-dose and high-dose acetylsalicyclic acid for patients undergoing carotid endarterectomy: a randomised controlled trial. *Lancet*, **353** (1999), 2179–84.
67. D. S. Baim & J. P. Carrozza, Stent thrombosis: closing in on the best preventative treatment. *Circulation*, **95** (1997), 1098–100.
68. M. Bourassa, L. Schwartz, J. Lesperance *et al.*, Prevention of acute complications after percutaneous transluminal coronary angioplasty. *Thrombosis Research*, **12** (1990), 51–8.
69. N. J. Lembo, A. J. Black, G. S. Roubin *et al.*, Effect of pretreatment with aspirin versus aspirin plus dipyridamole on frequency and type of acute complications of percutaneous transluminal coronary angioplasty. *American Journal of Cardiology*, **65** (1990), 422–6.
70. Antiplatelet Trialists' Collaboration II. Collaborative overview of randomised trials in antiplatelet therapy: maintenance of vascular graft or arterial patency by antiplatelet therapy. *British Medical Journal*, **308** (1994), 159–68.
71. European Stroke Prevention Study-2 Working Group. Second European stroke prevention study: antiplatelet therapy is effective regardless of age. *Acta Neurologica Scandinavia*, **99**(1) (1999), 54–60.
72. K. K. Wu, Inducible cyclooxygenase and nitric oxide synthase. *Advances in Pharmacology*, **33** (1995), 179–207.
73. J. A. Mitchell, P. Akarasereenont, C. Thiemermann *et al.*, Selectivity of nonsteroidal antiinflammatory drugs as inhibitors or constitutive and inducible cyclooxygenase. *Proceedings of the National Academy of Science*, **90**(24) (1993), 11693–7.
74. CAPRIE Steering Committee. A randomised, blinded trial of clopidogrel versus aspirin in patients at risk of ischaemic events (CAPRIE). *Lancet*, **348** (1996), 1329–39.
75. J. E. Tcheng, Glycoprotein IIb/IIIa receptor inhibitors: putting the EPIC, IMPACT II, RESTORE, and EPILOG trials into perspective. *American Journal of Cardiology*, **78**(3) (1996), 35–40.
76. S. G. Katz & R. D. Kohl, Does dextran-40 improve the early patency of autogenous infrainguinal bypass grafts? *Journal of Vascular Surgery*, **28** (1998), 23–6.
77. P. D. Hayes, A. J. Lloyd, N. Lennard *et al.*, Transcranial doppler-directed dextran 40 therapy is a cost-effective method of preventing carotid thrombosis after CEA. *European Journal of Vascular and Endovascular Surgery*, **19**(1) (2000), 56–61.
78. C. Levi, J. L. Stork, B. R. Chambers *et al.*, Dextran reduces embolic signbals after carotid endarterectomy. *Annals of Neurology*, **50** (2001), 544–7.
79. A. R. Naylor, P. D. Hayes, H. Allroggen *et al.*, Reducing the risk of carotid surgery: a 7-year audit of the role of monitoring and quality control assessment. *Journal of Vascular Surgery*, **32** (2000), 750–9.
80. T. Sudo, K. Tachibana, K. Toga *et al.*, Potent effects of novel anti-platelet aggregatory cilostamide analogues on recombinant cyclic nucleotide phosphodiesterase isozyme activity. *Biochemistry and Pharmacology*, **59** (2000), 347–56.
81. T. Igawa, T. Tani, T. Chijina *et al.*, Potentiation of anti-platelet aggregating activity of cilostazol with vascular endothelial cells. *Thrombosis Research*, **57** (1990), 617–23.

82. T. Tanaka, T. Ishikawa, M. Hagiwara *et al.*, Effect of cilostazol, a selective cAMP phosphodiesterase inhibitor on the contraction of vascular smooth muscle. *Pharmacology*, **36** (1998), 313–20.
83. A. Tsuchikane, A. Fukuhara, T. Kobayashi *et al.*, Impact of cilostazol on restenosis after percutaneous coronary balloon angioplasty. *Circulation*, **100** (1999), 21–6.
84. F. Gotoh, H. Tohgi, S. Hirai *et al.*, Cilostazol Stroke Prevention Study: a placebo-controlled double-blinded trial for secondary prevention of cerebral infarction. *Journal of Stroke and Cerebrovascular Disease*, **9** (2000), 147–57.
85. S. Money, A. Herd, J. L. Isaacsohn *et al.*, Effect of cilostazol on walking distances in patients with intermittent claudication caused by peripheral vascular disease. *Journal of Vascular Surgery*, **27** (1998), 267–75.
86. A. Lundell, D. Berguust & B. Lindblad, The uptake of platelets, fibrinogen and leucocytes in PTFE grafts. *European Journal of Vascular and Endovascular Surgery*, **7** (1993), 698–703.
87. R. Y. Rhee, P. Gloviczki, R. A. Cambria *et al.*, Experimental evaluation of bleeding complications, thrombogenicity and neointimal characteristics of patch materials used for carotid angioplasty. *Cardiovascular Surgery*, **4** (1996), 746–52.
88. A. I. Margovsky, M. S. Lord, A. C. Meek *et al.*, Artery wall damage and platelet uptake from so-called atraumatic clamps. *Cardiovascular Surgery*, **5** (1997), 42–7.

7 • Atherosclerosis

QINGBO XU

INTRODUCTION

Atherosclerosis, the principal cause of heart attack, stroke and gangrene of the extremities, remains a major contributor to morbidity and mortality in the western world. Although the aetiology and pathogenesis of atherosclerosis have been not fully elucidated, it is generally accepted that atherosclerosis is a multifactorial disease induced by the effects of various risk factors on appropriate genetic backgrounds [1]. Many factors, such as hypercholesterolaemia, modified lipoproteins, hypertension, diabetes mellitus, infections and smoking were identified in the development of atherosclerosis. Because this disease progresses slowly, begins in childhood and does not manifest until middle age or later [2], the mechanisms of atherogenesis are relatively difficult to study.

Atherosclerosis has been the subject of intense research for over 100 years. Since Anitschkow and Chalatow [3] reported for the first time that cholesterol can cause atherosclerosis, many investigators intensively studied the role of blood cholesterol in the pathogenesis of atherosclerosis. It was formerly considered a bland lipid storage disease. However, new insights into the pathogenesis of atherosclerosis have emerged during the last decades, due to the progress of cellular and molecular approaches to study cell interactions in the arterial wall as well as alterations of lipid metabolism. These were broadly summarized in three main theories, i.e. the 'response to injury' [4], 'oxidized low-density lipoprotein (LDL)' [5], and 'inflammation' [1] hypotheses.

The response to injury hypothesis [4] relies on the concept that the primary cause of atherosclerosis is an injury to the arterial endothelium induced by various factors, i.e. mechanical stress, oxidized-LDL, homocysteine, immunological events, toxins, viruses, etc. The oxidized-LDL hypothesis postulates that LDL oxidized by various factors including endothelial cells, macrophages and smooth muscle cells of the arterial wall, plays a key role in the development of atherosclerosis [5]. More recently, a widely accepted hypothesis is that atherosclerosis is an inflammatory disease, because recent advances in the basic science have established a fundamental role for inflammation in mediating all stages of this disease from initiation through progression and, ultimately, the thrombotic complications of atherosclerosis [1]. The insights provided by the intensive research have unravelled the molecular and mechanistic causes of lesion development and led to the identification of risk factors and therapeutic targets. The aim of the present chapter is to summarize the updated data from a variety of research areas providing an overview of atherosclerosis focusing on the mechanistic studies.

ATHEROSCLEROTIC LESIONS

The intima of large and medium sized arteries is composed of a monolayer of endothelial cells and matrix proteins, and a few smooth muscle cells under the endothelium (Figure 7.1a). The media of the vessel contains smooth muscle cells and the elastic lamina built by matrix proteins, while the main component of adventitia is connective tissue. With increasing age, the diseased arterial wall eventually thickens and develops focal lesions in the intima, which are early lesions, i.e. fatty streaks. These lesions can further develop into advanced lesions called atherosclerotic plaques or atheroma, which may lead to clinical symptoms in certain circumstances [6].

Fatty streaks

Fatty streaks are generally the lesion types found in children, although they may also occur in adults [2]. These lesions represent the very initial changes, and are recognized as an increase in the number of intimal macrophages and the appearance of macrophages

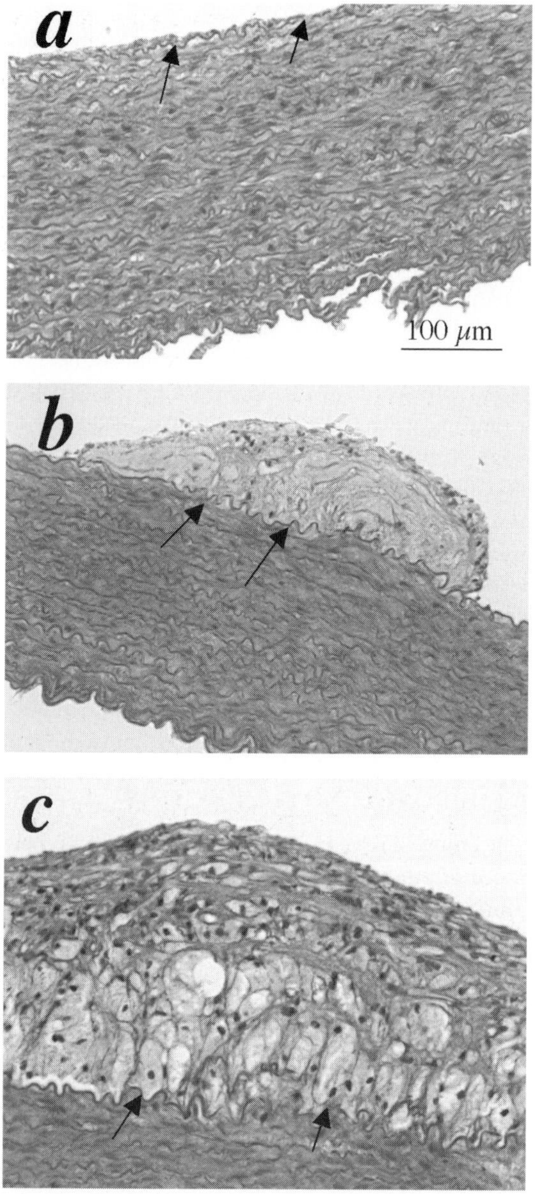

Fig. 7.1. Sections of the vessel wall. Rabbits were fed with: (a) a standard chow-diet; or (b) a cholesterol-enriched diet (0.2%) for three weeks; or (c) for 16 weeks. Their aortas were harvested, and sections prepared and stained with haematoxilin and eosin. Arrows indicate the internal elastic lamina, the border between the intima and media of the arterial wall (see colour plate section).

filled with lipid droplets (foam cells). A larger lesion can be grossly visible and characterized by layers of macrophage foam cells and lipid droplets within intimal smooth muscle cells, and minimal coarse-grained particles and heterogeneous droplets of extracellular lipid (Figure 7.1b). With the progression of lesion development, intermediate lesions as described by pathologists, are the morphological and chemical bridge between fatty streaks and advanced lesions. These lesions appear in some adaptive intimal thickenings (progression-prone locations) in young adults and are characterized by pools of extracellular lipid in addition to other components of fatty streak lesions. The fatty streak is itself clinically benign, but is the precursor to later, clinically relevant lesions [6].

Plaque or atheroma

The advanced lesion, a dense accumulation of extracellular lipid, occupies an extensive but well-defined region of the intima [7]. This type of extracellular lipid accumulation is known as the lipid core. There is no increase in fibrous tissue and complications such as defects of the lesion surface and thrombosis are not present. This atherosclerotic plaque is also known as atheroma (Figure 7.1c). The characteristic core appears to develop from an expansion and confluence of the small isolated pools of extracellular lipid that characterize atheroma. Between the lipid core and the endothelial surface, the intima contains macrophages, smooth muscle cells, lymphocytes and mast cells. Capillaries surround the lipid core, particularly at the lateral margins and facing the lumen. Frequently macrophages, macrophage foam cells and lymphocytes are more densely concentrated in the lesion periphery. Much of the tissue between the core and the surface endothelium corresponds to the proteoglycan-rich layer of the intima, although infiltrated with the cells just described. Lesions considered advanced by their histology may or may not narrow the arterial lumen, nor be visible by angiography, nor produce clinical manifestations. Such lesions may be clinically significant even though the arterial lumen is not narrowed, because complications may develop suddenly [7].

In addition, two types of atherosclerotic plaques, i.e. 'vulnerable' and 'stable' plaques, have been recognized [8]. Vulnerable plaques often have a well-preserved lumen, since plaques grow outward initially. The vulnerable plaque typically has a substantial lipid core and a thin fibrous cap separating the thrombogenic macrophages bearing tissue factor from the blood. At sites of lesion disruption, smooth muscle cells are often activated, as detected by their expression of the transplantation antigen HLA-DR. In contrast, the stable plaque has a relatively thick fibrous cap protecting the lipid core from contact with the blood. Clinical data suggest that stable plaques more often show luminal narrowing detectable by angiography than do vulnerable plaques, but with much less chance of rupture.

HYPERCHOLESTEROLAEMIA AND OXIDIZED-LDL

Accumulating evidence suggests a causal relationship between blood cholesterol and atherosclerosis. Blood cholesterol is carried by lipoproteins, including LDL, very low-density lipoprotein and high-density lipoprotein (HDL). Low-density lipoprotein is believed to be 'bad' lipoprotein, while HDL is 'good' and plays a protective role in atherogenesis [9]. It is established that family hypercholesterolaemia related to increased LDL levels causes premature atherosclerosis and heart disease [10], whereas non-genetic hypercholesterolaemia is also associated with the incidence of atherosclerosis [11]. The consensus of many trials using different cholesterol-lowering regimens indicate that for every 10% reduction in cholesterol level, the deaths of patients with coronary heart disease is reduced by at least 15% [12]. It has been assumed that the reduction in adverse clinical events when plasma cholesterol levels are decreased is directly related to the magnitude of the cholesterol lowering. That assumption is supported by the fact that the benefit relates to the change in cholesterol level in much the same way whether the cholesterol lowering is achieved with diet or with drugs [12]. These findings suggest that blood cholesterol exerts its role in the pathogenesis of atherosclerosis.

Low-density lipoprotein can be modified by oxidation *in vivo* and *in vitro* [13]. For instance, oxidized-LDL was generated by incubation of native LDL with cultured endothelial cells [13]. *In vivo*, presumably the rate of production of oxidized-LDL in the arterial intima is a function of the concentration of native LDL present. Oxidized-LDL is detectable in the circulation as well as in atherosclerotic lesions. Aortic wall concentrations of LDL in the rabbit are higher at lesion-susceptible sites than at lesion-resistant sites even before lesions appear [14].

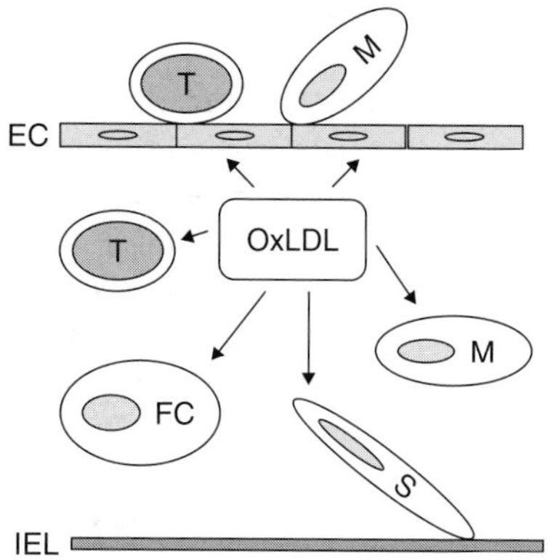

Fig. 7.2. Schematic representation of the role of oxidized-LDL (xLDL) in atherogenesis. Oxidized-LDL generated either locally or systemically stimulates endothelial cells (ECs) expressing adhesion molecules, including ICAM-1, VCAM-1 and E-selection, which are responsible for adhesion of blood mononuclear cells. Oxidized-LDL is a chemokine for T lymphocytes (T), monocytes (M) and smooth muscle cells (S), and promotes foam cell (FC) formation, which form the early lesion fatty streak. IEL = internal elastic lamina.

How does hypercholesterolaemia and oxidized-LDL trigger the event leading to the generation of the earliest lesion of atherosclerosis, the fatty streak (Figure 7.2)? Most of our knowledge concerning the pathogenesis of atherosclerosis caused by hyperlipidaemia has come from studies of animal models. Although rabbits were often used in studying this issue, the apolipoprotein (apo) E-deficient mouse [15] and the LDL receptor-deficient mouse [16] have become preferred animal models. Gene 'knock-outs' and 'knock-ins' are now the gold standard for critically testing the relevance of candidate genes in atherogenesis. By using these models, it was observed that one of the earliest responses induced by hypercholesterolaemia and oxidized-LDL is an increase in the expression of vascular cell adhesion molecule (VCAM) 1, a key adhesion molecule for monocytes and T cells, on the endothelial surface lining the major arteries [17]. Oxidized-LDL is itself directly chemotactic for monocytes and T cells [18]. Among other biological effects, oxidized-LDL is cytotoxic for endothelial cells [19], mitogenic for macrophages and smooth muscle cells [20], and stimulates the release of monocyte chemoattractant protein 1 and monocyte colony-stimulating factor from endothelial cells [21]. The oxidative modification hypothesis has been extensively reviewed [13; 22; 23].

Oxidized-LDL can account for the loading of macrophages with cholesterol. Here, monocytes undergo phenotypic modification and take up oxidized-LDL to become foam cells, loaded with multiple cytoplasmic droplets containing cholesterol esters [24]. Recently there has been considerable progress in identifying the components of oxidized-LDL that make it a ligand for scavenger receptors [25]. Extensive degradation of the polyunsaturated fatty acid in the *sn*-2 position of phospholipids by oxidation seems to be essential. Moreover, oxidized-LDL and apoptotic cells compete for binding to a macrophage scavenger receptor [26; 27]. This indicates that oxidized phospholipids in the membranes of apoptotic cells are involved in their binding to macrophage scavenger receptors. Therefore, oxidized-LDL promotes foam cell formation that forms the earliest lesions in the intima, which may progress to advanced lesions in the presence of other pro-atherogenic factors [23] (Figure 7.2).

HYPERTENSION AND BIOMECHANICAL STRESS

Hypertension is a well-established risk factor for atherosclerosis [28]. Clinical trials have shown that, in the highest quintile for diastolic pressure, even with the added risks of high cholesterol and smoking, hypertension still contributes significantly to the risk of atherosclerosis [29; 30]. Utilizing laboratory studies in which hypertension was induced in the Watanabe heritable hyperlipidaemic rabbit, Chobanian and his group [31] showed a synergistic effect that caused an intensification of atherosclerosis. In fact, atherosclerosis tends to occur only in those parts of the vascular system subjected to high pressure or biomechanical stress [32]. In other words, atherosclerotic lesions preferentially occur in the areas where haemodynamic or biomechanical stress is altered, e.g. bifurcation of the arteries. This suggests that hypertension exerts its role in the pathogenesis of atherosclerosis via altered mechanical stress to the vessel wall.

In vivo, the vessel wall is exposed to two main haemodynamic forces or biomechanical stress: shear stress, the dragging frictional force created by blood flow, and mechanical stretch, a cyclic strain stress created by blood pressure [32; 33]. Shear stress stimulates endothelial cells to release nitric oxide [34] and prostacyclin [35], resulting in vessel relaxation and protection of vascular cells, whereas smooth muscle cells are stimulated by cyclic strain stress [36]. In humans, atherosclerotic lesions occur predominantly at bifurcations and curvatures [37] where haemodynamic force is disturbed, i.e. lower shear stress and higher mechanical stretch [38]. Although veins do not develop spontaneous atherosclerosis-like lesions, accelerated atherosclerosis occurs rapidly in venous bypass grafts, which bear increased biomechanical forces due to alterations in blood pressure, i.e. vein (0–30 mm Hg) vs. artery (120 mm Hg). Therefore, mechanical stress could be a crucial factor in the pathogenesis of atherosclerosis.

Physical stimuli must be sensed by cells and transmitted through intracellular signal transduction pathways to the nucleus resulting in quantitative and qualitative changes in gene expression in the vessel wall. Recent evidence indicates that mechanical stretch initiates intracellular signal pathways, especially mitogen-activated protein kinase (MAPK) cascades [39]. Mitogen-activated protein kinases are thought to play a pivotal role in transmitting transmembrane signals required for cell proliferation, differentiation and apoptosis. Mitogen-activated protein kinases comprise a ubiquitous family of tyrosine/threonine kinases, and include extracellular signal-regulated kinases (ERKs), stress-activated protein kinases (SAPKs) or c-Jun NH^2-terminal kinases (JNKs) and p38 MAPKs [40]. They are highly activated or expressed in atherosclerotic lesions and vessel walls stimulated by acute hypertension [41; 42].

Biomechanical stress-induced cell death

While biomechanical force at physiological levels is essential to develop and maintain organic structure and function, at elevated levels mechanical stretch may result in cell death leading to pathological conditions [43]. In recent years, however, it has become widely recognized that cell death, namely apoptosis, is not just a response to injury but a highly regulated and controlled process [44]. Disturbances in the regulatory mechanisms of apoptosis often precede the development of atherosclerosis [44]. Exploration of the molecular signalling mechanisms leading to mechanical stress-induced apoptosis in cardiovascular disorders has revealed the crucial role of apoptosis in the pathogenesis of atherosclerosis [45]. Here recent data focusing on

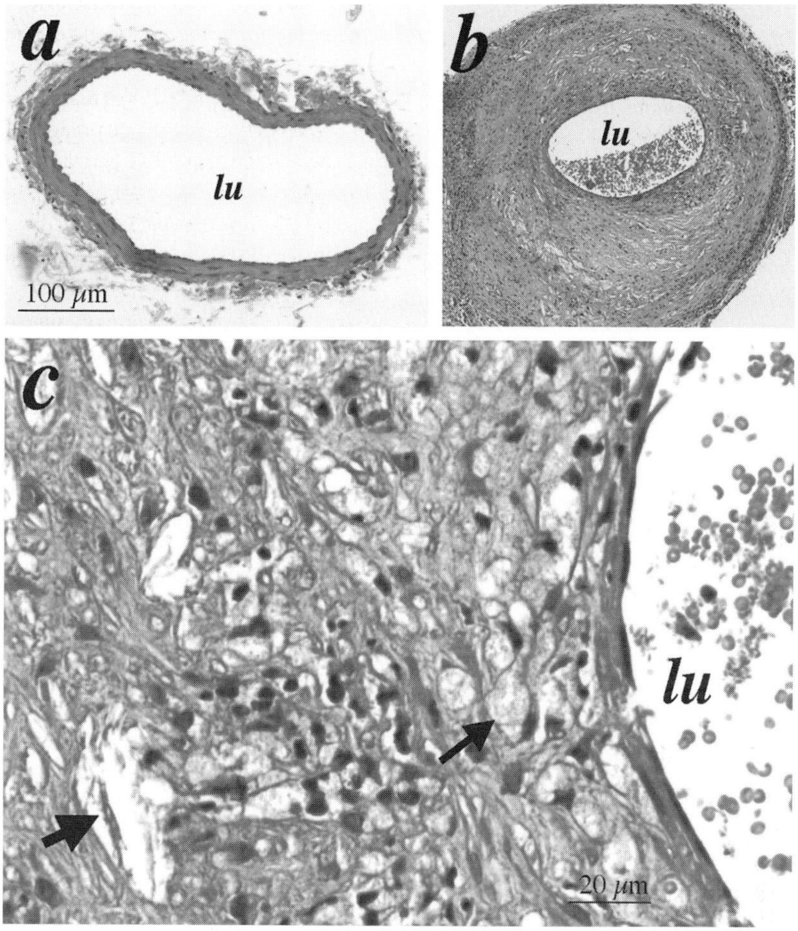

Fig. 7.3. Haematoxilin and eosin-stained sections of mouse vein grafts. Under anaesthesia, vena cava veins were removed and isografted into (a) carotid arteries of (b) apoE-/- mice. Animals were sacrificed eight weeks after surgery. The grafted tissue fragments were fixed in 4% phosphate phosphate-buffered (pH 7.2) formaldehyde, embedded in paraffin, sectioned and stained with haematoxilin-eosin. Panel (c) is a photograph of a vein graft section with higher magnification. Smaller arrow indicates a foam cell, whilst a larger one indicates a cholesterol crystal structure. The lumen of the vessel is inicated by *lu* (see colour plate section).

the molecular mechanisms of mechanical stress-induced apoptosis is summarized and the role of apoptosis in the development of atherosclerosis is highlighted.

Recently, the first mouse model of vein graft atherosclerosis was established by grafting autologous jugular vein or vena cava to carotid arteries in wild-type and apoE-deficient mice [46; 47]. In many respects, the morphological features of this murine vascular graft model resemble those of human graft atherosclerosis (Figure 7.3). Apoptosis occurred mainly in veins grafted to arteries, remaining unchanged in vein-to-vein grafts [48]. When mouse, rat and human arterial smooth muscle cells cultured on a flexible membrane were subjected to cyclic strain stress, apoptosis was observed in a time- and strength-dependent manner. Mechanical stretch resulted in p38 MAPK activation. Smooth muscle cell lines stably transfected with a dominant negative rac, an upstream signal transducer, or over-expressing MAPK phosphatase-1, a negative regulator for MAPKs, completely inhibited mechanical stress-stimulated p38 activation and abolished mechanical stress-induced apoptosis [49]. Interestingly, p53-deficient vein grafts had lower levels of apoptosis that correlated with increased atherosclerotic lesions [50].

Obviously, the grafted veins were subjected to increased biomechanical forces in the form of stretch stress due to blood pressure. The sudden elevation in mechanical forces could be a strong stimulus to the grafted vessel wall and may result in activation of intracellular signal pathways leading to gene expression and cell death. Thus, one of the earliest events in vein graft atherosclerosis is apoptosis, in which mechanical stress-induced p38 MAPK p53 activation is, at least in part, responsible for transducing signals leading to apoptosis.

Biomechanical stress and inflammation

Vein graft atherosclerosis has an inflammatory nature characterized by mononuclear cell infiltration followed by smooth muscle cell proliferation. It has been postulated that biomechanical stress plays a role in adhesion molecule expression via MAPK signal transduction pathways, leading to NF-κ B activation. Supporting this concept is the fact that neointimal lesions of vein grafts in intercellular adhesion molecule (ICAM)-1 −/− mice were reduced from 30% to 50% compared to wild-type controls. Intercellular adhesion molecule-1 is critical in the development of venous graft atherosclerosis [51]. It has been established that exposure of endothelial cells to shear (mechanical) stress results in increased expression of ICAM-1 and monocyte chemotactic protein-1 (MCP-1) via activation of transcription factor NF-κ B and AP-1 [52]. These molecules are essential for leucocyte-endothelial cell interaction and subsequently cell infiltration, which is characteristic of the early lesions of vein grafts that undergo elevated blood pressure. Interestingly, mechanical stress also leads to smooth muscle cells expressing ICAM-1 via activation of NF-κ B. In animal models smooth muscle cells express ICAM-1 which was associated with monocyte/macrophage accumulation in vein grafts. Smooth muscle cells of ICAM-1 −/− mice do not express ICAM-1 which correlated with reduced early lesions [51]. Mechanical stress-induced adhesion molecules and chemokine expression in the vessel wall could be important for the inflammatory response.

Biomechanical stress-induced smooth muscle cell proliferation

It has been established that mechanical stress stimulates DNA synthesis and the proliferation of *in vitro* cultured smooth muscle cells [53]. Hypertension increases mechanical force on the arterial wall up to 30%, resulting in marked alterations in signal transduction and gene expression in smooth muscle cells, which contribute to matrix protein synthesis, cell proliferation and differentiation [28]. Recently, several reports demonstrated that angioplasty resulted in stretching of the arterial wall leading to rapid activation of the MAPKs in the regenerating carotids [54; 55]. The magnitude of MAPK42 activation positively correlated with the degree of balloon injury to the arterial wall. *Ex vivo* stretching of the vessel wall also induced significant activation of MAPK42 kinases. These findings suggested that the kinase activation in the early phase following injury may be due to mechanical stimulation of the vessel wall.

In cultured smooth muscle cells, mechanical forces evoked ERK activation followed by enhanced DNA-binding activity of transcription factor AP-1 [56; 57]. Interestingly, physical forces rapidly result in phosphorylation of platelet-derived growth factor (PDGF) receptor [58], epithelial growth factor receptor [59] and vascular endothelial growth factor receptor [60]. Thus, mechanical stresses may directly perturb the cell surface or alter receptor conformation, thereby initiating signalling pathways normally used by growth factors. Suramin has been shown to be a growth factor receptor antagonist that inhibits cell proliferation. When vein isografts in mice were treated *ex vivo* and *in vivo* with suramin, intimal lesions were reduced by up to 70% compared to untreated controls [61]. The mechanism of suramin-inhibited neointima hyperplasia mainly involves inhibition of smooth muscle cell migration and proliferation via blocking PDGF receptor-MAPK-AP-1 signal pathways. Thus, research into biomechanical stress-regulated gene expression in atherosclerosis using these models could lead to a new therapeutic strategy in the treatment of this disease in humans.

INFECTIONS AND HEAT SHOCK PROTEINS

Whilst risk factors, such as high blood cholesterol, hypertension and smoking are well established as risk factors for atherosclerosis, they only explain a proportion of the incident cases of all atherosclerosis [62]. On the other hand, there is growing evidence that microorganisms play a role in the pathogenesis of atherosclerosis and may be a primary risk factor in people who do not suffer from other established risk factors [62]. Accumulating evidence suggests that infectious organisms reside in the wall of atherosclerotic vessels, including cytomegalovirus (CMV) and *Chlamydia* (*C*) *pneumoniae*, and seroepidemiological studies demonstrate an association between the pathogen-specific IgG antibodies and atherosclerosis [63; 64]. However, the data are inconsistent, with other studies showing no increased risk for atherosclerosis [65; 66]. One possible explanation for this disparity is that infections contributing to atherosclerosis risk may depend, at least in part, on the host response to the pathogen, i.e. inflammatory and immune reactions.

Infections

Several papers reviewing infections and atherosclerosis have been published [64; 67] and these will be summarized, i.e. regarding *C. pneumoniae, Helicobacter pylori* and CMV. Saikku *et al.* [68] were the first to show a link between *C. pneumoniae* infection, coronary artery disease and atherosclerosis. Since then, many studies have shown an association of *C. pneumoniae* with atherosclerosis. *In vitro* experiments have shown that *C. pneumoniae* infects macrophages, the vascular endothelium and vascular smooth muscle [69]. It is capable of replicating inside aortic endothelial cells [69]. *Chlamydia pneumoniae* may have a tropism for macrophages which in turn accumulate in atherosclerotic plaques. This is supported by studies of post-mortem specimens of vascular tissue which found a high correlation between the distribution of atherosclerosis and *C. pneumoniae* [70] as well as other organisms.

Another gram negative bacteria *H. pylori* typically infects human gastric epithelial cells and has been demonstrated in atherosclerotic plaques [65]. *Helicobacter pylori* seropositivity was implicated as a risk factor in coronary heart disease from the first report in 1994 [71]. However, a meta-analysis [66] of 18 studies failed to show any correlation between seropositivity against *H. pylori* and the presence or extent of coronary artery disease. Although the evidence supporting involvement of *H. pylori* in atherogenesis is not conclusive, it may be important to differentiate between virulent and avirulent strains of *H. pylori* to determine the effects on atherogenesis. Mayr *et al.* [72] conducted a population based study and investigated the effects of CagA (cytotoxin-associated gene A) positive and CagA negative strains of *H. pylori*. It is concluded that there was an increased risk of atherosclerosis in individuals who were infected with CagA positive strains of *H. pylori*. Another group has obtained similar results, indicating the role of this strain in the pathogenesis of atherosclerosis.

Heat shock proteins

The role of heat shock proteins (HSPs) in disease with regard to their physiological functions and pathological involvement have been described in excellent reviews [73; 74; 75; 76]. In short, the HSP family of proteins is subdivided into groups based on their molecular weight (e.g. HSP60 is a 60 kDa protein). They are produced by almost all cells and play an important role in the organism's general protective response to environmental and metabolic stresses (Table 7.1). They exist in all major cellular compartments [77]. For example, HSP10, HSP60 and HSP75 are mainly located in mitochondria, while others are found in different compartments throughout the cell. They have important physiological functions, primarily as a molecular chaperone [78]. HSPs also appear to be important in preventing cellular damage during repair processes following injury. Moreover, evidence indicates that HSPs may be autoantigens in some circumstances [79]. HSP47, HSP60 and HSP70 have been identified as being involved in the pathogenesis of atherosclerosis [80; 81; 82; 83].

Infections and HSP expression

Kleindienst *et al.* [84] demonstrated that increased HSP60 was detected on the endothelium, smooth muscle cells and mononuclear cells of all carotid and aortic specimens, whereas vessels with the normal intima showed no detectable expression of this HSP. The level of HSP60 expression correlated positively with atherosclerotic severity [85; 86]. Interestingly, Kol *et al.* [87] demonstrated the co-existence of chlamydial and human HSP60s in atherosclerotic lesions. These data support the concept that elevated HSP expression in lesions may be induced by the pathogen *Chlamydiae* spp. During its normal cycle generating infectious progeny, *Chlamydiae* express basal levels of HSP. During the lytic phases of chlamydial infection, host cells release their own HSP60 and chlamydial HSP60 that has been produced by these microorganisms. Xu *et al.* [88] demonstrated that soluble HSP60 (sHSP)

Table 7.1. *Heat shock protein families*

Family	Members/other names	Physiological function	Pathological involvement
HSP10	HSP10, HSP17	Promotes substrate release with HSP60	?
Small HSP	HSP20, HSP23, HSP27, HSP28	F-actin assembly; molecular chaperones	?
HSP40	HSP32, HSP40, HSP47	Guides protein folding; binding and transport of collagen	Atherosclerosis
HSP60	HSP58, GroEL HSP60, HSP65, Grp58	Assemble polypeptides; translocate proteins across membranes; accelerate protein folding and unfolding	Atherosclerosis, Rheumatoid arthritis, Adjuvant arthritis, Diabetes mellitus, Systemic sclerosis
HSP70	HSP68, Dnak, Hsc70, Hsx70, HSP72, HSP73, HSP75, Grp75, HSP78, Grp78	Molecular chaperone: assembly and transport newly synthesized proteins; fold or unfold polypeptides; remove denatured proteins; bind to specific polypeptides (e.g. p53); ATPase activity	Atherosclerosis Tuberculosis, Leprosy, Filariasis
HSP90	HSP83, HptG, HSP87, HSP90-α, Grp94, HSP90-β	Bind to specific polypeptide receptors (e.g. glucocorticoid receptor)	Schistosomiasis, Systemic lupus erythematosus

levels were significantly elevated in subjects with prevalent/incident carotid atherosclerosis and correlated to intima-media thickness independent of age, sex and other risk factors. Interestingly, sHSP60 was also correlated with anti-lipopolysaccharide, anti-*Chlamydia* and anti-HSP60 antibodies, inflammation markers and chronic infections [88].

Infections, sHSP and innate immunity

Infectious agents contribute to atherogenesis in a variety of ways. One mechanism is by triggering innate immune reactions leading to inflammatory responses. Innate immunity involves several different cell types, e.g. mononuclear phagocytes and endothelial cells. Both endothelial cells and macrophages express receptors that recognize molecular epitopes from a broad range of pathogens. These receptors include various scavenger and toll-like receptors (TLRs) [89]. So far, more than ten human TLRs have been identified. A variety of bacterial and fungal components are known TLR ligands, including peptidoglycan for TLR2, LPS for TLR4, flagellin for TLR5 and unmethylated CpG motifs in bacterial DNA for TLR9 [90]. It is possible that TLRs may be collectively responsible for detecting a large range of microbial pathogens. Toll-like receptors are evolutionarily conserved innate immune receptors that are shared by IL-1 receptor signalling to activate the NF-κ B pathway and release inflammatory cytokines [90]. Toll-like receptor ligation therefore induces expression of a wide variety of genes such as those encoding proteins involved in leucocyte recruitment, production of reactive oxygen species and phagocytosis. Activation of TLRs will also elicit the production of cytokines that augment local inflammation. Finally, TLR ligation may directly induce apoptosis, which is probably of key importance in the first line of defence [91].

In fact, the expression of TLR4 in atherosclerotic plaques has been found, preferentially in lipid-rich and macrophage-infiltrated areas of lesions [92]. This report has also demonstrated basal expression of TLR4 by macrophages, which was up-regulated by oxidized-LDL *in vitro*. These findings were confirmed by Edfeldt *et al.* [93] showing that of nine TLRs, the expression of TLR1, TLR2 and TLR4 was markedly enhanced in human atherosclerotic plaques. Furthermore, Kiechl *et al.* [94] provided the first evidence that a polymorphism or mutation of TLR4 was strongly correlated with the incidence and development of atherosclerosis in a large population study (Bruneck Study). Surprisingly, several groups reported that recombinant HSP60 and HSP70 from bacteria and humans specifically bind to TLR4 in macrophages, endothelial cells and smooth muscle cells [95; 96; 97]. Recombinant HSP60 binding to the TLR4/CD14 complex of macrophages and endothelial cells led to activation of MyD88-NF-κ B pathways. HSP70 and mycobacterial HSP65 have a similar binding activity to TLR4/CD14 that initiates MyD88-NF-κ B signal pathways [98]. These findings suggest that the TLR4/CD14 is a receptor for several HSPs that mediate the signal pathways leading to proinflammatory responses during infections.

In summary, infections with pro-atherogenic organisms may be important in individuals lacking these risk factors as well as acting synergistically with established risk factors. In this process, HSP may be a link between infections and the pathogenesis of atherosclerosis. Infectious agents may exert their role by producing their own HSPs and inducing host production which could be released into blood. The soluble form of HSPs contacts endothelial cells and immune cells where innate immune responses are initiated. Innate immune reactions to HSPs result in pro-inflammatory responses in the vessel wall. Together, infections via HSPs contribute to the development of atherosclerosis (Figure 7.4).

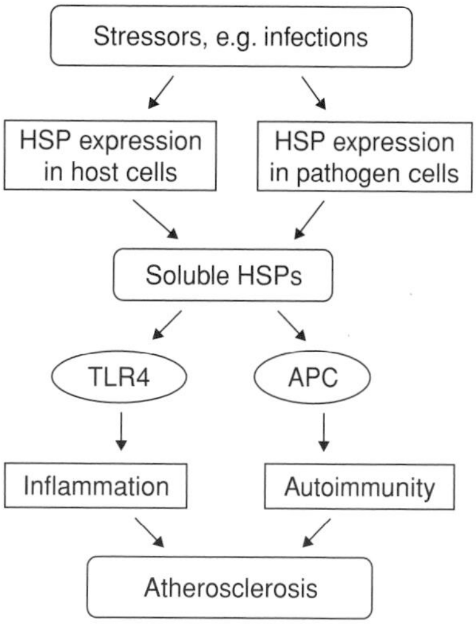

Fig. 7.4. Schematic representation of the model on the involvement of heat shock proteins (HSPs) in atherogenesis. TLR – Toll-like receptor; APC – antigen-presenting cells.

IMMUNE RESPONSES

The contribution of immune responses to the pathogenesis of atherosclerosis has been recognized and much progress in this research field has been achieved due to the participation of many investigators [91; 99; 100]. The involvement of the immune system in atherogenesis is supported by recent data, including the occurrence of granular deposits of immunoglobulins and co-distributed complement components, and increased expression of C3b receptors (CR1) and C3b1 receptors (CR3) on macrophages within atherosclerotic lesions, but not in unaltered vessels [101]. However, B cells are only found in very low numbers in various stages of atherosclerotic lesions and the site of production for these immunoglobulins must, therefore, be sought elsewhere. Other than these humoral immune phenomena, it is now clear that T cells are among the first cells infiltrating the intima of arteries during the earliest stages of atherosclerosis, most probably before the monocytes [102]. A majority of these early T cells are CD4+, HLA-DR+ and interleukin-2 receptor+ (IL-2R+), i.e. activated [103]. Other authors were able to show that T cells in late atherosclerotic plaques express the low molecular variant of the leucocyte common antigen (CD45RO) and the integrin very late activation antigen-1 (VLA-1) [104]. Hansson and his group [103] analysing the rearrangement of T cell receptor (TCR) genes in these latter cells derived from advanced lesions, showed that they represent a polyclonal population rather than displaying restricted TCR usage. These findings support the role of the immune system in atherogenesis.

Major histocompatibility complex (MHC) class II antigen and T cells

Regardless of which antigen these lymphocytes may recognize, it seems inprobable that endothelial cells which aberrantly express MHC class II antigens act as primary antigen-presenting cells for T cell sensitization. Xu *et al.* [105] were able to show MHC class II expression by endothelial cells at sites where T cell accumulations, and thus production of gamma-interferon (IFNγ), were present in the intima directly beneath these areas. Therefore, it can be concluded that the expression of MHC class II molecules by endothelial cells represents a secondary rather than a primary phenomenon. The large majority of $CD3^+$ cells in the mononuclear infiltrate in atherosclerotic lesions express the TCRα/β, but an unexpectedly high proportion also express TCRγ/δ [84]. While the latter type of cell only constitutes approximately 1% of leucocytes in peripheral blood, enrichment to 10% and more within early atherosclerotic lesions can be observed. The majority of these latter cells express the TCRγ 2 chain, i.e. resemble the TCRγ/δ+ population found in the intestinal mucosa. On the other hand, TCR Vγ9δ2+ cells characteristic of circulating TCRγ/δ + cells are not proportionally increased in the intima. Finally, it was possible to demonstrate on the protein- and mRNA-level that endothelial cells as well as leucocytes occurring in atherosclerotic lesions are able to produce a variety of immunological-inflammatory mediators. Among others, these include interleukin-1 (IL-1), tumor necrosis factor-α (TNFα), lymphotoxin, IL-2, IL-6, IL-8, monocyte-chemotactic peptide-1 and IFNγ [106; 107]. Together, these molecules can modulate the local cellular immune response within emerging atherosclerotic lesions.

Oxidized-LDL as a candidate antigen

T cells isolated from human atherosclerotic plaques were shown to be specifically reactive to oxidized-LDL [108]. One-fourth of all CD4+ T cells cloned from human plaques recognized oxidized-LDL in an HLA-DR-dependent manner. Oxidized-LDL-specific T cells are present in lymph nodes of apoE-knockout mice [109], which have strong humoral as well as cellular immune responses to such modified lipoproteins [110]. In humans, oxidized-LDL induces activation of a subset of peripheral T cells. In addition, antibodies to oxidized-LDL can be detected in atherosclerotic patients and experimental animals, and are present in atherosclerotic lesions, suggesting that it is a quantitatively important antigen [111]. The immune response to oxidized-LDL plays a pathogenetic role in atherosclerosis because lesion progression can be inhibited by immunization [112] or induction of neonatal tolerance to oxidized-LDL [109]. It seems paradoxical that both tolerization and hyperimmunization can reduce the extent of disease; this may be due to the different effector pathways activated by these two kinds of treatment.

HSP60 as a candidate antigen

As discussed above, HSPs have been implicated in the activation of innate immune responses involved in the pathogenesis of atherosclerosis [83]. Moreover, adaptive immune reactions to HSP60 have also been implicated in the development of atherosclerosis. For instance, Xu and coworkers [113] immunized rabbits with HSP65/60 and recorded induction of vascular inflammation, with endothelial activation and mononuclear cell adhesion. The developing lesions also contained T cells and cell lines derived from such infiltrates exhibited anti-HSP60 reactivity [85]. Anti-HSP60 antibodies occurred in peripheral blood [114], and immunization with HSP60 was found to increase fatty streak development in hypercholesterolaemic rabbits and mice [115; 116]. In humans, antibodies to HSP65/60 are elevated in early and late atherosclerosis [117; 118] and may predict the progression of atherosclerotic disease [119]. Because HSPs of humans and microbes are structurally and antigenically similar, it is possible that molecular mimicry between immune responses to microbial HSPs and homologues expressed by vascular cells could account for the association between infections and atherosclerosis [120]. Based on these findings, Maron *et al.* [121] provided the evidence that atherosclerotic lesions were reduced by nasal immunization with HSP65 in apoE-deficient mice, suggesting that atherosclerosis might be inhibited by vaccination against HSP65.

β2-glycoprotein Ib as a candidate antigen

A third autoantigen, β2-glycoprotein Ib (β2-GPI), is present on platelets but may also be expressed by endothelial cells. Autoantibodies to β2-GPI are produced in several inflammatory disorders, including atherosclerosis [122; 123]. The immune response to β2-GPI appears to be pro-atherogenic, because hyperimmunization with β2-GPI [116] or transfer of β2-GPI-reactive T cells aggravates fatty streak formation in LDL receptor −/− mice [124]. The pathogenic mechanism by which β2-GPI acts remains unclear, but it may be related to this protein's capacity to bind phospholipids.

In summary, adaptive immunity, with its T cells, antibodies and immunoregulatory cytokines, powerfully modulates the initiation and progression of atherosclerosis. Atherogenesis involves intercommunication between shared pathways involved in adaptive and innate immunity. Various established and emerging risk factors for atherosclerosis modulate aspects of immune responses, including lipoproteins and their modified products, HSPs, and infectious agents. As the molecular details become understood, new potential targets for therapies will doubtless emerge.

INFLAMMATION

It is generally accepted that atherosclerosis is an inflammatory disease [1], because new findings have provided important links between all risk factors and the mechanisms of atherogenesis. Clinical studies have shown that this emerging biology of inflammation in atherosclerosis applies directly to human patients. Elevation of markers for inflammation predicts the outcome in patients with acute coronary syndromes [8]. In addition, low-grade chronic inflammation, as indicated by levels of the inflammatory marker C-reactive protein (CRP), prospectively defines risk of atherosclerotic complications, thus adding to prognostic information provided by traditional risk factors [125]. Moreover, certain treatments that reduce atherosclerosis risk also limit inflammation. For example, statins, used for lipid lowering [8], have anti-inflammatory effects. How inflammation on the vessel wall is triggered has been intensively discussed above, i.e. hypercholesterolaemia, oxidized-LDL, hypertension, biomechanical stress and infection. These risk factors can directly or indirectly stimulate endothelial cells expressing adhesion molecules (VCAM-1, ICAM-1 and E-selectin) followed by mononuclear cell infiltration and foam cell formation in the subendothelial space [1]. In this section, some new findings that have not been described above will be summarized.

C-reactive protein

C-reactive protein is an acute-phase protein that is involved in inflammatory processes. Liuzzo *et al.* [126] demonstrated early on that elevated CRP correlated with an adverse short term prognosis in selected patients with coronary atherosclerosis. Half of the patients with coronary heart disease had persistently elevated CRP after discharge, a finding associated with recurrent episodes of instability and infarction [127]. Patients with severe coronary artery disease or atherosclerosis, had a very low incidence of elevated CRP, affirming the specificity of systemically detectable inflammation in coronary heart disease [128]. Wang *et al.* [129] demonstrated that levels of CRP were associated with subsequent measurements of carotid atherosclerosis in a large community-based cohort. An increased atherosclerotic burden may explain part of the increased risk of cardiovascular events in individuals, particularly women, with elevated CRP levels.

C-reactive protein may be not only a marker of inflammation and atherosclerosis, it may also be an active component participating in atherogenesis [130; 131; 132; 133]. It binds to lipoproteins and activates the complement system via the classical pathway. C-reactive protein deposits in the arterial wall early during lesion formation, which is co-localized with the terminal complement complex. This suggests that CRP may promote atherosclerotic lesion formation by activating the complement system and is involved in foam cell formation, which may be caused in part by the uptake of CRP-opsonized LDL [133].

CD40/CD40L

These antigens are present on the surface of endothelial cells, smooth muscle cells, macrophages, T lymphocytes and platelets within human atheroma [134; 135]. The pro-atherogenic functions of CD40 ligation include augmented expression of matrix metalloproteinases, procoagulant tissue factor, chemokines and cytokines [136; 137; 138]. Indeed, interruption of CD40 signalling not only reduced the initiation and progression of atherosclerotic lesions in hypercholesterolaemic mice *in vivo* [139; 140], but also modulated plaque architecture in ways that might lower the risk for causing thrombosis [141]. In addition to the 39-kDa cell membrane-associated form, CD40L also exists as a soluble protein, termed sCD40L [142]. Although lacking the cytoplasm, transmembrane region and parts of the extracellular domains, this, the soluble form of CD40L, is considered to possess biological activity. Of note, patients with unstable angina express higher sCD40L plasma levels than healthy individuals or patients with stable angina [143]. Moreover, it was recently demonstrated that elevated plasma concentrations of sCD40L predict a risk for future cardiovascular events [144]. Although *in vitro* and *in vivo* studies established that CD40 signalling participates in atherosclerosis, the initial trigger for CD40/CD40L expression within the atheroma may be regulated by oxidized-LDL. Thus CD40/CD40L may be a mediator in the inflammatory responses during the development of atherosclerosis.

SUMMARY AND PERSPECTIVES

Atherosclerosis is an inflammatory disease that is initiated by multiple risk factors, including hypercholesterolaemia, oxidized-LDL, altered biomechanical stress, smoking and infections. Due to research achievements in recent decades, atherogenesis is no longer an inevitable consequence of aging – the statin revolution has left this in no doubt. Better control of hypercholesterolaemia can clearly be achieved but many questions remain. For example, which factor is an initiator for the development of atherosclerotic lesions and how do other factors participate in the disease process. Currently, atherosclerosis research is highly topical. The mystery of the molecular mechanism in this disease will yield to the current multidisciplinary attack by academic institutions and the pharmaceutical industry using the powerful techniques of vascular biology and molecular approaches.

REFERENCES

1. R. Ross, Atherosclerosis – an inflammatory disease. *New England Journal of Medicine*, **340** (1999), 115–26.
2. H. C. Stary, Evolution and progression of atherosclerotic lesions in coronary arteries of children and young adults. *Arteriosclerosis*, **9** (1989), I19–32.
3. N. Anitschkow & S. Chalatow, Ueber expermentelle cholesterinsteatose und ihre bedeutehung einiger pathologischer prozesse. *Central Journal of Pathology and Anatomy*, **24** (1913) 1–9.
4. R. Ross, The pathogenesis of atherosclerosis – an update. *New England Journal of Medicine*, **314** (1986), 488–500.
5. D. Steinberg & J. L. Witztum, Lipoproteins and atherogenesis. Current concepts. *JAMA*, **264** (1990), 3047–52.
6. H. C. Stary, A. B. Chandler, S. Glagov *et al.*, A definition of initial, fatty streak, and intermediate lesions of atherosclerosis. A report from the Committee on Vascular Lesions of the Council on Arteriosclerosis, American Heart Association. *Circulation*, **89** (1994), 2462–78.
7. H. C. Stary, A. B. Chandler, R. E. Dinsmore *et al.*, A definition of advanced types of atherosclerotic lesions and a histological classification of atherosclerosis. A report from the Committee on Vascular Lesions of the Council on Arteriosclerosis, American Heart Association. *Arteriosclerosis, Thrombosis and Vascular Biology*, **15** (1995), 1512–31.
8. P. Libby, P. M. Ridker & A. Maseri, Inflammation and atherosclerosis. *Circulation*, **105** (2002), 1135–43.
9. C. K. Glass & J. L. Witztum, Atherosclerosis: the road ahead. *Cell*, **104** (2001), 503–16.
10. J. L. Goldstein, T. Kita & M. S. Brown, Defective lipoprotein receptors and atherosclerosis. Lessons from an animal counterpart of familial hypercholesterolemia. *New England Journal of Medicine*, **309** (1983), 288–96.
11. G. Brown, J. J. Albers, L. D. Fisher *et al.*, Regression of coronary artery disease as a result of intensive lipid-lowering therapy in men with high levels of apolipoprotein B. *New England Journal of Medicine*, **323** (1990), 1289–98.
12. A. L. Gould, J. E. Rossouw, N. C. Santanello *et al.*, Cholesterol reduction yields clinical benefit: impact of statin trials. *Circulation*, **97** (1998), 946–52.
13. J. A. Berliner & J. W. Heinecke, The role of oxidized lipoproteins in atherogenesis. *Free Radical Biology & Medicine*, **20** (1996), 707–27.
14. D. C. Schwenke & T. E. Carew, Initiation of atherosclerotic lesions in cholesterol-fed rabbits. II. Selective retention of LDL vs. selective increases in LDL permeability in susceptible sites of arteries. *Arteriosclerosis*, **9** (1989), 908–18.
15. S. H. Zhang, R. L. Reddick & J. A. Piedrahita *et al.*, Spontaneous hypercholesterolemia and arterial lesions in mice lacking apolipoprotein E. *Science*, **258** (1992), 468–71.
16. S. Ishibashi, J. L. Goldstein & M. S. Brown *et al.*, Massive xanthomatosis and atherosclerosis in cholesterol-fed low density lipoprotein receptor-negative mice. *Journal of Clinical Investigation*, **93** (1994), 1885–93.
17. H. Li, M. I. Cybulsky, M. A. Gimbrone, Jr. *et al.*, An atherogenic diet rapidly induces VCAM-1, a cytokine-

regulatable mononuclear leukocyte adhesion molecule, in rabbit aortic endothelium. *Arteriosclerosis and Thrombosis*, **13** (1993), 197–204.

18. M. T. Quinn, S. Parthasarathy, L. G. Fong *et al.*, Oxidatively modified low density lipoproteins: a potential role in recruitment and retention of monocyte/macrophages during atherogenesis. *Proceedings of the National Academy of Sciences of the USA*, **84** (1987), 2995–8.
19. J. R. Hessler, D. W. Morel, L. J. Lewis *et al.*, Lipoprotein oxidation and lipoprotein-induced cytotoxicity. *Arteriosclerosis*, **3** (1983), 215–22.
20. S. Yui, T. Sasaki, A. Miyazaki *et al.*, Induction of murine macrophage growth by modified LDLs. *Arterioscerosis and Thrombosis*, **13** (1993), 331–7.
21. S. Chatterjee & N. Ghosh, Oxidized low density lipoprotein stimulates aortic smooth muscle cell proliferation. *Glycobiology*, **6** (1996), 303–11.
22. M. Navab, J. A. Berliner, A. D. Watson *et al.*, The yin and yang of oxidation in the development of the fatty streak. A review based on the 1994 George Lyman Duff Memorial Lecture. *Arteriosclerosis, Thrombosis and Vascular Biology*, **16** (1996), 831–42.
23. D. Steinberg, Atherogenesis in perspective: hypercholesterolemia and inflammation as partners in crime. *Nature Medicine*, **8** (2002), 1211–17.
24. J. L. Witztum & D. Steinberg, The oxidative modification hypothesis of atherosclerosis: does it hold for humans? *Trends in Cardiovascular Medicine*, **11** (2001), 93–102.
25. A. Boullier, D. A. Bird, M. K. Chang *et al.*, Scavenger receptors, oxidized LDL, and atherosclerosis. *Annals of the New York Academy of Sciences*, **947** (2001), 214–22.
26. A. Boullier, K. L. Gillotte & S. Horkko *et al.*, The binding of oxidized low density lipoprotein to mouse CD36 is mediated in part by oxidized phospholipids that are associated with both the lipid and protein moieties of the lipoprotein. *Journal of Biological Chemistry*, **275** (2000), 9163–9.
27. E. A. Podrez, E. Poliakov, Z. Shen *et al.*, A novel family of atherogenic oxidized phospholipids promotes macrophage foam cell formation via the scavenger receptor CD36 and is enriched in atherosclerotic lesions. *Journal of Biological Chemistry*, **277** (2002), 38517–23.
28. R. W. Alexander, Theodore Cooper Memorial Lecture. Hypertension and the pathogenesis of atherosclerosis. Oxidative stress and the mediation of arterial inflammatory response: a new perspective. *Hypertension*, **25** (1995), 155–61.
29. J. Stamler, J. D. Neaton & D. N. Wentworth, Blood pressure (systolic and diastolic) and risk of fatal coronary heart disease. *Hypertension*, **13** (1989), 12–12.
30. W. B. Kannel, J. D. Neaton, D. Wentworth *et al.*, Overall and coronary heart disease mortality rates in relation to major risk factors in 325348 men screened for the MRFIT. Multiple Risk Factor Intervention Trial. *American Heart Journal*, **112** (1986), 825–36.
31. A. V. Chobanian, A. H. Lichtenstein, V. Nilakhe *et al.*, Influence of hypertension on aortic atherosclerosis in the Watanabe rabbit. *Hypertension*, **14** (1989), 203–9.
32. Q. Xu, Biomechanical-stress-induced signaling and gene expression in the development of arteriosclerosis. *Trends in Cardiovascular Medicine*, **10** (2000) 35–41.
33. P. F. Davies, Flow-mediated endothelial mechano-transduction. *Physiological Review*, **75** (1995), 519–60.
34. G. M. Rubanyi, J. C. Romero & P. M. Vanhoutte, Flow-induced release of endothelium-derived relaxing factor. *American Journal of Physiology*, **250** (1986), H1145–9.
35. A. Bhagyalakshmi & J. A. Frangos, Mechanism of shear-induced prostacyclin production in endothelial cells. *Biochemical and Biophysical Research Communications*, **158** (1989), 31–7.
36. A. Zampetaki, Z. Zhang, Y. Hu & Q. Xu, Biomechanical stress induces IL-6 expression in smooth muscle cells via Ras/Rac1-p38 MAPK-NF-kappaB signalling pathways. *American Journal of Heart and Circulatory Physiology*, **288** (2005), H2946–54.
37. H. F. Younis, M. R. Kaazempur-Mofrad, R. C. Chan *et al.*, Hemodynamics and wall mechanics in human carotid bifurcation and its consequences for atherogenesis: investigation of inter-individual variation. *Biomechanical Model and Mechanobiology*, **3** (2004), 17–32.
38. K. S. Cunningham & A.I. Gotlieb, The role of shear stress in the pathogenesis of atherosclerosis. *Laboratory Investigation*, **85** (2005), 9–23.
39. C. Li & Q. Xu, Mechanical stress-initiated signal transductions in vascular smooth muscle cells. *Cell Signal*, **12** (2000), 435–45.
40. R. Seger & E.G. Krebs, The MAPK signaling cascade. *FASEB Journal*, **9** (1995), 726–35.
41. Y. Hu, H. Dietrich, B. Metzler *et al.*, Hyperexpression and activation of extracellular signal-regulated kinases (ERK1/2) in atherosclerotic lesions of cholesterol-fed

rabbits. *Arteriosclerosis, Thrombosis and Vascular Biology*, **20** (2000), 18–26.

42. Q. Xu, Y. Liu, M. Gorospe *et al.*, Acute hypertension activates mitogen-activated protein kinases in arterial wall. *Journal of Clinical Investigation*, **97** (1996) 508–14.
43. F. Wernig & Q. Xu, Mechanical stress-induced apoptosis in the cardiovascular system. *Progress in Biophysics and Molecular Biology*, **78** (2002), 105–37.
44. Y. J. Geng & P. Libby, Progression of atheroma: a struggle between death and procreation. *Arteriosclerosis, Thrombosis and Vascular Biology*, **22** (2002), 1370–80.
45. M. Mayr & Q. Xu, Smooth muscle cell apoptosis in arteriosclerosis. *Experimental Gerontology*, **36** (2001), 969–87.
46. Y. Zou, H. Dietrich, Y. Hu *et al.*, Mouse model of venous bypass graft arteriosclerosis. *American Journal of Pathology*, **153** (1998), 1301–10.
47. H. Dietrich, Y. Hu, Y. Zou *et al.*, Rapid development of vein graft atheroma in ApoE-deficient mice. *American Journal of Pathology*, **157** (2000), 659–69.
48. M. Mayr, C. Li, Y Zou *et al.*, Biomechanical stress-induced apoptosis in vein grafts involves p38 mitogen-activated protein kinases. *FASEB Journal*, **14** (2000), 261–70.
49. M. Mayr, Y. Hu, H. Hainaut *et al.*, Mechanical stress-induced DNA damage and rac-p38 MAPK signal pathways mediate p53-dependent apoptosis in vascular smooth muscle cells. *FASEB Journal*, **16** (2002), 1423–5.
50. U. Mayr, M. Mayr, C. Li *et al.*, Loss of p53 accelerates neointimal lesions of vein bypass grafts in mice. *Circulation Research*, **90** (2002), 197–204.
51. Y. Zou, Y. Hu, M. Mayr *et al.*, Reduced neointima hyperplasia of vein bypass grafts in intercellular adhesion molecule-1-deficient mice. *Circulation Research*, **86** (2000), 434–40.
52. S. Jalali, Y. S. Li, M. Sotoudeh *et al.*, Shear stress activates p60src-Ras-MAPK signaling pathways in vascular endothelial cells. *Arteriosclerosis, Thrombosis and Vascular Biology*, **18** (1998), 227–234.
53. G. C. Cheng, P. Libby, A. J. Grodzinsky *et al.*, Induction of DNA synthesis by a single transient mechanical stimulus of human vascular smooth muscle cells. Role of fibroblast growth factor-2. *Circulation*, **93** (1996), 99–105.
54. T. Yamazaki, I. Komuro, S. Kudoh *et al.*, Mechanical stress activates protein kinase cascade of phosphorylation in neonatal rat cardiac myocytes. *Journal of Clinical Investigation*, **96** (1995), 438–46.
55. Y. Hu, L. Cheng, B. W. Hochleitner *et al.*, Activation of mitogen-activated protein kinases (ERK/JNK) and AP-1 transcription factor in rat carotid arteries after balloon injury. *Arteriosclerosis, Thrombosis and Vascular Biology*, **17** (1997), 2808–16.
56. C. Li, Y. Hu, M. Mayr *et al.*, Cyclic strain stress-induced mitogen-activated protein kinase (MAPK) phosphatase 1 expression in vascular smooth muscle cells is regulated by Ras/Rac-MAPK pathways. *Journal of Biological Chemistry*, **274** (1999), 25273–80.
57. D. F. Liao, J. L. Duff, G. Daum *et al.*, Angiotensin II stimulates MAP kinase kinase kinase activity in vascular smooth muscle cells, Role of Raf. *Circulation Research*, **79** (1996), 1007–14.
58. Y. Hu, B. Bock, G. Wick *et al.*, Activation of PDGF receptor alpha in vascular smooth muscle cells by mechanical stress. *FASEB Journal*, **12** (1998), 1135–42.
59. H. Iwasaki, S. Eguchi, H. Ueno *et al.*, Mechanical stretch stimulates growth of vascular smooth muscle cells via epidermal growth factor receptor. *American Journal of Heart and Circulatory Physiology*, **278** (2000), H521–9.
60. A. Shay-Salit, M. Shushy, E. Wolfovitz *et al.*, VEGF receptor 2 and the adherens junction as a mechanical transducer in vascular endothelial cells. *Proceedings of the National Academy of Sciences of the USA*, **99** (2002), 9462–7.
61. Y. Hu, Y. Zou, H. Dietrich *et al.*, Inhibition of neointima hyperplasia of mouse vein grafts by locally applied suramin. *Circulation*, **100** (1999), 861–8.
62. S. E. Epstein, Y. F. Zhou & J. Zhu, Infection and atherosclerosis: emerging mechanistic paradigms. *Circulation*, **100** (1999), e20–8.
63. S. E. Epstein, J. Zhu, M. S. Burnett *et al.*, Infection and atherosclerosis: potential roles of pathogen burden and molecular mimicry. *Arteriosclerosis, Thrombosis and Vascular Biology*, **20** (2000), 1417–20.
64. S. E. Epstein, The multiple mechanisms by which infection may contribute to atherosclerosis development and course. *Circulation Research*, **90** (2002), 2–4.
65. A. R. Folsom, F. J. Nieto, P. Sorlie *et al.*, *Helicobacter pylori* seropositivity and coronary heart disease incidence. Atherosclerosis Risk In Communities (ARIC) Study Investigators. *Circulation*, **98** (1998), 845–50.
66. J. Danesh & J. Peto, Risk factors for coronary heart disease and infection with *Helicobacter pylori*:

meta-analysis of 18 studies. *British Medical Journal*, **316** (1998), 1130–32.
67. J. Danesh, R. Collins & R. Peto, Chronic infections and coronary heart disease: is there a link? *Lancet*, **350** (1997), 430–6.
68. P. Saikku, M. Leinonen, K. Mattila *et al.*, Serological evidence of an association of a novel *Chlamydia*, TWAR, with chronic coronary heart disease and acute myocardial infarction. *Lancet*, **2** (1988), 983–6.
69. I. W. Fong, Value of animal models for *Chlamydia pneumoniae*-related atherosclerosis. *American Heart Journal*, **138** (1999), S512–13.
70. C. C. Kuo, A. M. Gown, E. P. Benditt *et al.*, Detection of *Chlamydia pneumoniae* in aortic lesions of atherosclerosis by immunocytochemical stain. *Arteriosclerosis and Thrombosis*, **13** (1993), 1501–4.
71. M. A. Mendall, P. M. Goggin, N. Molineaux *et al.*, Relation of *Helicobacter pylori* infection and coronary heart disease. *British Heart Journal*, **71** (1994), 437–9.
72. M. Mayr, S. Kiechl, J. Willeit *et al.*, Increased risk of atherosclerosis is confined to CagA positive *H. pylori* strains: prospective results from the Bruneck study. *Stroke*, **33** (2002), 2170–6.
73. W. J. Welch, How cells respond to stress. *Scientific American*, **268** (1993), 56–64.
74. M. J. Gething, Protein folding. The difference with prokaryotes. *Nature*, **388** (1997), 329, 331.
75. I. J. Benjamin, & D. R. McMillan, Stress (heat shock) proteins: molecular chaperones in cardiovascular biology and disease. *Circulation Research*, **83** (1998), 117–32.
76. L. H. Snoeckx, R. N. Cornelussen, F. A. Van Nieuwenhoven *et al.*, Heat shock proteins and cardiovascular pathophysiology. *Physiological Review*, **81** (2001), 1461–97.
77. E. A. Craig, B. D. Gambill & R. J. Nelson, Heat shock proteins: molecular chaperones of protein biogenesis. *Microbiological Review*, **57** (1993), 402–14.
78. E. A. Craig, J. S. Weissman & A. L. Horwich, Heat shock proteins and molecular chaperones: mediators of protein conformation and turnover in the cell. *Cell*, **78** (1994), 365–72.
79. J. Mollenhauer & A. Schulmeister, The humoral immune response to heat shock proteins. *Experientia*, **48** (1992), 644–9.
80. Q. Xu & G. Wick, The role of heat shock proteins in protection and pathophysiology of the arterial wall. *Molecular Medicine Today*, **2** (1996), 372–9.
81. P. Roma & A. L. Catapano, Stress proteins and atherosclerosis. *Atherosclerosis*, **127** (1996), 147–54.
82. A. G. Pockley, Heat shock proteins, inflammation, and cardiovascular disease. *Circulation*, **105** (2002), 1012–17.
83. Q. Xu, Role of heat shock proteins in atherosclerosis. *Arteriosclerosis, Thrombosis and Vascular Biology*, **22** (2002), 1547–59.
84. R. Kleindienst, Q. Xu, J. Willeit *et al.*, Immunology of atherosclerosis. Demonstration of heat shock protein 60 expression and T lymphocytes bearing alpha/beta or gamma/delta receptor in human atherosclerotic lesions. *American Journal of Pathology*, **142** (1993), 1927–37.
85. Q. Xu, R. Kleindienst, W. Waitz *et al.*, Increased expression of heat shock protein 65 coincides with a population of infiltrating T lymphocytes in atherosclerotic lesions of rabbits specifically responding to heat shock protein 65. *Journal of Clinical Investigation*, **91** (1993), 2693–702.
86. A. Hammerer-Lercher, J. Mair, J. Bonatti *et al.*, Hypoxia induces heat shock protein expression in human coronary artery bypass grafts. *Cardiovascular Research*, **50** (2001), 115–24.
87. A. Kol, G. K. Sukhova, A. H. Lichtman *et al.*, Chlamydial heat shock protein 60 localizes in human atheroma and regulates macrophage tumor necrosis factor-alpha and matrix metalloproteinase expression. *Circulation*, **98** (1998), 300–7.
88. Q. Xu, G. Schett, H. Perschinka *et al.*, Serum soluble heat shock protein 60 is elevated in subjects with atherosclerosis in a general population. *Circulation*, **102** (2000), 14–20.
89. P. Srivastava, Roles of heat-shock proteins in innate and adaptive immunity. *Nature Reviews Immunology*, **2** (2002), 185–94.
90. R. Medzhitov, Toll-like receptors and innate immunity. *Nature Reviews Immunology*, **1** (2001), 135–45.
91. G. K. Hansson, P. Libby, U. Schonbeck *et al.*, Innate and adaptive immunity in the pathogenesis of atherosclerosis. *Circulation Research*, **91** (2002), 281–91.
92. X. H. Xu, P. K. Shah, E. Faure *et al.*, Toll-like receptor-4 is expressed by macrophages in murine and human lipid-rich atherosclerotic plaques and upregulated by oxidized LDL. *Circulation*, **104** (2001), 3103–08.
93. K. Edfeldt, J. Swedenborg, G. K. Hansson *et al.*, Expression of toll-like receptors in human atherosclerotic lesions: a possible pathway for plaque activation. *Circulation*, **105** (2002), 1158–61.

94. S. Kiechl, E. Lorenz, M. Reindl *et al.*, Toll-like receptor 4 polymorphisms and atherogenesis. *New England Journal of Medicine*, **347** (2002), 185–92.
95. K. Ohashi, V. Burkart, S. Flohe *et al.*, Cutting edge: heat shock protein 60 is a putative endogenous ligand of the toll-like receptor-4 complex. *Journal of Immunology*, **164** (2000), 558–61.
96. A. Asea, M. Rehli, E. Kabingu *et al.*, Novel signal transduction pathway utilized by extracellular HSP70. *Journal of Biological Chemistry*, **277** (2002), 15028–34.
97. A. Kol, A. H. Lichtman, R. W. Finberg *et al.*, Cutting edge: heat shock protein (HSP) 60 activates the innate immune response: CD14 is an essential receptor for HSP60 activation of mononuclear cells. *Journal of Immunology*, **164** (2000), 13–17.
98. Y. Bulut, E. Faure, L. Thomas *et al.*, Chlamydial heat shock protein 60 activates macrophages and endothelial cells through Toll-like receptor 4 and MD2 in a MyD88-dependent pathway. *Journal of Immunology*, **168** (2002), 1435–40.
99. G. Wick, H. Perschinka & G. Millonig, Atherosclerosis as an autoimmune disease: an update. *Trends in Immunology*, **22** (2001), 665–9.
100. G. K. Hansson, Immune mechanisms in atherosclerosis. *Arteriosclerosis, Thrombosis and Vascular Biology*, **21** (2001), 1876–90.
101. P. S. Seifert, M. D. Kazatchkine, The complement system in atherosclerosis. *Atherosclerosis*, **73** (1988), 91–104.
102. G. Millonig, G. T. Malcom & G. Wick, Early inflammatory-immunological lesions in juvenile atherosclerosis from the Pathobiological Determinants of Atherosclerosis in Youth (PDAY)-study. *Atherosclerosis*, **160** (2002), 441–8.
103. S. Stemme, L. Rymo & G. K. Hansson, Polyclonal origin of T lymphocytes in human atherosclerotic plaques. *Laboratory Investigation*, **65** (1991), 654–60.
104. X. Zhou, S. Stemme & G. K. Hansson, Evidence for a local immune response in atherosclerosis. CD4+ T cells infiltrate lesions of apolipoprotein-E-deficient mice. *American Journal of Pathology*, **149** (1996), 359–66.
105. Q. B. Xu, G. Oberhuber, M. Gruschwitz *et al.*, Immunology of atherosclerosis: cellular composition and major histocompatibility complex class II antigen expression in aortic intima, fatty streaks, and atherosclerotic plaques in young and aged human specimens. *Clinical Immunology and Immunopathology*, **56** (1990), 344–59.
106. P. Libby & G. H. Hansson, Involvement of the immune system in human atherogenesis: current knowledge and unanswered questions. *Laboratory Investigation*, **64** (1991), 5–15.
107. J. L. Young, P. Libby & U. Schonbeck, Cytokines in the pathogenesis of atherosclerosis. *Thrombosis and Haemostosis*, **88** (2002), 554–67.
108. S. Stemme, B. Faber, J. Holm *et al.*, T lymphocytes from human atherosclerotic plaques recognize oxidized low density lipoprotein. *Proceedings of the National Academy of Sciences of the USA*, **92** (1995), 3893–97.
109. A. Nicoletti, G. Paulsson, G. Caligiuri *et al.*, Induction of neonatal tolerance to oxidized lipoprotein reduces atherosclerosis in ApoE knockout mice. *Molecular Medicine*, **6** (2000), 283–90.
110. W. Palinski, S. Horkko, E. Miller *et al.*, Cloning of monoclonal autoantibodies to epitopes of oxidized lipoproteins from apolipoprotein E-deficient mice. Demonstration of epitopes of oxidized low density lipoprotein in human plasma. *Journal of Clinical Investigation*, **98** (1996), 800–14.
111. J. Frostegard, R. Wu, R. Giscombe *et al.*, Induction of T-cell activation by oxidized low density lipoprotein. *Arteriosclerosis and Thrombosis*, **12** (1992), 461–7.
112. S. Ameli, A. Hultgardh-Nilsson, J. Regnstrom *et al.*, Effect of immunization with homologous LDL and oxidized LDL on early atherosclerosis in hypercholesterolemic rabbits. *Arteriosclerosis, Thrombosis and Vascular Biology*, **16** (1996), 1074–9.
113. Q. Xu, H. Dietrich, H. J. Steiner *et al.*, Induction of arteriosclerosis in normocholesterolemic rabbits by immunization with heat shock protein 65. *Arteriosclerosis and Thrombosis*, **12** (1992), 789–799.
114. Q. Xu, J. Willeit, M. Marosi *et al.*, Association of serum antibodies to heat-shock protein 65 with carotid atherosclerosis. *Lancet*, **341** (1993), 255–9.
115. Q. Xu, R. Kleindienst, G. Schett *et al.*, Regression of arteriosclerotic lesions induced by immunization with heat shock protein 65-containing material in normocholesterolemic, but not hypercholesterolemic, rabbits. *Atherosclerosis*, **123** (1996), 145–55.
116. J. George, A. Afek, B. Gilburd *et al.*, Induction of early atherosclerosis in LDL-receptor-deficient mice immunized with beta2-glycoprotein I. *Circulation*, **98** (1998), 1108–15.

117. J. Zhu, A. A. Quyyumi, D. Rott *et al.*, Antibodies to human heat-shock protein 60 are associated with the presence and severity of coronary artery disease: evidence for an autoimmune component of atherogenesis. *Circulation*, **103** (2001), 1071–5.
118. M. Mukherjee, C. De Benedictis, D. Jewitt *et al.*, Association of antibodies to heat-shock protein-65 with percutaneous transluminal coronary angioplasty and subsequent restenosis. *Thrombosis and Haemostasis*, **75** (1996), 258–60.
119. Q. Xu, S. Kiechl, M. Mayr *et al.*, Association of serum antibodies to heat-shock protein 65 with carotid atherosclerosis: clinical significance determined in a follow-up study. *Circulation*, **100** (1999), 1169–74.
120. M. Mayr, S. Kiechl, J. Willeit *et al.*, Infections, immunity, and atherosclerosis: associations of antibodies to *Chlamydia pneumoniae*, *Helicobacter pylori*, and cytomegalovirus with immune reactions to heat-shock protein 60 and carotid or femoral atherosclerosis. *Circulation*, **102** (2000), 833–9.
121. R. Maron, G. Sukhova, A. M. Faria *et al.*, Mucosal administration of heat shock protein-65 decreases atherosclerosis and inflammation in aortic arch of low-density lipoprotein receptor-deficient mice. *Circulation*, **106** (2002), 1708–15.
122. J. Frostegard, R. Wu, C. Gillis-Haegerstrand *et al.*, Antibodies to endothelial cells in borderline hypertension. *Circulation*, **98** (1998), 1092–8.
123. Y. Shoenfeld, D. Harats & J. George, Atherosclerosis and the antiphospholipid syndrome: a link unravelled? *Lupus*, **7** (Suppl 2) (1998), S140–3.
124. J. George, D. Harats, B. Gilburd *et al.*, Adoptive transfer of beta(2)-glycoprotein I-reactive lymphocytes enhances early atherosclerosis in LDL receptor-deficient mice. *Circulation*, **102** (2000), 1822–7.
125. P. M. Ridker, C. H. Hennekens, J. E. Buring *et al.*, C-reactive protein and other markers of inflammation in the prediction of cardiovascular disease in women. *New England Journal of Medicine*, **342** (2000), 836–43.
126. G. Liuzzo, L. M. Biasucci, A. G. Rebuzzi *et al.*, Plasma protein acute-phase response in unstable angina is not induced by ischemic injury. *Circulation*, **94** (1996), 2373–80.
127. P. M. Ridker, M. J. Stampfer & N. Rifai, Novel risk factors for systemic atherosclerosis: a comparison of C-reactive protein, fibrinogen, homocysteine, lipoprotein(a), and standard cholesterol screening as predictors of peripheral arterial disease. *JAMA*, **285** (2001), 2481–5.
128. P. M. Ridker, J. E. Buring, J. Shih *et al.*, Prospective study of C-reactive protein and the risk of future cardiovascular events among apparently healthy women. *Circulation*, **98** (1998), 731–3.
129. T. J. Wang, B. H. Nam, P. W. Wilson *et al.*, Association of C-reactive protein with carotid atherosclerosis in men and women: the Framingham Heart Study. *Arteriosclerosis, Thrombosis and Vascular Biology*, **22** (2002), 1662–7.
130. J. Torzewski, M. Torzewski, D. E. Bowyer *et al.*, C-reactive protein frequently colocalizes with the terminal complement complex in the intima of early atherosclerotic lesions of human coronary arteries. *Arteriosclerosis, Thrombosis and Vascular Biology*, **18** (1998), 1386–92.
131. I. W. Fong, B. Chiu, E. Viira *et al.*, Chlamydial heat-shock protein-60 antibody and correlation with *Chlamydia pneumoniae* in atherosclerotic plaques. *Journal of Infectious Disease*, **186** (2002),1469–73.
132. A. Klegeris, E. A. Singh & P. L. McGeer, Effects of C-reactive protein and pentosan polysulphate on human complement activation. *Immunology*, **106** (2002), 381–8.
133. T. P. Zwaka, V. Hombach & J. Torzewski, C-reactive protein-mediated low density lipoprotein uptake by macrophages: implications for atherosclerosis. *Circulation*, **103** (2001), 1194–7.
134. F. Mach, U. Schonbeck, G. K. Sukhova *et al.*, Functional CD40 ligand is expressed on human vascular endothelial cells, smooth muscle cells, and macrophages: implications for CD40-CD40 ligand signaling in atherosclerosis. *Proceedings of the National Academy of Sciences of the USA*, **94** (1997), 1931–6.
135. R. M. Reul, J. C. Fang, M. D. Denton *et al.*, CD40 and CD40 ligand (CD154) are coexpressed on microvessels *in vivo* in human cardiac allograft rejection. *Transplantation*, **64** (1997), 1765–74.
136. N. Malik, B. W. Greenfield, A. F. Wahl *et al.*, Activation of human monocytes through CD40 induces matrix metalloproteinases. *Journal of Immunology*, **156** (1996), 3952–60.
137. D. L. Miller, R. Yaron & M. J. Yellin, CD40L-CD40 interactions regulate endothelial cell surface tissue factor and thrombomodulin expression. *Journal of Leukocyte Biology*, **63** (1998), 373–9.

138. U. Schonbeck & P. Libby, The CD40/CD154 receptor/ligand dyad. *Cellular and Molecular Life Sciences*, **58** (2001), 4–43.
139. E. Lutgens, L. Gorelik, M. J. Daemen *et al.*, Requirement for CD154 in the progression of atherosclerosis. *Nature Medicine*, **5** (1999), 1313–16.
140. F. Mach, U. Schonbeck, G. K. Sukhova *et al.*, Reduction of atherosclerosis in mice by inhibition of CD40 signalling. *Nature*, **394** (1998), 200–3.
141. E. Lutgens, K. B. Cleutjens, S. Heeneman *et al.*, Both early and delayed anti-CD40L antibody treatment induces a stable plaque phenotype. *Proceedings of the National Academy of Sciences of the USA*, **97** (2000), 7464–9.
142. B. Ludewig, V. Henn, J. M. Schroder *et al.*, Induction, regulation, and function of soluble TRAP (CD40 ligand) during interaction of primary CD4+ CD45RA+ T cells with dendritic cells. *European Journal of Immunology*, **26** (1996), 3137–43.
143. P. Aukrust, F. Muller, T. Ueland *et al.*, Enhanced levels of soluble and membrane-bound CD40 ligand in patients with unstable angina. Possible reflection of T lymphocyte and platelet involvement in the pathogenesis of acute coronary syndromes. *Circulation*, **100** (1999), 614–20.
144. U. Schonbeck & P. Libby, CD40 signaling and plaque instability. *Circulation Research*, **89** (2001), 1092–103.

8 • Mechanisms of plaque rupture

KEVIN J. MOLLOY AND IAN M. LOFTUS

INTRODUCTION

Atherosclerosis continues to cause considerable morbidity and mortality, particularly in the western world. While risk factors have been clearly identified, their precise roles in early atherogenesis are complex. The early development of the plaque is dependent upon interactions between damaged endothelial cells, vessel wall smooth muscle cells and circulating inflammatory cells, mediated by the release of cytokines, growth factors and cell adhesion molecules. Plaque formation may represent a cell-mediated immune phenomenon, with a variety of potential antigenic agents identified. Shear stress and flow considerations also play a part.

Atherosclerosis begins in childhood, but it takes decades for atherosclerosis to evolve into the mature plaques responsible for the onset of ischaemic symptoms. Whilst plaque growth due to smooth muscle cell proliferation, matrix synthesis and lipid accumulation may narrow the arterial lumen and ultimately limit blood flow, uncomplicated atherosclerosis is essentially a benign disease. The final clinical outcome depends on whether a plaque becomes unstable, leading to acute disruption of its surface and exposure of its thrombogenic core to the luminal blood flow. The concept of a 'vulnerable plaque' was initially described in 1990 [1] and is now largely accepted [2].

The mature atherosclerotic plaque is composed of a lipid core that is separated from the vessel lumen by a cap composed of fibrillar collagen. Disruption of this cap exposes the plaque's underlying thrombogenic core to the bloodstream, resulting in thrombo-embolism. This process of 'plaque rupture' is responsible for the majority of acute coronary syndromes (unstable angina, MI) [3; 4; 5; 6] and ischaemic cerebral events (stroke, TIA, amaurosis fugax) [7; 8; 9].

Unravelling the complex biochemical and haemodynamic factors leading to plaque rupture is one of the greatest challenges facing contemporary medical research. The vital question in plaque pathogenesis is why, after years of indolent growth, life-threatening disruption and subsequent thrombosis should suddenly occur. Plaque stabilization may prove to be an important clinical strategy for preventing the development of complications [3]. By identifying 'vulnerable' plaques (i.e., those most at risk of rupture) we can more effectively direct pharmacotherapy to those most likely to benefit. Also, by understanding the mechanisms of plaque rupture we can strive to develop new treatments aimed at prevention.

EVIDENCE FOR THE 'PLAQUE RUPTURE' THEORY

Coronary circulation

Evidence that plaque rupture leads to acute coronary syndromes has been provided from a number of sources. Early pathological studies using post-mortem specimens from fatal cases of acute myocardial infarction have revealed that virtually all cases of coronary thrombosis are related to rupture or fissuring of atheromatous plaques, along with evidence of distal embolization [6; 10; 11; 12]. Angioscopic findings in patients with stable angina have identified smooth atheroma within their coronary arteries, but disrupted irregular atheroma in the arteries of those with unstable angina [13; 14].

Radiological and histological studies have demonstrated that patients with plaque morphology consisting of large lipid cores and thin fibrous caps are at an increased risk of cardiovascular events [15; 16; 17]. In addition, these 'unstable' plaques are not necessarily the ones causing severely stenotic lesions [18; 19; 20].

Cerebral circulation

A similar association between carotid plaque rupture and cerebrovascular events has been shown. In

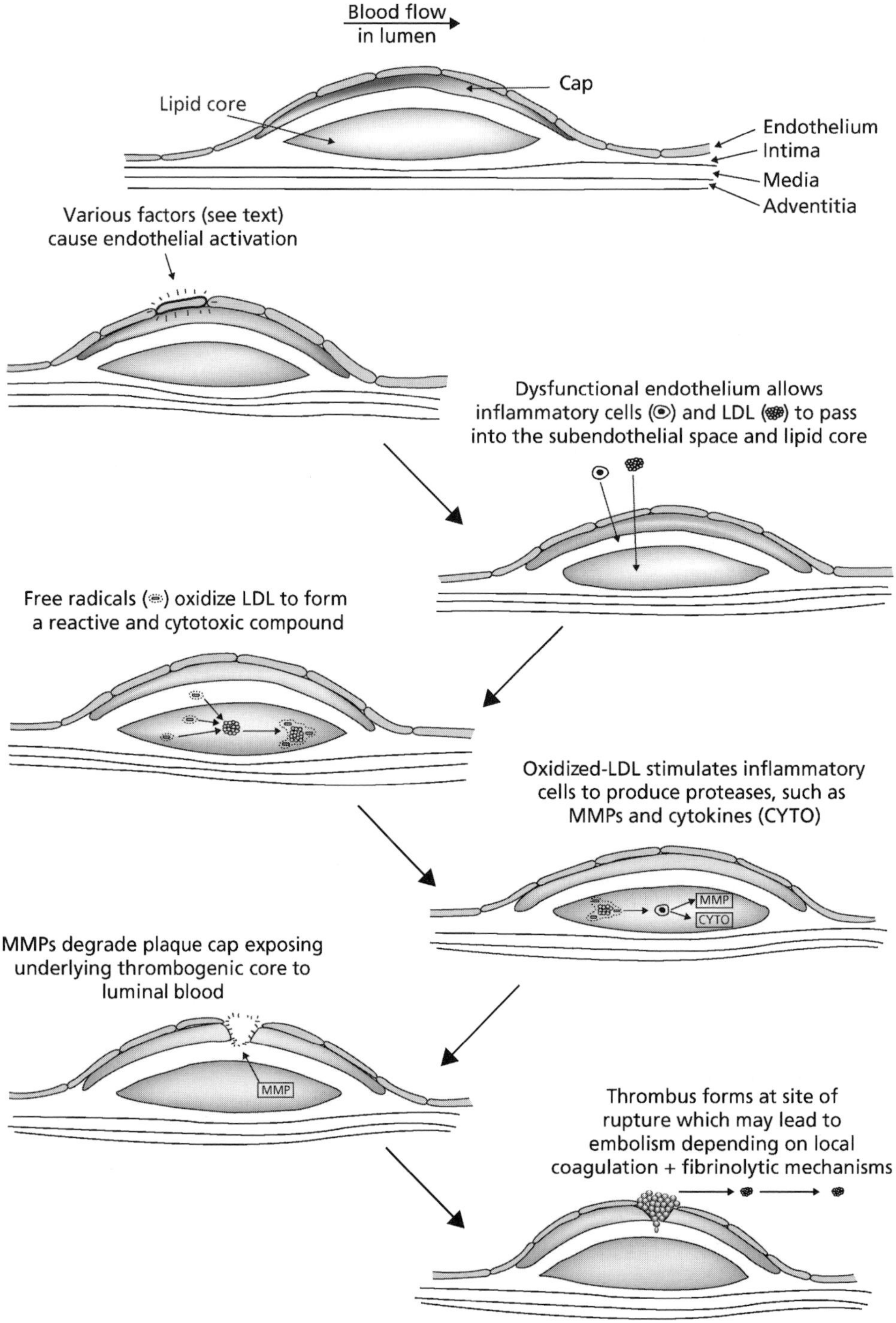

Fig. 8.1. The stages of plaque rupture.

patients undergoing multiple TIAs or stroke progression, microemboli can be detected in the middle cerebral artery by transcranial Doppler [7; 21]. Surface ulceration of carotid plaques seen on ultrasound imaging correlates well with symptoms [22] and echolucent (lipid-rich) plaques are at an increased risk of causing future cerebrovascular events.

Early work utilizing carotid plaques retrieved at carotid endarterectomy, highlighted the relationship between the presence of a thrombus and the clinical status of patients [23; 24]. This supported the theory that ischaemic attacks resulted from embolism rather than reduction in cerebral blood flow, particularly as few strokes occur in watershed areas [25].

A number of subsequent studies demonstrated a relationship between the presence of intraplaque haemorrhage and patient symptoms [26]. Persson *et al.* found that intraplaque haemorrhage appeared more frequently in symptomatic patients than asymptomatic patients [27], while Lusby *et al.* suggested a relationship between the onset of neurological symptoms and development of plaque haemorrhage [28]. Intraplaque haemorrhage may occur following cap rupture or disruption. Conversely, neovascularization identified in unstable plaques may result in plaque haemorrhage, since new vessels are more fragile and prone to haemorrhage [29]. The rapid expansion in the volume of the lipid core may increase the stress upon a weakened cap predisposing it to acute disruption.

The most compelling evidence for an association between carotid plaque rupture and ischaemic cerebral events, is that carotid endarterectomy specimens removed from symptomatic patients are more likely to show histological evidence of rupture, compared with those from asymptomatic patients [8; 9]. Van Damme and colleagues showed that 53% of complicated carotid plaques (intraplaque haemorrhage, haematoma, thrombus or ulceration) were symptomatic with a corresponding neurological deficit, compared to 21% of simple uncomplicated plaques [30].

THE ROLE OF INDIVIDUAL COMPONENTS OF THE ARTERIAL WALL

A number of intrinsic and extrinsic factors have been identified that determine plaque vulnerability: the size and consistency of the plaque core, the thickness and collagen content of the fibrous cap, and inflammation within the plaque. Further factors such as haemodynamic stress upon the plaque may ultimately contribute to cap disruption.

The evolution of a stable to an unstable plaque with cap rupture and thrombosis can be outlined in the following simplistic terms (Figure 8.1): endothelial damage allows passage of inflammatory cells and LDL into the vessel intima; free radicals are responsible for oxidation of the deposited LDL, and oxidized-LDL promotes cytokine and protease release from macrophages; proteases degrade the fibrous cap causing disruption, allowing exposure of thrombogenic material to the blood; and local thrombotic and fibrinolytic activity determine the degree of thrombus progression or dissolution.

Each component contributing to plaque rupture will be discussed in further detail. The relevant processes occur in the endothelium, the lipid core, the fibrous cap and the vessel lumen.

The endothelium

The origin of plaque destabilization can be traced back to endothelial dysfunction, or 'activation'. The endothelium is a single layer of highly specialized cells lining the vessel wall/lumen interface. It plays a vital role in modulating vascular permeability, perfusion, contraction and haemostasis (Chapter 1). Leucocytes do not bind to normal endothelium. However, endothelial activation leads to the early surface expression of cell adhesion molecules, including VCAM-1, ICAM-1, E-selectin and P-selectin, which permit leucocyte binding. Many of the known atherosclerosis risk factors (e.g., smoking, hyperlipidaemia, hyperglycaemia, hypertension, hyperhomocysteinaemia) exert their damaging effects by causing endothelial activation [31; 32; 33; 34; 35; 36].

Activated endothelial cells express chemoattractant cytokines such as MCP-1, MCSF, IL-1, IL-6 and TNF-α, as well as cell adhesion molecules. This pro-inflammatory environment, in conjunction with the altered permeability of the dysfunctional endothelium, mediates the migration and entry of leucocytes (mainly monocytes and lymphocytes) into the intima [37; 38; 39].

The degree of endothelial dysfunction depends upon the balance between endothelial activation and endothelial 'passivation' (Figure 8.2). Nitric oxide is

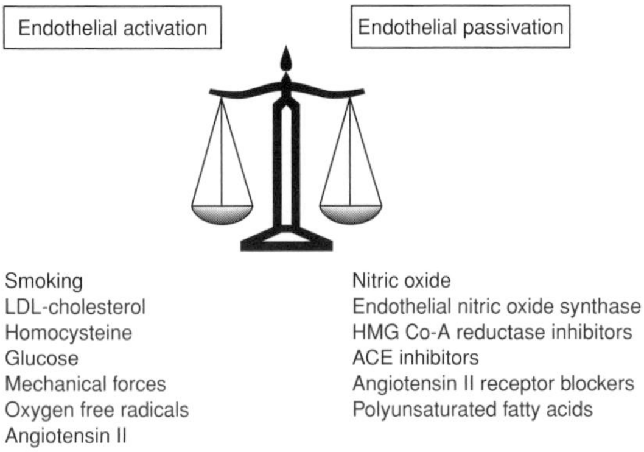

Fig. 8.2. Endothelial activation versus endothelial passivation.

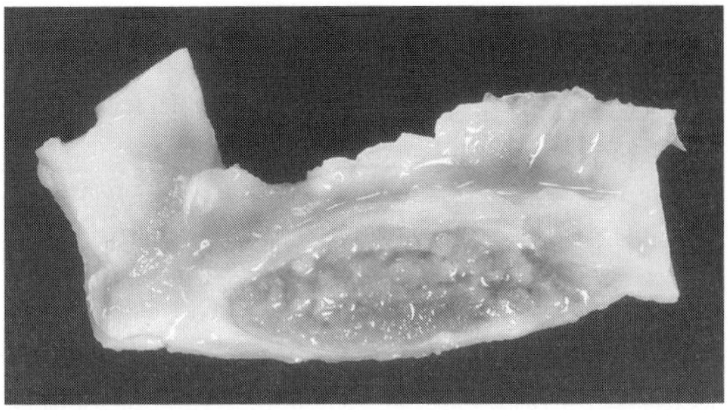

Fig. 8.3. Longitudinal section of carotid plaque demonstrating a large volume lipid core (see colour plate section).

the predominant molecule responsible for passivation and the endothelium acts as an autocrine organ in its production [40]. Nitric oxide is an antioxidant, but has other plaque-stabilizing properties, including reducing cell adhesion molecule expression [41], platelet aggregation and SMC proliferation. Endothelial nitric oxide synthase, the enzyme responsible for nitric oxide production, is increased in people undergoing regular physical exertion, which may partly explain the benefits of exercise in atherosclerosis prevention [42].

Endothelial cells are exposed to three different types of mechanical force. Hydrostatic forces (generated by the blood) and circumferential stress (generated by the vessel wall) are responsible for endothelial injury and activation. The third force is haemodynamic shear stress (generated by the flow of blood), which is inversely related to atherosclerosis formation – areas of high shear stress being relatively protected [43]. Despite the systemic nature of atherosclerosis, it is an anatomically focal disease with certain sites having a propensity for plaque formation. Arterial bifurcations exhibit slow blood flow, sometimes even bi-directional flow, resulting in decreased shear stress. The activity of endothelial nitric oxide synthase is decreased in these areas of non-laminar blood flow [44; 45]. In addition, there is increased oscillatory and turbulent shear stress at bifurcations, associated with an increase in oxygen free radical production [46] and monocyte adhesion [47].

According to Laplace's law, the higher the blood pressure and the larger the luminal diameter, the more circumferential tension develops in the wall [48]. This phenomenon combined with a radial compression of the vessel wall may lead to unbearable stress in vulnerable regions of the plaque, particularly the cap and shoulder [49]. For fibrous caps of the same tensile strength, those caps covering moderately stenotic plaques are probably more prone to rupture than those covering severely stenotic plaques, because the former have to bear a greater circumferential tension [50].

The propagating pulse wave causes cyclic changes in lumen size and shape with deformation and bending of plaques, particularly those with a large soft plaque core. Eccentric plaques typically bend at the junction between the relatively stiff plaque and the compliant vessel wall [51]. The force applied to this region is accentuated by changes in vascular tone.

High blood velocity within stenotic lesions may shear the endothelium away, but whether high wall stress alone may disrupt a stenotic plaque is questionable [5]. The absolute stresses induced by wall shear are usually much smaller than the mechanical stresses imposed by blood and pulse pressure [52].

It is clear that the endothelium is much more than an inert arterial wall lining. It is, in fact, a dynamic autocrine and paracrine organ responsible for the functional regulation of local haemodynamics. Factors that disturb this delicate balance are responsible for the initiation of a cascade of events eventually leading to plaque rupture.

The lipid core

The size and consistency of the atheromatous core is variable and critical to the stability of individual lesions, with a large volume lipid core being one of the constituents of the vulnerable plaque (Figure 8.3). It appears that the accumulation of lipids in the intima renders the plaque inherently unstable.

Although extremely variable, the 'average' coronary plaque is predominantly sclerotic with the atheromatous core making up <30% of the plaque volume [53]. The variability in plaque composition is poorly understood, with no relationship to any of the identified risk factors for atherosclerosis. Gertz and Roberts examined the histological composition of post-mortem plaques from 17 infarct-related coronary arteries [54]. They found much larger proportions of the disrupted plaques to be occupied by atheromatous gruel in comparison to the intact plaques. Davies *et al.* found a similar relationship in aortic lesions, with 91% of thrombosing plaques versus 11% of intact plaques exhibiting a lipid core that occupied >40% of the total plaque volume [55].

Histological data regarding the necrotic core of carotid plaques is limited. There is, however, considerable evidence to link ultrasound-detected echolucent plaques (deemed to contain more soft or amorphous tissue) with symptomatology [56; 57]. Feeley and colleagues demonstrated a significant increase in the proportion of symptomatic carotid plaques occupied by amorphous material compared with asymptomatic plaques [58], though other studies have failed to show such a relationship [8].

Low-density lipoprotein plays a more complex role in plaque instability than can be explained simply by the 'space-occupying' effect of accumulated lipid. A large core may produce a greater luminal narrowing, but plaque rupture sites are often characterized by 'outward remodelling' whereas those stenoses causing stable angina are more likely to be associated with 'inward remodelling' [59]. Indeed, it has been shown that in patients suffering acute coronary syndromes who had undergone angiography in the preceding months, the responsible lesion was recorded as causing a <70% stenosis in the majority of cases [18; 20; 59]. This is perhaps not surprising since, as mentioned earlier, a larger lumen places increased circumferential stress on the plaque, predisposing it to rupture.

As inflammatory cells cross the dysfunctional epithelium, cholesterol also enters in the form of LDL and becomes trapped in the subendothelial space. This LDL is oxidized by free radicals creating a pro-inflammatory compound [60]. Oxidized-LDL is taken up by intimal macrophages – the process being mediated via receptors expressed on the macrophage surface [61], although endocytosis of native LDL has also been demonstrated [62]. This process initially protects the surrounding smooth muscle and endothelial cells from the direct cytotoxic effects of oxidized-LDL, but leads to the formation of 'foam cells' (lipid-laden macrophages). Uptake of oxidized-LDL stimulates the expression of cytokines and proteolytic enzymes, propagating the cycle of inflammation.

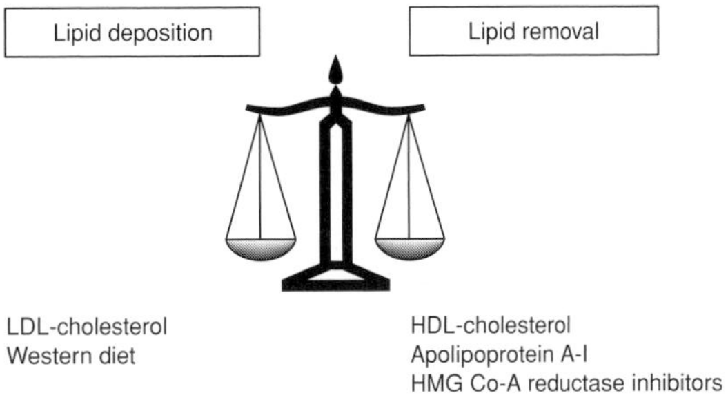

Fig. 8.4. Lipid deposition versus lipid removal.

The formation of a lipid core is a balance between LDL deposition of cholesterol in the damaged intima and removal by HDL (Figure 8.4). High density lipoprotein and its carrier, apolipoprotein A-I, are responsible for so-called 'reverse cholesterol transport' – moving cholesterol from cells into the blood (from where it can be transferred to the liver for excretion in the bile) [63]. However, it may also be capable of effecting lipid removal directly from the plaque, one of the possible explanations for plaque regression seen with increased HDL levels [64]. High density lipoprotein may have other beneficial effects also, such as improving endothelial function [65], decreasing cell adhesion molecule expression [66], and inhibiting oxidation of LDL [67].

The cap of the plaque

The cap of the atherosclerotic plaque plays a vital role in isolating the plaque's thrombogenic core from the bloodstream. The thickness and collagen content of the cap are important determinants of its strength, and therefore the overall stability of the plaque [50]. The cap is composed predominantly of fibrillar collagens, type I and type III [68]. The fibrillar collagens present in the cap have a lower thrombogenicity than the underlying core, but their exposure can be responsible for thrombus formation following erosion of the overlying endothelium [69; 70]. This phenomenon accounts for one-third

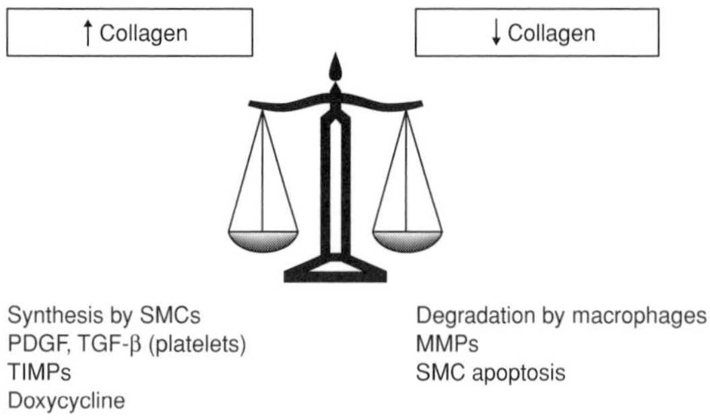

Fig. 8.5. Matrix production versus matrix degradation.

of acute coronary syndromes [71], and the subsequent healing process of erosions can account for rapid and step-wise progression in plaque growth, leading to sudden increases in stenosis or occlusion [72].

The most vulnerable area of the plaque is the shoulder region, where the cap is often at its thinnest [6]. Studies have shown a reduction in the collagen content of the cap around areas of plaque disruption, as well as steep transverse gradients of connective tissue constituents across ulcerated plaques [73]. This may result from a reduction in matrix production by smooth muscle cells, which exhibit diminished numbers in areas of plaque disruption [55], or from increased degradation of matrix by proteolytic enzymes. It is most likely, of course, that a combination of excessive matrix degradation and reduced matrix production are responsible for cap thinning (Figure 8.5). A reduction in SMCs within the fibrous cap would certainly undermine its strength [74]. Recently there has been interest in the role of SMC apoptosis in plaque cap weakening, caused by a combination of intrinsic and extrinsic factors, particularly macrophage and lipid derived products [75; 76].

Smooth muscle cells and collagen production

The SMC has a paradoxical role in plaque instability. On the one hand, SMCs are responsible for plaque matrix production and adverse arterial remodelling, while on the other, they produce collagens that give the plaque intrinsic strength. Smooth muscle cell inhibition therefore has potentially detrimental and beneficial effects.

In the normal arterial wall, SMCs are present in the media and express a differentiated phenotype. They are contractile and do not divide or migrate [77]. In atherosclerosis, when stimulated by the milieu of growth factors and cyokines, they 'dedifferentiate' and express a synthetic phenotype [78]. In the media, SMCs are surrounded by a basal lamina consisting of type IV collagen. Proteolytic enzymes secreted by macrophages are responsible for digestion of this supporting framework. The released SMCs are then able to migrate to the intima, where they secrete new extracellular matrix [79]. Smooth muscle cells play a crucial role in stabilizing atherosclerotic plaques, as they are responsible for the production of the cap fibrillar collagens [77]. Certain platelet factors, including PDGF and TGF-β, are felt to be particularly important in stimulating collagen synthesis by SMCs, whereas γ-interferon (from activated T cells) has the opposite effect [80].

Smooth muscle cell apoptosis may also be responsible for decreased plaque collagen [81; 82]. A recent, though small, study demonstrated that the proportion of SMCs undergoing apoptosis and the frequency of cytoplasmic remnants of apoptotic cells were significantly increased in unstable versus stable angina atherectomy specimens [83]. Apoptosis of SMCs and macrophages has been identified within plaques, but only in advanced disease with dense macrophage infiltration. Apoptotic cells are deemed to become susceptible to a special form of cell death (distinct from necrosis) characterized by a series of morphological changes, starting with shrinkage of the cell membrane and leading on to condensation of nuclear chromatin, cellular fragmentation and eventually engulfment of apoptotic bodies by the surrounding cells [76].

Pro-apoptotic proteins are present in advanced plaques, and it has been observed that cells derived from the plaque, but not the adjacent media, die when brought into culture [75; 84]. Intimal cell apoptosis may account for the low density of smooth muscle cells in unstable plaques and may contribute to the events leading up to plaque disruption. However, the converse relationship may also be true and the precise role of cellular apoptosis remains unclear.

Macrophages and collagen degradation

It is now known that inflammation plays a major role in plaque progression and especially in the period just prior to its rupture [85]. Macrophages control many of the inflammatory processes within the plaque [86], and are responsible for the production of proteolytic enzymes capable of degrading the extracellular matrix (ECM) [87; 88]. The predominant proteolytic enzymes involved

Table 8.1. *The MMP family*

MMP	Alternative names	Principal substrates
Collagenases		
MMP-1	Collagenase-1, Interstitial collagenase	Collagens I,II,III, gelatin, MMP-2 & 9
MMP-8	Collagenase-2, Neutrophil collagenase	Collagens I,II,III, gelatin
MMP-13	Collagenase-3	Collagens I,II,III, gelatin, PAI-2
MMP-18	Collagenase-4, Xenopus collagenase	Collagen I
Gelatinases		
MMP-2	Gelatinase-A, 72 kDa gelatinase	Gelatin, collagens, IV, V,VII,X,XI,XIV, elastin, fibronectin, aggrecan
MMP-9	Gelatinase-B, 92 kDa gelatinase	Gelatin, collagens IV,V,VII,X, elastin
Stromelysins		
MMP-3	Stromelysin-1	Collagens III,IV,IX,X, gelatin, aggrecan, MMP-1,7,8,9 & 13
MMP-10	Stromelysin-2	Collagens III,IV,V, gelatin, MMP-1 & 8
MMP-11	Stromelysin-3	
Matrilysins		
MMP-7	Matrilysin-1, Pump-1	
MMP-26	Matrilysin-2, Endometase	
Membrane types		
MMP-14	MT1-MMP	Collagens I,II,III, gelatin, MMP-2 & 13
MMP-15	MT2-MMP	MMP-2, gelatin
MMP-16	MT3-MMP	MMP-2
MMP-17	MT4-MMP	
MMP-24	MT5-MMP	
MMP-25	MT6-MMP	
Others		
MMP-12	Macrophage elastase	
MMP-19	No trivial name	
MMP-20	Enamelysin	
MMP-21	XMMP (Xenopus)	
MMP-23		
MMP-27		
MMP-28	Epilysin	

in plaque disruption are the matrix metalloproteinases or MMPs [89].

The MMPs are a family of proteolytic enzymes characterized by the presence of zinc ions at their active sites. All degrade components of the extracellular matrix, and are divided into four main classes on the basis of their substrate specificity (Table 8.1).

The MMPs are essential in normal healthy individuals, playing a key role in processes such as wound healing [90; 91]. However, there is growing interest in a role in disease states where ECM breakdown plays a predominant role [92]. Early interest focused on a pathological role for MMPs in the resorption of periodontal structures in periodontal disease [93], the destruction of joints in rheumatoid arthritis [94], and the local invasive behaviour of malignancies [95]. In vascular disease, they have been implicated in many of the stages of atherosclerosis but most particularly in acute plaque disruption [96]. The site of rupture is characterized by an intense inflammatory infiltrate consisting predominantly of macrophages [88], that undergoes activation resulting in increased MMP expression. This shifts the delicate equilibrium towards proteolysis and away from matrix accumulation, making plaque disruption more likely (Figure 8.5).

Matrix metalloproteinase activity is tightly controlled at several levels. Firstly, expression of MMPs is determined at the transcriptional level by various cytokines and growth factors [97]. In a variety of tissue types, IL-1, PDGF and TNF-α stimulate expression [98; 99], while heparin, TGF-β and corticosteroids inhibit expression [100; 101]. Secondly, MMPs are secreted as latent inactive proenzymes and converted to the active state by cleavage of a propeptide domain [102]. The major physiological activator is plasmin, which in turn is regulated by PAI [103]. Thrombin has been shown to activate MMP-2 *in vitro* [104] and could provide a mechanism for MMP activation at sites of vascular injury. Reactive oxygen species also modulate enzyme activation [105; 106]. Thirdly, the existence of naturally occurring MMP inhibitors, or tissue inhibitors of metalloproteinases (TIMP)s, provides a further level of control [107]. Overall proteolytic activity depends on the ratio of activated MMPs to TIMPs.

Early studies showed that MMPs were present at increased levels in atherosclerotic arteries. Raised levels of gelatinase activity were demonstrated in the aortas of patients with occlusive disease compared with healthy controls and zymography revealed that this was predominantly MMP-9 [108]. Subsequently, quantitative studies using ELISA revealed a six-fold increase in MMP-9 levels in atherosclerotic aortas [109]. The level and expression of MMP-2 is also increased in atherosclerotic aortic tissue compared with normal aorta [110]. While expression of MMP-2 has been detected in normal arteries, it appears that most MMPs are expressed only in atherosclerotic tissue [111]. The colocalization of MMP-1, -2, -3 and -9 to the vulnerable shoulder of the plaque provided further evidence of their potential role in acute disruption [111].

More recent studies have demonstrated an association between MMP levels and markers of plaque instability. Increased immunostaining for MMP-9 was seen in 12 atherectomy specimens retrieved from patients with unstable angina compared with the stable form [112]. A larger study, involving 75 carotid endarterectomy specimens, demonstrated a close association between raised plaque levels of MMP-9 and a number of indicators of plaque instability, including symptomatology, cerebral embolization and histological features of plaque rupture [9].

Convincing evidence therefore exists of increased levels of MMP-2 and -9 in unstable plaques. However, intact type I and type III collagen molecules, which account for the load-bearing strength of the plaque cap, are not substrates for MMP-2 and -9. While it has been reported that high concentrations of MMP-2 can degrade type I collagen in an *in vitro* environment devoid of TIMPs [113], it is likely that *in vivo* only the collagenases MMP-1, -8 and -13 are capable of degrading fibrillar collagens.

The MMP-1 and -13 levels are higher in 'atheromatous' compared with 'fibrous' plaques [114], and MMP-8 has been demonstrated in atheroma but not normal arteries [115]. The expression of MMP-1 is increased in areas of high circumferential stress [116]. It is likely that both mechanics and proteolysis play a role in the degradation and weakening of the collagen-rich extracellular matrix, and understanding their interaction may be crucial [117].

Recent evidence from our laboratories [197] suggests that active MMP-8 is significantly raised in unstable plaques retrieved at carotid endarterectomy (Figure 8.6). The ratio of active MMP-8 to TIMP-1 and -2 (its naturally occurring inhibitors) were also significantly higher in the more unstable plaques of the 159 specimens collected in this study. This implies net proteolysis of the types of collagen found in the cap of the plaque by MMP-8. Immunohistochemistry confirmed the presence of MMP-8 protein within the plaque, which co-localized with macrophages (Figure 8.7).

Genetic variation in the genes controlling MMPs could theoretically be responsible for the susceptibility of some individuals to atherosclerotic plaque rupture. Early work has identified a number of polymorphisms that may be influential in this regard. Price *et al.* have identified a novel genetic variation in the MMP-2 gene [118]. Ye and colleagues detected a polymorphism in the promoter region of the MMP-3 gene that may lead to increased systemic levels [119]. This polymorphism was subsequently found to be more common in patients suffering from MI, compared with a control group [120]. A single nucleotide polymorphism (C to T transition at position –1562) has been shown to influence MMP-9

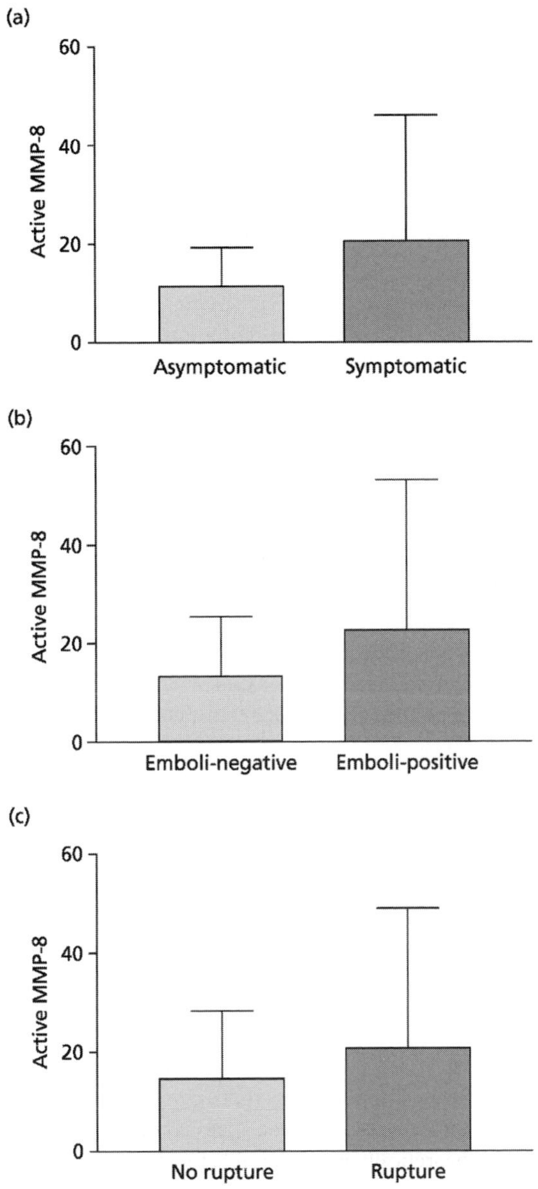

Fig. 8.6. Plaque concentrations of active MMP-8 are significantly higher in the carotid plaques: (a) from patients suffering carotid territory symptoms in the six months prior to surgery, (b) from patients with pre-operative cerebral embolization detected by transcranial Doppler, and (c) showing histological evidence of plaque rupture. Median values and interquartile ranges (in ng/g net weight of plaque) are shown.

transcription [121]. In this study by Zhang and coworkers, triple-vessel coronary artery disease was detected by angiography in 26% of patients with this polymorphism compared with 15% of those without [121]. Presenting a coherent picture of the interactions between various polymorphisms and the corresponding gene expression is difficult, and further complicated by environmental effects. However, it is clear that the potential exists to identify 'at risk' individuals in such a manner.

The vessel lumen

Disruption alone would not precipitate ischaemic syndromes without thrombus formation on the plaque surface, so plaque instability and thrombogenicity in tandem predispose to acute clinical events. Platelet adherence to the subendothelium after surface disruption leads to activation, with ADP and serotonin release stimulating further platelet recruitment and activation.

Once formed, the thrombus can behave in three ways, dependent on the physical nature of the rupture, and the balance between local fibrinolytic and coagulation processes (see Figure 8.8). Firstly, the initial thrombus may progress to cause occlusion of the vessel. Secondly, the thrombus may disintegrate resulting in distal embolization. Thirdly, the clot can undergo rapid dissolution, with the healed rupture resulting in a variable decrease in vessel lumen diameter [72].

Tissue factor is a major regulator of haemostasis [122]. It is the most thrombogenic component of atherosclerotic plaques [123] and is expressed by numerous cell types, including endothelial cells. The level of tissue factor in coronary plaques from patients with unstable angina is more than twice the value observed in those plaques from stable angina patients [124]. Positive immunostaining for tissue factor correlates with areas of intense macrophage infiltration and SMCs, suggesting a cell-mediated increased thrombogenicity in unstable plaques. The increase in tissue factor levels seems to be linked to expression of the CD40 receptor on the macrophage cell surface. The CD40 ligand is expressed on activated T lymphocytes, and other atheroma-associated cells [125], which can therefore induce tissue factor production by macrophages via this signalling system. Expression is also regulated by cytokines and oxidized-LDL [126; 127]. It has been recently reported that a blood-borne pool of tissue

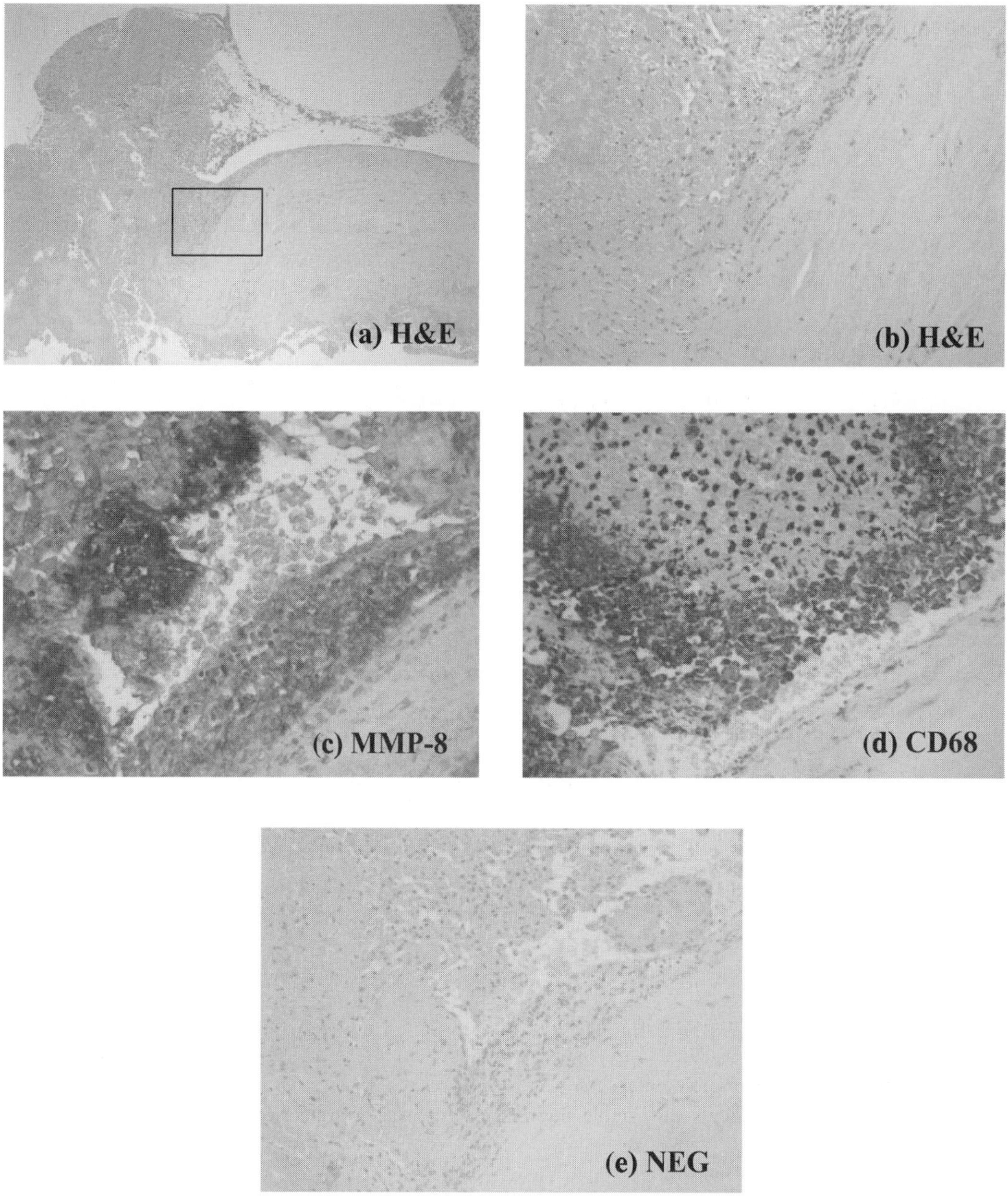

Fig. 8.7. Histological sections taken from the shoulder region of a symptomatic carotid plaque. Some sections show disruption of the friable plaque. (a) Low power haematoxilin and eosin (H&E) section with boxed area delineating high power view shown in (b–e). (b) High power H&E section demonstrating a cellular infiltrate. (c) Strong reactivity for MMP-8 in cells. (d) Positive staining for CD68. (d) Negative immunochemistry control (see colour plate section).

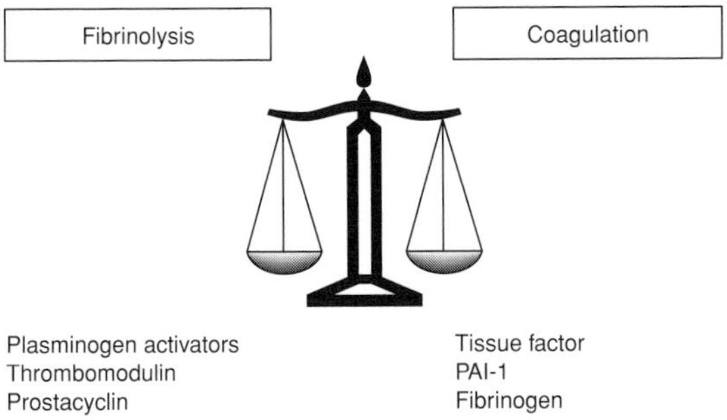

Fig. 8.8. Fibrinolysis versus coagulation.

factor exists [128], though in the context of plaque disruption, macrophage production of tissue factor is predominantly responsible for plaque thrombogenicity [124; 129; 130]. It is interesting to note that many of the recognized cardiovascular risk factors increase the expression of tissue factor [131; 132].

THE ROLE OF ANGIOGENESIS IN PLAQUE RUPTURE

Angiogenesis is essential for normal growth and development. Neovascularization has been observed in plaques [133] and it is postulated that it may play a role in atherosclerosis (by providing growth factors and cytokines to regions of plaque development). In addition, angiogenesis may be involved in plaque destabilization (by promoting intraplaque haemorrhage from fragile newly formed vessels) and atherosclerotic plaque rupture (by recruiting inflammatory cells into vulnerable areas of the lesion).

A study of coronary atherectomy specimens revealed the presence of neovascularization in 50% of specimens from patients with unstable angina compared to 10% of specimens from patients with stable angina [29], suggesting a possible role in plaque instability. Also, a recent histological study of plaques showed a significant increase in microvessel density in lipid-rich compared with fibrous plaques [134]. Perhaps more importantly, most of these vessels were located in the vulnerable shoulder area of the plaque. Immunostaining for inflammatory cells showed a close association between angiogenesis and inflammatory infiltration. In addition, a parallel increase in the expression of leucocyte adhesion molecules in the same vulnerable areas was demonstrated [134].

Angiogenesis involves interactions between endothelial cells and components of the basement membrane matrix. Matrix metalloproteinase activity is required for such interactions, especially MMP-2 and MT1-MMP [135]. Tissue inhibitors of metalloproteinases have been shown to reduce angiogenesis, while up-regulation of MMP activity stimulates its increase [136].

It is presently unclear as to whether angiogenesis is a cause or an effect of plaque destabilization. Whilst neovascularization may promote and sustain inflammatory infiltration, the converse may also be true, whereby changes in the plaque associated with inflammation may themselves promote angiogenesis.

THE ROLE OF INFECTIOUS AGENTS IN PLAQUE RUPTURE

The role of infectious agents in atherosclerosis and plaque rupture is controversial. Definitive proof of a causal relationship is lacking, although studies have reported associations between plaque development and *Chlamydia pneumoniae* [137; 138; 139], *Helicobacter pylori* [140] and cytomegalovirus [141; 142].

Certain infectious agents can evoke cellular and molecular changes supportive of a role in atherogenesis [143]. Work has shown that chlamydial interaction with monocytes results in up-regulation of TNF-α and IL-1β [144; 145] both of which are associated with plaque development. Chlamydial production of the HSP60 antigen activates human vascular endothelium, and increases TNF-α and MMP expression in macrophages [146; 147].

There is some doubt about the methods employed for *Chlamydia* detection [148], and the role of potential confounding factors in epidemiological studies [149]. A large-scale prospective study of 15 000 healthy men in the USA which was controlled for age, smoking, socio-economic status and other cardiovascular risk factors, failed to show any association between *Chlamydia* seropositivity and the risk of MI [150].

The recent STAMINA trial [151] demonstrated that eradication therapy (amoxicillin/azithromycin, metronidazole and omeprazole) administered for one week after an acute coronary syndrome, significantly reduced cardiac death and acute coronary syndrome readmission rates over the following 12 months. These effects were unrelated to *Chlamydia pneumoniae* or

Helicobacter pylori seropositivity, however, suggesting that the trial therapy prevented lesion progression by a mechanism unrelated to its antibiotic action.

RISK PREDICTION OF PLAQUE INSTABILITY

Imaging

Angiography can demonstrate ulceration [152] but does not appear to be able to adequately distinguish between stable and unstable plaques [153]. In addition, the degree of stenosis detected by angiography does not correlate well with the future risk of events [18; 19; 20]. Ultrasound studies have shown an association between carotid plaque morphology and neurological symptoms [154] but have been unable to predict the risk of future events [22]. More promisingly, intravascular ultrasound (IVUS) studies have shown an increase in the incidence of ulcerated and ruptured plaques in patients with acute coronary syndromes [155].

Increased inflammatory activity occurs prior to plaque rupture and attempts have been made to detect this increase using local temperature measurements. Thermography studies have shown that temperature correlates well with macrophage cell density in human carotid plaques [156]. The temperature of coronary vessels in patients with ischaemic heart disease, in particular acute coronary syndromes, is higher than in normal controls [157]. In addition, increased local plaque temperature has been shown to be an independent predictor of adverse clinical outcome [158].

High-resolution MRI appears to characterize the atherosclerotic plaque better than other imaging techniques [159]. It is more accurate than angiography for measuring the degree of stenosis and, unlike angiography and intravascular ultrasound (IVUS), is non-invasive. Technically, images are limited by small vessel size and movement artefact, and studies have not yet demonstrated the ability to predict the risk of future cardiovascular events. However, advances in the technique suggest a potential future role for MRI in detection of the high-risk plaque.

Blood markers

It has long been established that adverse lipid profiles correlate with increased risk of MI and stroke. C-reactive protein levels are also associated with increased cardiovascular risk in apparently healthy patients [160; 161], and enough evidence now exists to incorporate their use in generating individual risk assessment profiles.

MMP-2 and MMP-9 are raised in the peripheral blood of patients suffering from acute coronary syndromes [162], while plasma MMP-9 is raised in patients with unstable carotid plaques [163]. A recent study of 1127 patients with coronary artery disease identified baseline plasma MMP-9 levels to be a novel predictor of cardiovascular mortality [164]. Further work is required to identify the nature and source of these elevated MMPs, but clearly the potential for risk prediction exists.

THERAPY AIMED AT PLAQUE STABILIZATION

Pharmacotherapy to induce plaque stabilization could be targeted at different aspects of the complex pathway leading to plaque rupture, in particular:

(1) The endothelium – by increasing endothelial passivation
(2) The lipid core – by reducing LDL deposition/augmenting LDL removal
(3) The fibrous cap – by increasing collagen deposition/preventing collagen degradation
(4) The vessel lumen – by altering the thrombogenicity of the local environment

Most recent interest has focused on the role of hydroxymethylglutaryl coenzyme-A (HMG Co-A) reductase inhibitors, which appear capable of influencing plaque stabilization at all these levels.

HMG CO-A REDUCTASE INHIBITORS

The HMG Co-A reductase inhibitors, or statins, are well known for their lipid-lowering action. They are the most effective group of therapeutic agents for lowering LDL and raising HDL levels. However, recent evidence suggests that they are also capable of decreasing cardiovascular events in those with normal cholesterol levels [165; 166]. The Oxford Heart Protection Study [165] was a randomized controlled trial of simvastatin vs. placebo in 20 536 individuals at high risk of cardiovascular disease. Coronary death rate and other vascular events were significantly reduced in the simvastatin groups, even in patients with lipid levels below currently recommended targets (<5 mmol/l total cholesterol and <3 mmol/l LDL-cholesterol).

In the lipid lowering arm of the Anglo-Scandinavian Cardiac Outcomes Trial (ASCOT) [166], 10 305 individuals with total cholesterol levels <6.5 mmol/l were randomized to either atorvastatin or placebo. The trial was stopped 1.7 years before the planned 5-year follow-up target was reached, as there were significantly fewer cardiovascular events in the atorvastatin group. The observed clinical benefit is probably a combination of lipid lowering below levels previously considered 'normal' and additional lipid-independent plaque stabilizing actions. Several studies have reported effects other than lipid-lowering properties, including anti-proteolytic and anti-inflammatory mechanisms [167; 168].

Statins increase nitric oxide synthase activity [169] and encourage endothelial passivation (Figure 8.2). As discussed earlier, nitric oxide causes vasodilatation, inhibition of SMC proliferation and platelet aggregation, and has widespread anti-inflammatory and antioxidant properties. Statins also reduce the expression of cell adhesion molecules [170], interfering with the adherence of monocytes to the endothelium.

Statins may also have direct anti-inflammatory and anti-proteolytic actions, which contribute to increased plaque stability. In experimental and animal models, statins have been shown to reduce macrophage secretion of MMP-1, -2, -3 and -9 [171], and increase the collagen content of the plaque [172]. Also, CRP levels are decreased by statins in a lipid-independent manner [168; 173].

Work from our laboratories suggests that statin therapy stabilizes carotid plaques by lowering the levels of MMP-1, MMP-9 and IL-6 [198]. In an observational non-randomized study of 137 patients, we found that patients on statin therapy were significantly less likely to have suffered carotid territory symptoms within the month prior to carotid endarterectomy. The number of patients undergoing spontaneous pre-operative cerebral embolization was also significantly lower in the statin group.

The HMG Co-A reductase inhibitors also have the potential to reduce thrombogenicity by decreasing tissue factor activity [174] and lowering levels of PAI-1 [175; 176].

MMP INHIBITION

The realization that tissue remodelling due to increased MMP activity plays a key role in disease states has led to considerable interest in the potential for MMP inhibition. Most clinical and pre-clinical data regarding therapeutic manipulation of the extracellular matrix has been in the fields of arthritis, periodontal disease and cancer [96]. Matrix metalloproteinase inhibition aimed at plaque stabilization aims to redress the imbalance between enzymes and inhibitors, which causes excessive tissue degradation. Potential methods of MMP inhibition include the administration of TIMPs, synthetic MMP inhibitors or doxycycline.

TIMPs

The level of TIMPs can be increased either by the exogenous administration of recombinant TIMPs or by stimulating their local production through gene therapy. Increased TIMP-1 raised the collagen, elastin and smooth muscle content of atherosclerotic lesions in animal models [177], while local gene transfer of TIMP-2 has been shown to decrease vascular remodelling in conjunction with lowered MMP activity (experimental models) [178].

It is difficult to extrapolate these data to potential applications in humans. The major drawback associated with TIMPs would be tissue delivery, since exogenous products would be metabolized and denatured with minimal tissue penetration at the intended site of action. Systemic stimulation of TIMPs would almost certainly have significant side effects precluding clinical use. Therefore, treatment would have to take the form of local tissue delivery or gene therapy. Clearly either system will be very expensive to develop, so more interest has concentrated on the development of synthetic MMP inhibitors.

Synthetic MMP inhibitors

Synthetic peptides work by binding to the zinc ion at the active site of the MMP, thus preventing cleavage of substrate collagen molecules [179]. Batimastat showed promise in decreasing tumour development and metastasis (animal models) [180], and limiting aneurysm expansion (experimental models) [181], but is not available in an oral form. Marimastat, which is available orally, was shown to limit intimal hyperplasia [182] and aneurysm expansion *in vivo* [183]. It also showed promise in early human cancer studies, but caused significant musculoskeletal side effects in 30% of patients [184]. Recent studies of MMI270, a more specific inhibitor (of MMP-2, MMP-8 and MMP-9), have shown a similar side effect profile [185].

Doxycycline

Doxycycline, a member of the tetracycline antibiotic family, is also a non-selective MMP inhibitor [186], with a proven safety profile. Clinical trials have shown that doxycycline is capable of decreasing cartilage MMP levels when given to patients prior to hip surgery [187]. It has also been shown to limit intimal hyperplasia [188] and aneurysm expansion *in vivo* [189], by reducing MMP-9 activity. Furthermore, when given to patients prior to AAA repair the expression of MMP-2 and MMP-9 was reduced in the aortic wall [190].

A randomized clinical trial of doxycycline versus placebo in patients prior to carotid endarterectomy demonstrated decreased plaque MMP-1 levels and a potential for clinical benefit [191]. A phase II study of doxycycline administration to patients with small AAAs recently showed that it was reasonably well-tolerated (92% completed the six-month course) and reduced plasma MMP-9 levels [192]. Further studies are on going to evaluate its effects on small aneurysm expansion.

ACE INHIBITORS

ACE inhibitors and angiotensin II receptor antagonists decrease cardiovascular events, independently of their effects on blood pressure control. The ACE inhibitor, trandalopril, and the experimental angiotensin receptor antagonist, HR720, decrease the area of atherosclerotic lesions in the thoracic aorta of cholesterol-fed monkeys [193]. This was achieved without alteration of mean blood pressure or cholesterol levels. The Heart Outcomes Prevention Evaluation (HOPE) study demonstrated a decrease in cardiovascular events in high-risk patients given ramipril as opposed to placebo [194]. This effect could only be partly explained by the modest decrease in mean blood pressure seen between the two groups (3/2 mm Hg).

Angiotensin II promotes endothelial activation [195], and therefore the mechanism of action of ACE inhibitors could be through endothelial passivation (leading to a reduction in cell adhesion molecule expression and macrophage infiltration). This therapy is also capable of decreasing oxygen free radicals and performing other regulatory processes in the extracellular matrix. Navalkar *et al.* provided biochemical evidence to support these hypotheses by demonstrating that irbesartan (an angiotensin II receptor blocker) can decrease plasma levels of VCAM-1, TNF-α and superoxide [196].

SUMMARY

Acute plaque disruption precedes the onset of clinical ischaemic syndromes. Exposure of the highly thrombogenic core to luminal blood results in platelet adherence and thrombosis. Inflammation is clearly involved in the process of plaque development and acute disruption, though the precise mechanism by which the inflammatory process is initiated remains unclear. The roles of angiogenesis, cellular apoptosis and infectious agents also require further clarification. Unstable plaques have a large lipid core and a thin fibrous cap with reduced collagen content. A major component of plaque destabilization appears to be increased matrix degradation, the primary regulators of which are the MMPs and their inhibitors. There are a number of potential therapeutic options aimed at preventing plaque disruption. In particular, MMP inhibition is an attractive target for such pharmacotherapy.

ABBREVIATIONS

AAA = abdominal aortic aneurysm
ACE = angiotensin converting enzyme
ADAMTS = A disintegrin and metalloproteinase with thrombospondin motifs
CD = cluster of differentiation
CEA = carotid endarterectomy
CRP = C-reactive protein
ECM = extracellular matrix
ELISA = enzyme-linked immunosorbent assay
HDL = high-density lipoprotein
HMG Co-A = hydroxymethylglutaryl coenzyme-A
HSP = heat shock protein
ICAM = intercellular adhesion molecule

IHD = ischaemic heart disease
IL = interleukin
LDL = low-density lipoprotein
MCSF = macrophage colony stimulating factor
MCP = monocyte chemoattractant protein
MI = myocardial infarction
MMP = matrix metalloproteinase
MRI = magnetic resonance imaging
MT-MMP = membrane-type MMP
PAI = plasminogen activator inhibitor
PDGF = platelet-derived growth factor
PPAR = peroxisomal proliferation activating receptor
SMC = smooth muscle cell
TGF-β = transforming growth factor-beta
TIA = transient ischaemic attack
TIMP = tissue inhibitor of metalloproteinase
TNF-α = tumour necrosis factor-alpha
VCAM = vascular cell adhesion molecule

REFERENCES

1. W. C. Little, Angiographic assessment of the culprit coronary artery lesion before acute myocardial infarction. *American Journal of Cardiology*, **66** (1990), 44G–47G.
2. W. Casscells, M. Naghavi & J. T. Willerson, Vulnerable atherosclerotic plaque: a multifocal disease. *Circulation*, **107** (2003), 2072–5.
3. P. K. Shah, Plaque disruption and thrombosis: potential role of inflammation and infection. *Cardiology Review*, **8** (2000), 31–9.
4. P. Libby, Current concepts of the pathogenesis of the acute coronary syndromes. *Circulation*, **104** (2001), 365–72.
5. E. Falk, P. K. Shah & V. Fuster, Coronary plaque disruption. *Circulation*, **92** (1995), 657–71.
6. E. Falk, Unstable angina with fatal outcome: dynamic coronary thrombosis leading to infarction and/or sudden death. Autopsy evidence of recurrent mural thrombosis with peripheral embolization culminating in total vascular occlusion. *Circulation*, **71** (1985), 699–708.
7. M. Sitzer, W. Muller, M. Siebler *et al.*, Plaque ulceration and lumen thrombus are the main sources of cerebral microemboli in high-grade internal carotid artery stenosis. *Stroke*, **26** (1995), 1231–3.
8. S. Carr, A. Farb, W. H. Pearce, R. Virmani & J. S. Yao, Atherosclerotic plaque rupture in symptomatic carotid artery stenosis. *Journal of Vascular Surgery*, **23** (1996), 755–65.
9. I. M. Loftus, A. R. Naylor, S. Goodall *et al.*, Increased matrix metalloproteinase-9 activity in unstable carotid plaques. A potential role in acute plaque disruption. *Stroke*, **31** (2000), 40–7.
10. M. J. Davies & A. Thomas, Thrombosis and acute coronary-artery lesions in sudden cardiac ischemic death. *New England Journal of Medicine*, **310** (1984), 1137–40.
11. E. Falk, Plaque rupture with severe pre-existing stenosis precipitating coronary thrombosis. Characteristics of coronary atherosclerotic plaques underlying fatal occlusive thrombi. *British Heart Journal*, **50** (1983), 127–34.
12. M. Friedman, Pathogenesis of coronary thrombosis, intramural and intraluminal hemorrhage. *Advances in Cardiology*, **4** (1970), 20–46.
13. J. S. Forrester, F. Litvack, W. Grundfest & A. Hickey, A perspective of coronary disease seen through the arteries of living man. *Circulation*, **75** (1987), 505–13.
14. C. T. Sherman, F. Litvack, W. Grundfest *et al.*, Coronary angioscopy in patients with unstable angina pectoris. *New England Journal of Medicine*, **315** (1986), 913–9.
15. F. D. Kolodgie, A. P. Burke, A. Farb, H. K. Gold, J. Yuan, J. Narula, A. V. Finn, R. Virmani, The thin-cap fibroatheroma: a type of vulnerable plaque: the major precursor lesion to acute coronary syndromes. *Current Opinion in Cardiology*, **16** (2001), 285–92.
16. M. J. Davies, The pathophysiology of acute coronary syndromes. *Heart*, **83** (2000), 361–6.
17. C. V. Felton, D. Crook, M. J. Davies & M. F. Oliver, Relation of plaque lipid composition and morphology to the stability of human aortic plaques. *Arteriosclerosis, Thrombosis and Vascular Biology*, **17** (1997), 1337–45.
18. J. A. Ambrose, S. L. Winters, A. Stern *et al.*, Angiographic morphology and the pathogenesis of unstable angina pectoris. *Journal of the American College of Cardiology*, **5** (1985), 609–16.
19. D. Hackett, G. Davies & A. Maseri, Pre-existing coronary stenoses in patients with first myocardial infarction are not necessarily severe. *European Heart Journal*, **9** (1988), 1317–23.
20. D. Giroud, J. M. Li, P. Urban, B. Meier & W. Rutishauer, Relation of the site of acute myocardial infarction to the most severe coronary arterial stenosis

at prior angiography. *American Journal of Cardiology*, **69** (1992), 729–32.

21. H. S. Markus, N. D. Thomson & M. M. Brown, Asymptomatic cerebral embolic signals in symptomatic and asymptomatic carotid artery disease. *Brain*, **118** (4) (1995), 1005–11.
22. J. Golledge, R. Cuming, M. Ellis, A. H. Davies & R. M. Greenhalgh, Carotid plaque characteristics and presenting symptom. *British Journal of Surgery*, **84** (1997), 1697–701.
23. M. J. Harrison & J. Marshall, The finding of thrombus at carotid endarterectomy and its relationship to the timing of surgery. *British Journal of Surgery*, **64** (1997), 511–12.
24. A. J. Gunning, G. W. Pickering, A. H. Robb-Smith & R. R. Russell, Mural thrombosis of the internal carotid artery and subsequent embolism. *Quarterly Journal of Medicine*, **33** (1964), 155–95.
25. J. Bogousslavsky, G. Van Melle & F. Regli, The Lausanne Stroke Registry: analysis of 1,000 consecutive patients with first stroke. *Stroke*, **19** (1988), 1083–92.
26. A. M. Imparato, T. S. Riles & M. D. Gorstein, The carotid bifurcation plaque: pathological findings associated with cerebral ischaemia. *Stroke*, **10** (1979), 238–45.
27. A. V. Persson, W. T. Robichaux & M. Silverman, The natural history of carotid plaque development. *Archives of Surgery*, **118** (1983), 1048–52.
28. R. J. Lusby, L. D. Ferrell, W. K. Ehrenfeld, R. J. Stoney & E. J. Wylie, Carotid plaque haemorrhage: its role in the production of cerebral ischaemia. *Archives of Surgery*, **117** (1982), 1479–88.
29. A. N. Tenaglia, K. G. Peters, M. H. Sketch & B. H. Annex, Neovascularisation in atherectomy specimens from patients with unstable angina: implications for pathogenesis of unstable angina. *American Heart Journal*, **135** (1998), 10–14.
30. H. V. M. Van Damme, Pathologic aspects of carotid plaques: surgical and clinical significance. *International Angiology*, **12** (1993), 299–311.
31. T. F. Luscher, F. C. Tanner & G. Noll, Lipids and endothelial function: effects of lipid-lowering and other therapeutic interventions. *Current Opinion in Lipidology*, **7** (1996), 234–40.
32. R. S. Barua, J. A. Ambrose, S. Srivastava, M. C. DeVoe & L. J. Eales-Reynolds, Reactive oxygen species are involved in smoking-induced dysfunction of nitric oxide biosynthesis and upregulation of endothelial nitric oxide synthase: an *in vitro* demonstration in human coronary artery endothelial cells. *Circulation*, **107** (2003), 2342–7.
33. R. S. Barua, J. A. Ambrose, D. C. Saha & L. J. Eales-Reynolds, Smoking is associated with altered endothelial-derived fibrinolytic and antithrombotic factors: an *in vitro* demonstration. *Circulation*, **106** (2002), 905–8.
34. I. P. Salt, V. A. Morrow, F. M. Brandie, J. M. Connell & J. R. Petrie, High glucose inhibits insulin-stimulated nitric oxide production without reducing endothelial nitric-oxide synthase ser1177 phosphorylation in human aortic endothelial cells. *Journal of Biological Chemistry*, **278** (2003), 18791–7.
35. S. Taddei, A. Virdis, L. Ghiadoni, I. Sudano & A. Salvetti, Endothelial dysfunction in hypertension. *Journal of Cardiovascular Pharmacology*, **38** (Suppl 2) (2001), S11–4.
36. C. G. Hanratty, L. T. McGrath, D. F. McAuley, I. S. Young & G. D. Johnston, The effects of oral methionine and homocysteine on endothelial function. *Heart*, **85** (2001), 326–30.
37. M. I. Cybulsky & M. A. Gimbrone, Jr., Endothelial expression of a mononuclear leukocyte adhesion molecule during atherogenesis. *Science*, **251** (1991), 788–91.
38. A. C. van der Wal, P. K. Das, A. J. Tigges & A. E. Becker, Adhesion molecules on the endothelium and mononuclear cells in human atherosclerotic lesions. *American Journal of Pathology*, **141** (1992), 1427–33.
39. P. M. Vanhoutte, Endothelial dysfunction and atherosclerosis. *European Heart Journal*, **18** (Suppl E) (1997), E19–29.
40. R. De Caterina, P. Libby, H. B. Peng *et al.*, Nitric oxide decreases cytokine-induced endothelial activation. Nitric oxide selectively reduces endothelial expression of adhesion molecules and proinflammatory cytokines. *Journal of Clinical Investigation*, **96** (1995), 60–8.
41. S. Moncada & A. Higgs, The L-arginine-nitric oxide pathway. *New England Journal of Medicine*, **329** (1993), 2002–12.
42. B. A. Kingwell, B. Sherrard, G. L. Jennings, A. M. Dart, Four weeks of cycle training increases basal production of nitric oxide from the forearm. *American Journal of Physiology*, **272** (1997), 1070–77.
43. A. M. Malek, S. L. Alper & S. Izumo, Hemodynamic shear stress and its role in atherosclerosis. *JAMA*, **282** (1999), 2035–42.

44. M. A. Gimbrone, Jr, N. Resnick, T. Nagel *et al.*, Hemodynamics, endothelial gene expression, and atherogenesis. *Annals of the New York Academy of Sciences*, **811** (1997), 1–10.
45. S. Nadaud, M. Philippe, J. F. Arnal, J. B. Michel & F. Soubrier, Sustained increase in aortic endothelial nitric oxide synthase expression *in vivo* in a model of chronic high blood flow. *Circulation Research*, **79** (1996), 857–63.
46. G. W. De Keulenaer, D. C. Chappell, N. Ishizaka *et al.*, Oscillatory and steady laminar shear stress differentially affect human endothelial redox state: role of a superoxide-producing NADH oxidase. *Circulation Research*, **82** (1998), 1094–101.
47. D. C. Chappell, S. E. Varner, R. M. Nerem, R. M. Medford & R. W. Alexander, Oscillatory shear stress stimulates adhesion molecule expression in cultured human endothelium. *Circulation Research*, **82** (1998), 532–39.
48. R. T. Lee & R. D. Kamm, Vascular mechanisms for the cardiologist. *Journal of the American College of Cardiology*, **23** (1994), 1289–95.
49. G. C. Cheng, H. M. Loree, R. D. Kamm, M. C. Fishbein & R. T. Lee, Distribution of circumferential stress in ruptured and stable atherosclerotic lesions: a structural analysis with histopathological correlation. *Circulation*, **87** (1993), 1179–87.
50. H. M. Loree, R. D. Kamm, R. G. Stringfellow & R. T. Lee, Effects of fibrous cap thickness on peak circumferential stress in model atherosclerotic vessels. *Circulation Research*, **71** (1992), 850–58.
51. A. I. MacIsaac, J. D. Thomas & E. J. Topol, Toward the quiescent coronary plaque. *Journal of the American College of Cardiology*, **22** (1993), 1228–41.
52. M. L. Gronholdt, S. Dalager-Pedersen & E. Falk, Coronary atherosclerosis: determinants of plaque rupture. *European Heart Journal* (Suppl C) (1998), C24–9.
53. A. H. Kragel, S. G. Reddy, J. T. Wittes & W. C. Roberts, Morphometric analysis of the composition of atherosclerotic plaques in the four major epicardial coronary arteries in acute myocardial infarction and in sudden coronary death. *Circulation*, **80** (1989), 1747–56.
54. S. D. Gertz & W. C. Roberts, Haemodynamic shear force in rupture of coronary arterial atherosclerotic plaques. *American Journal of Cardiology*, **66** (1990), 1368–72.
55. M. J. Davies, P. D. Richardson, N. Woolf, D. R. Katz & J. Mann, Risk of thrombosis in human atherosclerotic plaques: role of extracellular lipid, macrophage, and smooth muscle cell content. *British Heart Journal*, **69** (1993), 377–81.
56. L. M. Reilly, R. J. Lusby, L. Hughes *et al.*, Carotid plaque histology using real-time ultrasonography. *American Journal of Surgery*, **146** (1983), 188–93.
57. N. El-Barghouti, A. N. Nicolaides, T. Tegos & G. Geroulakos, The relative effect of carotid plaque heterogeneity and echogenicity on ipsilateral cerebral infarction and symptoms of cerebrovascular disease. *International Angiology*, **15** (1996), 300–6.
58. T. M. Feeley, E. J. Leen, M. P. Colgan *et al.*, Histologic characteristics of carotid artery plaque. *Journal of Vascular Surgery*, **13** (1991), 719–24.
59. M. Takano, K. Mizuno, K. Okamatsu *et al.*, Mechanical and structural characteristics of vulnerable plaques: analysis by coronary angioscopy and intravascular ultrasound. *Journal of the American College of Cardiology*, **38** (2001), 99–104.
60. D. Steinberg, Low density lipoprotein oxidation and its pathobiological significance. *Journal of Biological Chemistry*, **272** (1997), 20963–6.
61. A. C. Nicholson, J. Han, M. Febbraio, R. L. Silversterin & D. P. Hajjar, Role of CD36, the macrophage class B scavenger receptor, in atherosclerosis. *Annals of the New York Academy of Sciences*, **947** (2001), 224–8.
62. H. S. Kruth, W. Huang, I. Ishii & W. Y. Zhang, Macrophage foam cell formation with native low density lipoprotein. *Journal of Biological Chemistry*, **277** (2002), 34573–80.
63. M. de la Llera Moya, V. Atger, P. L. Paul *et al.*, A cell culture system for screening human serum for ability to promote cellular cholesterol efflux. Relations between serum components and efflux, esterification, and transfer. *Arteriosclerosis and Thrombosis*, **14** (1994), 1056–65.
64. J. J. Badimon, L. Badimon & V. Fuster, Regression of atherosclerotic lesions by high density lipoprotein plasma fraction in the cholesterol-fed rabbit. *Journal of Clinical Investigation*, **85** (1990), 1234–41.
65. L. E. Spieker, I. Sudano, D. Hurlimann *et al.*, High-density lipoprotein restores endothelial function in hypercholesterolemic men. *Circulation*, **105** (2002), 1399–402.
66. P. J. Barter, Inhibition of endothelial cell adhesion molecule expression by high-density lipoproteins. *Clinical and Experimental Pharmacology and Physiology*, **24** (1997), 286–7.

67. K. Y. Lin, Y. L. Chen, C. C. Shih *et al.*, Contribution of HDL-apolipoproteins to the inhibition of low density lipoprotein oxidation and lipid accumulation in macrophages. *Journal of Cellular Biochemistry*, **86** (2002), 258–67.
68. S. Katsuda, Y. Okada, T. Minamoto *et al.*, Collagens in human atherosclerosis. Immunohistochemical analysis using collagen type-specific antibodies. *Arteriosclerosis and Thrombosis*, **12** (1992), 494–502.
69. A. C. van der Wal, A. E. Becker, C. M. van der Loos & P. K. Das, Site of intimal rupture or erosion of thrombosed coronary atherosclerotic plaques is characterized by an inflammatory process irrespective of the dominant plaque morphology. *Circulation*, **89** (1994), 36–44.
70. A. Farb, A. P. Burke, A. L. Tang *et al.*, Coronary plaque erosion without rupture into a lipid core. A frequent cause of coronary thrombosis in sudden coronary death. *Circulation*, **93** (1996), 1354–63.
71. R. Virmani, F. D. Kolodgie, A. P. Burke, A. Farb & S. M. Schwartz, Lessons from sudden coronary death: a comprehensive morphological classification scheme for atherosclerotic lesions. *Arteriosclerosis, Thrombosis and Vascular Biology*, **20** (2000), 1262–75.
72. A. P. Burke, F. D. Kolodgie, A. Farb *et al.*, Healed plaque ruptures and sudden coronary death: evidence that subclinical rupture has a role in plaque progression. *Circulation*, **103** (2001), 934–40.
73. M. C. Burleigh, A. D. Briggs, C. L. Lendon *et al.*, Collagen types I and III, collagen content, GACs and mechanical strength of human atherosclerotic plaque caps: span-wise variations. *Atherosclerosis*, **96** (1992), 71–81.
74. M. J. Davies, Stability and instability: two faces of coronary atherosclerosis. *Circulation*, **94** (1996), 2013–20.
75. M. M. Kockx, M. G. De, J. Muhring *et al.*, Apoptosis and related proteins in different stages of human atherosclerotic plaques. *Circulation*, **97** (1998), 2307–15.
76. M. M. Kockx, Apoptosis in the atherosclerotic plaque. *Arteriosclerosis, Thrombosis and Vascular Biology*, **18** (1999), 1519–22.
77. M. J. Barnes & R. W. Farndale, Collagens and atherosclerosis. *Experimental Gerontology*, **34** (1999), 513–25.
78. R. J. Dilley, J. K. McGeachie & F. J. Prendergast, A review of the proliferative behaviour, morphology and phenotypes of vascular smooth muscle. *Atherosclerosis*, **63** (1987), 99–107.
79. A. C. Newby, Molecular and cell biology of native coronary and vein-graft atherosclerosis: regulation of plaque stability and vessel-wall remodelling by growth factors and cell-extracellular matrix interactions. *Coronary Artery Disease*, **8** (1997), 213–24.
80. E. P. Amento, N. Ehsani, H. Palmer & P. Libby, Cytokines and growth factors positively and negatively regulate interstitial collagen gene expression in human vascular smooth muscle cells. *Arteriosclerosis and Thrombosis*, **11** (1991), 1223–30.
81. Y. J. Geng & P. Libby, Evidence for apoptosis in advanced human atheroma. Colocalization with interleukin-1 beta-converting enzyme. *American Journal of Pathology*, **147** (1995), 251–66.
82. Y. J. Geng, Biologic effect and molecular regulation of vascular apoptosis in atherosclerosis. *Current Atherosclerosis Reports*, **3** (2001), 234–42.
83. G. Bauriedel, R. Hutter, U. Welsch *et al.*, Role of smooth muscle cell death in advanced coronary primary lesions: implications for plaque instability. *Cardiovascular Research*, **41** (1999), 480–8.
84. M. R. Bennett, G. I. Evan & S. M. Schwartz, Apoptosis of human vascular smooth muscle cells derived from normal vessels and coronary atherosclerotic plaques. *Journal of Clinical Investigation*, **95** (1995), 2266–74.
85. L. M. Buja & J. T. Willerson, Role of inflammation in coronary plaque disruption. *Circulation*, **89** (1994), 503–5.
86. P. Libby & D. I. Simon, Inflammation and thrombosis: the clot thickens. *Circulation*, **103** (2001), 1718–20.
87. P. K. Shah, E. Falk, J. J. Badimon *et al.*, Human monocyte-derived macrophages induce collagen breakdown in fibrous caps of atherosclerotic plaques. Potential role of matrix-degrading metalloproteinases and implications for plaque rupture. *Circulation*, **92** (1995), 1565–9.
88. P. R. Moreno, E. Falk, I. F. Palacios *et al.*, Macrophage infiltration in acute coronary syndromes. Implications for plaque rupture. *Circulation*, **90** (1994), 775–8.
89. I. M. Loftus, A. R. Naylor, P. R. Bell & M. M. Thompson, Matrix metalloproteinases and atherosclerotic plaque instability. *British Journal of Surgery*, **89** (2002), 680–94.
90. A. B. Wysocki, L. Staiano- Coico, F. Grinnell, Wound fluid from chronic leg ulcers contains elevated levels of

metalloproteinases MMP-2 and MMP-9. *Journal of Investigative Dermatology*, **101** (1993), 64–8.
91. M. S. Agren, L. N. Jorgensen, M. Andersen, J. Viljanto & F. Gottrup, Matrix metalloproteinase 9 level predicts optimal collagen deposition during early wound repair in humans. *British Journal of Surgery*, **85** (1998), 68–71.
92. S. Krane, Clinical importance of metalloproteinases and their inhibitors. *Annals of the New York Academy of Sciences*, **732** (1994), 1–10.
93. R. C. Page, The role of inflammatory mediators in the pathogenesis of periodontal disease. *Journal of Periodontal Research*, **26** (1991), 230–42.
94. E. D. Harris, Jr., Rheumatoid arthritis. Pathophysiology and implications for therapy. *New England Journal of Medicine*, **322** (1990), 1277–89.
95. S. L. Parsons, S. A. Watson, P. D. Brown, H. M. Collins & R. J. Steele, Matrix metalloproteinases. *British Journal of Surgery*, **84** (1997), 160–6.
96. C. M. Dollery, J. R. McEwan & A. M. Henney, Matrix metalloproteinases and cardiovascular disease. *Circulation Research*, **77** (1995), 863–8.
97. A. Mauviel, Cytokine regulation of metalloproteinase gene expression. *Journal of Cellular Biochemistry*, **53** (1993), 288–95.
98. T. B. Rajavashisth, X. P. Xu, S. Jovinge *et al.*, Membrane type 1 matrix metalloproteinase expression in human atherosclerotic plaques: evidence for activation by proinflammatory mediators. *Circulation*, **99** (1999), 3103–9.
99. C. F. Singer, E. Marbaix, P. Lemoine, P. J. Courtoy & Y. Eeckhout, Local cytokines induce differential expression of matrix metalloproteinases but not their tissue inhibitors in human endometrial fibroblasts. *European Journal of Biochemistry*, **259** (1999), 40–5.
100. B. Gogly, W. Hornebeck, N. Groult, G. Godeau & B. Pellat, Influence of heparin(s) on the interleukin-1-beta-induced expression of collagenase, stromelysin-1, and tissue inhibitor of metalloproteinase-1 in human gingival fibroblasts. *Biochemical Pharmacology*, **56** (1998), 1447–54.
101. H. Chen, D. Li, T. Saldeen & J. L. Mehta, TGF-beta 1 attenuates myocardial ischemia-reperfusion injury via inhibition of upregulation of MMP-1. *American Journal of Heart and Circulatory Physiology*, **284** (2003), H1612–7.
102. H. Nagase, Activation mechanisms of matrix metalloproteinases. *Biological Chemistry*, **378** (1997), 151–60.
103. H. R. Lijnen, Plasmin and matrix metalloproteinases in vascular remodeling. *Thrombosis and Haemostasis*, **86** (2001), 324–33.
104. Z. S. Galis, R. Kranzhofer, J. W. Fenton, 2nd & P. Libby, Thrombin promotes activation of matrix metalloproteinase-2 produced by cultured vascular smooth muscle cells. *Arteriosclerosis, Thrombosis and Vascular Biology*, **17** (1997), 483–9.
105. X. P. Xu, S. R. Meisel, J. M. Ong *et al.*, Oxidized low-density lipoprotein regulates matrix metalloproteinase-9 and its tissue inhibitor in human monocyte-derived macrophages. *Circulation*, **99** (1999), 993–8.
106. S. Rajagopalan, X. P. Meng, S. Ramasamy, D. G. Harrison & Z. S. Galis, Reactive oxygen species produced by macrophage-derived foam cells regulate the activity of vascular matrix metalloproteinases *in vitro*. Implications for atherosclerotic plaque stability. *Journal of Clinical Investigation*, **98** (1996), 2572–9.
107. D. E. Gomez, D. F. Alonso, H. Yoshiji, U. P. Thorgeirsson, Tissue inhibitors of metalloproteinases: structure, regulation and biological functions. *European Journal of Cell Biology*, **74** (1997), 111–22.
108. N. Vine & J. T. Powell, Metalloproteinases in degenerative aortic disease. *Clinical Science (London)*, **81** (1991), 233–9.
109. R. W. Thompson, D. R. Holmes, R. A. Mertens *et al.*, Production and localization of 92-kilodalton gelatinase in abdominal aortic aneurysms. An elastolytic metalloproteinase expressed by aneurysm-infiltrating macrophages. *Journal of Clinical Investigation*, **96** (1995), 318–26.
110. Z. Li, L. Li, H. R. Zielke *et al.*, Increased expression of 72-kd type IV collagenase (MMP-2) in human aortic atherosclerotic lesions. *American Journal of Pathology*, **148** (1996), 121–8.
111. Z. S. Galis, G. K. Sukhova, M. W. Lark & P. Libby, Increased expression of matrix metalloproteinases and matrix degrading activity in vulnerable regions of human atherosclerotic plaques. *Journal of Clinical Investigation*, **94** (1994), 2493–503.
112. D. L. Brown, M. S. Hibbs, M. Kearney, C. Loushin & J. M. Isner, Identification of 92-kD gelatinase in human coronary atherosclerotic lesions. Association of active enzyme synthesis with unstable angina. *Circulation*, **91** (1995), 2125–31.
113. R. T. Aimes & J. P. Quigley, Matrix metalloproteinase-2 is an interstitial collagenase. Inhibitor-free enzyme

catalyzes the cleavage of collagen fibrils and soluble native type I collagen generating the specific 3/4- and 1/4-length fragments. *Journal of Biological Chemistry*, **270** (1995), 5872–6.

114. G. K. Sukhova, U. Schonbeck, E. Rabkin *et al.*, Evidence for increased collagenolysis by interstitial collagenases-1 and -3 in vulnerable human atheromatous plaques. *Circulation*, **99** (1999), 2503–9.
115. M. P. Herman, G. K. Sukhova, P. Libby *et al.*, Expression of neutrophil collagenase (matrix metalloproteinase-8) in human atheroma: a novel collagenolytic pathway suggested by transcriptional profiling. *Circulation*, **104** (2001), 1899–904.
116. R. T. Lee, F. J. Schoen, H. M. Loree, M. W. Lark & P. Libby, Circumferential stress and matrix metalloproteinase 1 in human coronary atherosclerosis. Implications for plaque rupture. *Arteriosclerosis, Thrombosis and Vascular Biology*, **16** (1996), 1070–3.
117. L. H. Arroyo & R. T. Lee, Mechanisms of plaque rupture: mechanical and biologic interactions. *Cardiovascular Research*, **41** (1999), 369–75.
118. S. J. Price, D. R. Greaves & H. Watkins, Identification of novel, functional genetic variants in the human matrix metalloproteinase-2 gene: role of Sp1 in allele-specific transcriptional regulation. *Journal of Biological Chemistry*, **276** (2001), 7549–58.
119. S. Ye, G. F. Watts, S. Mandalia, S. E. Humphries & A. M. Henney, Preliminary report: genetic variation in the human stromelysin promoter is associated with progression of coronary atherosclerosis. *British Heart Journal*, **73** (1995), 209–15.
120. M. Terashima, H. Akita, K. Kanazawa *et al.*, Stromelysin promoter 5A/6A polymorphism is associated with acute myocardial infarction. *Circulation*, **99** (1999), 2717–19.
121. B. Zhang, S. Ye, S. M. Herrmann *et al.*, Functional polymorphism in the regulatory region of gelatinase B gene in relation to severity of coronary atherosclerosis. *Circulation*, **99** (1999), 1788–94.
122. Y. Nemerson, Tissue factor and hemostasis. *Blood*, **71** (1988), 1–8.
123. A. Fernandez-Ortiz, J. J. Badimon, E. Falk *et al.*, Characterization of the relative thrombogenicity of atherosclerotic plaque components: implications for consequences of plaque rupture. *Journal of the American College of Cardiology*, **23** (1994), 1562–9.
124. P. R. Moreno, V. H. Bernardi, J. Lopez-Cuellar *et al.*, Macrophages, smooth muscle cells, and tissue factor in unstable angina. Implications for cell-mediated thrombogenicity in acute coronary syndromes. *Circulation*, **94** (1996), 3090–7.
125. F. Mach, U. Schonbeck & P. Libby, CD40 signaling in vascular cells: a key role in atherosclerosis? *Atherosclerosis*, **137** (Suppl) (1998), S89–95.
126. M. P. Bevilacqua, R. R. Schleef, M. A. Gimbrone, Jr. & D. J. Loskutoff, Regulation of the fibrinolytic system of cultured human vascular endothelium by interleukin 1. *Journal of Clinical Investigation*, **78** (1986), 587–91.
127. M. Aikawa, S. J. Voglic, S. Sugiyama *et al.*, Dietary lipid lowering reduces tissue factor expression in rabbit atheroma. *Circulation*, **100** (1999), 1215–22.
128. P. L. Giesen, U. Rauch, B. Bohrmann *et al.*, Blood-borne tissue factor: another view of thrombosis. *Proceedings of the National Academy of Sciences of the USA*, **96** (1999), 2311–5.
129. V. Toschi, R. Gallo, M. Lettino *et al.*, Tissue factor modulates the thrombogenicity of human atherosclerotic plaques. *Circulation*, **95** (1997), 594–9.
130. S. R. Meisel, X. P. Xu, T. S. Edgington *et al.*, Differentiation of adherent human monocytes into macrophages markedly enhances tissue factor protein expression and procoagulant activity. *Atherosclerosis*, **161** (2002), 35–43.
131. A. Sambola, J. Osende, J. Hathcock *et al.*, Role of risk factors in the modulation of tissue factor activity and blood thrombogenicity. *Circulation*, **107** (2003), 973–7.
132. S. Matetzky, S. Tani, S. Kangavari *et al.*, Smoking increases tissue factor expression in atherosclerotic plaques: implications for plaque thrombogenicity. *Circulation*, **102** (2000), 602–4.
133. A. C. Barger, R. Beeuwkes, 3rd, L. L. Lainey & K. J. Silverman, Hypothesis: vasa vasorum and neovascularization of human coronary arteries. A possible role in the pathophysiology of atherosclerosis. *New England Journal of Medicine*, **310** (1984), 175–7.
134. O. J. de Boer, A. C. van der Wal, P. Teeling & A. E. Becker, Leucocyte recruitment in rupture prone regions of lipid-rich plaques: a prominent role for neovascularization? *Cardiovascular Research*, **41** (1999), 443–9.
135. T. L. Haas & J. A. Madri, Extracellular matrix-driven matrix metalloproteinase production in endothelial

cells: implications for angiogenesis. *Trends in Cardiovascular Medicine*, **9** (1999), 70–77.
136. G. Kostoulas, A. Lang, H. Nagase & A. Baici, Stimulation of angiogenesis through cathepsin B inactivation of the tissue inhibitors of matrix metalloproteinases. *FEBS Letters*, **455** (1999), 286–90.
137. P. Saikku, M. Leinonen, L. Tenkanen *et al.*, Chronic *Chlamydia pneumoniae* infection as a risk factor for coronary heart disease in the Helsinki Heart Study. *Annals of Internal Medicine*, **116** (1992), 273–8.
138. P. Saikku, K. Mattila, M. S. Nieminen *et al.*, Serological evidence of an association of a novel chlamydia, TWAR, with chronic coronary heart disease and acute myocardial infarction. *Lancet*, **2** (1988), 983–6.
139. J. B. Muhlestein, J. L. Anderson, E. H. Hammond *et al.*, Infection with *Chlamydia pneumoniae* accelerates the development of atherosclerosis and treatment with azithromycin prevents it in a rabbit model. *Circulation*, **97** (1998), 633–6.
140. N. Ossei-Gerning, P. Moayyedi, S. Smith *et al.*, *Helicobacter pylori* infection is related to atheroma in patients undergoing coronary angiography. *Cardiovascular Research*, **35** (1997), 120–4.
141. F. J. Nieto, E. Adam, P. Sorlie *et al.*, Cohort study of cytomegalovirus infection as a risk factor for carotid intimal-medial thickening, a measure of subclinical atherosclerosis. *Circulation*, **94** (1996), 922–7.
142. A. H. M. Span, G. Grauls, F. Bosman, C. P. A. Van Boven & C. A. Bruggerman, Cytomegalovirus infection induces vascular injury in the rat. *Atherosclerosis*, **93** (1992), 41–52.
143. S. E. Epstein, J. Zhu, M. S. Burnett *et al.*, Infection and atherosclerosis: potential roles of pathogen burden and molecular mimicry. *Arteriosclerosis, Thrombosis and Vascular Biology*, **20** (2000), 1417–20.
144. S. S. Kaukoranta-Tolvanen, T. Ronni, M. Leinonen, P. Saikku & K. Laitinen, Expression of adhesion molecules on endothelial cells stimulated by *Chlamydia pneumoniae*. *Microbiology and Pathology*, **21** (1996), 407–11.
145. M. Heinemann, M. Susa, U. Simnacher, R. Marre & A. Essig, Growth of *Chlamydia pneumoniae* induces cytokine production and expression of CD14 in a human monocytic cell line. *Infection and Immunity*, **64** (1996), 4872–5.
146. A. Kol, G. K. Sukhova, A. H. Lichtman & P. Libby, Chlamydial heat shock protein 60 localizes in human atheroma and regulates macrophage tumor necrosis factor-alpha and matrix metalloproteinase expression. *Circulation*, **98** (1998), 300–7.
147. A. Kol, T. Bourcier, A. H. Lichtman & P. Libby, Chlamydial and human heat shock protein 60 activates human vascular endothelium, smooth muscle cells, and macrophages. *Journal of Clinical Investigation*, **103** (1999), 571–7.
148. S. M. Weiss, P. M. Roblin, C. A. Gaydos *et al.*, Failure to detect *Chlamydia pneumoniae* in coronary atheromas of patients undergoing atherectomy. *Journal of Infectious Diseases*, **173** (1996), 957–62.
149. D. L. Hahn & R. Golubjatnikov, Smoking is a potential confounder of the *Chlamydia pneumoniae*-coronary artery disease association. *Arteriosclerosis and Thrombosis*, **12** (1992), 945–7.
150. P. M. Ridker, R. B. Kundsin, M. J. Stampfer, S. Poulin & C. H. Hennekens, Prospective study of *Chlamydia pneumoniae* IgG seropositivity and risks of future myocardial infarction. *Circulation*, **99** (1999), 1161–4.
151. A. F. Stone, M. A. Mendall, J. C. Kaski *et al.*, Effect of treatment for *Chlamydia pneumoniae* and *Helicobacter pylori* on markers of inflammation and cardiac events in patients with acute coronary syndromes: South Thames Trial of Antibiotics in Myocardial Infarction and Unstable Angina (STAMINA). *Circulation*, **106** (2002), 1219–23.
152. M. Eliasziw, J. Y. Streifler, A. J. Fox *et al.*, Significance of plaque ulceration in symptomatic patients with high-grade carotid stenosis. North American Symptomatic Carotid Endarterectomy Trial. *Stroke*, **25** (1994), 304–8.
153. P. M. Rothwell, R. Salinas, L. A. Ferrando, J. Slattery & C. P. Warlow, Does the angiographic appearance of a carotid stenosis predict the risk of stroke independently of the degree of stenosis? *Clinical Radiology*, **50** (1995), 830–3.
154. M. L. Gronholdt, Ultrasound and lipoproteins as predictors of lipid-rich, rupture-prone plaques in the carotid artery. *Arteriosclerosis, Thrombosis and Vascular Biology*, **19** (1999), 2–13.
155. G. Rioufol, G. Finet, I. Ginon *et al.*, Multiple atherosclerotic plaque rupture in acute coronary syndrome: a three-vessel intravascular ultrasound study. *Circulation*, **106** (2002), 804–8.
156. W. Casscells, B. Hathorn, M. David *et al.*, Thermal detection of cellular infiltrates in living atherosclerotic

plaques: possible implications for plaque rupture and thrombosis. *Lancet*, **347** (1996), 1447–51.
157. C. Stefanadis, L. Diamantopoulos, C. Vlachopoulos *et al.*, Thermal heterogeneity within human atherosclerotic coronary arteries detected *in vivo*: a new method of detection by application of a special thermography catheter. *Circulation*, **99** (1999), 1965–71.
158. C. Stefanadis, K. Toutouzas, E. Tsiamis *et al.*, Increased local temperature in human coronary atherosclerotic plaques: an independent predictor of clinical outcome in patients undergoing a percutaneous coronary intervention. *Journal of the American College of Cardiology*, **37** (2001), 1277–83.
159. R. M. Botnar, M. Stuber, K. V. Kissinger *et al.*, Noninvasive coronary vessel wall and plaque imaging with magnetic resonance imaging. *Circulation*, **102** (2000), 2582–7.
160. P. M. Ridker, J. E. Buring, J. Shih, M. Matias & C. H. Hennekens, Prospective study of C-reactive protein and the risk of future cardiovascular events among apparently healthy women. *Circulation*, **98** (1998), 731–3.
161. P. M. Ridker, M. Cushman, M. J. Stampfer, R. P. Tracy & C. H. Hennekens, Inflammation, aspirin, and the risk of cardiovascular disease in apparently healthy men. *New England Journal of Medicine*, **336** (1997), 973–9.
162. H. Kai, H. Ikeda, H. Yasukawa *et al.*, Peripheral blood levels of matrix metalloproteases-2 and -9 are elevated in patients with acute coronary syndromes. *Journal of the American College of Cardiology*, **32** (1998), 368–72.
163. I. M. Loftus, A. R. Naylor, P. R. Bell & M. M. Thompson, Plasma MM-9 – a marker of carotid plaque instability. *European Journal of Vascular and Endovascular Surgery*, **21** (2001), 17–21.
164. S. Blankenberg, H. J. Rupprecht, O. Poirier *et al.*, Plasma concentrations and genetic variation of matrix metalloproteinase 9 and prognosis of patients with cardiovascular disease. *Circulation*, **107** (2003), 1579–85.
165. MRC/BHF Heart Protection Study of cholesterol lowering with simvastatin in 20 536 high-risk individuals: a randomised placebo-controlled trial. *Lancet*, **360** (2002), 7–22.
166. P. S. Sever, B. Dahlof, N. R. Poulter *et al.*, Prevention of coronary and stroke events with atorvastatin in hypertensive patients who have average or lower-than-average cholesterol concentrations, in the Anglo-Scandinavian Cardiac Outcomes Trial-Lipid Lowering Arm (ASCOT-LLA): a multicentre randomised controlled trial. *Lancet*, **361** (2003), 1149–58.
167. S. Bellosta, D. Via, M. Canavesi *et al.*, HMG-CoA reductase inhibitors reduce MMP-9 secretion by macrophages. *Arteriosclerosis, Thrombosis and Vascular Biology*, **18** (1998), 1671–8.
168. R. Scalia, M. E. Gooszen, S. P. Jones *et al.*, Simvastatin exerts both anti-inflammatory and cardioprotective effects in apolipoprotein E-deficient mice. *Circulation*, **103** (2001), 2598–603.
169. M. Endres, U. Laufs, Z. Huang *et al.*, Stroke protection by 3-hydroxy-3-methylglutaryl (HMG)-CoA reductase inhibitors mediated by endothelial nitric oxide synthase. *Proceedings of the National Academy of Sciences of the USA*, **95** (1998), 8880–5.
170. O. Shovman, Y. Levy, B. Gilburd & Y. Shoenfeld, Antiinflammatory and immunomodulatory properties of statins. *Immunology Research*, **25** (2002), 271–85.
171. Z. Luan, A. J. Chase & A. C. Newby, Statins inhibit secretion of metalloproteinases-1, -2, -3, and -9 from vascular smooth muscle cells and macrophages. *Arteriosclerosis, Thrombosis and Vascular Biology*, **23** (2003), 769–75.
172. M. Crisby, G. Nordin- Fredriksson, P. K. Shah *et al.*, Pravastatin treatment increases collagen content and decreases lipid content, inflammation, metalloproteinases, and cell death in human carotid plaques: implications for plaque stabilization. *Circulation*, **103** (2001), 926–33.
173. P. M. Ridker, N. Rifai & S. P. Lowenthal, Rapid reduction in C-reactive protein with cerivastatin among 785 patients with primary hypercholesterolemia. *Circulation*, **103** (2001), 1191–3.
174. M. Aikawa, E. Rabkin, S. Sugiyama *et al.*, An HMG-CoA reductase inhibitor, cerivastatin, suppresses growth of macrophages expressing matrix metalloproteinases and tissue factor *in vivo* and *in vitro*. *Circulation*, **103** (2001), 276–83.
175. T. Bourcier & P. Libby, HMG CoA reductase inhibitors reduce plasminogen activator inhibitor-1 expression by human vascular smooth muscle and endothelial cells. *Arteriosclerosis, Thrombosis and Vascular Biology*, **20** (2000), 556–62.

176. P. Libby & M. Aikawa, Effects of statins in reducing thrombotic risk and modulating plaque vulnerability. *Clinical Cardiology*, **26** (2003), I11–4.
177. M. Rouis, C. Adamy, N. Duverger *et al.*, Adenovirus-mediated overexpression of tissue inhibitor of metalloproteinase-1 reduces atherosclerotic lesions in apolipoprotein E- deficient mice. *Circulation*, **100** (1999), 533–40.
178. Y. Hu, A. H. Baker, Y. Zou, A. C. Newby & Q. Xu, Local gene transfer of tissue inhibitor of metalloproteinase-2 influences vein graft remodeling in a mouse model. *Arteriosclerosis, Thrombosis and Vascular Biology*, **21** (2001), 1275–80.
179. M. A. Schwartz, S. Venkataraman, M. A. Ghaffari *et al.*, Inhibition of human collagenases by sulfur-based substrate analogs. *Biochemical and Biophysical Research Communications*, **176** (1991), 173–9.
180. S. A. Watson, T. M. Morris, S. L. Parsons, R. J. Steele & P. D. Brown, Therapeutic effect of the matrix metalloproteinase inhibitor, batimastat, in a human colorectal cancer ascites model. *British Journal of Cancer*, **74** (1996), 1354–8.
181. D. A. Bigatel, J. R. Elmore, D. J. Carey *et al.*, The matrix metalloproteinase inhibitor BB-94 limits expansion of experimental abdominal aortic aneurysms. *Journal of Vascular Surgery*, **29** (1999), 130–8.
182. K. E. Porter, I. M. Loftus, M. Peterson *et al.*, Marimastat inhibits neointimal thickening in a model of human vein graft stenosis. *British Journal of Surgery*, **85** (1998), 1373–7.
183. G. D. Treharne, J. R. Boyle, S. Goodall *et al.*, Marimastat inhibits elastin degradation and matrix metalloproteinase 2 activity in a model of aneurysm disease. *British Journal of Surgery*, **86** (1999), 1053–8.
184. D. C. Talbot & P. D. Brown, Experimental and clinical studies on the use of matrix metalloproteinase inhibitors for the treatment of cancer. *European Journal of Cancer*, **32A** (1996), 2528–33.
185. N. C. Levitt, F. A. Eskens, K. J. O'Byrne *et al.*, Phase I and pharmacological study of the oral matrix metalloproteinase inhibitor, MMI270 (CGS27023A), in patients with advanced solid cancer. *Clinical Cancer Research*, **7** (2001), 1912–22.
186. R. A. Greenwald, L. M. Golub, N. S. Ramamurthy *et al.*, *In vitro* sensitivity of the three mammalian collagenases to tetracycline inhibition: relationship to bone and cartilage degradation. *Bone*, **22** (1998), 33–8.
187. G. N. Smith, Jr., L. P. Yu, Jr., K. D. Brandt & W. N. Capello, Oral administration of doxycycline reduces collagenase and gelatinase activities in extracts of human osteoarthritic cartilage. *Journal of Rheumatology*, **25** (1998), 532–5.
188. I. M. Loftus, K. Porter, M. Peterson *et al.*, MMP inhibition reduces intimal hyperplasia in a human vein graft stenosis model. *Annals of the New York Academy of Sciences*, **878** (1999), 547–50.
189. D. Petrinec, S. Liao, D. R. Holmes *et al.*, Doxycycline inhibition of aneurysmal degeneration in an elastase-induced rat model of abdominal aortic aneurysm: preservation of aortic elastin associated with suppressed production of 92 kD gelatinase. *Journal of Vascular Surgery*, **23** (1996), 336–46.
190. R. W. Thompson & B. T. Baxter, MMP inhibition in abdominal aortic aneurysms. Rationale for a prospective randomized clinical trial. *Annals of the New York Academy of Sciences*, **878** (1999), 159–78.
191. B. Axisa, I. M. Loftus, A. R. Naylor *et al.*, Prospective, randomized, double-blind trial investigating the effect of doxycycline on matrix metalloproteinase expression within atherosclerotic carotid plaques. *Stroke*, **33** (2002), 2858–64.
192. B. T. Baxter, W. H. Pearce, E. A. Waltke *et al.*, Prolonged administration of doxycycline in patients with small asymptomatic abdominal aortic aneurysms: report of a prospective (phase II) multicenter study. *Journal of Vascular Surgery*, **36** (2002), 1–12.
193. M. Miyazaki, H. Sakonjo, S. Takai, Anti-atherosclerotic effects of an angiotensin converting enzyme inhibitor and an angiotensin II antagonist in cynomolgus monkeys fed a high-cholesterol diet. *British Journal of Pharmacology*, **128** (1999), 523–9.
194. S. Yusuf, P. Sleight, J. Pogue *et al.*, Effects of an angiotensin-converting-enzyme inhibitor, ramipril, on cardiovascular events in high-risk patients. The Heart Outcomes Prevention Evaluation Study Investigators. *New England Journal of Medicine*, **342** (2000), 145–53.
195. P. E. Tummala, X. L. Chen, C. L. Sundell *et al.*, Angiotensin II induces vascular cell adhesion molecule-1 expression in rat vasculature: a potential link between the renin-angiotensin system and atherosclerosis. *Circulation*, **100** (1999), 1223–9.
196. S. Navalkar, S. Parthasarathy, N. Santanam & B. V. Khan, Irbesartan, an angiotensin type 1 receptor

inhibitor, regulates markers of inflammation in patients with premature atherosclerosis. *Journal of the American College of Cardiology*, **37** (2001), 440–4.

197. K. J. Molloy, M. M. Thompson, J. L. Jones *et al.*, Unstable carotid plaques exhibit raised MMP-8 activity. *Circulation*, **110** (2004), 337–43.

198. K. J. Molloy, M. M. Thompson, J. L. Jones *et al.*, Comparison of levels of matrix metalloproteinases, tissue inhibitor of metalloproteinases, interleukins and tissue necrosis factor in carotid endarterectomy Specimens from patients. On – vs. – not on statins pre-operatively. *American Journal of Cardiology*, **94** (2004), 144–6.

9 • Current and emerging therapies in atheroprotection

STEPHEN J. NICHOLLS AND PHILIP J. BARTER

BACKGROUND

Atherosclerotic cardiovascular disease is a leading cause of morbidity and mortality in the western world. The increasing prevalence of atherosclerotic risk factors (Table 9.1) in the developing world will see the global burden of vascular disease continue to rise. A greater understanding of both the pathogenesis of atherosclerosis and the critical role played by various risk factors has led to the development of potent therapeutic approaches to prevent both the development of atheroma and its complications.

Patients with established clinical vascular disease, regardless of the territory involved, have the highest ongoing risk of cardiovascular events. Those with peripheral arterial disease have a probability of death due to coronary artery or cerebrovascular disease of 55% and 10%, respectively [1]. Given the large event rate, therapeutic interventions have the potential to result in the greatest absolute reduction in clinical events.

Atherosclerosis is a chronic inflammatory condition, characterized by the accumulation of inflammatory cells, lipid and apoptotic material within the arterial wall. The driving forces underlying this process include the accumulation of atherogenic lipoproteins, inflammatory cells and oxidative stress [2]. The earliest changes occur in the endothelial cell layer. This single cell layer lining the lumen of the vasculature serves to regulate permeability of the arterial wall, vascular tone and tendency to thrombus formation. Dysfunction of the endothelial layer results in the expression of cell surface adhesion molecules (vascular cell adhesion molecule-1 (VCAM-1), intercellular adhesion molecule-1 (ICAM-1) and E-selectin), prothrombotic substances (von Willebrand factor (vWF) and plasminogen activator inhibitor-1 (PAI-1)) and impaired vascular reactivity. These abnormalities appear to be related to a reduction in the bioavailability of nitric oxide, the principal product of the endothelium [3].

The expression of cellular adhesion molecules anchors circulating monocytes to the endothelium and promotes their transmigration into the subendothelial space, in concert with chemokines such as monocyte chemoattractant protein-1 (MCP-1). Migrated monocytes undergo morphologic changes to become macrophages, which engulf extracellular lipid, to become foam cells, the hallmark of the atherosclerotic plaque. Foam cells produce various pro-inflammatory cytokines leading to the increasing accumulation of inflammatory and foam cells. This accumulation results in the formation of the fatty streak, the earliest morphologic change of atherogenesis [2].

Smooth muscle cells migrate into the area and produce collagen, which is laid down to form the fibrous cap. This separates the enlarging inflammatory and lipid milieu from the circulating blood stream. The accumulation of inflammatory cells, lipid and apoptotic ma-terial, covered by a strong fibrous cap, represents the mature atherosclerotic plaque [2]. Most atherosclerotic plaques remain clinically quiescent. However, some plaques progress to an advanced stage, characterized by the development of aneurysms or plaque rupture. Both of these complications relate to the degeneration of the extracellular collagen matrix, due to the production of various matrix metalloproteinases [4].

Degradation of collagen within the fibrous cap leads to a reduction in its tensile strength, and subject to the mechanical stress of blood flow, can lead to erosion or rupture [5]. This exposes the circulating bloodstream to the plaque contents including inflammatory cells, lipid, apoptotic material and the prothrombotic tissue factor (TF). This initiates the aggregation of platelets and activation of both further platelets and the coagulation cascade, leading to thrombus formation. It is the formation of a thrombus, overlying the atheroma, which leads to the occlusion of the arterial lumen and subsequent ischaemia [6].

Atherosclerotic prophylactic therapies can therefore be targeted at either primary or secondary prevention. Primary prevention aims to inhibit the development of atherosclerotic disease in the first instance. Secondary prevention, meanwhile, aims to prevent the occurrence of further clinical events and plaque complications, in those with established clinical atherosclerotic disease. This chapter will review the role of current pharmacologic agents and emerging therapies, their ability to regulate the fundamental processes of inflammation, oxidative stress and nitric oxide production, and their overall role in the prevention of atherosclerotic cardiovascular disease (Table 9.2).

Table 9.1. *Modifiable atherogenic risk factors*

- Elevated atherogenic lipoproteins
  - LDL cholesterol
  - Triglyceride
  - Lipoprotein (a)
  - Chylomicron remnant particles
- Reduced HDL cholesterol
- Hypertension
- Diabetes mellitus
- Obesity
- Cigarette smoking

RISK FACTOR MODIFICATION

Population studies have established an association of numerous factors, which can be modified, with an increased risk for the development of atherosclerotic disease [7; 8; 9]. These risk factors include: (i) elevated plasma concentrations of atherogenic lipoproteins, including low-density lipoprotein cholesterol (LDL-C), lipoprotein (a), triglyceride containing lipoproteins (such as chylomicrons), very low-density lipoprotein cholesterol (VLDL-C) and their remnant particles, and small, dense forms of LDL-C; (ii) reduced plasma concentrations of high-density lipoprotein cholesterol (HDL-C); (iii) hypertension; (iv) diabetes and impaired glycaemic control; (v) smoking; and (vi) obesity. Many of these factors, in particular the presence of small, dense LDL-C, reduced HDL-C, hypertension, impaired glycaemic control and obesity appear to be associated in the metabolic syndrome, with the pathogenic consequence insulin resistance. This syndrome is a strong stimulus of the inflammatory cascade in the vascular wall [10].

Primary and secondary intervention studies have demonstrated marked benefits for the therapeutic reduction of pro-atherogenic lipoproteins, the elevation of anti-atherogenic lipoproteins, aggressive control of blood pressure and the reduction of platelet activity. The results, however, of aggressive glycaemic control, hormone replacement and antioxidants have been disappointing.

Table 9.2. *Established agents which modify atherogenic and anti-atherogenic lipoproteins*

- Hypercholesterolaemia
  - Statins
  - Bile acid sequestrants
  - Nicotinic acid
- Hypertriglyceridaemia
  - Fibrates
  - Fish oil
  - Nicotinic acid
- Elevated lipoprotein (a)
  - Nicotinic acid
- Reduced HDL cholesterol
  - Fibrates

Modification of atherogenic lipoproteins

Population studies have demonstrated an unequivocal relationship between the plasma concentration of atherogenic lipoproteins and future risk of cardiovascular disease [7]. The atherogenic lipoproteins include LDL-C, triglycerides, remnant particles, lipoprotein (a), and the small, dense form of LDL-C associated with diabetes and the metabolic syndrome. Animal models [11; 12] and intervention studies [13], aimed at the therapeutic modulation of these lipoproteins, have resulted in marked reductions in both atherosclerotic burden and clinical cardiovascular events. Established therapies aimed at the reduction of these atherogenic lipoproteins include hydroxymethylglutaryl Co-A reductase inhibition, fibric acid derivatives, bile acid sequestrants, nicotinic acid, fish oils, LDL-C apheresis and ileal bypass surgery.

Hydroxymethylglutaryl Co-A reductase inhibition

Hydroxymethylglutaryl coenzyme-A (HMG Co-A) reductase is the rate limiting enzyme in the pathway leading to the endogenous synthesis of cholesterol by the liver (Table 9.3). Inhibition of this enzyme leads to the up-regulation of hepatic LDL receptors with subsequent removal of LDL-C from the circulating plasma [14]. Enzyme inhibition by the 'statin' agents leads to substantial reductions in LDL-C, in association with moderate reduction in triglyceride and modest elevation of HDL-C [15]. The agents are well tolerated, with small numbers developing an elevation of hepatic transaminases [16] and myositis [17]. Fulminant rhabdomyolysis is a rare complication of statin therapy [18].

Studies of both primary [19; 20] and secondary [21; 22; 23] prevention have established relative risk reductions of 20%–40% with statin therapy. The Scandinavian Simvastatin Survival Study (4S) [21] randomized 4444 patients, aged 35–70 years, with established coronary artery disease and fasting total cholesterol (TC) between 5.5 and 8 mmol/l, to treatment with simvastatin or placebo. After 5.4 years the primary end point of all-cause mortality was reduced by 30% with simvastatin. Similarly recurrent myocardial infarction, stroke and revascularization were reduced by 30%–40%. The Cholesterol and Recurrent Events (CARE) study [22] randomized 4159 patients, aged 21–75 years, with previous myocardial infarction and plasma TC of less than 6.2 mmol/l to pravastatin or placebo. Coronary end points of mortality, myocardial infarction and revascularization were reduced by 20%–30% over a five year follow-up. The Long-term Intervention with Pravastatin in Ischaemic Disease (LIPID) [23] study randomized 9014 patients, aged 31–75 years, with a history of an acute coronary syndrome and baseline TC between 4 and 7 mmol/l, to pravastatin or placebo. After 6.1 years pravastatin reduced coronary and all-cause mortality by 22% and 23%, respectively.

The West Of Scotland Coronary Prevention Study (WOSCOPS) [19] was a primary prevention study, which randomized 6595 middle aged males, with TC greater than 6.5 mmol/l, to pravastatin or placebo. A 4.9 year follow-up demonstrated that pravastatin reduced fatal and non-fatal coronary events by 31% and 33%, respectively. The AFCAPS/TexCAPS trial [20] randomized 6605 patients, with relatively 'average' total plasma cholesterol, between 4.6 and 6.8 mmol/l, to lovastatin or placebo. During a 5.2 year follow-up lovastatin reduced the combined end point of sudden death, myocardial infarction and unstable angina by 33%.

The Heart Protection Study (HPS) [24] randomized 20 536 patients, aged 40–80 years, with established atherosclerotic cardiovascular disease, or determined to be at high risk on the basis of diabetes mellitus, and TC greater than 3.5 mmol/l, to treatment with simvastatin or placebo. Significant reductions in clinical events, including all-cause mortality by 13%, cardiovascular mortality by 17%, coronary events by 27% and stroke by 25% were found with simvastatin therapy.

Sub-group analyses of the statin trials have failed to demonstrate a group with established atherosclerotic disease who do not derive benefit from this therapy. In particular, age, gender, baseline LDL-C and renal function did not affect the likelihood of response to statin initiation [24]. The clinical benefit found in the secondary prevention trials of statin therapy has not been paralleled by evidence of plaque regression on angiographic follow-up [25], although recent studies using intravascular ultrasound have demonstrated marked plaque remodelling within the arterial wall in response to statin therapy [26].

Whilst the clinical benefit found in the statin trials can be predicted from the degree of LDL-C lowering [27], *in vitro* and *in vivo* studies have supported the idea that statin agents have, in addition to the reduction of LDL-C, many potential anti-atherogenic effects. These pleiotropic effects include the reversal of endothelial dysfunction, increased production of nitric oxide, reduced reactive oxygen species, inhibition of adhesion molecule expression, inhibition of smooth muscle cell proliferation and apoptosis, reduced inflammatory infiltrate and metalloproteinase production, and inhibition of the pro-thrombogenic state, including reduced platelet aggregation, promotion of endogenous anticoagulants and reduced expression of the fibrinolytic inhibitor, PAI-1. Inhibition of mevalonic acid synthesis and its products may contribute to these non-lipid lowering effects [28].

The major benefit of statins is found in those patients with a high inflammatory state. *Post hoc* analysis of the CARE study demonstrated that those with circulating inflammatory markers greater than the 90th percentile had the greatest risk of recurrent events. In addition the greatest benefit from pravastatin, in terms of a reduction in the recurrent event rate, occurred in this group [29].

These pleiotropic effects can potentially result in stabilization of the established plaque, which becomes less likely to rupture and lead to clinical events. This has the potential to result in early benefits in terms of reduced events during periods of acute plaque ***rupture***. Evidence to support this theory is limited. A Swedish registry [30] of 19 599 patients admitted to hospital with acute myocardial infarction analysed the outcome according to statin administration at the time of hospital discharge. Those patients receiving therapy at discharge demonstrated a 25% reduction in mortality at 12 months. The Myocardial Ischaemia Reduction with Aggressive Cholesterol Lowering (MIRACL) study [31] randomized 3086 patients, older than 18 years, presenting to hospital with unstable angina or a non-Q-wave myocardial infarction, to receive high dose atorvastatin or placebo commencing 24–96 hours after admission. After 16 weeks, the atorvastatin group demonstrated a 14% reduction in the composite clinical end point of death, myocardial infarction, resuscitated cardiac arrest or admission for suspected ischaemia. This benefit resulted entirely due to a significant reduction in hospital admissions.

Thus the use of statin agents is well established in all patients with established vascular disease. The benefit of initiating therapy during the acute clinical event remains to be categorically demonstrated. Whilst a LDL-C threshold, below which no further benefit exists, has not been demonstrated, this is the subject of ongoing trials [32]. Given the low clinical event rate in those without established vascular disease, the empirical use of statins in those with elevated LDL-C cannot be supported. The use of statins for primary prevention is restricted to those with other vascular risk factors or marked elevations of LDL-C.

Table 9.3. *Statin summary points*

- Inhibit the rate limiting enzyme in cholesterol synthesis
- Up-regulate hepatic expression of LDL receptors
- Substantial reduction of plasma LDL cholesterol
- Modest reduction of plasma triglyceride
- Minor elevation of plasma HDL cholesterol
- 20%–30% reduction of events in primary prevention studies
- 30%–40% reduction of events in secondary prevention studies
- Clinical benefit proportionate to degree of LDL lowering
- Pleiotropic effects may contribute to clinical benefit
- Potential benefit from administration during acute ischaemic syndromes
- Benefit for all patients with established atherosclerosis

Fibric acid derivatives

These agents, known as fibrates, result in marked reductions in plasma triglyceride and elevation of HDL-C, with only modest reductions in LDL-C [15] (Table 9.4). Their mechanism of action remains unclear, but is thought to operate through the activation of the nuclear hormone receptor, peroxisome proliferator-activator receptor-α (PPAR-α) [33]. These agents are similarly associated with a small incidence of transaminase elevation and myositis. The combination of fibrate and statin therapy is associated with a greater incidence of rhabdomyolysis than either agent alone, although this seemed to be more of a problem with the use of cerivastatin [34].

Studies of both primary [35] and secondary [36; 37] prevention resulted in significant (20%–30%) reductions in clinical ischaemic events in patients with low concentrations of plasma HDL-C and relatively normal concentrations of LDL-C. The Helsinki heart study [35] was a primary prevention study of 4081 middle aged males with plasma non-HDL-C concentrations greater than 5.2 mmol/l, who were randomized to gemfibrozil or placebo. Treatment with gemfibrozil resulted in a 34% reduction in cardiac end points during a five year follow-up. *Post hoc* analysis revealed that in subjects with baseline plasma triglyceride greater than 2.3 mmol/l, in association with HDL-C less than 1.0 mmol/l, a much greater (68%) reduction in events was demonstrated with gemfibrozil [38].

The Veterans Affairs High-density Lipoprotein Intervention Trial (VA-HIT) [36] randomized 2531 males, younger than 74 years with coronary artery disease and plasma HDL-C concentration less than 1.0 mmol/l, LDL-C less than 3.6 mmol/l and triglyceride less than 3.4 mmol/l to treatment with gemfibrozil or placebo. After 5.1 years of follow-up study, gemfibrozil resulted in a 20% reduction in cardiac events. The

Table 9.4. *Summary of fibric acid derivatives*

- Agonists for the nuclear receptor PPAR-α
- Marked reduction of plasma triglyceride
- Marked elevation of plasma HDL cholesterol
- Potential anti-inflammatory actions
- 34% reduction in events in primary prevention trials
- 20% reduction in events in secondary prevention trials
- Greatest clinical benefit seen in those with hypertriglyceridaemia and elevated body mass index
- Predominant role in patients with established atherosclerosis and the metabolic syndrome

HDL-C concentration on therapy accurately predicted events.

The Bezafibrate Infarction Prevention (BIP) trial [37] randomized 3090 patients, aged 45–74 years, with existing coronary artery disease, HDL-C less than 1.16 mmol/l, triglyceride less than 3.4 mmol/l and TC between 4.7 and 6.5 mmol/l, to treatment with bezafib-rate or placebo. There was no significant reduction in clinical events with fibrate therapy during a 6.2 year follow-up period. Although a substantial number of patients in this study were subsequently prescribed statin therapy during the trial. Substudy analysis did however reveal a 31% reduction in events with fibrate therapy, in those with baseline plasma triglyceride concentrations in excess of 2.25 mmol/l.

Thus the major benefit in fibrate trials of both primary and secondary prevention, involving patients with reduced plasma HDL-C and relatively normal LDL-C, has been demonstrated in those with elevated plasma triglyceride, elevated body mass index and features of insulin resistance. In established atherosclerosis, their use should be primarily for those with hypertriglyceridaemia and low HDL-C, despite established statin therapy.

Bile acid sequestrants

The bile acid resins act to bind bile acids in the intestinal lumen, leading to the inhibition of enterohepatic recycling. The subsequent increase in hepatic bile acid synthesis is associated with a reduction in the plasma concentration of LDL-C and increases in plasma triglyceride [15]. These agents are not absorbed into the systemic circulation and therefore do not appear to have any pleiotropic effects. Clinical trials have demonstrated a reversal of endothelial dysfunction [39], and reduced clinical events [40; 41], in addition to the promotion of atherosclerotic regression and inhibition of progression on an angiographic follow-up [42]. Despite their efficacy in lowering LDL-C and ischaemic events, both alone and in combination with other lipid-lowering agents, their benefit is limited by their low tolerability due to gastrointestinal side effects [40].

Nicotinic acid

This class of agents has numerous effects on plasma lipoproteins secondary to a reduction of hepatic VLDL-C production, inhibition of peripheral lipolysis and an increased circulating concentration of apolipoprotein A-I, the predominant protein of HDL-C. This leads to reductions of plasma LDL-C, triglyceride and lipoprotein (a), in addition to the elevation of HDL-C [15]. Trials of nicotinic acid, alone [43] or in combination with other lipid lowering agents [44; 45], reduce clinical events, in addition to promoting atherosclerotic regression and inhibiting progression [44; 46; 47]. Its use is limited by intolerance, particularly flushing, hyperuricaemia, hepatic dysfunction and hyperglycaemia [15].

Lipoprotein (a), a variant of LDL-C, is potently atherogenic due to its high cholesterol ester content in addition to its plasminogen like structure, which leads to competitive inhibition of the fibrinolytic system [48]. The plasma concentration of lipoprotein (a) is an independent risk factor for the development of clinical atherosclerotic events [49]. Despite the ability of nicotinic acid to decrease lipoprotein (a), there have been no large clinical trials to demonstrate benefit in terms of reduced clinical events.

Fish oils

Population studies have demonstrated an inverse correlation between dietary consumption of fish and the incidence of cardiovascular disease [50; 51]. The ω-3 fatty acids have anti-inflammatory, antiplatelet and antiarrhythmic effects which potentially contribute to a reduction of cardiovascular events [15]. In addition, the plasma triglyceride concentration is decreased [15]. Fish oil supplementation in secondary intervention studies reduces clinical events [52].

LDL apheresis

The removal of LDL-C from the circulating plasma is usually reserved for those with familial hypercholesterolaemia, with marked elevation in LDL-C, despite maximal medical therapy. Its use on a periodic basis leads to a marked reduction in plasma LDL-C. Studies in patients with established coronary artery disease have demonstrated a variable ability to inhibit plaque progression [53], and in some cases to promote the regression of an atherosclerotic burden on angiographic [54; 55] and intravascular ultrasound [56] analysis. In association with these findings are improvements in symptoms [53; 54; 57], exercise tolerance [58], regional myocardial perfusion [59] and coronary event rates [60].

Partial ileal bypass

This surgical procedure aims to reduce the plasma concentration of TC via inhibition of the enterohepatic recycling of bile salts. This has secondary effects through an increase in bile salt production by the liver, with a concomitant increase in LDL receptor expression and consequent reduction in plasma LDL-C [15]. The Program on the Surgical Control of the Hyperlipidemias (POSCH) [61] randomized subjects with a previous myocardial infarction to diet or diet combined with partial ileal bypass. During long term follow-up patients assigned to the surgical arm demonstrated significant reductions in TC and LDL-C, an elevation in HDL-C and less progression of coronary artery disease on the basis of angiographic follow-up. Extended post-trial follow-up of patients demonstrated significant reductions in mortality, non-fatal myocardial infarction, coronary revascularization and clinical onset of peripheral arterial disease in the surgical arm [62].

Elevation of HDL cholesterol

The plasma concentration of HDL-C is inversely correlated with the incidence of cardiovascular events (Table 9.5). Multivariate analysis of Framingham data demonstrated that HDL-C was the strongest independent predictor of future events [63]. For every 1 mg/dl increase in plasma HDL-C concentration, cardiovascular risk reduces by 2% in males and 3% in females. Similarly, baseline HDL-C is a strong predictor of events in the statin trials [20].

This atheroprotective property has been subsequently confirmed both in animal models [64; 65; 66; 67; 68] involving the administration, or transgenic expression, of HDL-C or its major protein, apolipoprotein A-I and in human intervention studies [35; 36; 37] aimed at its therapeutic elevation. High-density lipoprotein cholesterol has numerous potential atheroprotective functions. These include the promotion of reverse cholesterol transport [69], protection of both LDL-C and endothelial cells from oxidative change [70; 71], inhibition of the cytokine induced expression of endothelial cell surface adhesion molecules [72] and subsequent monocyte migration [73], and inhibition of the prothrombogenic milieu associated with atheroma [68].

High-density lipoprotein cholesterol is produced in a lipid depleted form of circulating apolipoprotein A-I, the major protein of HDL-C, in both the liver and small intestine. Lipid poor apolipoprotein A-I comes into contact with cell membranes and accepts both effluxed cholesterol and phospholipid. Efflux is promoted by a family of transmembrane associated proteins, which utilize ATP as an energy source [74]. Cholesterol taken up by the HDL-C particle is quickly esterified by the enzyme lecithin:cholesterol acyltransferase (LCAT) and stored in the core of the particle. This maintains the free cholesterol gradient promoting further efflux of cholesterol from the cell to HDL-C [75].

High-density lipoprotein cholesterol has two pathways by which it disposes of this effluxed cholesterol. It can deliver cholesterol directly to the liver, where it is internalized through interaction with the scavenger receptor-BI, (SR-BI), where it is excreted in the form of bile acids. Alternatively cholesterol can be transferred from HDL-C to LDL-C particles, via the enzyme cholesterol ester transfer protein (CETP), which is then transported to the liver, via the LDL receptor [76; 77; 78]

Numerous strategies have been proposed to increase the circulating plasma concentration of HDL-C, through either an increase in production or reduced catabolism. Non-pharmacologic options include weight loss, smoking cessation and mild alcohol consumption [15]. Established pharmacologic agents, including fibrates, statins and nicotinic acid, increase HDL-C by 10%–35%, 5%–15% and 15%–35%, respectively [15].

Primary [35] and secondary [36; 37] prevention trials of fibrates, in conditions of low HDL-C, alone and in combination with nicotinic acid [45], lead to reduced cardiovascular events. Sub-group analysis has demonstrated the greatest benefit in those with

Table 9.5. *Summary of HDL cholesterol*

- Strongest independent predictor of cardiovascular events
- Atheroprotective through numerous actions
  - Promotes cholesterol efflux
  - Anti-inflammatory actions
  - Reduces oxidation of LDL
  - Reduces cytotoxicity of oxidized LDL
  - Inhibits thromogenicity
- Potential to stabilize atherosclerotic plaque
- Elevated by weight loss, cigarette smoking cessation and mild alcohol consumption
- Therapeutically elevated by fibrates and nicotinic acid
- Enzymes that remodel HDL cholesterol are attractive targets for therapeutic manipulation

hypertriglyceridaemia and increased body mass index [38]. Angiographic studies in diabetic patients have shown reduced atherosclerotic progression [79]. Clinical trials of fibrate therapy in diabetic patients are currently in progress [80]. These trials strongly support the use of fibrates in those patients with established cardiovascular disease, low HDL-C and concomitant insulin resistance.

Similarly, the combination of nicotinic acid and statin therapy in patients with established coronary artery disease, low HDL-C and normal LDL-C leads to a significant reduction of LDL-C, elevation of HDL-C and regression of atherosclerosis on follow-up angiography. This benefit is attenuated with the addition of antioxidants [44].

Various developments in the understanding of both the function and metabolism of HDL-C highlight potential therapeutic options to enhance its atheroprotection. Recent animal studies have demonstrated the rapid depletion of lipid and inflammatory cells from established atheroma following a single infusion of apolipoprotein A-I_{Milano}, a variant of apolipoprotein A-I. This highlights the potential for acute elevation of HDL-C to stabilize an established plaque [81]. In addition, oral peptides which stimulate the production of apolipoprotein A-I and elevate HDL-C, are atheroprotective in animal models [82]. Circulating HDL-C is subject to numerous plasma factors which contribute to remodelling of the particle in terms of size and composition. These include the enzymes LCAT, CETP, hepatic lipase and phospholipid transfer protein, and represent potential therapeutic targets for the elevation of HDL-C and atheroprotection [83].

Hypertension

Epidemiologic studies have established a direct relationship between both systolic and diastolic blood pressure and cardiovascular events [84] (Table 9.6). The strength of this relationship varies throughout the vascular tree, being greatest for cerebrovascular disease. Observational data revealed that 25% of the US adult population have hypertension, the incidence increasing with age [85]. Framingham data predict the lifetime risk of developing hypertension to be about 90% by the age 65 [86]. The Multiple Risk Factors Intervention Trial (MRFIT) demonstrated a continuous and graded relationship between both systolic and diastolic blood pressure and death due to both coronary heart disease and stroke [87]. The strength of these relationships is greater for systolic blood pressure. In addition, isolated systolic hypertension, the most common form of hypertension results in a 2.5-fold greater risk of cardiovascular disease compared with matched patients with normal blood pressure [88].

Hypertension alters shear forces in the vascular lumen, and promotes structural and biochemical changes at the level of the endothelial cell, leading to dysfunction and the initiation of the atherosclerotic process [89]. Steady laminar flow stimulates endothelial cellular functions which maintain appropriately regulated permeability, thrombogenicity and vascular tone. These changes in flow are commonly seen at bifurcations and curved regions of arteries, the sites predisposed to atheroma formation [90].

Conditions leading to a reduction in mean shear stress, oscillatory flow and reversal of flow result in various changes to endothelial cell function promoting the inflammatory cascade of atherogenesis [91]. These include an increase in the permeability and retention of atherogenic lipoproteins by the arterial wall, in addition to an increased production of cell surface adhesion molecules, and chemotactic and growth factors, promoting the accumulation of an inflammatory infiltrate.

The cellular, biochemical and structural changes result from changes to vascular regulatory substances, including nitric oxide, endothelin, intracellular calcium and angiotensin II. In addition, chronic shear alteration promotes changes in gene expression, including endothelial nitric oxide synthase. These changes occur in response to the mechanotransduction of signals, from the endothelial surface, in response to altered shear stress [92].

The use of anti-hypertensive therapy for primary prevention reduces cardiovascular events. A meta-analysis of randomized controlled trials involving the reduction of systemic hypertension in primary prevention revealed a 21% risk reduction in events due to coronary heart disease and a 37% reduction in the incidence of stroke [93].

A substudy of the United Kingdom Prospective Diabetes Study (UKPDS) randomized diabetics with hypertension to conventional or aggressive blood pressure lowering arms. An incremental 13 mm Hg reduction in systolic blood pressure in the aggressive arm was associated with a 44% reduction in the incidence of stroke when compared with the conventional group [94].

The Hypertension Optimisation Trial (HOT) study randomized patients with hypertension to therapy aiming at three groups of blood pressure targets. Analysis revealed the lowest incidence of cardiovascular events in those with a mean diastolic blood pressure on therapy of 82.6 mm Hg. Thus the data support an aggressive lowering of blood pressure into the 'normal' range to reduce events [95].

The Heart Outcome Prevention Evaluation (HOPE) study supports the use of angiotensin converting enzyme (ACE) inhibition in all high risk patients. Despite the minimal blood pressure reduction seen in the ramipril arm, treatment with the ACE inhibitor reduced the composite vascular end point by 22%. This supports the critical role played by the renin-angiotensin system in the promotion of the atherosclerotic process [96].

The recently published Antihypertensive and Lipid-Lowering Treatment to prevent Heart Attack Trial (ALLHAT) demonstrated no difference in ischaemic cardiovascular event rates in patients with hypertension treated with a thiazide diuretic, ACE inhibitor or calcium channel antagonist. In addition, the diuretic arm was associated with a significant reduction in hospitalization for heart failure. This highlights the benefit of the cost effective thiazide diuretics, which should be considered front line agents and essential components of combination therapy for hypertension [97].

Table 9.6. *Summary of hypertension*

- Strong independent risk factor
- Small reductions in blood pressure result in marked reduction in clinical events
- Reduction of blood pressure to the normal range results in the least number of clinical events
- ACE inhibition reduces events in all high risk patients, regardless of baseline blood pressure
- Thiazide diuretics should be considered first line agents and be part of all combination regimens

Glycaemic control

Diabetes mellitus and impaired fasting glucose promote the atherosclerotic process (Table 9.7). More than 90% of clinical cardiovascular disease in diabetics is found in those with the adult onset form [98]. The presence of diabetes increases the risk of incident coronary, cerebrovascular and peripheral arterial disease by two- to four-fold compared with matched non-diabetic controls [99; 100; 101]. In patients with established clinical events, the incidence of diabetes increases morbidity and mortality related to the acute event, and in the long term increases the likelihood of recurrent ischaemic events and mortality [102; 103; 104; 105]. In addition, the relative protection from clinical cardiovascular disease in premenopausal women, is attenuated in the presence of diabetes [106]. In light of these findings, the newly released National Cholesterol Education Program-Adult Treatment Panel III (NCEP-ATP III) risk factor modification guidelines consider the presence of diabetes mellitus to be an atherosclerosis equivalent and suggest that patients with diabetes should be treated the same as those with established clinical cardiovascular disease in terms of risk factor modification [15].

Numerous factors contribute to atherogenesis in diabetes. These include chronic hyperglycaemia, advanced glycation end products, oxidative stress, dyslipidaemia and insulin resistance [98]. The resultant reduced bioavailability of nitric oxide [98], increased production of reactive oxygen species [107] and endothelin [108], and liberation of free fatty acids [109] promote functional and structural changes in the endothelial cell, including the activation of NF-κ β. These changes promote the adhesion and transmigration of inflammatory cells, vasoconstriction and thrombogenicity characteristic of endothelial dysfunction. In addition, advanced glycated end products promote the migration [110] and subsequent apoptosis of vascular smooth muscle cells [111]. Hyperglycaemia is associated with increased metalloprotease production [112]. The prothrombogenic state is further promoted through increased platelet activation and tissue factor accumulation, in addition to the inhibition of fibrinolysis and anticoagulation [113]. Thus hyperglycaemia contributes to all stages of atherogenesis.

Given the strong relationship between diabetes, dyslipidaemia, hypertension and obesity as part of the metabolic syndrome, the anti-atherosclerotic therapeutic approach is multifactorial. Weight loss and lifestyle modification are an integral approach to the management of each of these components, and thus form the first stage approach in management.

Despite the strong relationship between increasing plasma glucose concentration and cardiovascular risk [114], intervention studies of glycaemic control have been disappointing. Despite the use of aggressive glycaemic control leading to a significant reduction in the incidence of microvascular complications, the United Kingdom Prospective Diabetes Study (UKPDS) failed to demonstrate a reduction in macrovascular events, regardless of the agent used. A sub-group with obesity and insulin resistance did demonstrate a reduction in events with metformin [115].

Few studies have assessed the benefit of aggressive glycaemic control in secondary prevention. In patients with acute myocardial infarction and elevated plasma glucose concentration, aggressive glycaemic control with an insulin infusion followed by multiple daily doses of insulin for three months led to reduced clinical events over a five year period compared with conventional therapy [116]. A larger study is currently in progress.

The peroxisome proliferator-activated receptor-γ (PPAR-γ) agonists have the potential to improve glycaemic control and reduce events. These agents, represented by the thiazolidinediones, improve insulin sensitivity [117] and inhibit the pro-inflammatory cascade in the vascular wall [118], contributing to the atherosclerotic process, and are thus of potential benefit in both primary and secondary prevention. The results of large scale trials are awaited.

Table 9.7. *Summary of Diabetes*

- Diabetes and insulin resistance are both strong risk factors
- Increases morbidity and mortality in those with established atherosclerosis
- Glycaemic control correlates with clinical outcome
- Aggressive glycaemic control reduces microvascular complications
- Trials involving aggressive glycaemic control and macrovascular complications have been disappointing
- Strongest evidence for risk reduction via aggressive control of blood pressure and lipids
- PPAR-γ agonists have the potential to reduce events through their ability to improve glycaemic control and reduce vascular inflammation

The greatest benefit for diabetic patients, in terms of event reduction, has resulted from aggressive modification of plasma lipoproteins and blood pressure. Diabetic dyslipidaemia, characterized by elevated triglyceride, reduced HDL-C and the presence of small, dense LDL-C particles, represents a potent atherogenic stimulus. Weight loss and aggressive glycaemic control lead to an improvement in this lipid profile [15]. The statin [21] and fibrate [36] trials demonstrated greater relative risk reduction in the diabetic sub-groups. Similarly, aggressive blood pressure control results in greater benefit in terms of risk reduction when compared with non-diabetics [119]. The blood pressure lowering substudy of the UKPDS confirmed a reduction in cerebrovascular events in those with aggressive blood pressure lowering [94]. The HOPE data suggested a similar benefit for the use of ramipril in patients with diabetes at baseline, compared with those with established vascular disease [96]. In accordance with these findings the American Diabetes Association recommends a target blood pressure of 130/80 mm Hg for cardiovascular risk reduction [120].

ANTIPLATELET THERAPY

The platelet plays a critical role in thrombus formation, the pathological cause of ischaemic cardiovascular events. Platelet activation and aggregation is potently stimulated in the setting of rupture or erosion of the fibrous cap, exposing the atheromatous core of lipid, necrotic material, inflammatory cells and tissue factor. Thrombus formation either leads to luminal occlusion or is covered by a fibrous cap and integrated into an enlarging plaque. Therapies directed at the prevention of thrombosis and dissolution of the thrombus are critical in the management of atherosclerotic cardiovascular disease.

The platelet is now thought to play an important role in the early stages of atherogenesis [121]. Through the surface expression of P-selectin and CD40 ligand, and aggregation with von Willebrand factor on the surface of dysfunctional endothelial cells, the platelet contributes to the adhesion and subsequent transmigration of inflammatory cells into the arterial wall. Thus antiplatelet therapies have the potential to inhibit the atherosclerotic process at a much earlier stage than rupture of the fibrous cap.

The role of antiplatelet agents in the secondary prevention of cardiovascular disease, regardless of vascular territory, is well established. Meta-analysis demonstrated a 22% reduction in recurrent events, regardless of the agent used [122]. The evidence for primary prevention is not as strong. The Physician's Health Study demonstrated that clinical benefit of the primary use of aspirin in middle aged men was restricted to those with an elevation of high sensitivity C-reactive protein at baseline [123]. This result supports a potential anti-inflammatory benefit of antiplatelet agents.

Aspirin, the most commonly used antiplatelet agent, is limited by gastrointestinal toxicity and variable platelet resistance [124]. This has stimulated the search for other antiplatelet targets to extend therapeutic benefit. The thienopyridines target the platelet surface ADP receptor. They are not associated with significant gastrointestinal toxicity. The use of clopidogrel in established cardiovascular disease led to an 8% relative risk reduction of ischaemic events in comparison to aspirin [125].

The glycoprotein IIb/IIIa receptor on the platelet surface represents the final common pathway leading to platelet aggregation. It therefore represents an ideal therapeutic target to inhibit thrombus formation [126]. The use of intravenous antagonists of this receptor have led to benefits in terms of reduced clinical events, in the setting of both acute coronary syndromes [127] and percutaneous intervention [128]. However, trials of oral formulations have been disappointing [129].

HORMONE REPLACEMENT THERAPY

Clinical atherosclerotic disease begins at a later age in females. This gender difference in clinical events narrows following the onset of the menopause and is attributed to the effects of oestrogen [130]. Oestrogen has numerous potential atheroprotective actions. These include the promotion of a favourable lipid profile with (i) reduced LDL-C, (ii) reduced lipoprotein (a) and (iii) elevation of HDL-C, as well as improved vascular tone, reduced oxidative stress and a reduction in vascular inflammation [131].

The administration of synthetic oestrogen analogues leads to a reduction in the atherosclerotic burden in animal models [132]. When combined with progestins, this benefit is reduced [133]. Oestrogen administration also leads to improvements in non-invasive markers of vascular risk including flow mediated dilatation [134] and arterial compliance [135]. Population studies have supported a role for hormone replacement therapy in reducing clinical events by 40%–50% [136].

Despite this potential benefit, intervention studies of hormone replacement therapy, in both the primary and secondary prevention of cardiovascular events, have been disappointing. The Women's Health Initiative (WHI) demonstrated a 29% increase in cardiovascular events during five year follow-up with the combination of oestrogen and medroxyprogesterone acetate [137]. Similarly the Heart and Estrogen/Progestin Replacement Study (HERS) of women with established vascular disease demonstrated no benefit after five years of the combination of oestrogen and medroxyprogesterone acetate, following an initial increase in events during the first 12 months [138].

Randomized, placebo controlled studies of hormone replacement therapy in women with established coronary artery disease [138] or increased carotid intimal medial thickness [139] have failed to demonstrate any benefit for hormone replacement in terms of atherosclerosis regression. These disappointing results parallel the lack of clinical benefit.

The reasons underlying these results remain unclear. An increase in thrombotic events secondary to supplemental oestrogen administration may explain part of these findings. Hormone replacement has varying effects on inflammatory markers [140]. It may be that an early increase in inflammation and thrombogenicity with hormone replacement led to the increase in events during the first 12 months of the HERS trial. The subsequent reduction in events may reflect the more long term improvement in plasma lipoproteins, with its concomitant reductions in inflammation and thrombogenicity. Different progesterone formulations have varying effects on vascular tone. For example, oestrogen appears to promote a greater improvement in vascular reactivity when used in combination with micronized progestin, compared with medroxyprogesterone acetate [131; 141]. Regardless, whether it be for primary or secondary prophylaxis, the routine use of hormone replacement therapy for the indication of the prevention of cardiovascular events can not be recommended at this time.

ANTIOXIDANT VITAMINS

Oxidative stress plays a fundamental role in the development of the atherosclerotic plaque. It promotes dysfunction of the endothelial cell and propagation of the pro-inflammatory cascade, leading to the accumulation of lipid, inflammatory cells and necrotic material in the evolving plaque. Animal models have demonstrated a reduction of the atherosclerotic burden following administration of antioxidants [142; 143; 144]. Population studies have demonstrated an inverse correlation between the intake of vitamin E and the incidence of clinical cardiovascular events [145; 146].

Unfortunately, intervention studies have failed to demonstrate a benefit for the administration of these antioxidants in both primary and secondary prevention. The clinical use of probucol, a potent antioxidant, is associated with a reduction of plasma HDL-C concentration and progression of coronary atherosclerosis [147]. The beta carotene study revealed no reduction in the primary occurrence of cardiovascular events [148]. The antioxidant arm of the HOPE study revealed no benefit with vitamin E in patients with established vascular disease or diabetes [96]. Similarly the antioxidant of the Heart Protection Study revealed no benefit with the antioxidant cocktail of vitamin E, vitamin C and beta carotene [149]. The HATS trial found no benefit for an antioxidant cocktail of vitamin E, vitamin C, beta carotene and selenium in terms of lipid profile, clinical events and atherosclerotic progression. In addition, their concomitant use attenuated the benefit found with the combination of statin and niacin [44].

These strategies sought to include a broad range of natural antioxidants at sufficient doses to have an effect. The reason for this consistent lack of benefit remains unclear. Some potential antioxidant strategies do appear to work. For example, HDL-C can inhibit the oxidation of lipoproteins in the arterial wall, through the action of enzymes such as paraoxonase [70]. Given the established role for oxidative stress in the early stages of atherogenesis, it may be that the intervention studies have targeted patients at too late a stage to have a major impact. In addition, oral vitamin supplementation may not efficiently penetrate the arterial wall, where its action would be of greatest benefit.

ANTIBIOTIC THERAPY

Infection has been proposed to promote the inflammatory cascade in the arterial wall. The histologic [150] and serologic [151] association of various infectious organisms with the presence of atherosclerosis and clinical cardiovascular disease suggests a possible role for antimicrobial therapy in the therapeutic prevention of atherosclerosis and its complications. Early studies of anti-chlamydial antibiotics reduced clinical events [152]. However, larger randomized studies have been disappointing [153]. Recent data suggest that the extent of atherosclerotic disease and clinical outcome are correlated with the extent of infectious burden, represented by the number of serologic responses to various infectious organisms [154]. This supports a role for the overall infectious exposure contributing to inflammation in the arterial wall and would suggest that agents targeted against specific organisms are of limited use in atheroprotection.

DIET

Population studies have correlated the dietary intake of saturated fat with the incidence of atherosclerotic cardiovascular disease [155]. Similarly, diets enriched in polyunsaturated fatty acids appear to confer some protection from clinical events [156]. Dietary intervention trials involving a reduction in the content of saturated fat led to a reduction in both the plasma concentration of atherogenic lipoproteins and incidence of cardiovascular events [157]. These results support the findings of animal studies which demonstrate a reduction in atherosclerotic burden with diets, deplete of saturated fat and enriched with polyunsaturated fat [158].

Secondary dietary intervention studies have also demonstrated a profound benefit for reductions in saturated fat and enriched polyunsaturated fatty acids in terms of decreased cardiovascular mortality. The benefit seen in the DART [159] and GISSI-Prevenzione [52] studies was limited to significant reductions in sudden cardiac death. This was consistent with the known antiarrhythmic actions of ω 3 fatty acids. The Lyon Diet Heart Study [160] demonstrated reductions in both recurrent ischaemia and sudden cardiac death with the use of a Mediterranean diet, enriched with monounsaturated fat and deplete in saturated fat, following acute myocardial infarction.

In light of these findings, the American Heart Association (AHA) guidelines for dietary recommendations in the setting of established atherosclerotic disease have been updated [161]. Emphasis has been placed on severe restrictions of both total and saturated fat, in addition to dietary cholesterol.

FOLIC ACID

The plasma concentration of homocysteine is directly correlated with the incidence of cardiovascular events on meta-analysis, although the association is weaker for prospective studies [162; 163]. Homocysteine has been demonstrated to have many potential pro-atherogenic actions in both *in vitro* and *in vivo* models [164]. These include the promotion of inflammation, oxidative stress and thrombogenicity. Folic acid is a water soluble, B-complex vitamin, which through its reduced forms acts as co-factors and substrates for various metabolic enzymes. The main dietary sources of folic acid include green leafy vegetables, fruit and fortified cereal. One of the effects of folic acid is to inhibit the production of homocysteine.

The Homocysteine Lowering Trialist's Collaboration reported analysis of 12 trials demonstrating a 25% reduction in the plasma concentration of homocysteine following the dietary supplementation of 0.5–5 mg folic acid [165]. High dose folic acid administration, in the setting of hyperhomocysteinaemia, has been demonstrated to reduce plasma homocysteine concentration and improve endothelial function, as measured by vascular reactivity [166]. In addition to reduced homocysteine, folic acid may also have direct beneficial actions at the level of the endothelial cell [167]. The ability of folic acid to reduce clinical end points is unknown, but is the subject of numerous ongoing randomized controlled trials [164].

OTHER EMERGING THERAPIES

It remains unclear whether a LDL-C threshold exists, below which no further risk reduction occurs. In addition to more powerful statin agents, other modalities are under development to lower LDL-C. Inhibition of the enzyme acyl:cholesterol acyltransferase [168] and the low intestinal absorption of dietary cholesterol [169] leads to a further reduction in LDL-C and atheroprotection in animal models. The ability to combine these agents with established lipid-lowering agents is under investigation.

The peroxisome proliferator-activator receptors (PPAR) are a family of nuclear receptors which co-ordinate multiple effector pathways regulating metabolism and the inflammatory cascade. The early generation of therapeutic agonists of these receptors include the fibric acid derivatives and the thiazolidinediones. These agents are relatively weak receptor agonists. In addition to their ability to regulate free fatty acid metabolism, plasma HDL concentration and glycaemic control, these agents have been demonstrated in animal models to have potent anti-inflammatory actions. The therapeutic benefit with relatively weak agonists would suggest that more powerful agonists have the potential to exert a profound anti-atherosclerotic effect. In addition, the development of compounds which target more than one class of PPAR are of immense interest in light of the high prevalence of concomitant metabolic abnormalities [170].

The inflammatory cascade is promoted by a complex network of adhesion molecules, chemokines, cytokines and growth factors. These pro-inflammatory factors each represent potential targets for atheroprotection. There is, however, a relative degree of redundancy in the promotion of this cascade, and therefore the key unifying factors such as NF-κ β and CD40 ligand may be more attractive targets as they are potent regulators of this complex process [171].

In the event of established atheroma, the stabilization of a plaque may be a more important therapeutic target than the promotion of plaque regression. In addition to a reduction of plaque inflammation, inhibition of metalloproteases and a reduction in plaque thrombogenicity contribute to plaque stability. Specific metalloproteinase inhibitors have been trialled in various inflammatory conditions, but are associated with substantial toxicity [172]. The benefit of antiplatelet [122], antithrombotic [173] and fibrinolytic [174] therapies in the treatment of cardiovascular events is well established. The development of more specific modalities which target the factors co-ordinating the thrombogenic state of complicated atheroma will result in further reductions in clinical events.

MONITORING THERAPY

The emergence of new anti-atherosclerotic therapies has coincided with the development of novel strategies to monitor atheroma and the underlying inflammatory process (Table 9.8). The evolution of these modalities has resulted from the inability of the traditional cardiovascular risk factors to accurately predict the risk of clinical events in all patients. These modalities can be divided into three broad categories: (i) serum or plasma markers, (ii) non-invasive analysis of atheroma, and (iii) invasive plaque imaging.

Various circulating inflammatory markers have been correlated with the risk of cardiovascular events. In addition, their response to known anti-atherosclerotic therapies, appears to predict the clinical benefit of these agents. High sensitivity C-reactive protein predicts future cardiovascular events in subjects with and without established atherosclerotic disease [175; 176]. In addition, elevated concentrations predict those likely to receive the greatest relative risk reduction from treatment with aspirin [123] and statins [29].

The endothelial cell surface adhesion molecules appear in the circulating plasma in elevated concentrations in those with atheroma [177] and acute coronary syndromes [178]. The relationship between soluble adhesion molecules and cardiovascular risk assessment varies among studies [179]. Other possible inflammatory markers include circulating interleukins and metalloproteinases.

Given the close association between inflammation, thrombogenicity and atherogenesis, various haemostatic markers in the plasma may be of use in the assessment of risk and monitoring therapy. These include fibrinogen [180], PAI-1 [181] and soluble forms of the CD40 ligand [182]. The pivotal role of oxidative stress in the promotion of the inflammatory cascade highlights a role for monitoring plasma concentrations of oxidative markers such as oxidized LDL-C [183].

Dysfunctional endothelium is characterized by reduced bioavailability of nitric oxide and impaired vascular reactivity, in response to acetylcholine and ischaemic stress. The use of brachial artery ultrasonography to measure the change in arterial diameter and flow following the infusion of acetylcholine or inflation of blood pressure cuffs to suprasystolic levels is well correlated with the presence of atherosclerotic risk factors [184] and established vascular disease [185]. As a research tool, flow mediated dilatation improves in response to risk factor modification.

The ankle brachial index predicts future cardiovascular events and mortality [186], in addition to the severity of vascular disease within the leg [187]. The measurement of intimal medial thickness of the carotid artery is now used as a research tool as a surrogate marker of atheroma. It appears to be well correlated with the plasma concentration of inflammatory markers [188] and predicts clinical cardiovascular events [189]. It may be of use in monitoring the response of anti-atherosclerotic therapies.

Calcification of the coronary arteries, demonstrated by electron beam computerized tomography, predicts not only the presence and overall burden of atherosclerosis within the coronary tree [190], but is also able to predict the risk of clinical events [191]. This modality has entered the clinical spectrum, although controversy exists as to in whom it should be used. The ability of coronary calcification to predict future events in superiority to traditional risk factor assessment has not been clearly established [192]. Statin therapy attenuates the rise in calcium score on follow-up imaging [193].

Whilst each of these modalities can assess the plaque in terms of its burden, calcification or physiologic effect, they lack the ability to assess plaque composition with a view to predicting the likelihood of rupture. In addition to the assessment of overall atherosclerotic burden, magnetic resonance imaging, can visualize the plaque with resolution to characterize lipidic, inflammatory and fibrocellular areas. These findings correlate with histologic assessment in animal models and allow for a non-invasive measure of plaque stability [194]. Statin therapy increases the fibrocellular component of the plaque, consistent with stabilization [195].

Table 9.8. *Monitoring therapy*

- Circulating markers
  - High sensitivy C-reactive protein
  - Cell adhesion molecules
  - Interleukins
  - Metalloproteinases
  - Fibrinogen
  - Plasminogen activator inhibitor-1
  - CD40 and CD40 ligand
  - Oxidized LDL-C
- Non-invasive assessment of the endothelium and atheroma
  - Flow mediated dilatation
  - Ankle brachial index
  - Carotid intimal medial thickness
  - Coronary artery calcification
  - Magnetic resonance imaging
- Invasive plaque imaging
  - Angiography
  - Intravascular ultrasound
  - Intravascular thermography
  - Optical coherence tomography

Angiography is the accepted gold standard modality in the assessment of atherosclerosis. However, this assessment of luminal stenosis is limited by its inability to assess plaque composition and to identify the plaque in the remodelled wall of an arterial segment that retains its normal sized vascular lumen. Various intravascular strategies have been developed that allow for imaging of the plaque and assessment of its inflammatory potential. Intravascular ultrasound can assess plaque volume, composition and associated vascular remodelling [196]. Preliminary studies have demonstrated plaque regression following statin therapy [26]. In a similar fashion, intravascular optical coherence tomography can image the plaque through the analysis of reflected light, rather than sound [197]. Thermographic catheters can assess the heat emitted from the plaque, consistent with the inflammatory content of the atheroma [198].

CONCLUSION

Atherogenesis represents the culmination of a complex series of cellular and humoral events that promote the inflammatory cascade and thrombogenicity. The therapeutic approach to both the primary and secondary prevention of atherosclerotic disease has now broadened beyond the traditional approach of modification of conventional cardiovascular risk factors. Established therapies can now be interpreted in terms of their ability to switch off vascular inflammation. Emerging modalities aim to target specific aspects of the inflammatory process. The development of more powerful plasma and imaging markers of atherosclerotic burden and its inflammatory content will improve risk prediction for cardiovascular events, and the ability to monitor the response to anti-atherosclerotic therapies.

Table 9.9. *Summary points*

- Strongest evidence for risk reduction for therapeutic reduction of atherogenic lipoproteins
- All patients with established atherosclerosis should receive a statin
- Those with insulin resistance should receive a fibrate
- Elevation of plasma HDL-C is an attractive target
- Aggressive blood pressure control reduces events
- The greatest reduction in events in diabetics results from aggressive blood pressure and lipid control
- Fundamental role of the platelet in all stages of atherogenesis
- Dietary modification to reduce saturated fatty acids and increase unsaturated fatty acids reduce events
- Trials of antioxidant vitamins, hormone replacement and antibiotics have been disappointing
- All therapeutic modalities should be considered by their ability to reduce vascular inflammation

REFERENCES

1. TransAtlantic Inter-Society Consensus (TASC). Management of peripheral arterial disease. *Journal of Vascular Surgery*, **1**(Suppl) (2001), 1–296.
2. R. Ross, Atherosclerosis – an inflammatory disease. *New England Journal of Medicine*, **340** (1999), 115–26.
3. D. Behrendt, Endothelial function. From vascular biology to clinical applications. *American Journal of Cardiology*, **90** (10C) (2002), 40L–48L.
4. H. Lijnen, Extracellular proteolysis in the development and progression of atherosclerosis. *Biochemical Society Transactions*, **30** (2002), 163–7.

5. L. Arroyo, Mechanisms of plaque rupture: mechanical and biologic interactions. *Cardiovascular Research*, **41** (1999), 369–75.
6. P. Libby, Current concepts of the pathogenesis of the acute coronary syndromes. *Circulation*, **104** (2001), 365–72.
7. M. Martin, Serum cholesterol, blood pressure, and mortality: implications from a cohort of 361 662 men. *Lancet*, **2** (1986), 933–6.
8. K. Anderson, Cholesterol and mortality. 30 years of followup from the Framingham Study. *JAMA*, **257** (1987), 2176–80.
9. G. Assmann, The Munster heart study (Procam). Results of follow-up at 8 years. *European Heart Journal*, **19** (Suppl A) (1998), A2–11.
10. A. Raji, Insulin resistance, diabetes, and atherosclerosis: thiazolidinediones as therapeutic interventions. *Current Cardiology Reports*, **4** (2002), 514–21.
11. R. Rosenson, Antiatherothrombotic properties of statins: implications for cardiovascular event reduction. *JAMA*, **279** (1998), 1643–50.
12. J. Fruchart, The role of fibric acids in atherosclerosis. *Current Atherosclerosis Reports*, **3** (2001), 83–92.
13. C. Sirtori, Cardiovascular risk changes after lipid lowering medications: are they predictable? *Atherosclerosis*, **152** (2000), 1–8.
14. A. Endo, The discovery and development of HMG-CoA reductase inhibitors. *Journal of Lipid Research*, **33** (1992), 1569–82.
15. National Cholesterol Education Program. Detection, evaluation, and treatment of high blood cholesterol in adults (Adult Treatment Panel III). *Circulation*, **106** (2002), 3143–421.
16. R. Bradford, Expanded Clinical Evaluation of Lovastatin (EXCEL) study results. I. Efficacy in modifying plasma lipoproteins and adverse event profile in 8245 patients with moderate hypercholesterolemia. *Archives of Internal Medicine*, **151** (1991), 43–9.
17. M. Davidson, Lipid-altering efficacy and safety of simvastatin 80mg/day: worldwide long-term experience in patients with hypercholesterolemia. *Nutrition, Metabolism and Cardiovascular Diseases*, **10** (2001), 253–62.
18. R. Pasternak, ACC/AHA/NHLBI clinical advisory in the use and safety of statins. *Circulation*, **106** (2002), 253–62.
19. J. Shepherd, Prevention of coronary heart disease with pravastatin in men with hypercholesterolemia. *New England Journal of Medicine*, **333** (1995), 1301–7.
20. J. Downs, Primary prevention of acute coronary events with lovastatin in men and women with average cholesterol levels. *JAMA*, **279** (1998), 1615–22.
21. Randomised trial of cholesterol lowering in 4444 patients with coronary heart disease: the Scandinavian Simvastatin Survival Study (4S). *Lancet*, **344** (1994), 1383–9.
22. F. Sacks, The effect of pravastatin on coronary events after myocardial infarction in patients with average cholesterol levels. *New England Journal of Medicine*, **335** (1996), 1001–9.
23. The Long-term Intervention with Pravastatin in Ischaemic Disease (LIPID) Study Group. Prevention of cardiovascular events and death with pravastatin in patients with coronary heart disease and a broad range of initial cholesterol levels. *New England Journal of Medicine*, **339** (1998), 1349–57.
24. Heart Protection Study Group. MRC/BHF Heart Protection Study of cholesterol lowering with simvastatin in 20536 high-risk individuals: a randomized placebo-controlled trial. *Lancet*, **360** (2002), 7–22.
25. R. Archbold, Modification of coronary artery disease progression by cholesterol-lowering therapy: the angiographic studies. *Current Opinion in Lipidology*, **10** (1999), 527–34.
26. T. Hagenaars, Early experience with intravascular ultrasound in evaluating the effect of statins on femoralpopliteal arterial disease: hypothesis-generating observations in humans. *Cardiovascular Drugs Therapy*, **14** (2000), 635–41.
27. A. Gould, Cholesterol reduction yields clinical benefit: impact of statin trials. *Circulation*, **98** (1998), 839–44.
28. M. Takemoto, Pleiotropic effects of 3-hydroxy-3-methylglutaryl coenzyme a reductase inhibitors. *Arteriosclerosis, Thrombosis and Vascular Biology*, **21** (2001), 1712–9.
29. P. Ridker, Inflammation, pravastatin, and the risk of coronary events after myocardial infarction in patients with average cholesterol levels. Cholesterol and Recurrent Events (CARE) Investigators. *Circulation*, **98** (1998), 839–44.
30. U. Stenestrand & L. Wallentin, Swedish Register of cardiac Intensive Care (RIKS-HIA). Early statin treatment following acute myocardial infarction and 1-year survival. *JAMA*, **285** (2001), 430–6.

31. G. Schwartz, Effects of atorvastatin on early recurrent ischemic events in acute coronary syndromes: the MIRACL study: a randomized controlled trial. *JAMA*, **295** (2001), 1711–8.
32. C. Cannon, Design of the Pravastatin or Atorvastatin Evaluation and Infection Therapy (PROVE IT)-TIMI 22 trial. *American Journal of Cardiology*, **89** (2002), 860–1.
33. K. Schoonjans, Role of the peroxisome proliferator-activated receptor (PPAR) in mediating the effects of fibrates and fatty acids on gene expression. *Journal of Lipid Research*, **37** (1996), 907–25.
34. C. Bolego, Safety considerations for statins. *Current Opinion in Lipidology*, **13** (2002), 637–44.
35. M. Frick, Helsinki heart study: primary-prevention trial with gemfibrozil in middle-aged men with dyslipidemia. *New England Journal of Medicine*, **317** (1987), 1237–45.
36. H. Rubins, Gemfibrozil for the secondary prevention of coronary heart disease in men with low levels of high-density lipoprotein cholesterol. *New England Journal of Medicine*, **341** (1999), 410–8.
37. The Bezafibrate Infarction Prevention (BIP) Study Group. Secondary prevention by raising HDL cholesterol and reducing triglycerides in patients with coronary heart disease. The bezafibrate infarction prevention (BIP) study. *Circulation*, **102** (2000), 21–7.
38. V. Manninen, Joint effects of serum triglyceride and LDL cholesterol and HDL cholesterol concentrations on coronary heart disease risk in Helsinki heart study. Implications for treatment. *Circulation*, **85** (1992), 37–45.
39. W. Leung, Beneficial effect of cholesterol-lowering therapy on coronary endothelium-dependent relaxation in hypercholesterolaemic patients. *Lancet*, **341** (1993), 1496–500.
40. Lipid Research Clinics Program. The Lipid Research Clinics Coronary Primary Prevention Trial results. I: reduction in the incidence of coronary heart disease. *JAMA*, **251** (1984), 351–64.
41. Lipid Research Clinics Program. The Lipid Research Clinics Coronary Primary Prevention Trial results. II: the relationship of reduction in incidence of coronary heart disease to cholesterol lowering. *JAMA*, **251** (1984), 365–74.
42. G. Watts, Effects on coronary artery disease of lipid-lowering diet, or diet plus cholestyramine, in the St Thomas' Atherosclerosis Regression Study (STARS). *Lancet*, **339** (1992), 563–9.
43. Coronary Drug Project Research Group. Clofibrate and niacin in coronary heart disease. *JAMA*, **231** (1975), 360–81.
44. B. Brown, Simvastatin and niacin, antioxidant vitamins, or the combination for the prevention of coronary disease. *New England Journal of Medicine*, **345** (2001), 1583–92.
45. L. Carlson, Reduction of mortality in the Stockholm Ischaemic Heart Disease Secondary Prevention Study by combined treatment with clofibrate and nicotinic acid. *Acta Medica Scandinavica*, **223** (1988), 405–18.
46. D. Blankenhorn, Beneficial effects of combined colestipol-niacin therapy on coronary atherosclerosis and coronary venous bypass grafts. *JAMA*, **257** (1987), 3233–40.
47. G. Brown, Regression of coronary artery disease as a result of intensive lipid-lowering therapy in men with high levels of apolipoprotein B. *New England Journal of Medicine*, **323** (1990), 1289–98.
48. S. Ishibashi, Lipoprotein (a) and atherosclerosis. *Arteriosclerosis, Thrombosis and Vascular Biology*, **21** (2001), 1–2.
49. J. Danesh, Lipoprotein (a) and coronary heart disease: meta-analysis of prospective studies. *Circulation*, **102** (2000), 1082–5.
50. C. Albert, Fish consumption and risk of sudden cardiac death. *JAMA*, **279** (1998), 23–8.
51. M. Daviglus, Fish consumption and the 30-year risk of fatal myocardial infarction. *New England Journal of Medicine*, **336** (1997), 1046–53.
52. GISSI-Prevenzione Investigators. Dietary supplementation with n-3 polyunsaturated fatty acids and vitamin E after myocardial infarction: results of the GISSI-Prevenzione Trial. *Lancet*, **354** (1999), 447–55.
53. T. Waidner, The effect of LDL apheresis on progression of coronary artery disease in patients with familial hypercholesterolemia: results of a multicenter LDL apheresis study. *Clinical Investigation*, **72** (1994), 858–63.
54. P. Schuff-Werner, The HELP-LDL-Apheresis multicentre study, an angiographically assessed trial on the role of LDL-apheresis in the secondary prevention of coronary heart disease, II: final evaluation of the effect of regular treatment on LDL-cholesterol plasma concentrations and the course of coronary heart disease. *European Journal of Clinical Investigation*, **24** (1994), 724–32.

55. R. Tatami, Regression of coronary atherosclerosis by combined LDL-apheresis and lipid-lowering drug therapy in patients with familial hypercholesterolemia: a multicenter study. *Atherosclerosis*, **95** (1992), 1–13.
56. M. Matsuzaki, Intravascular ultrasound evaluation of coronary plaque regression by low density lipoprotein-apheresis in familial hypercholesterolemia: the Low Density Lipoprotein-Apheresis Coronary Morphology and Research Trial (LACMART). *Journal of the American College of Cardiology*, **40** (2002), 220–7.
57. S. Mii, LDL apheresis for arteriosclerosis obliterans with occluded bypass graft: change in prostacyclin and effect on ischemic symptoms. *Angiology*, **49** (1998), 175–80.
58. A. Kroon, LDL-Apheresis Atherosclerosis Regression Study (LAARS): effect of aggressive versus conventional lipid lowering treatment on coronary atherosclerosis. *Circulation*, **93** (1996), 1826–35.
59. W. Aengevaeren, Low density lipoprotein apheresis improves regional myocardial perfusion in patients with hypercholesterolaemia and extensive coronary artery disease: LDL-Apheresis Atherosclerosis Regression Study (LAARS). *Journal of the American College of Cardiology*, **28** (1996), 1696–704.
60. H. Mabuchi, Long-term efficacy of low density lipoprotein apheresis on coronary heart disease. *American Journal of Cardiology*, **82** (1998), 1489–95.
61. H. Buchwald, Effect of partial ileal bypass surgery on mortality and morbidity from coronary heart disease in patients with hypercholesterolemia. Report of the Program on the Surgical Control of the Hyperlipidemias (POSCH). *New England Journal of Medicine*, **323**(14) (1990), 946–55.
62. H. Buchwald, Effective lipid modification by partial ileal bypass reduced long-term coronary heart disease mortality and morbidity: five-year posttrial followup report from the POSCH. Program on the Surgical Control of the Hyperlipidemias. *Archives of Internal Medicine*, **158**(11) (1998), 1253–61.
63. D. Gordon, High-density lipoprotein cholesterol and cardiovascular disease. Four prospective American studies. *Circulation*, **79** (1989), 8–15.
64. N. Duverger, Inhibition of atherosclerosis development in cholesterol-fed human apolipoprotein A-I-transgenic rabbits. *Circulation*, **94** (1996), 713.
65. C. Paszty, Apolipoprotein AI transgene corrects apolipoprotein E deficiency-induced atherosclerosis in mice. *Journal of Clinical Investigation*, **94** (1994), 899–903.
66. E. Rubin, Inhibition of early atherogenesis in transgenic mice by human apolipoprotein AI. *Nature*, **353** (1991), 265–67.
67. J. Badimon, Regression of atherosclerotic lesions by high density lipoprotein plasma fraction in the cholesterol-fed rabbit. *Journal of Clinical Investigation*, **85** (1990), 1234–41.
68. J. Rong, Elevating high-density lipoprotein cholesterol in apolipoprotein E-deficient mice remodels advanced atherosclerotic lesions by decreasing macrophage and increasing smooth muscle cell content. *Circulation*, **104** (2001), 2447–52.
69. C. Fielding, Molecular physiology of reverse cholesterol transport. *Journal of Lipid Research*, **36** (1995), 211.
70. S. Parthasarathy, High-density lipoprotein inhibits the oxidative modification of low-density lipoprotein. *Biochimica et Biophysica Acta*, **1044** (1990), 275–83.
71. C. Banka, High density lipoprotein and lipoprotein oxidation. *Current Opinion in Lipidology*, **7** (1996), 139.
72. G. Cockerill, High-density lipoproteins inhibit cytokine-induced expression of endothelial cell adhesion molecules. *Arteriosclerosis Thrombosis and Vascular Biology*, **15** (1995), 1987–94.
73. M. Navab, Monocyte transmigration induced by modification of low density lipoprotein in cocultures of human aortic wall cells is due to induction of monocyte chemotactic protein 1 synthesis and is abolished by high density lipoprotein. *Journal of Clinical Investigation*, **88** (1991), 2039–46.
74. S. Santamarina-Fojo, & Regulation and intracellular trafficking of the ABCA1 transporter. *Journal of Lipid Research*, **42** (2001), 1339–45.
75. S. Santamarina-Fojo, Lecithin-cholesterol acyltransferase: role in lipoprotein metabolism, reverse cholesterol transport and atherosclerosis. *Current Opinion in Lipidology*, **11** (2000), 267–75.
76. P. Barter, Cholesteryl ester transfer protein, high density lipoprotein and arterial disease. *Current Opinion in Lipidology*, **12** (2001), 377–82.
77. P. Barter, CETP and atherosclerosis. *Arteriosclerosis, Thrombosis and Vascular Biology*, **20** (2000), 2029–31.
78. S. Acton, The HDL receptor SR-BI: a new therapeutic target for athersclerosis? *Molecular Medicine Today*, **5** (1999), 518–24.
79. DAIS Investigators. Effects of fenofibrate on progression of coronary-artery disease in type 2

diabetes: the Diabetes Atherosclerosis Intervention Study, a randomised study. *Lancet*, **357** (2001), 905–10.
80. G. Steiner, Lipid intervention trials in diabetes. *Diabetes Care*, **23**(Suppl 2) (2000), B49–53.
81. P. Shah, High-dose recombinant apolipoprotein A-Imilano mobilizes tissue cholesterol and rapidly reduces plaque lipid and macrophage content in apolipoprotein E-deficient mice. *Circulation*, **103** (2001), 3047–50.
82. B. van Lenten, Influenza infection promotes macrophage traffic into arteries of mice that is prevented by D-4F, an apo A-I mimetic peptide. *Circulation*, **106** (2002), 1127–32.
83. K. Rye, Remodelling of high density lipoproteins by plasma factors. *Atherosclerosis*, **145** (1999), 227–38.
84. The Framingham Study, An epidemiological investigation of cardiovascular disease. Section 34. Some risk factors related to the annual incidence of cardiovascular disease and death using pooled repeated biennial measurements: *Framingham Heart Study, 30-year Follow-up*. (Bethesda, MD: National Heart, Lung, and Blood Institute, 1987).
85. The sixth report of the Joint National Committee on prevention, detection, evaluation, and treatment of high blood pressure. *Archives of Internal Medicine*, **157** (1997), 2413–46.
86. R. Vasan, Residual lifetime risk for developing hypertension in middle-aged women and men: The Framingham Heart Study. *JAMA*, **287** (2002), 1003–10.
87. J. Stamler, Blood pressure, systolic and diastolic, and cardiovascular risks. US population data. *Archives of Internal Medicine*, **153** (1993), 598–615.
88. S. Wilking, Determinants of isolated systolic hypertension. *JAMA*, **260** (1988), 3451–5.
89. A. Fisher, Endothelial cellular response to altered shear stress. *American Journal of Physiology – Lung Cellular and Molecular Physiology*, **281** (2001), L529–33.
90. C. Zarins, Carotid bifurcation atherosclerosis. Quantitative correlation of plaque localization with flow velocity profiles and wall shear stress. *Circulation Research*, **53** (1983), 502.
91. O. Traub, Laminar shear stress: mechanisms by which endothelial cells transduce an atheroprotective force. *Arteriosclerosis, Thrombosis and Vascular Biology*, **18** (1998), 677.
92. P. Davies, Flow-mediated endothelial mechanotransduction. *Physiological Review*, **75** (1995), 519.
93. J. He, Elevated systolic blood pressure and risk of cardiovascular and renal disease: overview of evidence from observational epidemiologic studies and randomised controlled trials. *American Heart Journal*, **138** (1999), 211–9.
94. UK Prospective Diabetes Study Group. Tight blood pressure control and risk of macrovascular and microvascular complications in type 2 diabetes: UKPDS 38. *British Medical Journal*, **317** (1998), 703–13.
95. L. Hansson, Effects of intensive blood-pressure lowering and low-dose aspirin in patients with hypertension. *Lancet*, **351** (1998), 1755–62.
96. S. Yusuf, Effects of an angiotensin-converting-enzyme inhibitor, ramipril, on cardiovascular events in high-risk patients. The Heart Outcomes Prevention Evaluation Study Investigators. *New England Journal of Medicine*, **342** (2000), 145–53.
97. ALLHAT Collaborative Research Group, Major outcomes in high-risk hypertensive patients randomised to angiotensin-converting enzyme inhibitor or calcium channel blocker versus diuretic: the Antihypertensive and Lipid-Lowering Treatment to prevent Heart Attack Trial (ALLHAT). *JAMA*, **288** (2002), 2981–97.
98. J. Beckman, Diabetes and atherosclerosis. Epidemiology, pathophysiology, and management. *JAMA*, **287** (2002), 2570–81.
99. E. Feskens, Glucose tolerance and the risk of cardiovascular disease: the Zutphen Study. *Journal of Clinical Epidemiology*, **45** (1992), 1327–34.
100. A. Newman, Ankle-arm index as a marker of atherosclerosis in the Cardiovascular Health Study. *Circulation*, **88** (1993), 837–45.
101. J. Stamler, Diabetes, other risk factors, and 12-yr cardiovascular mortality for men screened in the Multiple Risk Factor Intervention Trial. *Diabetes Care*, **16** (1993), 434–44.
102. F. Hu, The impact of diabetes mellitus on mortality from all causes and coronary heart disease in women. *Archives of Internal Medicine*, **161** (2001), 1717–23.
103. S. Kjaergaard, In-hospital outcome for diabetic patients with acute myocardial infarction in the thrombolytic era. *Scandinavian Cardiovascular Journal*, **33** (1999), 166–70.
104. K. Malmberg, Impact of diabetes on long-term prognosis in patients with unstable angina and non-Q-wave myocardial infarction: results of the OASIS (Organization to Assess Strategies for Ischemic Syndromes) Registry. *Circulation*, **102** (2000), 1014–9.

105. G. Zuanetti, Influence of diabetes on mortality in acute myocardial infarction. *Journal of the American College of Cardiology*, **22** (1993), 1788–94.
106. D. Shindler, Diabetes mellitus in cardiogenic shock complicating acute myocardial infarction. **36** (2000), 1097–103.
107. A. De Vriese, Endothelial dysfunction in diabetes. *British Journal of Pharmacology*, **130** (2000), 963–74.
108. P. Quehenberger, Endothelin 1 transcription is controlled by nuclear factor-kappa B in AGE-stimulated cultured endothelial cells. *Diabetes*, **49** (2000), 1561–70.
109. M. Hennes, Insulin resistant lipolysis in abdominally obese hypertensive individuals. *Hypertension*, **28** (1996), 120–6.
110. L. Suzuki, Diabetes accelerates smooth muscle accumulation in lesions of atherosclerosis. *Diabetes*, **50** (2001), 851–60.
111. S. Taguchi, A comparative study of cultured smooth muscle cell proliferation and injury, utilizing glycated low density lipoproteins with slight oxidation, auto-oxidation, or extensive oxidation. *Journal of Atherosclerosis and Thrombosis*, **7** (2000), 132–7.
112. S. Uemura, Diabetes mellitus enhances vascular matrix metalloprotease activity. *Circulation Research*, **88** (2001), 1291–8.
113. A. Ceriello, Hyperglycemia-induced thrombin formation in diabetes. *Diabetes*, **44** (1995), 924–8.
114. R. Turner, The UK Prospective Diabetes Study: a review. *Diabetes Care*, **21**(Suppl 3) (1998), C35–8.
115. UK Prospective Diabetes Study Group. Intensive blood-glucose control with sulphonlyureas or insulin compared with conventional treatment and risk of complications in patients with type 2 diabetes (UKPDS33). *Lancet*, **352** (1998), 837–53.
116. K. Malmberg, Randomized trial of insulin-glucose infusion followed by subcutaneous insulin treatment in diabetic patients with acute myocardial infarction (DIGAMI study): effects of mortality at 1 year. *Journal of the American College of Cardiology*, **26** (1995), 57–65.
117. S. Aronoff, Pioglitazone hydrocholoride monotherapy improves glycemic control in the treatment of patients with type 2 diabetes. *Diabetes Care*, **23** (2000), 1605–11.
118. J. Plutzky, Peroxisome proliferator-activated receptors in vascular biology and atherosclerosis. *Current Atherosclerosis Reports*, **2** (2000), 327–35.
119. J. Tuomilehto, Effects of calcium-channel blockade in older patients with diabetes and systolic hypertension. *New England Journal of Medicine*, **340** (1999), 677–84.
120. J. Sowers, Diabetes, hypertension, and cardiovascular disease. *Hypertension*, **37** (2001), 1053–9.
121. S. Prescott, Sol Sherry lecture in thrombosis: molecular events in inflammation. *Arteriosclerosis, Thrombosis and Vascular Biology*, **22** (2002), 727–33.
122. Antithrombotic Trialest's Collaboration, Collaborative meta-analysis of randomised trials of antiplatelet therapy for prevention of death, myocardial infarction, and stroke in high risk patients. *British Medical Journal*, **324** (2002), 71–86.
123. P. Ridker, Inflammation, aspirin, and the risk of cardiovascular disease in apparently healthy men. *New England Journal of Medicine*, **336** (1997), 973–9.
124. P. Mehta, Aspirin in the prophylaxis of coronary artery disease. *Current Opinion in Cardiology*, **17** (2002), 552–8.
125. CAPRIE Steering Committee, A randomised blinded trial of clopidogrel versus aspirin in patients at risk of ischaemic events (CAPRIE). *Lancet*, **348** (1996), 1329–39.
126. D. Kereiakes, Preferential benefit of platelet glycoprotein IIb/IIIa receptor blockade: specific considerations by device and disease state. *American Journal of Cardiology*, **81**(Suppl 7) (1998), 49E–54E.
127. Inhibition of the platelet glycoprotein IIb/IIIa receptor with tirofiban in unstable angina and non-Q-wave myocardial infarction. Platelet receptor inhibition in ischaemic syndrome management in patients limited by unstable signs. *New England Journal of Medicine*, **338** (1998), 1488–97.
128. The EPISTENT (Evaluation of Platelet IIb/IIIa inhibition for Stenting) Investigators, Randomised placebo-controlled and balloon-angioplasty-controlled trial to assess safety of coronary stenting with use of platelet glycoprotein-IIb/IIIa blockade. *Lancet*, **352** (1998), 87–92.
129. D. Chew, Oral glycoprotein IIb/IIIa antagonists in coronary artery disease. *Current Cardiology Reports*, **3** (2001), 63–71.
130. N. Wenger, Coronary heart disease: an older woman's major health risk. *British Medical Journal*, **315** (1997), 1085–90.
131. P. Collins, Clinical cardiovascular studies of hormone replacement therapy. *American Journal of Cardiology*, **90**(Suppl) (2002), 30F–34F.
132. J. Stamler, Prevention of coronary atherosclerosis by estrogen-androgen administration in the cholesterol fed chick. *Circulation Research*, **1** (1953), 94.

133. R. Levine, Medroxyprogesterone attenuates estrogen-mediated inhibition of neointima formation after balloon injury of the rate carotid artery. *Circulation*, **94** (1996), 2221–7.
134. P. Ganz, Vasomotor and vascular effects of hormone replacement therapy. *American Journal of Cardiology*, **90**(Suppl) (2002), 11F–16F.
135. K. Kawecka-Jaszcz, The effect of hormone replacement therapy on arterial blood pressure and vascular compliance in postmenopausal women with arterial hypertension. *Journal of Human Hypertension*, **16** (2002), 509–16.
136. D. Grady, Hormones to prevent coronary disease in women: when are observational studies adequate evidence? *Annals of Internal Medicine*, **133** (2000), 999–1001.
137. J. Rossouw, Risks and benefits of estrogen plus progestin in healthy postmenopausal women: principal results from the Women's Health Initiative randomised controlled trial. *JAMA*, **288** (2002), 321–33.
138. S. Hulley, Randomized trial of estrogen plus progestin for secondary prevention of coronary heart disease in postmenopausal women. *JAMA*, **280** (1998), 605–13.
139. R. Byington, C. Furberg, D. Herrington *et al.*, Effect of estrogen progestin on progression of carotid atherosclerosis in postmenopausal women with heart disease: HERS B-mode substudy. *Arteriosclerosis, Thrombosis and Vascular Biology*, **22** (2002), 1692–7.
140. M. Cushman, Hormone replacement therapy, inflammation, and hemostasis in elderly women. *Arteriosclerosis, Thrombosis and Vascular Biology*, **19** (1999), 893–9.
141. A. A. Faludi, J. M. Aldrighi, M. C. Bertolami *et al.*, Progesterone abolishes estrogen and/or atorvastatin endothelial dependent vasodilatory effects. *Atherosclerosis*, **177** (2004), 89–96.
142. C. Sparrow, Low density lipoprotein is protected from oxidation and the progression of atherosclerosis is slowed in cholesterol-fed rabbits by the antioxidant N,N'-diphenyl-phenylenediamine. *Journal of Clinical Investigation*, **89** (1992), 1885–91.
143. T. Carew, Antiatherogenic effect of probucol unrelated to its hypocholesterolemic effect: evidence that antioxidants *in vivo* can selectively inhibit low density lipoprotein degradation in macrophage-rich fatty streaks and slow the progression of atherosclerosis in the Watanabe heritable hyperlipidemic rabbit. *Proceedings of the National Academy of Sciences of the USA*, **84** (1987), 7725–9.
144. M. Sasahara, Inhibition of hypercholesterolemia-induced atherosclerosis in the nonhuman primate by probucol, I: is the extent of atherosclerosis related to resistance of low density lipoprotein to oxidation? *Journal of Clinical Investigation*, **94** (1994), 155–64.
145. M. Stampfer, Vitamin E consumption and the risk of coronary disease in women. *New England Journal of Medicine*, **328** (1993), 1444–9.
146. E. Rimm, Vitamin E consumption and the risk of coronary heart disease in men. *New England Journal of Medicine*, **328** (1993), 1450–6.
147. J. Johansson, Lowering of HDL2b by probucol partly explains the failure of the drug to affect femoral atherosclerosis in subjects with hypercholesterolemia: the Probucol Quantitative Regression Swedish Trial (PQRST). *American Journal of Cardiology*, **74** (1994), 875–83.
148. C. Hennekens, Lack of effect of long-term supplementation with beta carotene on the incidence of malignant neoplasms and cardiovascular disease. *New England Journal of Medicine*, **334** (1996), 1145–9.
149. Heart Protection Study Group. MRC/BHF Heart Protection Study of antioxidant vitamin supplementation in 20536 high-risk individuals: a randomised placebo-controlled trial. *Lancet*, **360** (2002), 23–33.
150. M. Kalayoglu, *Chlamydia pneumoniae* as an emerging risk factor for cardiovascular disease. *JAMA*, **288** (2002), 2724–31.
151. J. Danesh, *Chlamydia pneumoniae* IgG titres and coronary heart disease: prospective study and meta-analysis. *British Medical Journal*, **321** (2000), 208–13.
152. S. Gupta, Elevated *Chlamydia pneumoniae* antibodies, cardiovascular events, and azithromycin in male survivors of myocardial infarction. *Circulation*, **96** (1997), 404–7.
153. J. Muhlestein, Randomized secondary prevention trial of azithromycin in patients with coronary artery disease: primary clinical results of the ACADEMIC study. *Circulation*, **102** (2000), 1755–60.
154. C. Espinola-Klein, Impact of infectious burden on extent and long-term prognosis of atherosclerosis. *Circulation*, **105** (2002), 15–21.

155. F. Hu, Dietary fat intake and the risk of coronary heart disease in women. *New England Journal of Medicine*, **337** (1997), 1491–9.
156. E. Dewailly, Relations between n-3 fatty acid status and cardiovascular disease risk factors among Quebecers. *American Journal of Clinical Nutrition*, **74** (2000), 603–11.
157. R. Singh, Randomised controlled trial of cardioprotective diet in patients with recent acute myocardial infarction: results of one year followup. *British Medical Journal*, **304** (1992), 1015–9.
158. L. Rudel, Compared with dietary monounsaturated and saturated fat, polyunsaturated fat protects African green monkeys from coronary artery atherosclerosis. *Arteriosclerosis, Thrombosis and Vascular Biology*, **15** (1995), 2101–10.
159. M. Burr, Effects of changes in fat, fish and fibre intakes on death and myocardial reinfarction: Diet and Reinfarction Trial (DART). *Lancet*, **2** (1989), 757–61.
160. M. De Lorgeril, Mediterranean diet, traditional risk factors, and the rate of cardiovascular complications after myocardial infarction: final report of the Lyon Diet Heart Study. *Circulation*, **99** (1999), 779–85.
161. R. Krauss, AHA dietary guidelines. Revision 2000: a statement for healthcare professionals from the Nutrition Committee of the American Heart Association. *Circulation*, **102** (2000), 2284–99.
162. C. Boushey, A quantitative assessment of plasma homocysteine as a risk factor for vascular disease. Probable benefits of increasing folic acid intake. *JAMA*, **274** (1995), 1049–57.
163. J. Danesh, Plasma homocysteine and coronary heart disease: systematic review of published epidemiological studies. *Journal of Cardiovascular Risk*, **5** (1998), 229–32.
164. I. Graham, The role of folic acid in the prevention of cardiovascular disease. *Current Opinion in Lipidology*, **11** (2000), 577–87.
165. R. Clarke, Homocysteine Lowering Trialist's Collaboration. Lowering blood homocysteine with folic acid based supplements: meta-analysis of randomised trials. *British Medical Journal*, **316** (1998), 894–8.
166. M. Bellamy, Oral folate enhances endothelial function in hyperhomocysteinemia subjects. *European Journal of Clinical Investigation*, **29** (1999), 659–62.
167. M. Verhaar, Future for folates in cardiovascular disease. *European Journal of Clinical Investigation*, **29** (1999), 657–8.
168. Y. Tauchi, Inhibitory effect of acyl-CoA:cholesterol acyltransferase inhibitor-low density lipoprotein complex on experimental atherosclerosis. *Biological and Pharmaceutical Bulletin*, **26** (2003), 73–8.
169. C. Dujovne, Efficacy and safety of a potent nex selective cholesterol absorption inhibitor, ezetimibe, in patients with primary hypercholesterolemia. *American Journal of Cardiology*, **90** (2002), 1092–7.
170. G. Etgen, A tailored therapy for the metabolic syndrome: the dual peroxisome proliferator-activated receptor-alpha/gamma agonist LY465608 ameliorates insulin resistance and diabetic hyperglycemia while improving cardiovascular risk factors in preclinical models. *Diabetes*, **51** (2002), 1083–7.
171. P. Andre, Platelet-derived CD40L: the switch-hitting player of cardiovascular disease. *Circulation*, **106** (2002), 896–9.
172. I. Benjamin, Matrix metalloproteinases: from biology to therapeutic strategies in cardiovascular disease. *Journal of Investigative Medicine*, **49** (2001), 381–97.
173. A. Makin, Antithrombotic therapy in peripheral vascular disease. *British Medical Journal*, **325** (2002), 1101–4.
174. P. Sinnaeve, Thrombolytic therapy. State of the art. *Thrombosis Research*, **103**(Suppl 1) (2001), S91–6.
175. P. Ridker, High-sensitivity C-reactive protein. Potential adjunct for global risk assessment in the primary prevention of cardiovascular disease. *Circulation*, **103** (2001), 1813–8.
176. R. Rosenson, High-sensitivity C-reactive protein and cardiovascular risk in patients with coronary heart disease. *Current Opinion in Cardiology*, **17** (2002), 325–31.
177. C. Ballantyne, Soluble adhesion molecules and the search for biomarkers for atherosclerosis. *Circulation*, **106** (2002), 766–7.
178. C. Parker, III, Soluble adhesion molecules and unstable coronary artery disease. *Atherosclerosis*, **157** (2001), 417–24.
179. P. Ridker, Role of inflammatory biomarkers in prediction of coronary heart disease. *Lancet*, **358** (2001), 946–8.
180. P. Ridker, Novel risk factors for systemic atherosclerosis. A comparison of C-reactive protein, fibrinogen, homocysteine, lipoprotein (a), and standard cholesterol screening as predictors of peripheral arterial disease. *JAMA*, **285** (2001), 2481–5.

181. J. Fareed, Useful laboratory tests for studying thrombogenesis in acute coronary syndromes. *Clinical Chemistry*, **44** (1998), 1845–53.

182. U. Schonbeck, Soluble CD40L and cardiovascular risk in women. *Circulation*, **104** (2001), 2266–8.

183. K. Nishi, Oxidized LDL in carotid plaques and plasma associates with plaque instability. *Arteriosclerosis, Thrombosis and Vascular Biology*, **22** (2002), 1649–54.

184. D. Celermajer, Non-invasive detection of endothelial dysfunction in children and adults at risk of atherosclerosis. *Lancet*, **8828** (1992), 1111–15.

185. J. Vita, Endothelial function: a barometer for cardiovascular risk? *Circulation*, **106** (2002), 640–2.

186. J. Dormandy, Ankle:arm blood pressure index as a predictor of atherothrombotic events: evidence from CAPRIE. *Cerebrovascular Disease*, **9**(Suppl 1) (1999), 1–128.

187. K. Ouriel, Doppler ankle pressure: an evaluation of three methods of expression. *Archives of Surgery*, **117** (1982), 1297–300.

188. L. Rohde, Circulating cell adhesion molecules are correlated with ultrasound-based assessment of carotid atherosclerosis. *Arteriosclerosis, Thrombosis and Vascular Biology*, **18** (1998), 1765–70.

189. D. O'Leary, Intima-media thickness: a tool for atherosclerosis imaging and event prediction. *American Journal of Cardiology*, **90**(Suppl 10C) (2002), 18L–21L.

190. D. Baumgart, Comparison of electron beam computer tomography with intracoronary ultrasound and coronary angiography for detection of coronary atherosclerosis. *Journal of the American College of Cardiology*, **30** (1997), 57–64.

191. Y. Arad, Prediction of coronary events with electron beam computer tomography. *Journal of the American College of Cardiology*, **36** (2000), 1253–60.

192. R. O'Rourke, ACC/AHA expert consensus document on electron-beam computer tomography for the diagnosis and prognosis of coronary artery disease. *Circulation*, **102** (2000), 126–40.

193. M. Budoff, Rates of progression of coronary calcium by electron beam computer tomography. *American Journal of Cardiology*, **86** (2000), 8–11.

194. Z. Fayad, Clinical imaging of the high-risk or vulnerable atherosclerotic plaque. *Circulation Research*, **89** (2001), 305–16.

195. R. Corti, Effects of lipid lowering by simvastatin on human atherosclerotic lesions. A longitudinal study by high-resolution, non-invasive magnetic resonance imaging. *Circulation*, **104** (2001), 249–52.

196. S. Nissen, Intravascular ultrasound: novel pathophysiological insights and current clinical applications. *Circulation*, **103** (2001), 604–16.

197. M. Brezinski, Characterizing arterial plaque with optical coherence tomography. *Current Opinion in Cardiology*, **17** (2002), 648–55.

198. A. Zarrabi, Intravascular thermography: a novel approach for detection of vulnerable plaque. *Current Opinion in Cardiology*, **17** (2002), 656–62.

10 • Molecular approaches to revascularization in peripheral vascular disease

MARK J. McCARTHY AND NICHOLAS P.J. BRINDLE

INTRODUCTION

Current treatment options for peripheral vascular disease include angioplasty and reconstructive surgery. An attractive potential alternative is the possibility of being able to revascularize ischaemic tissue by the induction of vascular growth. Such a strategy would be less invasive than surgical intervention. It would also be particularly welcome for patients in whom current approaches are difficult or prone to failure, including those with conditions that would make surgical intervention unsafe, patients with diffuse occlusive disease and those in which there is significant downstream microvascular disease. In recent years there have been major advances in understanding the molecular mechanisms of vascular formation and remodelling as well as identification of key molecules controlling this process. Based on this work, the therapeutic induction of new vessel formation in ischaemic tissue has progressed to pre-clinical studies and clinical trials. Most work has focused on the induction of new vessel formation by stimulating angiogenesis and this has been the goal of the clinical trials directed at peripheral vascular disease. Whilst stimulation of angiogenesis may be appropriate for the relief of microvascular defects, bypass of occluded conduit vessels in peripheral vascular disease patients will require the formation of more substantial collateral vessels by the process of arteriogenesis. In this review we will outline current understanding of the mechanisms controlling angiogenesis and arteriogenesis, approaches that are and could be pursued to induce vessel growth in peripheral vascular disease, as well as summarizing the current status of clinical trials, and the limitations and directions for future work.

MECHANISMS OF VASCULAR GROWTH

Strategies currently being developed for the therapeutic induction of vessel growth have evolved, largely, from knowledge of the physiological mechanisms of developmental vascularization. In development, blood vessels arise initially by the process of vasculogenesis in which precursor cells, known as angioblasts, differentiate into endothelial cells and organize into primitive vessels [1]. These vessels expand by angiogenesis, which includes both sprouting growth and non-sprouting remodelling.

Vasculogenesis

The angioblasts that give rise to endothelial cells in the first stages of developmental vascularization originate in the mesoderm under the influence of fibroblast growth factor-2 (FGF-2) [2]. These angioblasts differentiate into endothelial cells that proliferate and aggregate into cords, and become lumenized to form primitive vascular plexuses [1]. Signalling through vascular endothelial growth factor receptor-2 (VEGF-R2) is crucial for angioblast survival and establishment of these first vessels [3].

Endothelial cell formation from precursor cells and *in situ* differentiation into vessels, was thought to be confined to developmental vascularization. However, recent work has shown that circulating endothelial progenitor cells (EPCs) exist in the adult and that they can contribute to vessel formation [4]. These cells originate in the bone marrow and express CD34 and VEGF-R2 as well as the orphan receptor AC133 [5; 6]. Endothelial progenitor cells can incorporate into neovessels formed in healing wounds, ischaemic tissue and tumours [7; 8]. The mechanisms controlling the incorporation of EPCs into neovessels are at present poorly defined although a number of growth factors, including VEGF, FGF2, granulocyte-macrophage colony stimulating factor (GMCSF) and angiopoietins have been shown to increase the mobilization of EPCs from bone marrow [8; 9]. Crude cell fractions that include EPCs can be expanded *ex vivo* and transplanted into ischaemic tissue in animal models where they have been reported to incorporate into neovessels [4; 8]. Importantly, in some situations neovessels comprising only of EPC-derived cells were observed. This raises the possibility that EPCs, or EPC-derived cells, can form vessels *in situ*, by a process similar to vasculogenesis.

Angiogenesis

Establishment of the vascular network in development, as well as new vessel formation in the adult, requires angiogenesis. Two types of angiogenesis have been defined, sprouting angiogenesis and non-sprouting angiogenesis [1]. These two processes are responsible for remodelling of the primitive vascular plexus into a complex functional network. In sprouting angiogenesis, endothelial cells are activated by growth factors to undergo migration, proliferation and morphogenesis into new vessels. Vascular endothelial growth factor is the major physiological activator of sprouting angiogenesis, although as discussed below angiogenesis can be directly or indirectly stimulated by many factors.

Ischaemia is the primary initiator of sprouting angiogenic growth. Low oxygen tension activates expression of a wide range of angiogenic factors including VEGF, VEGF receptors, angiopoietin-2 and platelet-derived growth factor (PDGF). Genes for these factors contain hypoxia responsive elements in their promoters and some, like VEGF, have been shown to be direct targets of the transcriptional regulator hypoxia inducible factor (HIF). Hypoxia inducible factor-1 is a heterodimer composed of HIFα and HIFβ subunits [10]. Under normoxic conditions HIF-1α is held at low intracellular concentrations by proteosomal degradation. With decreased oxygen tension HIF-1α becomes hydroxylated on key proline residues preventing its association with the von Hippel-Lindau ubiquitin ligase complex that is responsible for directing HIF-1α for degradation [11]. Hypoxia inducible factor-1α then accumulates in the cell allowing it to activate transcription of hypoxia-inducible genes via the HIFα:β dimer.

Vascular endothelial growth factor expressed in response to HIF is secreted by ischaemic cells and acts on endothelial cells in adjacent microvessels. In these previously quiescent microvessels, endothelial activation, proliferation and migration are normally suppressed by signals from abluminal perivascular support cells, pericytes. This suppression needs to be relieved before angiogenesis can proceed [12]. The close interaction between endothelial cells and pericytes is promoted by the ligand angiopoietin-1, which is produced by the pericyte and acts on the endothelial receptor Tie2 [13]. Disruption of this signalling interaction is likely to involve angiopoietin-2, another hypoxia-responsive molecule [14]. Angiopoietin-2 can act to inhibit angiopoietin-1-induced activation of Tie2 [15]. Once released from the pro-stabilizing effects of pericytes the endothelial cells are free to invade the perivascular space, aided by proteases that degrade extracellular matrix. Many metalloproteinases have been implicated in angiogenic sprouting, including matrix metalloproteinases 2, 3, 7, and 9 as well as other proteolytic enzymes such as urokinase-type plasminogen activator [16]. Migration of the activated endothelial cells is aided by plasma proteins that extravasate from the activated microvessels in response to the vasodilatory and permeabilizing effects of VEGF. This growth factor is a potent chemoattractant and mitogen for endothelial cells, and directs their migration and proliferation. Interestingly, *in vivo* endothelial cells in the developing vascular sprouts respond differentially to VEGF, with the cells at the tip migrating and those behind the tip proliferating [17]. Migration and proliferation give rise to endothelial cords that become lumenized. The mechanism of lumen formation is poorly understood, though it is known that lumen formation is enhanced by angiopoietin-1 [18].

Neovessel maturation

Whether created by vasculogenesis or angiogenesis, newly formed blood vessels are highly unstable, and may haemorrhage, thrombose and undergo spontaneous regression in the absence of elevated growth factors [19; 20; 21]. Such vessels are characteristically found in pathological vascularization and their phenotype can directly contribute to the disease process [22; 23; 24; 25]. Newly formed primitive vascular channels are maintained by local high concentrations of VEGF, withdrawal of which leads to endothelial apoptosis and neovessel regression [26]. Transformation to a functional vessel requires interaction of endothelial cells in the nascent vessel with perivascular cells [1; 16]. These perivascular cells originate as mesenchymal cells that are recruited to the developing vessel and differentiate into pericytes on contact with the endothelium [27; 28]. Proliferation and migration of partially or fully differentiated pericytes along established microvessels also contribute to mural cell acquisition by sprouting neovessels, and sprouts can themselves recruit mesenchymal cells [19; 27; 28; 29]. Migration and proliferation of pericytes is regulated mainly by platelet-derived growth factor-B (PDGFB) secreted by endothelial cells. Interaction between mesenchymal cells and endothelial cells in a developing vessel produces phenotypic changes in both cell types. The mesenchymal cell is directed toward a pericyte or smooth muscle phenotype and the endothelial cell adopts the phenotype required for formation of a stabilized microvessel [1; 30]. Pericytes supply anti-apoptotic ligands, including angiopoietin-1 [31], to underlying endothelial cells allowing neovessels to survive the decrease in VEGF concentrations that occur as the ischaemia is relieved by increased perfusion. In addition, pericytes suppress endothelial proliferation and migration, and increase deposition of the perivascular basement membrane, all of which contribute to switching the fragile nascent vessel into a quiescent functional microvessel [32]. Transforming growth factor-β, produced by proteolytic cleavage from a precursor form as a result of endothelial:pericyte interaction [33], has a central role in these effects.

Microvascular network maturation

Maturation of vascular channels into functional vessels is accompanied by maturation of the neovessel network. This involves optimization of the new vessel configuration, density, branching pattern and vessel hierarchy. Spatial distributions of angiogenic initiators, like VEGF, have a major influence on the direction of the initial branches. There are six members of the VEGF family and VEGF-A is expressed as a number of alternatively spliced variants; in humans these are mainly forms with 121, 165, 189 and 206 amino acids [34]. VEGF165, 189 and 206 possess heparin-binding domains that allow these forms to interact with the extracellular matrix. The ability of VEGF isoforms to be retained by the matrix is important in regulating the spatial organization of vessel branching [35].

Patterning also occurs through selective loss of certain vessels by regression. Another major determinant of network maturation is the branching and 'splitting' of vessels by non-sprouting angiogenesis. This occurs by the process of intussusception in which vessel lumens are internally divided by insertion, and subsequent growth and stabilization, of transcapillary tissue pillars [36]. The mechanism of intussusception and factors that regulate it are poorly understood, though the Tie receptors are known to have a role [37].

Arteriogenesis

Further expansion and muscularization of vessels occurs by the process of arteriogenesis. This involves recruitment of additional mural cells and their proliferation, as well as expansion of the abluminal extracellular matrix. Despite the importance of this process, the mechanisms involved and factors controlling it are poorly understood. Platelet-derived growth factor-B with its effects on smooth muscle cell recruitment and proliferation, and TGFβ, a known regulator of vascular extracellular matrix synthesis, are likely to be key regulators.

Importantly, remodelling of pre-existing small arteriole resistance vessels into conductance vessels by arteriogenesis can be triggered in the adult. Induction of arteriogenesis in collateral vessels offers the most promise as a therapeutic target for the relief of tissue ischaemia in peripheral vascular disease.

Arteriogenesis of collateral vessels has been demonstrated in a number of animal models following the occlusion of major vessels [38]. In humans, well-developed collateral vessels that bypass occluded arteries have been found frequently and those patients with the best developed collaterals often have minimal symptoms [39]. Arteriogenesis of collaterals in response to the occlusion of primary supply vessels occurs in two phases, an initial increase in lumen size occurs within a few days and this is followed by a slower remodelling of smooth muscle cell and extracellular matrix cover [38]. The early phase of this adaptive arteriogenesis is associated with inflammation. There is monocyte attachment to endothelium, as well as extravasation and accumulation in the adventitia and perivascular space, with mast cells and T lymphocytes [40; 41; 42]. Monocytes have a critical role in adaptive arteriogenesis as experimental suppression of monocyte numbers decreases arteriogenesis [42]. These cells are likely to provide growth factors to stimulate vessel enlargement and proteases that can act on the extracellular matrix to accommodate increased vessel size. Changes to the wall of the vessel, involve remodelling of the media, with increased turnover of medial smooth muscle cells and a shift towards a synthetic phenotype [43]. A new internal elastic lamina is established and vessel wall thickening results from increased extracellular matrix deposition.

THERAPEUTIC INDUCTION OF VASCULAR GROWTH

Most studies on the therapeutic induction of vessel growth at a pre-clinical level, and all clinical trials, have focused on angiogenesis. Clinical trials aimed at relieving peripheral vascular disease by therapeutic angiogenesis have had limited success. This is perhaps not surprising given the very limited ability of angiogenic growth to compensate for the loss of conductance vessels. It is now being generally recognized that revascularization in peripheral vascular disease, as in coronary heart disease, would be best achieved by the therapeutic activation of collateral arteriogenesis. Nevertheless the ability to activate angiogenesis therapeutically would be valuable where significant microvascular disease exists, such as in Buerger's disease [44]. In addition, the early work on therapeutic angiogenesis has provided data and approaches that may be valuable in future studies aimed at the activation of arteriogenesis.

Delivery of molecular activators of vascular growth

Induction of angiogenesis in the appropriate ischaemic areas and in future local arteriogenesis at suitable sites for collateral development, requires activating agents to be delivered in a manner that ensures controllable local activity and minimizes systemic side effects. Growth factors are readily degraded and if administered systemically would have to be used at high concentrations in order to ensure enough active growth factor reaches the appropriate site. There are risks associated with non-local delivery, for example, systemically delivered VEGF produces severe hypotension in animal models [45]. In addition to localization, activators must be present for sufficient time to induce optimal vascular growth.

The two principal methods used to deliver angiogenic activators in pre-clinical studies as well as clinical trials have been as recombinant proteins or as the genes that encode these proteins. Activators can be delivered locally via intravascular catheters, direct injection into the muscle or use of coated stents. An important consideration in the use of peptide growth factors is ensuring sufficient longevity of the molecules at the desired site. Where recombinant proteins are injected this would necessitate multiple injections during the course of treatment. An alternative strategy is the use of local reservoirs of recombinant protein, such as biodegradable microspheres [46]. A major limitation to the use of recombinant protein is the expense and difficulty in obtaining large enough quantities of appropriate purity, especially when cocktails of growth factors are required.

Delivery of angiogenic factors by gene transfer has significant advantages over the administration of recombinant protein. It is relatively easy to produce high purity DNA in large quantities and the transfected genes remain active over a period of several days to two to three weeks. Use of gene transfer for angiogenic clinical trials has been approved in many countries. In contrast to gene therapy aimed at correcting genetic diseases, gene transfer as a means of providing short term local expression of therapeutic proteins has been successful. Surprisingly, small amounts of DNA plasmid vectors can be taken up by muscle cells *in vivo* and are reported to result in significant gene expression in humans [47]. Improvements in transfer efficiency have been sought by the use of liposomal carriers and viral vectors. Adenovirus is the most common viral vector used for the delivery of angiogenic genes. Genes transferred via adenovirus do not integrate into chromosomes of transduced cells and provide transient expression.

There have been reports of an inflammatory reaction to adenoviral vectors in human trials, but no long term safety problems at doses appropriate for angiogenic therapy. Second generation adenoviral vectors with deletions of E1 and E4 regions have better transfection efficiency and elicit a decreased inflammatory response [48] and further improved adenoviral vectors can be expected [49]. The adeno-associated viruses (AAV) offer an alternative viral means for gene delivery. Adeno-associated viruses efficiently transduce skeletal muscle and vasculature [50]. However, along with retroviruses and lentiviruses, AAV integrate into the recipient genome requiring the development of regulatory systems if they are to provide controllable expression of vascular growth genes. As with recombinant protein, local delivery of genes can be accomplished by direct intramuscular injection, implantation of coated stents or catheter. It may also be possible to utilize tissue-specific endothelial surface molecules for targeting vectors to particular vascular beds. Implantation of cells transfected *ex vivo* offer an additional route of local delivery.

Angiogenic activators

Perhaps the simplest approach to activating angiogenesis is the administration of a soluble angiogenic activator. Vascular endothelial growth factor is relatively specific for endothelial cells and physiologically relevant. Although VEGF-A, -B, -C, -D and -E, as well as the VEGF-R1 ligand placental growth factor, have all been shown to activate angiogenesis when administered in animal models, most studies have concentrated on VEGF-A. Administration of VEGF alone results in a high percentage of malformed capillaries in animal models [51]. This growth factor also induces vessel permeability resulting in local hypotension and oedema [45]. Neovessels induced by VEGF are transient, with regression occurring on growth factor withdrawal [52]. Importantly, however, it was observed that if stimulation with VEGF extended beyond a critical time period in the mouse model, the neovessels appeared to become resistant to loss of the growth factor [52]. These data indicate formation of a sustained microvessel network may require relatively long term exposure to the angiogenic initiator.

The fibroblast growth factors have also been examined as potential therapeutic agents to induce angiogenesis in clinical trials. There are 23 members of the FGF family and FGF-2 and FGF-4 have been used in clinical trials. Fibroblast growth factor-1, -2, -4 and -9 are highly mitogenic for endothelial cells, although these growth factors are also active on non-endothelial cells [53]. Another growth factor that induces angiogenesis and is in early trials is hepatocyte growth factor; again its effects are not confined to endothelial cells [54].

With the recognition that physiological angiogenesis requires a spatially and temporally co-ordinated repertoire of signals, attempts have been made to improve capillary formation by providing cocktails of growth factors. Indeed combination of VEGF with the pro-stabilizing Tie2 agonist angiopoietin-1 in a mouse model does produce microvessels with increased lumen size, less thrombosis and increased perfusion compared with VEGF alone [18]. These vessels are also less leaky than those formed in response to VEGF alone [55]. Another approach aimed at providing a more physiological range of angiogenic factors is the targeting of HIF. Expression of a form of HIF-1α that is resistant to oxygen-induced degradation in mouse skin led to up-regulation of HIF-sensitive angiogenic genes and the stimulation of microvessel formation [56]. Again the vessels produced were not associated with oedema. The cell permeable peptide, PR39, inhibits proteosomal degradation and can stabilize HIF-1α [57]. PR39 stimulates angiogenesis in mouse heart, although further studies are required to determine its specificity [57].

An additional potential therapeutic approach to stimulate angiogenic growth is the manipulation of EPCs. These cells can be expanded *ex vivo* and used for autologous transplantation. With the appropriate stimuli endogenous EPCs could also be mobilized, directed to the appropriate area and induced to differentiate and contribute to neovessel formation.

Pre-clinical and early clinical studies have shown that angiogenesis can be induced *in vivo* by a variety of approaches. The challenge now is to devise a means to stimulate the conversion of these neovessels into optimally organized, persistent and functional microvascular networks.

Arteriogenic activators

Little is known about the molecular mechanisms of arteriogenesis. In contrast to the ischaemic tissue microenvironment in which angiogenesis occurs, collateral arteriogenesis in the limb takes place in normoxic conditions [58]. In adaptive arteriogenesis studied in animal models, the biomechanical effects of the increased flow that the collaterals experience as a result of occlusion of conductance vessels plays a major role. These effects include increased wall shear stress as well as tangential and axial stresses. Increased shear can up-regulate adhesion molecules, such as intercellular adhesion molecule-1, as well as monocyte chemoattractant protein-1 which contribute to monocyte recruitment [59; 60]. Growth factors are undoubtedly involved in adaptive arteriogenesis, but again more work is required to identify the key factors and their roles. In animal models FGF-1 and FGF-2 were found to be unchanged during adaptive arteriogenesis, although there was a transient increase in expression of FGF-receptor-1 [61].

TGFβ is increased during collateral development and can enhance arteriogenesis in animal models. Several factors have been found to enhance arteriogenesis when administered to animals, including

FGF-2, VEGF, placental growth factor, angiopoietin-1 and monocyte chemoattractant protein-1 [38]. The mechanisms by which these factors regulate arteriogenesis need to be defined. Many appear to have indirect actions, for example, VEGF and placental growth factor infusions are likely to enhance arteriogenesis via their monocyte chemoattractive activity. Given the great potential of therapeutic induction of collateral arteriogenesis for the treatment of peripheral vascular disease, it is important that we gain a better understanding of the molecular mechanisms controlling this process. Identification of key regulators that can induce or enhance arteriogenesis of collaterals is a priority.

Clinical trials for angiogenic therapy of peripheral vascular disease

There have been a number of phase 2 and 3 clinical trials aimed at relieving peripheral vascular disease by angiogenic therapy. The TRAFFIC study used single or repeated doses of recombinant FGF-2 delivered by arterial puncture and cross-over catheter in patients with intermittent claudication. Patients receiving a single FGF-2 dose showed a significant improvement in peak walking time at 90 days [62]. In another trial, the Regional Angiogenesis with Vascular Endothelial Growth Factor (RAVE) study, VEGF121 gene transfer by adenovirus was utilized but failed to produce a significant improvement in peak walking time at 12 weeks [63]. In contrast, in a different study adenoviral delivered VEGF165 given during angioplasty did produce an increased vascularity at three months as assessed by angiography [64].

Although these trials have met with limited success, together with phase 1 studies and earlier small trials, they demonstrate the feasibility and safety of molecular approaches to therapeutic modulation of vascular growth. The trials have also been valuable in aiding development of techniques for delivering therapeutic agents, as well as helping clinicians refine aspects of trial design for future clinical work on arteriogenesis and angiogenesis.

The realization that therapeutic induction of collateralization by arteriogenesis would be most appropriate for occlusive disease, whilst angiogenic therapy would benefit patients with microvascular defects, should help improve selection of the most appropriate populations for use in future trials. Clear clinical endpoints are required in such work. Where angiogenesis is the aim, establishment of optimal treatment modalities will depend on further pre-clinical work focused on determining ways to establish mature, correctly patterned vascular networks. This may involve defined cocktails of stimulators, or activation of transcriptional factors triggering co-ordinated expression of stimulators. In both cases distinct spatial and temporal expression patterns are likely to be required.

CONCLUSIONS

The prospects for a molecular approach to stimulate vascular growth as a means of relieving tissue ischaemia in peripheral vascular disease and coronary heart disease are promising. Whilst the rush to clinical trials has been premature, this early clinical work, together with a better understanding of vascular growth mechanisms, has allowed us to recognize the key areas in which progress is required in order to bring therapeutic vascular growth to the clinic. Bypassing the occluded conductance vessels is now recognized to require collateral growth by arteriogenesis, rather than angiogenesis. In comparison to angiogenesis our understanding of arteriogenesis is rudimentary. Significant work is needed therefore to understand the mechanisms regulating physiological arteriogenesis as well as adaptive arteriogenesis, and to identify key molecular regulators. Activation of angiogenic growth will be valuable where microvascular disease is prevalent. Indeed situations in which activation of arteriogenesis to restore conductance level flow together with activation of angiogenesis to relieve microvascular defects can be envisaged. It is clear that optimum microvascular growth will require correctly patterned, functional and persistent mature microvessel networks. Further work on the basic biology of angiogenesis is needed to determine the best means of inducing this therapeutically. Although significant challenges remain they are far outweighed by the enormous potential benefits of treating ischaemic disease by molecular activation of therapeutic revascularization.

REFERENCES

1. W. Risau, Mechanisms of angiogenesis. *Nature*, **386** (1997), 671–4.
2. T. J. Poole, E. B. Finkelstein & C. M. Cox, The role of FGF and VEGF in angioblast induction and migration

during vascular development. *Developmental Dynamics*, **220** (2001), 1–17.
3. F. Shalaby, J. Rossant, T. Yamaguchi *et al.*, Failure of blood-island formation and vasculogenesis in Flk-1-deficient mice. *Nature*, **376** (1995), 62–6.
4. T. Asahara, T. Murohara, A. Sullivan *et al.*, Isolation of putative progenitor endothelial cells for angiogenesis. *Science*, **275** (1997), 964–7.
5. U. M. Gehling, S. Ergun, U. Schumacher *et al.*, *In vitro* differentiation of endothelial cells from AC133-positive progenitor cells. *Blood*, **95** (2000), 3106–12.
6. M. Peichev, A. J. Naiyer, D. Pereira *et al.*, Expression of VEGFR-2 and AC133 by circulating human CD34(+) cells identifies a population of functional endothelial precursors. *Blood*, **95** (2000), 952–8.
7. T. Asahara, H. Masuda, T. Takahashi *et al.*, Bone marrow origin of endothelial progenitor cells responsible for postnatal vasculogenesis in physiological and pathological neovascularization. *Circulation Research*, **85** (1999), 221–8.
8. T. Takahashi, C. Kalka, H. Masuda *et al.*, Ischemia- and cytokine-induced mobilization of bone marrow-derived endothelial progenitor cells for neovascularization. *Nature Medicine*, **5** (1999), 434–8.
9. T. Asahara, T. Takahashi, H. Masuda, VEGF contributes to postnatal neovascularization by mobilizing bone marrow-derived endothelial progenitor cells. *EMBO Journal*, **18** (1999), 3964–72.
10. G. L. Semenza, Transcriptional regulation by hypoxia-inducible factor 1. *Trends in Cardiovascular Medicine*, **6** (1996), 151–7.
11. C. W. Pugh & P. J. Ratcliffe, Regulation of angiogenesis by hypoxia: role of the HIF system. *Nature Medicine*, **9** (2003), 677–84.
12. D. C. Darland & P. A. D'Amore, Cell-cell interactions in vascular development. *Current Topics in Developmental Biology*, **52** (2001), 107–49.
13. C. Suri, P. F. Jones, S. Patan *et al.*, Requisite role of angiopoietin-1, a ligand for the TIE2 receptor, during embryonic angiogenesis. *Cell*, **87** (1996), 1171–80.
14. H. Oh, H. Takagi, K. Suzuma *et al.*, Hypoxia and vascular endothelial growth factor selectively up-regulate angiopoietin-2 in bovine microvascular endothelial cells. *Journal of Biological Chemistry*, **274** (1999), 15732–9.
15. P. C. Maisonpierre, C. Suri, P. F. Jones *et al.*, Angiopoietin-2, a natural antagonist for Tie2 that disrupts *in vivo* angiogenesis. *Science*, **277** (1997), 55–60.
16. P. Carmeliet, Mechanisms of angiogenesis and arteriogenesis. *Nature Medicine*, **6** (2000), 389–95.
17. H. Gerhardt, M. Golding, M. Fruttiger *et al.*, VEGF guides angiogenic sprouting utilizing endothelial tip cell filopodia. *Journal of Cell Biology*, **161** (2003), 1163–77.
18. T. Asahara, D. Chen, T. Takahashi *et al.*, Tie2 receptor ligands, angiopoietin-1 and angiopoietin-2, modulate VEGF-induced postnatal neovascularization. *Circulation Research*, **83** (1998), 233–40.
19. L. E. Benjamin, I. Hemo & E. Keshet, A plasticity window for blood vessel remodelling is defined by pericyte coverage of the preformed endothelial network and is regulated by PDGF-B and VEGF. *Development*, **125** (1998), 1591–8.
20. L. E. Benjamin, D. Golijanin, A. Itin, D. Pode & E. Keshet, Selective ablation of immature blood vessels in established human tumors follows vascular endothelial growth factor withdrawal. *Journal of Clinical Investigation*, **103** (1999), 159–65.
21. D. C. Darland & P. A. D'Amore, Blood vessel maturation: vascular development comes of age. *Journal of Clinical Investigation*, **103** (1999), 157–8.
22. O. J. de Boer, A. C. van der Wal, P. Teeling & A. E. Becker, Leucocyte recruitment in rupture prone regions of lipid-rich plaques: a prominent role for neovascularization? *Cardiovascular Research*, **41** (1999), 443–9.
23. A. N. Tenaglia, K. G. Peters, M. H. Sketch, Jr. & B. H. Annex, Neovascularization in atherectomy specimens from patients with unstable angina: implications for pathogenesis of unstable angina. *American Heart Journal*, **135** (1998), 10–14.
24. E. O 'Brien, M. R. Garvin, R. Dev *et al.*, Angiogenesis in human coronary atherosclerotic plaques. *American Journal of Pathology*, **145** (1994), 883–94.
25. P. Carmeliet & R. K. Jain, Angiogenesis in cancer and other diseases. *Nature*, **407** (2000), 249–57.
26. T. Alon, I. Hemo, A. Itin *et al.*, Vascular endothelial growth factor acts as a survival factor for newly formed retinal vessels and has implications for retinopathy of prematurity. *Nature Medicine*, **1** (1995), 1024–8.
27. L. Beck, P. A. D'Amore, Vascular development: cellular and molecular regulation. *FASEB Journal*, **11** (1997), 365–73.
28. M. Hellstrom, M. Kalen, P. Lindahl, P. Abramsson & C. Betsholtz, Role of PDGF-B and PDGFR-beta in recruitment of vascular smooth muscle cells and

pericytes during embryonic blood vessel formation in the mouse. *Development*, **126** (1999), 3047–55.
29. P. Lindahl, B. R. Johansson, P. Levéen & C. Betsholtz, Pericyte loss and microaneurysm formation in PDGF-B-deficient mice. *Science*, **277** (1997), 242–5.
30. P. Carmeliet & D. Collen, Genetic analysis of blood vessel formation. *Trends in Cardiovascular Medicine*, **7** (1997), 271–81.
31. I. Kim, H. G. Kim, J. S. So *et al.*, Angiopoietin-1 regulates endothelial cell survival through the phosphatidylinositol 3′-kinase/Akt signal transduction pathway. *Circulation Research*, **86** (2000), 24–9.
32. K. K. Hirschi & P. A. D'Amore. Pericytes in the microvasculature. *Cardiovascular Research*, **32** (1996), 687–98.
33. A. Antonelli-Orlidge, K. B. Saunders, S. R. Smith & P. A. D'Amore, An activated form of transforming growth factor beta is produced by co-cultures of endothelial cells and pericytes. *Proceedings of National Academy of Sciences of the USA*, **86** (1989), 4544–8.
34. N. Ferrara, H. P. Gerber & J. LeCouter, The biology of VEGF and its receptors. *Nature Medicine*, **9** (2003), 669–76.
35. C. Ruhrberg, H. Gerhardt, M. Golding *et al.*, Spatially restricted patterning cues provided by heparin-binding VEGF-A control blood vessel branching morphogenesis. *Genes and Development*, **16** (2002), 2684–98.
36. V. Djonov, M. Schmid, S. A. Tschanz & P. H. Burri, Intussusceptive angiogenesis its role in embryonic vascular network formation. *Circulation*, **86** (2000), 286–92.
37. S. Patan, TIE1 and TIE2 receptor tyrosine kinases inversely regulate embryonic angiogenesis by the mechanism of intussusceptive microvascular growth. *Microvascular Research*, **56** (1998), 1–21.
38. W. Schaper & D. Scholz, Factors regulating arteriogenesis. *Arteriosclerosis, Thrombosis and Vascular Biology*, **23** (2003), 1143–51.
39. A. Maseri, L. Araujo & M. L. Finocchiaro, Collateral development and function in man. In *Collateral Circulation: Heart, Brain, Kidney, Limbs*, ed. W. Schaper and J. Schaper. (Boston, MA: Kluwer Academic, 1993), pp. 381–402.
40. M. Arras, W. D. Ito, D. Scholz *et al.*, Monocyte activation in angiogenesis and collateral growth in the rabbit hindlimb. *Journal of Clinical Investigation*, **101** (1998), 40–50.
41. C. Wolf, W. J. Cai, R. Vosschulte *et al.*, Vascular remodeling and altered protein expression during growth of coronary collateral arteries. *Journal of Molecular and Cellular Cardiology*, **30** (1998), 2291–305.
42. M. Heil, T. Ziegelhoeffer, F. Pipp *et al.*, Blood monocyte concentration is critical for enhancement of collateral artery growth. *American Journal of Heart and Circulatory Physiology*, **283** (2002), H2411–19.
43. D. Scholz, W. Ito, I. Fleming *et al.*, Ultrastructure and molecular histology of rabbit hind-limb collateral artery growth (arteriogenesis). *Virchows Archiver*, **436** (2000), 257–70.
44. J. M. Isner, I. Baumgartner, G. Rauh *et al.*, Treatment of thromboangiitis obliterans (Buerger's disease) by intramuscular gene transfer of vascular endothelial growth factor: preliminary clinical results. *Journal of Vascular Surgery*, **28** (1998), 964–73.
45. M. D. Hariawala, J. J. Horowitz, D. Esakof *et al.*, VEGF improves myocardial blood flow but produces EDRF-mediated hypotension in porcine hearts. *Journal of Surgical Research*, **63** (1996), 77–82.
46. M. Arras, H. Mollnau, R. Strasser, The delivery of angiogenic factors to the heart by microsphere therapy. *Nature Biotechnology*, **16** (1998), 159–62.
47. S. K. Tripathy, E. C. Svensson, H. B. Black *et al.*, Long-term expression of erythropoietin in the systemic circulation of mice after intramuscular injection of a plasmid DNA vector. *Proceedings of the National Academy of Sciences of the USA*, **93** (1996), 10876–80.
48. H. S. Qian, K. Channon, V. Neplioueva *et al.*, Improved adenoviral vector for vascular gene therapy: beneficial effects on vascular function and inflammation. *Circulation Research*, **88** (2001), 911–17.
49. D. Maione, C. D. Rocca, P. Giannetti *et al.*, An improved helper-dependent adenoviral vector allows persistent gene expression after intramuscular delivery and overcomes preexisting immunity to adenovirus. *Proceedings of the National Academy of Sciences of the USA*, **98** (2001), 5986–91.
50. P. E. Monahan & R. J. Samulski, Adeno-associated virus vectors for gene therapy: more pros than cons? *Molecular Medicine Today*, **6** (2000), 433–40.
51. C. J. Drake & C. D. Little, Exogenous vascular endothelial growth factor induces malformed and hyperfused vessels during embryonic neovascularization. *Proceedings of the National Academy of Sciences of the USA*, **92** (1995), 7657–61.

52. Y. Dor, V. Djonov, R. Abramovitch *et al.*, Conditional switching of VEGF provides new insights into adult neovascularization and pro-angiogenic therapy. *EMBO Journal*, **21** (2002), 1939–47.
53. S. Javerzat, P. Auguste & A. Bikfalvi, The role of fibroblast growth factors in vascular development. *Trends in Molecular Medicine*, **8** (2002), 483–9.
54. R. Morishita, S. Nakamura, S. Hayashi *et al.*, Therapeutic angiogenesis induced by human recombinant hepatocyte growth factor in rabbit hind limb ischemia model as cytokine supplement therapy. *Hypertension*, **33** (1999), 1379–84.
55. G. Thurston, C. Suri, K. Smith *et al.*, Leakage-resistant blood vessels in mice transgenically overexpressing angiopoietin-1. *Science*, **286** (1999), 2511–14.
56. D. A. Elson, G. Thurston, L. E. Huang *et al.*, Induction of hypervascularity without leakage or inflammation in transgenic mice overexpressing hypoxia-inducible factor-1alpha. *Genes and Development*, **15** (2001), 2520–32.
57. J. Li, M. Post, R. Volk *et al.*, PR39, a peptide regulator of angiogenesis. *Nature Medicine*, **6** (2000), 49–55.
58. W. D. Ito, M. Arras, D. Scholz *et al.*, Angiogenesis but not collateral growth is associated with ischemia after femoral artery occlusion. *American Journal of Heart and Circulatory Physiology*, **273** (1997), H1255–65.
59. P. L. Walpola, A. I. Gotlieb, M. I. Cybulsky & B. L. Langille, Expression of ICAM-1 and VCAM-1 and monocyte adherence in arteries exposed to altered shear stress. *Arteriosclerosis, Thrombosis and Vascular Biology*, **15** (1995), 2–10.
60. Y. J. Shyy, H. J. Hsieh, S. Usami & S. Chien, Fluid shear stress induces a biphasic response of human monocyte chemotactic protein 1 gene expression in vascular endothelium. *Proceedings of the National Academy of Sciences of the USA*, **91** (1994), 4678–82.
61. E. Deindl, I. E. Hoefer, B. Fernandez *et al.*, Involvement of the fibroblast growth factor system in adaptive and chemokine-induced arteriogenesis. *Circulation Research*, **92** (2003), 561–8.
62. R. J. Lederman, F. O. Mendelsohn, R. D. Anderson *et al.*, Therapeutic angiogenesis with recombinant fibroblast growth factor-2 for intermittent claudication (the TRAFFIC study): a randomised trial. *Lancet*, **359** (2002), 2053–8.
63. S. Rajagopalan, E. R. Mohler, 3rd, R. J. Lederman *et al.*, Regional angiogenesis with vascular endothelial growth factor in peripheral arterial disease: a phase II randomized, double-blind, controlled study of adenoviral delivery of vascular endothelial growth factor 121 in patients with disabling intermittent claudication. *Circulation*, **108** (2003), 1933–8.
64. K. Makinen, H. Manninen, M. Hedman, Increased vascularity detected by digital subtraction angiography after VEGF gene transfer to human lower limb artery: a randomized, placebo-controlled, double-blinded phase II study. *Molecular Therapy*, **6** (2002), 127–33.

11 • Raynaud's phenomenon and the vasculitides

DEAN PATTERSON, DONALD J. ADAM, ROBERT A. FITRIDGE AND JILL J. F. BELCH

INTRODUCTION

One of the first types of small vessel disease to be described was *'local asphyxia and symmetrical gangrene of the extremities'* in 1862 by Maurice Raynaud, while the first account of a systemic vasculitic disease was made in 1866 by Kussmaul and Maier (later referred to as polyarteritis nodosa). Since then many other disorders, some primarily vascular in origin have been described that can contribute to small vessel disease (SVD). Vasculitis is not necessarily restricted by vessel calibre (Figure 11.1). Any vascular bed can be affected and the pattern of organ involvement often aids in diagnosis. The causes of SVD are multiple, and hence the mechanisms involved are varied and disease dependent.

Some disorders like primary Raynaud's predominantly involve vascular malfunction while others like secondary vasculitides have additional underlying pathology. Vascular malfunction may consist of alterations of neurogenic vasotonic control mechanisms and/or endothelial nitric oxide bioactivity. Some diseases present with finger or toe ischaemia alone while others may compromise circulation to the internal organs, including the brain, kidney, heart and eyes, sometimes leading to significant delays before clinical manifestations become apparent. This chapter includes a brief summary of conditions that involve Raynaud's, arteritis or small vessel disease which can present with disturbed blood flow to an extremity. As can be seen in Table 11.1 there are many conditions with one or more of these characteristics and, as some are multisystem disorders, specific reference will be made to major organ involvement where relevant.

SMALL VESSEL DISEASE

The clinical presentation of the numerous causes of SVD listed in Table 11.1a, b and c can vary from cold intolerance to more advanced ischaemic sequelae and tissue loss. A normal pulse at the level of the wrist with ischaemic lesions on the hands confirms the presence of small artery obstruction (permanent obstruction or temporary vasospasm), yet it does not exclude an embolic source from the heart or proximal arteries. Possible symptoms and signs include Raynaud's phenomenon (RP), cold peripheries despite the presence of good pulses, haematuria, retinal infarcts and haemorrhages, ulceration and small infarcts of the extremities, stroke, peripheral neuropathy, and hypertension.

RAYNAUD'S PHENOMENON

Raynaud's phenomenon is characterized by recurrent episodic attacks of digital ischaemia on exposure to cooling, emotional stress, tobacco smoke, hormones or trauma [2]. It occurs due to episodic vasospasm of the small muscular arteries, precapillary arterioles and cutaneous arteriovenous shunts of the digits. The fact that this process can also affect the circulation of the nose, tongue and ear lobes as well as viscera such as the myocardium, lung and oesophagus suggests that RP is a systemic disease. Raynaud's phenomenon can be classified into primary Raynaud's disease (RD) which occurs in isolation and secondary Raynaud's syndrome (RS) which is associated with another disease, usually connective tissue disease.

Normal regulation of vascular tone involves complex interactions between endothelial cells (ECs), vascular smooth muscle cells, and the autonomic and sensory nerves which supply the blood vessel. Endothelial cells synthesize and release cytokines, growth factors, prostaglandins such as the vasodilator prostacyclin (PGI_2), and other molecules such as the vasodilator nitric oxide (NO) and the vasoconstrictor endothelin (ET)-1. Neurotransmitters such as substance P, calcitonin gene-related peptide and acetylcholine act as vasodilators. Physiological cold-induced vasoconstriction of cutaneous arteries is mediated predominantly

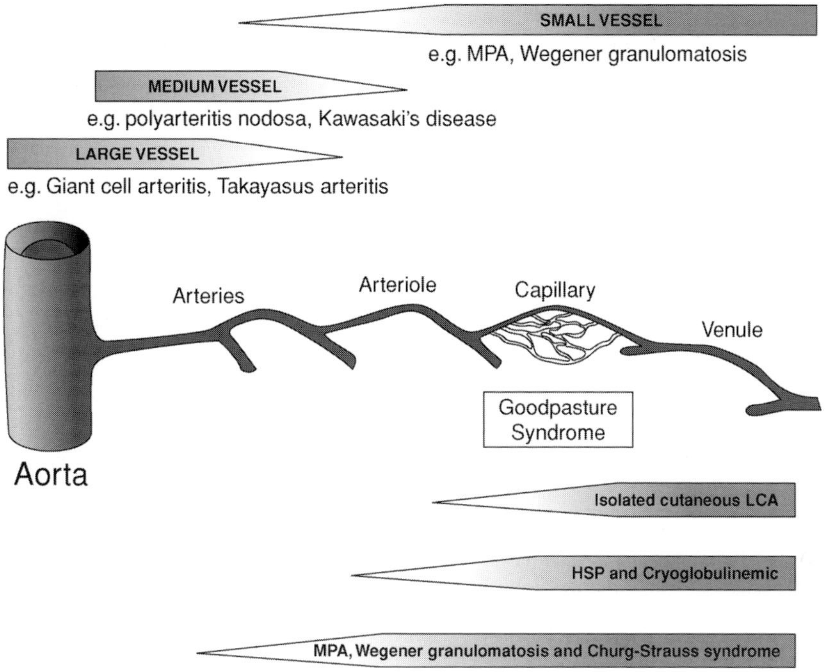

Fig. 11.1. Distribution of vasculitis by vessel size (adapted from Jennette & Falk) [1]. The width and colour gradient of the trapezoids indicates the frequencies of involvement of the vasculature. LCV = leucocytoclastic vasculitis; HSP = Henoch-Schönlein purpura; MPA = Microscopic polyangitis.

via the post-junctional α_2-adrenergic receptors on vascular smooth muscle cells.

Endothelium-dependent mechanisms

Although elevated plasma levels of ET and reduced NO release have been demonstrated in RP, there is no evidence that these EC responses contribute to the pathophysiology of RP [3; 4; 5]. Furthermore, the cutaneous arteries of unaffected skin of patients with RP demonstrate a normal vascular response to ET [4], and arterioles from unaffected skin of patients with scleroderma-associated RS retain normal endothelium-mediated vasodilatory capacity [6]. A reduced NO-mediated vasodilatation response to body cooling has been demonstrated in RD suggesting that seasonal variations in environmental temperature may be a contributory factor [7]. Oestrogen is an endothelium-dependent vasodilator, and women with RD may have blunted core temperature responses after ovulation when oestrogen and progesterone levels are elevated, and may also exhibit cyclical alterations in digital blood flow [8].

Endothelial cell activation and injury may compromise perfusion by:

(a) exacerbating vasospasm
(b) mediating proliferation and contraction of vascular smooth muscle cells
(c) inducing a procoagulant and hypofibrinolytic state [9; 10] with resultant microvascular thrombosis
(d) releasing chemokines and adhesion molecules which lead to leucocyte activation, inflammation and tissue injury [11]

Endothelium-independent mechanisms

Calcitonin gene-related peptide has a direct vasodilatory effect on vascular smooth muscle. Reduced levels of calcitonin gene-related peptide have been demonstrated in the peripheral circulation of patients with RP, especially those with scleroderma-associated RS [12]. This may occur due to loss of sensory calcitonin gene-related peptide-releasing nerves in affected arteries or reduced levels of the peptide in intact neurones [12]. There is evidence of increased α_2-adrenergic receptor sensitivity and density, and increased β-presynaptic

Table 11.1a. *Vascular conditions that may present with limb ischaemia and/or Raynaud's phenomenon (RP), and the association with small vessel disease (SVD)*

Condition	RP	SVD	Limb ischaemia
Obstructive vascular disease			
Arterial thrombo-embolism	✓		✓
Atherosclerosis	✓	✓	✓
Aneurysm	✓		✓
Thromboangiitis obliterans (Buerger's)	✓	✓	✓
Vascular malfunction			
Primary Raynaud's disease	✓	✓	✓
Erythromelalgia	✓	✓	

receptor responsiveness in the peripheral nerves of patients with RP. Dermal arterioles from patients with scleroderma-associated RS exhibit an exaggerated response to α_2-agonists 6, and α_2-receptor blockade reduces vasospasm in RD [13]. Evidence for the role of the central nervous system in RP includes the observations that vibration affecting one hand leads to vasoconstriction in the contralateral hand which is abolished by proximal nerve blockade, and body cooling without peripheral cooling leads to digital vasospasm.

Changes in blood rheology occur in RP. Elevated fibrinogen levels, increased plasma viscosity, stiffer red and white blood cells, and platelet activation and aggregation, lead to reduced blood flow in the microcirculation. There is no evidence that platelet release of thromboxane A2 and serotonin are important in the pathophysiology of RP.

Ischaemia-reperfusion injury occurs in exacerbations of RP and probably has an important role in the progressive tissue damage seen in scleroderma-associated RS. Activated white blood cells aggregate and adhere to the endothelium, and generate oxygen free radicals. Blood flow in the microcirculation is reduced, ECs are activated with a resultant procoagulant state and tissue damage occurs with a local inflammatory response.

Emotional stress may have a role as indicated by the finding that cutaneous arteries of patients with RD demonstrate a failure of habituation of their vasomotor response to stressful noise [14]. Finally, five candidate regions of potential genome linkage have been demonstrated in familial RP [15].

Table 11.1b. *Vasculitic and immune complex disease that may present with limb ischaemia and/or Raynaud's phenomenon (RP) and the association with small vessel disease (SVD)*

Condition	RP	SVD	Limb Ischaemia
Vasculitis			
Takayasu's arteritis (TA)	✓	✓	✓
Giant cell arteritis (GCA)	✓	✓	✓
Wegener granulomatosis		✓	
Churg-Strauss syndrome		✓	✓
Polyarteritis nodosa (PAN)	✓	✓	
Kawasaki disease		✓	
Immune complex vasculitis			
Goodpasture syndrome	✓	✓	
Henoch-Schönlein purpura	✓	✓	
IgA nephropathy	✓	✓	
Systemic lupus erythematosus (SLE)*	✓	✓	✓
Rheumatoid arthritis*	✓	✓	✓
Polymyositis/dermatomyositis	✓	✓	✓
Scleroderma	✓	✓	✓
Mixed connective tissue disease	✓	✓	✓
Antiphospholipid antibody syndrome	✓	✓	✓
Sjogren's syndrome	✓	✓	✓
Inflammatory bowel disease	✓	✓	✓
Essential cryoglobulinemia	✓	✓	✓
Cold agglutinins	✓	✓	✓
Drug-induced vasculitis	✓	✓	✓
Serum sickness	✓	✓	✓
Lympho/myelo-proliferative*, carcinoma	✓	✓	✓
Behçet disease	✓	✓	✓

*may be associated with erythromelalgia.

Clinical features of Raynaud's phenomenon

Classical colour changes in the skin associated with RP are distinctive blanching (ischaemia), then blue (deoxygenation of static blood), then red (reactive

Table 11.1c. *Medical, environmental and pharmacological disorders that may present with limb ischaemia and/or Raynaud's phenomenon (RP) and the association with small vessel disease (SVD)*

Condition	RP	SVD	Limb ischaemia
Haematological			
Myeloma/macroglobulinaemia	✓	✓	✓
Polycythaemia*	✓	✓	✓
Neurological			
Syringomyelia	✓		✓
Poliomyelitis	✓		✓
Multiple sclerosis	✓		✓
Hemiplegia	✓		✓
Thoracic outlet syndrome	✓		✓
Carpal tunnel syndrome	✓		✓
Cervical spondylosis	✓		✓
Endocrine disorders			
Hypothyroidism	✓	✓	
Phaeochromocytoma	✓	✓	
Carcinoid	✓	✓	
Diabetes mellitus*	✓	✓	
Environmental and occupational			
Sports activities weightlifting, rowing, etc.			✓
Vibration syndrome	✓	✓	✓
Electrical or thermal injury		✓	✓
Hypothenar hammer syndrome	✓		✓
PVC exposure	✓	✓	✓
Complex regional pain syndrome	✓	✓	✓
Frozen food and ammunition workers	✓	✓	
Pharmacological			
Propylthiouracil, phenytoin		✓	
B-blockers, cocaine, amphetamine,	✓	✓	✓
Vinblastine, bleomycin, cis-platinium	✓	✓	✓
Heavy metals, and β interferon	✓	✓	✓
Overdose, dopamine, ergotamine	✓	✓	✓
Infection induced			
Hepatitis B & C, parvovirus, *Helicobacter pylori*	✓	✓	✓

*may be associated with erythromelalgia.

hyperaemia), which may be accompanied by throbbing pain, swelling and hyperhidrosis. These triphasic changes are not essential for the diagnosis as cold induced digital blanching can still reflect significant vasospasm. Attacks varying from minutes to hours commonly affect the fingers and toes but occasionally the lips, mouth, tip of the nose, and in women rarely the nipples. Raynaud's phenomenon can be associated with cerebral (migraine), coronary (Prinzmetal angina) and oesophageal vasospasm indicating the potential

Table 11.2. *Differentiating primary from secondary Raynaud's phenomenon*

	Primary	Secondary
Associated diseases	No	Yes
Age at onset	Younger (<30 y)	Older (>30 y)
Nail fold capillaries	Normal	Abnormal
Autoantibodies	Negative	Frequent
Endothelial cell activation	Yes	Yes
Endothelial damage	No	Frequent
Structural occlusion	No	Yes
Digital gangrene	Never	Can occur
Carotid artery stiffness	Normal	Increased

systemic nature to the disease. It has a prevalence of 5%–10% in the adult population worldwide with a predisposition to younger women and a familial link that is more common in those with early disease onset. Repeated attacks of RP occur only in about 30%, the majority of which are classified as primary RP (Raynaud's disease). Less commonly if an underlying disorder causing a lesion in the capillary wall is diagnosed, subjects are classified as secondary RP which can be complicated by trophic changes (skin atrophy, clubbing and deformity of nails, scarring, and sclerodactyly). Primary RP is not associated with a specific disease entity but some (~10%) of these subjects later develop connective tissue disease (CTD).

Treatment

Conservative measures:

- Thermal underwear, body warmers, hand muffs, ski-glove, boot liners, electrically heated gloves and socks
- Withdrawal of aggravating drugs, such as beta-blockers
- Change of occupation
- Biofeedback techniques
- Physical exercise

Drug therapy:

Scleroderma patients with Raynaud's and SVD suffering intense pain with functional impairment or tissue ischaemia require drug therapy [16]. Response to drugs is idiosyncratic, so it is worth trying more than one drug within a particular class. In general the use of vasodilator therapy is more effective in primary rather than secondary RP.

Table 11.3. *Differentiation of primary and secondary EM*

	Primary	Secondary
Symmetry	bilateral	unilateral
Age	young	older
Sex	male	both
Family history	yes	no
Lab tests	normal	abnormal

Options include:

- Calcium antagonists – nifedipine is the drug of choice (others are also effective), reducing the severity and frequency of attacks. These drugs are in general limited by side effects of dizziness, palpitations, headache, flushing and ankle swelling, which can be limited by using low dosages and sustained release formulations
- Naftidrofuryl oxalate – may produce symptomatic improvement after three months
- Iloprost – a synthetic prostacyclin analogue administered through a peripheral vein over a 6–8 hour period once a day for 3–5 days. Additional advantages include inhibition of platelet aggregation and increased red cell deformability. It raises the temperature of the hands and fingers, brings about pain relief but requires hospitalization for intravenous administration. The effects however can last for up to 16 weeks [17]

Alternatives:

- Nitrates, a topical 2% ointment can be useful for localized disease
- Ginko biloba [18]
- Fluoxetine, an SSRI has some vasodilator and antiplatelet action [19]
- Evening primrose oil (concentrated linoleic and gamolenic acids) and fish oil (omega-3 marine triglycerides) are metabolized to prostaglandin and prostacyclin-like elements. Their efficacy is unproven

Surgery:

A last resort in severe disease, cervical sympathectomy produces only a short lived improvement, lumbar sympathectomy is more longlasting and digital

Table 11.4. *Type of vasculitis and size of blood vessel commonly involved*

Type of vasculitis	Size of blood vessel: Aorta and branches	Large- and medium-sized vessels	Medium-sized muscular arteries
Giant cell arteritis	YES	YES	
Takayasu's arteritis	YES		
Thromboangiitis obliterans	YES	YES	
Polyarteritis nodosa		YES	YES

sympathectomy relieves severe pain and heals ulcers in patients with critical ischaemia. Adventitial stripping of palmar arteries, a radical alternative, has been shown to help [20].

ERYTHROMELALGIA (EM)

Erythromelalgia is characterized by a sensation of heat and intense burning pain in the skin particularly of the lower limbs associated with hyperaemia. These symptoms can be precipitated by exercise, dependency and exposure to heat, and partial relief may be obtained by elevation of the affected part or by cooling. The attacks can last from minutes to days and are heralded by an itching/pricking sensation which develops into burning pain of a severe and distressing nature, later accompanied by erythema, warmth and on occasions swelling of the affected part. Patients are often driven to extreme measures to obtain relief such as sleeping with feet out the window, in the fridge and walking barefoot in the snow [3]. Like RP there are primary and secondary forms of EM. Differentiation between them (Table 11.3) is useful as secondary forms are more amenable to treatment.

Treatment

Secondary EM is more amenable to treatment, hence 75 mg aspirin benefits those with thrombocythaemia, venesection helps in polycythaemia and steroids may be beneficial in connective tissue disease.

VASCULITIS

Vasculitis is characterized by histologic evidence of blood vessel inflammation. When such inflammation occurs, it can lead to blood vessel stenosis/occlusion with resultant tissue ischaemia, as well as thinning or rupture, resulting in aneurysms or haemorrhage. Although vasculitis is usually classified as a small, medium or large vessel disease, some vasculitic processes are not limited by vessels calibre (Figure 11.1). The classical '*primary*' vasculitides are rare, with an incidence of 20–100/million [21]. The signs and symptoms of vasculitis overlap with the much more common disorders of infection, connective tissue disease and malignancy, and this together with the variability in presentation often lead to delays in establishing a final diagnosis. Additionally, identifying the cause of deterioration in the patient known to have vasculitis can be extremely difficult because of the overlap between active disease, infection or complications of drug therapy.

Vasculitis secondary to connective tissue disease

Rheumatoid arthritis (RA)

Vasculitis may affect the skin, gastrointestinal tract, central and peripheral nervous system, and heart. The features of cutaneous rheumatoid vasculitis overlap with the characteristics of both cutaneous necrotizing venulitis and cutaneous polyarteritis nodosa. These different types of vasculitis can co-exist in the same or different lesional skin leading to diverse cutaneous vasculitic manifestations of RA. Perivascular infiltrates are diagnostic of vasculitis in RA. Dermal venulitis (leucocytoclastic vasculitis) is the most common presentation of vasculitis and when associated with extra-articular involvement may follow a poor prognosis.

Systemic lupus erythematosus (SLE)

Vasculitis secondary to SLE is characterized by immune dysregulation, which results in the production of

Table 11.5. *Common antibodies in connective tissue disease*

	SLE	Sjogren's	Systemic Sclerosis	MCTD	PM/DM
Nuclear Ab	ANA several	ANA speckled	ENA nucleolar (D) centromere (L)	ANA speckled	ANA several
DsDNA	60%				
SsA	35%	70%			
SsB		30%			
RNP				95%	
SCL-70			35% (D)		
JO1					40%
RF	+	++		++	
Histone	20% (95%*)				
Sm	20%				

PM = polymyositis; DM = dermatomyositis; *drug induced SLE.

autoantibodies (see Table 11.3), activation of the complement system and immune complex generation. One of the most characteristic lesions of SLE is vascular injury, which has wide ranging clinical manifestations including cutaneous vasculitis, glomerulonephritis, as well as cardiopulmonary, cerebrovascular and, less commonly, gastrointestinal damage. Inflammatory and/or thrombotic endothelial activation and damage are central to the pathogenesis of vascular disease [22].

Systemic sclerosis (SSc)

Systemic sclerosis is characterized by extensive cutaneous and visceral fibrosis, and small vessel vasculopathy. The pathogenesis is unknown, however, autoimmune mechanisms directed against self-fibroblasts are considered pivotal. Three autoantigens are specifically expressed at significantly higher levels in fibroblasts from scleroderma patients: fibrillarin, centromeric autoantigen p27 and RNA polymerase II [23]. Vascular function is abnormal in SSc with both large and small vessel endothelial and neurogenic control mechanism disturbances leading to vasoconstriction. Although some of the results are conflicting, the balance of evidence is suggests a greater impairment in endothelial-dependent function compared to endothelial-independent mechanisms [24]. Some 2% of women and 6% of men with RP develop SSc.

Mixed connective tissue disease

This syndrome with associated positive anti-RNP (see Table 11.5) consists of oedema of the hands, RP, acrosclerosis, synovitis and myositis (laboratory or biopsy evidence). The main cause of death is pulmonary hypertension. On rare occasions when there is associated vasculitis the prognosis is usually poor.

Antiphospholipid antibody syndrome (APLS)

A syndrome that includes a hypercoagulable state, thrombocytopenia, fetal loss, dementia, strokes (see Sneddon's syndrome), optic changes, Addison's disease and skin rashes. About 30%–50% of patients with SLE will have APLS. Antiphospholipid antibodies (APL-Ab) can also be found in patients with other autoimmune diseases. Children will often develop transient APL-Ab after viral infections and ~30% of patients with human immunodeficiency virus (HIV) infection will also develop them. Infection associated APL-Ab are not associated with thrombosis. Medications like chlorpromazine, procainamide and quinidine may also induce APL-Ab [25]. In screening studies of blood donors, up to 8% of normal people may have a low APL-Ab titre usually in young women.

Treatment

Therapy aimed at treating the disease itself is usually sufficient to treat the vasculitic omponent although a more intensive approach is often needed. Therapies for

SSc such as iloprost and hyperbaric oxygen are used in the research setting.

Behçet disease

Behçet disease is a multisystem inflammatory disease with vascular manifestations that can affect vessels of all sizes. It is most prevalent in 20- to 35-year-old people of Asian and eastern Mediterranean descent. It is characterized by recurrent aphthous oral ulcers and at least two or more of the following: recurrent genital ulceration, eye lesions' cutaneous lesions or a positive pathergy test. Among the most severe manifestations are gastrointestinal inflammation and ulceration, ocular inflammation that may lead to blindness, and CNS disease with meningoencephalitis. Large venous or arterial lesions occur in 7% to 38% of patients and may include vessel thrombosis and occlusion, as well as pulmonary or peripheral artery aneurysms. Behçet disease may remit and relapse frequently. Death occurs in 4% of cases, generally as the result of gastrointestinal perforation, vascular rupture and CNS disease [26]. Many patients develop lesions that clinically resemble erythema nodosum but have different microscopic features.

Treatment

Treatment is based on the disease manifestations. Aphthous lesions and mucocutaneous disease may be treated with topical or intralesional glucocorticoids, dapsone or colchicine. Thalidomide has been used with success but side effects prevent prolonged use.

Large-vessel and medium-sized-vessel vasculitides

Systemic vasculitis is categorized as large-vessel, medium-sized-vessel and small-vessel vasculitis based on the predominant vascular distribution of the lesions (Table 11.4). The large- and medium-sized-vessel vasculitides only affect arteries while the small-vessel vasculitides mainly affect capillaries and venules. The large- and medium-sized-vessel vasculitides may be infective or non-infective. Mycotic aneurysm is the commonest presentation of vasculitis secondary to an infectious agent. Kawasaki's disease is a medium-sized-vessel arteritis commonly affecting coronary and iliac arteries, and there is some evidence that toxic shock syndrome toxin-1 (TSST-1) positive *Staphylococcus aureus* may be responsible [27]. Giant cell arteritis (GCA) and Takayasu's arteritis (TA) are the commonest non-infective vasculitides presenting to the vascular surgeon.

Giant cell arteritis

Giant cell arteritis principally affects the extracranial carotid, vertebral, subclavian, axillary and proximal brachial arteries. Transmural inflammation leads to intimal hyperplasia which causes arterial occlusion and end-organ ischaemia. Giant cell arteritis of the thoracic aorta and to a lesser extent the abdominal aorta can lead to aneurysm formation, dissection and rupture.

Common clinical manifestations include headache, jaw claudication, polymyalgia rheumatica and visual symptoms. Early diagnosis and treatment with prednisolone can prevent blindness. The risk of developing a thoracic aortic aneurysm is increased approximately 20-fold in these patients.

Giant cell arteritis is diagnosed by histological examination of a temporal artery biopsy. The characteristic features are panarteritis with mononuclear infiltrates penetrating all layers of the blood vessel wall, activated T cells and macrophages arranged in granulomas, multinucleated giant cells in close proximity to fragmented internal elastic lamina, and intimal hyperplasia with concentric occlusion of the vessel lumen. Vessel wall necrosis is not a feature of GCA.

Giant cell arteritis is a T cell-dependent disease requiring the presence of CD4+ T cells [28]. The antigen which is recognized by and stimulates the CD4+ T cells has not been identified and infectious agents have not been isolated.

Dendritic cells are antigen-presenting cells and they play a crucial role in the pathophysiology of GCA. Activated dendritic cells are trapped at the adventitia-media border of medium-sized inflamed arteries, and they produce chemokines which recruit CD4+ T cells and macrophages into the arterial wall. Once recruited, the dendritic cells initiate and maintain CD4+ T cell activation. Adventitial CD4+ T cells secrete cytokines, especially interferon (IF)-γ, which regulate macrophage differentiation into effector cells with tissue-destructive potential, and maintains inflammatory cellular infiltrates which organize into granulomas in the arterial media. These mulitnucleated giant cells cause fragmentation of the internal elastic lamina. Macrophage function depends on their site in the arterial wall. Adventitial macrophages release IL-1β and IL-6, and may contribute to antigen presentation and

T cell activation. Adventitial macrophages also synthesize transforming growth factor (TGF)-β which may contribute to the mobilization and hyperproliferation of myofibroblasts, and matrix deposition essential for intimal hyperplasia. Medial macrophages secrete metalloproteinases and produce oxygen free radicals which are responsible for tissue injury.

Oxygen free radicals from medial macrophages cause lipid peroxidation of cell membranes of the medial vascular smooth muscle cells with resultant structural disintegration and cell death. Another mechanism of injury appears to be as a consequence of the accumulation of nitrated proteins which stimulate endothelial nitric oxide synthase and this, in combination with oxygen free radical production, causes activation and injury to the ECs which line the inflammation-induced neocapillaries in the media.

Macrophages and vascular smooth muscle cells also produce platelet-derived growth factor (PDGF) and vascular endothelial growth factor (VEGF). Platelet-derived growth factor is required for the proliferation of intimal myofibroblasts, and VEGF stimulates neoangiogenesis in the media and intima, both of which are essential for intimal hyperplasia.

The blood vessel wall components, especially ECs, amplify the inflammatory response by three mechanisms:

(a) Adhesion molecule expression and function is essential for immune complex and complement-mediated injury to blood vessels. Endothelial cells are more commonly a target for injury in small-vessel vasculitis. However, circulating anti-endothelial cell antibodies have been detected in GCA, Takayasu's arteritis and thromboangiitis obliterans but the antigens recognized by these antibodies and their pathogenetic role have not been well characterized. Anti-endothelial cell antibody which binds to ECs and complement activation products (including C5a and C1q) induce adhesion molecule expression by ECs. C5a up-regulates P-selectin expression and C1q induces E-selectin, intracellular adhesion molecule (ICAM)-1 and vascular cell adhesion molecule (VCAM)-1. Activated lymphocytes and macrophages produce IL-1, tumour necrosis factor (TNF)-α and IF-γ which induce adhesion molecule expression by ECs. Adhesion molecules mediate leucocyte interactions such as adhesion and migration into the vessel wall. Infiltrating leucocytes release inflammatory mediators which cause a vascular response to inflammation. In large-vessel vasculitis, adhesion molecule expression occurs in neovessels in the adventitia and within the inflammatory lesion mainly at the intima-media junction. This suggests that infiltrating leucocytes penetrate the blood vessel from peri-arterial tissues via adventitial vasa vasora and neovessels rather than from the lumen.

(b) Cytokines produced by ECs contribute to the systemic acute phase protein response (IL-1α, IL-6) and selectively attract leucocyte subpopulations, T cells and macrophages. They also assist in tissue targeting (IL-8 and other chemokines) and prolong the half life of infiltrating leucocytes (colony stimulating factor, CSF). The cytokines IL-1 and TNFα, and various growth factors may contribute to a procoagulant state. IL-1, TGF-β, PDGF and fibroblast growth factor (FGF)-β stimulate myointimal cell proliferation and matrix deposition which lead to intimal hyperplasia.

(c) Angiogenesis occurs in inflammatory lesions especially in the adventitial layer or peri-arterial tissues and, in large-vessel vasculitis, within the inflammatory infiltrates at the intima-media junction. In the medium-sized-vessel and large-vessel vasculitides, neovessels express leucocyte adhesion molecules and provide an increased surface area of activated ECs which help to amplify the inflammatory response by increased cytokine, chemokine and growth factor production. In GCA, VEGF, IL-8 and FGF-2 are angiogenic factors while TNFα, and TGF-β may have indirect angiogenic activity.

Takayasu's arteritis (TA)

Takayasu's arteritis is a chronic inflammatory disease of large elastic arteries including the aorta, carotid, pulmonary, coronary and renal arteries. Diffuse dilatation, aneurysm formation and thrombotic occlusion are commoner in TA than GCA.

Takayasu's arteritis predominantly affects women under 40 years of age and usually presents with non-specific constitutional symptoms such as fevers, myalgia, fatigue and weight loss. Carotodynia (pain over the carotid arteries) is a particularly suggestive but uncommon complaint. Later symptoms result from vessel stenosis or occlusion such as hypertension, claudication, syncope and visual disturbances.

The microscopic features of TA and GCA are similar [29]. The acute phase is characterized by panarteritis. There is inflammation of the adventitial vasa vasora which precedes and may induce inflammation in the adventitia where an inflammatory infiltrate of T cells and dendritic cells occurs. There is infiltration of lymphocytes and occasional multinucleated giant cells in the media with neovascularization. The intima is invaded by vascular smooth muscle cells and fibroblasts which produce excess mucopolysaccharides and cause intimal thickening. The chronic phase is characterized by destruction of the collagen and elastin layers in the media with fibrosis of all three layers of the blood vessel wall which leads to segmental luminal narrowing. In cases of rapid disease progression, the fibrotic reaction may be inadequate and this leads to aneurysm formation.

CD4+ and CD8+ T cells and natural killer cells play a major role in the vascular injury. The CD4+ T cells respond to the 65 kDa heat shock protein and this is strongly expressed in the aortic tissues of patients with TA. Stimulated T cells lead to macrophage activation and release of proteins which damage the aortic wall.

Autoimmune abnormalities may contribute to TA but as yet no specific antigen has been identified. Anti-endothelial cell antibodies are elevated, and these antibodies activate ECs and increase complement-dependent cytotoxicity *in vitro* [30; 31; 32]. The disease is associated with an increased incidence of HLA alleles in different populations. The finding of similar vascular lesions in animals with various viral infections suggests that viral infection may also be important [33].

Thromboangiitis obliterans (Buerger's disease)

Thromboangiitis obliterans (TAO) is a segmental inflammatory disease of small and medium-sized arteries, veins and nerves. It is more common in the lower than the upper limbs but may affect almost any vascular bed in the body. The acute phase of the disease is associated with a highly cellular and inflammatory occlusive thrombus containing polymorphonuclear leucocytes, mulinucleated giant cells and microabscesses. However, it differs from the other vasculitides in that there is relative sparing of the blood vessel wall architecture with preservation of the internal elastic lamina and no evidence of vessel necrosis. Vessel wall calcification, atheromatous plaque and aneurysm formation are also absent.

Although there is little doubt that persistent tobacco use is a major risk factor for disease onset and progression, the precise mechanism of TAO is unknown. There is no evidence that a procoagulant state is responsible but some evidence exists that it may be an immunological condition, although the responsible antigen has not yet been identified. An increased cell-mediated immune response to type I and/or type III collagen (which are normal arterial constituents) [34] and increased levels of anti-endothelial cell antibodies have been demonstrated in patients with the disease [35]. While vessel wall architecture is preserved, immunocytochemical analysis of acute lesions has identified T cells, macrophages and dendritic cells within the intima, and immunoglobulins and complement factors along the intact internal elastic lamina [36]. Abnormal regulation of vascular tone may also contribute to the development of TAO. Impaired endothelium-dependent vasorelaxation in response to intra-arterial infusion of acetylcholine has been demonstrated in the peripheral blood vessels of diseased and non-diseased limbs with preservation of a normal endothelium-independent vasorelaxation response to intra-arterial sodium nitroprusside.

Polyarteritis nodosa (PAN)

Polyarteritis nodosa is a medium-sized-vessel vasculitis which presents with hypertension, fever, and musculoskeletal, gut and renal symptoms. Lung involvement is extremely rare and suggests an alternative diagnosis. Five year survival with treatment is approximately 80%.

The acute phase is characterized by segmental necrotizing arteritis with neutrophil and monocyte infiltration, and occasional vessel thrombosis. Neutrophil and monocyte activation occurs at the blood-artery interface, and leads to transmural cell infiltration and necrosis which may track longitudinally in the medial or adventitial plane. This inflammatory reaction may progress to circumferential transmural fibrinoid necrosis and ultimately the vessel wall is replaced by a collagenous scar. Extensive destruction of the vessel wall and peri-arterial tissues may result in inflammatory pseudoaneurysm formation. Medium-sized-vessel vasculitis such as PAN occurs preferentially at arterial branch points and it has been speculated that high shear stress may initiate the inflammatory process [37]. Increased shear stress induces up-regulation of endothelial adhesion molecules (such as ICAM-1) and pro-inflammatory transcription factors (such as NF-κ B) [38]. Increased concentrations of intimal macrophages are also present at sites of increased shear stress [39].

FIBROMUSCULAR DYSPLASIA (FMD)

This is a non-inflammatory, non-atherosclerotic arteriopathy. It can affect any small and medium-sized artery, but is most commonly seen in the renal, internal carotid and external iliac arteries. Presenting symptoms are due to reduced perfusion, embolism, dissection and aneurysm formation.

The cause of FMD is unknown but there are several hypotheses. There is some evidence that the disease may have a genetic basis with autosomal dominant inheritance [40]. The renal, internal carotid and external iliac arteries are long arteries which are free of branches. Vasa vasora usually originate at branch points and thus ischaemia may be a contributory factor in the development of FMD. In animal studies, injury to the vasa vasorum has led to dysplastic arterial lesions, and perimedial and medial dysplasia occur in the media-adventitia junction where the vasa vasorum are most important [41]. The renal and internal carotid arteries are exposed to repetitive stretching during head movement and respiration, and this may lead to increased production of collagen, hyaluronate and chondroitin sulphate in the arterial wall [42].

The lesions are classified according to the layer of the arterial wall which is affected [43]. Medial fibroplasia accounts for over 80% of cases. Pathological findings consist of alternating areas of thickened and thinned media, fibrous tissue in the outer media and ground substance and collagen separating smooth muscle cells in the inner media, and normal intima and adventitia. Perimedial fibroplasia accounts for over 10% of cases and is characterized by increased elastic tissue between the adventitia and medial layers with normal intima. In cases of intimal fibroplasia, there is subendothelial collagen deposition in the intima with disruption of the internal elastic lamina, and normal media and adventitia. In medial hyperplasia there is isolated vascular smooth muscle cell hyperplasia.

DIAGNOSTIC APPROACH TO LIMB ISCHAEMIA WHEN A NON-ATHEROSCLEROTIC CAUSE SUSPECTED

History

The differential diagnosis for patients presenting with possible limb ischaemia includes clinically complex entities, such as collagen-vascular diseases and endocarditis. Careful attention must be paid to seemingly unrelated issues, such as rash, photosensitivity, ulcers, changes in skin texture, dryness of eyes, calcinotic deposits, difficulty swallowing, breathlessness, neuropathy, visual disturbances, ear nose and throat symptoms, weight loss, fatigue, myalgias, and arthralgias. A thorough medical history is necessary to elucidate predisposing factors, e.g. systemic sclerosis, family history, drug exposure (such as ergotamine, beta-blockers or oral contraceptives), use of vibrating machinery, and work in a cold environment (for example, the fishing industry).

Examination

Palpation and auscultation of the limb pulses, and measurement of blood pressure in both arms is required bearing in mind that unilateral Raynaud's phenomenon can indicate local pathology, e.g. an aneurysm. Examination of the hands should include an Allen test and nail fold capillaroscopy with an ophthalmoscope at +20 dioptres. Normally nail fold capillaries are regular loops but an underlying connective tissue disease can be indicated by the presence of dilated and tortuous capillary loops.

Investigations

Non-invasive tests such as segmental and digital pressures, and Doppler are helpful in documenting the distal nature of disease when assessing a patient with possible limb ischaemia (Figure 11.2). Abnormal segmental pressure is indicative of proximal large artery disease but does not necessarily exclude the possibility of co-existing small vessel disease and hence objective measures of blood flow are needed.

Segmental pressure measurements

Examination of the patient should begin with the segmental pressure measurements test. The pressure

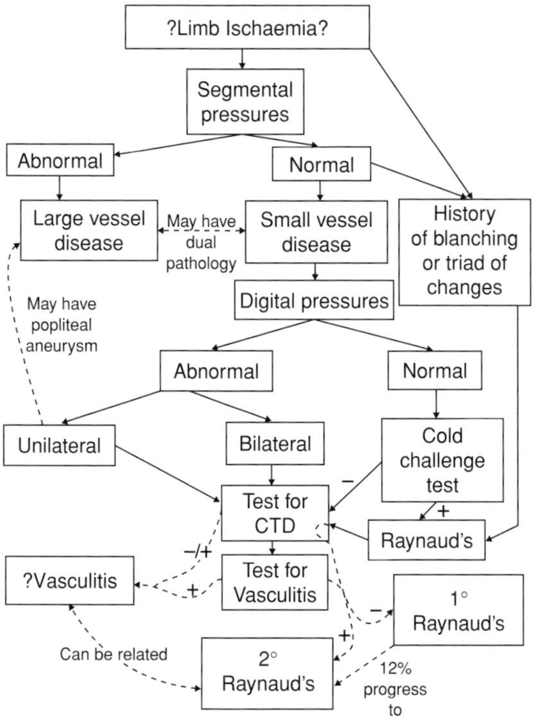

Fig. 11.2. General schema for evaluating patients with suspected limb arterial disease. CTD-Connective tissue disease.

differential between adjacent levels or when compared with the identical level on the contralateral extremity seldom exceeds 5 to 7 mm Hg. Wrist:brachial or forearm:brachial ratios are usually less than 1.0; ratios below 0.70 are abnormal. In contrast ankle:brachial pressure index is normally >0.9; in claudication 0.5–1; with rest pain 0.3–0.5 and impending gangrene <0.2 (critical ischaemia), although subjects have been known to claudicate at 0.9 or not at 0.5.

Digital pressures

The finger ipsilateral brachial index normally averages 0.97 and ranges from 0.80 to 1.27. Values are typically in the normal range in individuals with primary RD performed when the patient is warm and vasodilated. A cold challenge test is usually performed in such cases by cooling of the hand in water at 10–12 °C for five minutes and digital pressures are reassessed. All vasoactive drugs should be stopped 24 hours prior to testing. If the subject attends during a vasospastic attack and if the pressures normalize on rewarming, one can be confident that vasospasm is playing an important role in the ischaemic process, whereas if there is little change, fixed obstruction or continuing vasospasm is likely present. In the presence of proximal palmar or digital disease without inflow disease, the finger ipsilateral index is markedly decreased to <0.70. Because the measurement of pressures is performed in the base of the phalanx, obstruction in the distal portions of the vessels might have no perceptible change in digital pressures.

Pulse volume and wave forms

When using Doppler, one normally encounters triphasic signals. Dampened or monophasic signals indicate a significant proximal occlusion. Because of the extensive collateral networks in the palm and wrist, one can detect normal Doppler flow signals at these levels even in the presence of a complete occlusion. By compressing one of the vessels, one can bring out a loss of signal akin to an Allen's test. Alternatively, one can detect a reversal of flow in the radial or ulnar arteries if there is a proximal occlusion involving either artery.

Radiography

A chest X-ray should be performed in all patients with upper limb ischaemic phenomena to detect bony abnormalities such as those of the thoracic outlet, and this can be followed by magnetic resonance imaging (MRI) in select cases. Hand radiographs can also be useful to detect soft tissue calcification in scleroderma and mixed connective tissue disease, while a barium swallow can also be useful for detecting oesophageal hypomobility syndrome. Chest radiographs and computed tomography (CT) scanning often reveal lung involvement in many of the primary and secondary vasculitides even in the absence of pulmonary symptoms. Computed tomography scanning is usually performed after an abnormal pulmonary function test result. Magnetic resonance imaging angiography of upper extremity vessels including the aortic arch should be performed when the diagnosis is unclear and primary Raynaud's has been excluded. This should be performed bilaterally even if only one extremity is symptomatic, because of the bilateral nature of diffuse small artery obstructive disease and the need to differentiate it from the unilateral diffuse small artery obstruction, produced by embolism. In addition, certain diseases such as thromboangiitis

Table 11.6. *Laboratory evaluation of limb ischaemia*

FBC	Immunology screeen (see below)
PV	Cryoglobulins
CRP	Complement
Chemistry profile	Serum protein electrophoresis
Lipid profile	Hepatitis screen
Urinalysis	Plasma homocysteine (fasting)
Blood glucose	Antiphospholipid antibodies

obliterans can demonstrate clinical disease in one limb, but angiographic involvement in multiple limbs. If MRI angiography or CT angiography fails to reveal any proximal embolic source in the presence of characteristic distal findings, transoesophageal echocardiography may detect ulcerated atherosclerotic plaques in the aortic arch at the innominate or left subclavian artery origins that cannot otherwise be detected.

Pulmonary assessment

Formal pulmonary function testing is useful in giving a sensitive measure of disease activity in the connective tissue diseases, pulmonary renal syndromes and other vasculitides. Bronchoscopy can be used to assess for infection, alveolar hemorrhage, and biopsy or lavage of endobronchial lesions.

Body fluid analyses

Investigations to be performed in the evaluation of limb vascular involvement are listed in Table 11.6. Extensive cultures and urinalysis including microscopy should be performed in all patients with suspected or proven vasculitis. In cases of unexplained limb ischaemia blood levels for ergotamine and a urine screen for cannabis, cocaine, amphetamines and nicotine may be helpful.

Immunology

Rheumatoid factor, antinuclear and anticardiolipin antibodies may be positive in primary vasculitis, although high titres and specific antibodies (Table 11.6) clearly favour connective tissue disease. Complement (C3 and C4) should be obtained whenever SLE remains in the differential. Hepatitis B and C serologies may also be indicated because hepatitis B is associated with PAN and hepatitis C is associated with cryoglobulinaemia.

Biopsy

Biopsy remains a mainstay of diagnosis of vasculitis, and easily accessible sites, such as skin or ENT lesions, are preferred.

CONCLUSION

The diagnosis of acute, severe or global limb ischaemia is usually straightforward, but when symptoms of altered blood flow are gradual in onset or subtle in nature then one should be aware of the multitude of conditions that can contribute to vascular instability. Multiple pathologies need to be considered and indeed do sometimes co-exist, further complicating the diagnostic challenge. The strategy outlined above should hopefully assist in clarify the management of more difficult cases.

REFERENCES

1. J. C. Jennette & R. J. Falk, Small-vessel vasculitis. *New England Journal of Medicine*, **337**(21) (1997), 1512–23.
2. F. M. Wigley, Clinical practice. Raynaud's phenomenon. *New England Journal of Medicine*, **347**(13) (2002), 1001–8.
3. A. E. Smyth, L. Bell, I. N. Bruce, S. McGrann & J. A. Allen, Digital vascular responses and serum endothelin-1 concentrations in primary and secondary Raynaud's phenomenon. *Annals of Rheumatic Diseases*, **59** (2000), 870–74.
4. P. J. W. Smith, C. J. Ferro, D. S. McQueen & D. J. Webb, Functional studies in small arteries do not support a primary role for endothelin in the pathogenesis of Raynaud's disease. *Journal of Cardiovascular Pharmacology*, **31**(Suppl) (1998), S473–76.
5. F. Khan, S. J. Litchfield, M. McLaren *et al.*, Oral L-arginine supplementation and cutaneous vascular responses in patients with primary Raynaud's phenomenon. *Arthritis and Rheumatism*, **40** (1997), 352–57.
6. N. A. Flavahan, S. Falavahan, Q. Liu *et al.*, Increased α_2-adrenergic constriction of isolated arteries in diffuse scleroderma. *Arthritis and Rheumatism*, **43** (2000), 1886–990.
7. J. Leppert, A. Ringqvist, J. Ahlner *et al.*, Seasonal variations in cyclical GMP response on whole-body

cooling in women with primary Raynaud's phenomenon. *Clinical Science*, **93** (1997), 175–9.
8. D. Greenstein, N. Jeffcote, D. Ilsley & R. C. Kester, The menstrual cycle and Raynaud's phenomenon. *Angiology*, **47** (1996), 427–36.
9. C. S. Lau, M. McLaren & J. J. F. Belch, Factor VIII von Willebrand factor antigen levels correlate with symptom severity in patients with Raynaud's phenomenon. *British Journal of Rheumatology*, **30** (1991), 433–6.
10. C. S. Lau, M. McLaren, I. Mackay & J. J. F. Belch, Baseline plasma fibrinolysis and its correlation with clinical manifestations in patients with Raynaud's phenomenon. *Annals of Rheumatic Diseases*, **52** (1993), 443–8.
11. C. S. Lau, A. O'Dowd & J. J. F. Belch, White blood cell activation in Raynaud's phenomenon of systemic sclerosis and vibration induced white finger syndrome. *Annals of Rheumatic Diseases*, **51** (1992), 249–52.
12. C. B. Bunker, G. Terenghi, D. R. Springall, J. M. Polak & P. M. Dowd, Deficiency of calcitonin gene-related peptide in Raynaud's phenomenon. *Lancet*, **336** (1990), 1530–33.
13. R. R. Freedman, R. P. Baer & M. D. Mayes, Blockade of vasospastic attacks by α_2-adrenergic but not α_1-adrenergic antagonists in idiopathic Raynaud's disease. *Circulation*, **92** (1995), 1448–51.
14. C. M. Edwards, J. M. Marshall & M. Pugh, Lack of habituation of the pattern of cardiovascular response evoked by sound in subjects with primary Raynaud's disease. *Clinical Science*, **95** (1998), 249–60.
15. E. Susol, A. J. MacGregor, J. H. Barrett *et al.*, A two-stage genome-wide screen for susceptibility loci in primary Raynaud's phenomenon. *Arthritis and Rheumatism*, **43** (2000), 1641–6.
16. S. D. Sule & F. M. Wigley, Treatment of scleroderma: an update. *Expert Opinion on Investigational Drugs*, **12** (3) (2003), 471–82.
17. C. M. Black, L. Halkier-Sorensen, J. J. Belch *et al.*, Oral iloprost in Raynaud's phenomenon secondary to systemic sclerosis: a multicentre, placebo-controlled, dose-comparison study. *British Journal of Rheumatology*, **37**(9) (1998), 952–60.
18. A. H. Muir, R. Robb, M. McLaren, F. Daly, J. J. Belch, The use of Ginkgo biloba in Raynaud's disease: a double-blind placebo-controlled trial. *Vascular Medicine*, 7(4) (2002), 265–7.
19. I. A. Jaffe, Serotonin reuptake inhibitors in Raynaud's phenomenon. *Lancet*, **345**(8961) (1995), 1378.
20. B. Balogh, W. Mayer, M. Vesely *et al.*, Adventitial stripping of the radial and ulnar arteries in Raynaud's disease. *Journal of Hand Surgery (American)*, **27**(6) (2002), 1073–80.
21. R. A. Watts, M. A. Gonzalez-Gay, S. E. Lane *et al.*, Geoepidemiology of systemic vasculitis: comparison of the incidence in two regions of Europe. *Annals of Rheumatic Diseases*, **60**(2) (2001), 170–2.
22. D. D'Cruz, Vasculitis in systemic lupus erythematosus. *Lupus*, **7**(4) (1998), 270–4.
23. N. A. Flavahan, S. Flavahan, S. Mitra & M. A. Chotani, The vasculopathy of Raynaud's phenomenon and scleroderma. *Rheumatic Disease Clinics of North America*, **29**(2) (2003), 275–91, vi.
24. A. L. Herrick, Vascular function in systemic sclerosis. *Current Opinion in Rheumatology*, **12**(6) (2000), 527–33.
25. J. S. Levine, D. W. Branch & J. Rauch, The antiphospholipid syndrome. *New England Journal of Medicine*, **346**(10) (2002), 752–63.
26. H. Yazici, S. Yurdakul & V. Hamuryudan, Behçet disease. *Current Opinion Rheumatology*, **13**(1) (2001), 18–22.
27. J. W. Cohen Tervaert, E. R. Popa & N. A. Bos, The role of superantigens in vasculitis. *Current Opinion in Rheumatology*, **11** (1999), 24–33.
28. C. M. Wyand & J. J. Goronzy, Pathogenic mechanisms in giant cell arteritis. *Cleveland Clinic Journal of Medicine*, **69** (Suppl II) (2002), 28–32.
29. S. J. Inder, Y. V. Boryshev, S. M. Cherian *et al.*, Accumulation of lymphocytes, dendritic cells, and granulocytes in the aortic wall affected by Takayasu's disease. *Angiology*, **51** (2000), 565–79.
30. M. Blank, I. Krause, T. Godkorn *et al.*, Monoclonal anti-endothelial cell antibodies from a patient with Takayasu arteritis activate endothelial cells from large vessels. *Arthritis and Rheumatism*, **42** (1999), 1421–32.
31. J. Eichhorn, D. Sima, B. Thiele *et al.*, Anti-endothelial cell antibodies in Takayasu arteritis. *Circulation*, **94** (1996), 2396–401.
32. N. K. Tripathy, S. Upadhyaya, N. Sinha *et al.*, Complement and cell mediated cytotoxicity by antiendothelial cell antibodies in Takayasu's arteritis. *Journal of Rheumatology*, **28** (2001), 805–8.
33. A. J. Dal & H. W. Canto, Virgin, Animal models of infection-mediated vasculitis: implications for human disease. *International Journal of Cardiology*, **75** (2000), S37–S45.

34. R. Adar, M. Z. Papa, Z. Halpern *et al.*, Cellular sensitivity to collagen in thromboangiitis obliterans. *New England Journal of Medicine*, **308** (1983), 1113–16.
35. J. Eichhorn, D. Sima, C. Lindschau *et al.*, Antiendothelial cell antibodies in thromboangiitis obliterans. *American Journal of the Medical Sciences*, **315** (1998), 17–23.
36. M. Kobayashi, M. Ito, A. Nakagawa *et al.*, Immunohistochemical analysis of arterial wall cellular infiltration in Buerger's disease (endarteritis obliterans). *Journal of Vascular Surgery*, **29** (1999), 451–5.
37. J. C. Jennette, Implications for pathogenesis of patterns of injury in small- and medium-sized-vessel vasculitis. *Cleveland Clinic Journal of Medicine*, **69** (Suppl II) (2002), 33–8.
38. T. Nagel, N. Resnick, C. F. Dewey & M. A. Gimbrone, Vascular endothelial cells respond to spatial gradients in fluid shear stress by enhanced activation of transcription factors. *Arteriosclerosis, Thrombosis and Vascular Biology*, **19** (1999), 1825–34.
39. H. C. Stary, Macrophages, macrophage foam cells, and eccentric intimal thickening in the coronary arteries of young children. *Atherosclerosis*, **64** (1987), 91–108.
40. A. R. Rushton, The genetics of fibromuscular dysplasia. *Archives of Internal Medicine*, **140** (1980), 233–6.
41. V. Sottiurai, W. J. Fry & J. C. Stanley, Ultrastructural characteristics of experimental arterial medial fibroplasia induced by vasa vasorum occlusion. *Journal of Surgical Research*, **24** (1978), 169.
42. D. Y. M. Leung, S. Glagov & M. B. Matthews, Cyclical stretching stimulates synthesis of matrix components by arterial smooth muscle cells in vitro. *Science*, **191** (1976), 475–7.
43. J. C. Stanley, B. L. Gewerts, E. L. Bove *et al.*, Arterial fibroplasia, histopathologic character and current etiologic concepts. *Archives of Surgery*, **110** (1975), 561–6.

12 • Vascular biology of restenosis

RICHARD D. KENAGY, PATRICK C.H. HSIEH AND
ALEXANDER W. CLOWES

INTRODUCTION

A major limitation of all forms of vascular intervention for the treatment of ischaemic lesions is that they inevitably damage vessels. This is true for direct repair (patch angioplasty, endarterectomy), bypass grafting (vein, synthetic) and for intraluminal approaches (balloon angioplasty, atherectomy, stent angioplasty). Lumen enlargement after angioplasty or stenting is the result of a combination of plaque reduction (compression and embolization), plaque redistribution within or outside the lesion area and vessel expansion [1; 2]. These effects determine the success of the intervention, but also contribute to restenosis, usually defined as a renarrowing of the arterial lumen, as each represents aspects of injury. Greater than 20% of all interventions fail because of restenosis. Failure occurs early due to technical problems and later (1–12 months) because of injury-induced scarring [3]. At much later periods (>12 months), failure results from the underlying atherosclerotic process. Although restenosis occurs within the context of atherosclerosis, the clinical features, fundamental mechanisms, and genetic control of atherosclerosis and restenosis are different [4]. Atherosclerosis is a multifactoral, inflammatory disease [5] that develops slowly, usually taking decades, while restenosis results from the wound healing response to arterial injury and occurs within months [6].

Restenosis has great clinical significance. The morbidity and expense of further treatment is considerable, since adjuvant therapies to prevent luminal renarrowing are only now being realized in the limited context of stent angioplasty with drug coated stents. The ultimate goal of research in this area is to develop pharmacological strategies to modify vascular scarring so that zones of injury are repaired without luminal narrowing. The objectives of this chapter are to review the mechanisms of restenosis and treatment strategies currently used or under investigation. For a more detailed discussion of therapy the reader is referred to Chapter 13.

MECHANISMS OF RESTENOSIS

Restenosis is the result of the following processes, which contribute to varying degrees depending on the intervention employed (e.g. angioplasty vs. stenting).

- elastic recoil
- arterial remodelling
- reorganization of thrombus
- intimal hyperplasia

Elastic recoil

The elastic properties of elastin in the vessel wall cause recoil of the artery after the overstretch caused by inflation of the balloon catheter. Recoil occurs within minutes after deflation of the balloon and produces a significant degree of restenosis (defined as ≥50% loss of gain in lumen area) within one day [7]. Stenting greatly reduces elastic recoil [8].

Arterial remodelling

The bulk of research on the arterial response to injury over the last few decades has focused on intimal hyperplasia. Intimal hyperplasia is the principal mechanism of luminal narrowing in stented arteries. However, remodelling is the major factor in restenosis after angioplasty. Remodelling refers to a change in the luminal dimensions of the blood vessel, not attributable to vasospasm, vasodilation or changes in wall area. While it can refer to a change in constituents without a change in size, the term generally refers to changes in diameter and, thus, terms such as geometric remodelling are commonly used. Remodelling can be favourable (outward, positive, compensatory or adaptive) or unfavourable (inward, negative or maladaptive). Using post-mortem samples, Glagov [9] first described positive remodelling during the early stages of atherosclerosis when lumen size was maintained in the face of increasing intimal lesion size by expansion of the entire vessel. This observation has been confirmed prospectively using ultrasound [10]. Negative remodelling refers to a loss of total arterial area (generally measured as a loss of the area within the external elastic lamina). Kimura *et al.* [11] reported that arteries showed further gains in lumen area between one day and one month after angioplasty. While all arteries lost some vessel area thereafter, the restenotic arteries showed a greater loss than non-restenotic arteries. In confirmation of studies in pigs [12], rabbits [13] and non-human primates [14]. Mintz and coworkers [15] found that negative remodelling contributed more to restenosis after angioplasty in humans than did intimal hyperplasia. In contrast, in rigid artificial grafts and stented arteries, which are unable to change their overall size, intimal hyperplasia is the primary mechanism of restenosis [16].

Mechanisms of arterial remodelling are poorly understood. For example, the relative roles of the adventitial and medial layers of the artery are unclear. Some data suggest that adventitial fibrosis contributes to negative remodelling [17] and the macrophage content of the lesion correlates with positive remodelling [18]. Although it is intuitively obvious that extracellular matrix attachments to cells must be broken and reformed to change the geometry of the vessel, the mechanisms and factors involved have not been well characterized. The possible roles of matrix degrading proteinases, such as matrix metalloproteinases and extracellular matrix components will be discussed below.

Reorganization of thrombus

Balloon injury denudes the vessel of endothelium and can cause medial dissection. Subsequent exposure of the subendothelium and medial layers to blood can lead to thrombus formation, key components of which are fibrin and platelets. Tissue factor, which is exposed in the subendothelium, is an essential mediator of thrombin and fibrin generation [19]. Adherence of platelets is mediated by receptors such as the integrin, glycoprotein IIb/IIIa. Aggregation of platelets causes the release into the wall of numerous factors, including thromboxane A2, ADP, serotonin, and matrix metalloproteinases 2 and 9, that further stimulate platelet adherence and/or aggregation. Platelets also release a variety of growth and chemotactic factors. Antiplatelet therapy, particularly inhibitors of IIb/IIIa in both animals and humans [20; 21; 22; 23], has demonstrated the importance of platelets to the restenotic process. Leucocyte attachment and migration after arterial injury appears to depend on adherent platelets [24; 25]. Also a thrombus can act as a scaffold upon which smooth muscle cells (SMCs) migrate, and synthesize and degrade extracellular matrix components [26; 27], thus reorganizing the thrombus.

Intimal hyperplasia

Most of our understanding of the underlying cellular mechanisms of intimal hyperplasia comes from animal models of vascular injury. In some, but not all, respects these model the clinical situation. For example, most animal models have employed a partially inflated Fogarty embolectomy catheter with lower inflation pressures than used in clinical percutaneous transluminal angioplasty. A percutaneous transluminal coronary angioplasty (PTCA) catheter is placed in a lesion and inflated to avoid removing the endothelium elsewhere, while the Fogarty balloon is usually repeatedly drawn through a vessel to completely remove the endothelium and damage the media. Because the PTCA catheter is used in a diseased segment, plaque fissure, intimal tears and tangential medial splitting frequently occur. A direct comparison of the two methods in rats demonstrated that, in contrast to the Fogarty balloon, the PTCA catheter causes intimal hyperplasia only when the internal elastic lamina is ruptured [28]. Despite these differences there are many common features shared between the two procedures. Both damage the endothelium followed by platelet adherence and activation. Arteries damaged by Fogarty balloon or PTCA show intimal and medial remodelling, production of extracellular matrix, endothelial cell regrowth, and intimal and medial cell proliferation. Thus, despite their limitations, animal models of vascular injury have provided useful insights, particularly when the ability to study the human response prospectively at the cellular and biochemical level has been limited. Only now are non-invasive methods like magnetic resonance imaging [29; 30] being developed for the detailed analysis of the human response to injury.

The sequence of events after arterial injury that leads to intimal hyperplasia are summarized in Figure 12.1 and illustrated in Figure 12.2. An immediate event is a stretch or shear injury that within 30 minutes kills up to 70% of medial SMCs via apoptosis [31]. Preparation and placement of a vein graft into the arterial circulation [32] and placement of stents [33; 34] also cause substantial apoptosis. Of interest, the rates of apoptosis in SMCs and macrophages in restenotic lesions are less than those in the primary atherosclerotic lesion [35], although this is an observation of a late event. The medial SMC proliferation rate jumps from 0.06% before injury to 10%–40% in the injured arteries of rats [36], rabbits [37] and non-human primates [38] during the first two days. Animal studies [39] and clinical studies with stents [40] indicate that intimal hyperplasia is generally correlated with the degree of injury. Smooth muscle cell growth returns to baseline in the media at four weeks and by eight weeks in endothelialized intima, but SMCs at the luminal surface in de-endothelialized areas continue to proliferate at a low rate [36].

Migration of medial SMCs into the rat neointima occurs as early as four days after injury [36]. About half of these SMCs undergo two rounds of proliferation in the intima [41]. The role of SMC migration in human vessels is unknown [42]. This is because the presence of intimal SMCs in normal arteries of species other than rat and mouse, and the presence of intimal SMCs in arterial lesions, makes the measurement of migration impossible by currently available methods. In addition, the long term significance of medial SMC migration is uncertain, since in some instances, pharmacological inhibition of migration causes only transient inhibition of intimal hyperplasia. For example, matrix metalloproteinase inhibitors [43] and heparin [44] inhibit migration of SMCs to the intima, and inhibit short term intimal hyperplasia. However, in both cases a counter regulatory mechanism (different for each) in the intima results in no therapeutic effect on intimal hyperplasia at later times. Thus, when there are pre-existing intimal SMCs the impact of medial SMC migration is not clear.

Other cells can contribute to the formation of the intima after vessel injury (see Figure 12.3 for possible sources of the major cells of the intima). Studies in the rat [45], pig [46] and rabbit [47] indicate that to varying degrees adventitial fibroblasts dedifferentiate into myofibroblasts and migrate into the intima [48]. Although this appears to require significant damage and even fracture of the medial layer, some investigators did not find evidence for significant adventitial involvement in intima formation even with complete interruption of the media [49]. In addition, studies of arterial injury in chimeric mice [50] and rats [51] indicate that a significant number of non-leucocyte intimal cells are derived from blood-borne progenitors of bone marrow origin [52]. Finally, evidence from studies of embryonic development and with cultured endothelial cells demonstrate that endothelial cells can undergo a phenotypic transition to SMCs [53].

Animal studies demonstrate that both SMC proliferation and extracellular matrix (ECM) production contribute to intimal hyperplasia [44]. However, post-angioplasty restenotic tissue from humans demonstrates substantial amounts of matrix and little proliferation [54; 55; 56]. It is probable that SMC replication does not play a major role in restenosis after angioplasty. Data obtained using restenotic tissue from patients with stable angina [35] support the idea proposed by O'Brien *et al.* [54] that decreased rates of apoptosis, rather than increased proliferation, cause increased cell density in restenotic tissue. Of interest, Koyama and Reidy found that re-injury to the rat carotid artery one month after the first balloon injury led to an increase in intimal lesion size that was entirely the result of an increase in ECM [57; 58].

Inflammation has been implicated in restenosis [59]. There is a strong correlation between inflammation and restenosis in stented arteries [40], between macrophages in the primary lesion and the occurrence of restenosis after angioplasty [60], and between pre- and post-procedural serum levels of C-reactive protein and restenosis [61]. The data suggest inflammation acts primarily by stimulating intimal hyperplasia. Leucocyte recruitment to the injured vascular wall occurs via binding to adherent platelets [62] and to cell adhesion molecules that are up-regulated by injury, such as vascular cell adhesion molecule-1 and intercellular adhesion molecule-1 [63]. Neutrophil binding leads to integrin activation and chemokine secretion [25]. Monocytes play a major role in intimal hyperplasia after angioplasty in rats, non-human primates [64] and hypercholesterolaemic rabbits [65], as demonstrated by the inhibition of intimal hyperplasia by a dominant-negative mutant of monocyte chemoattractant protein-1 (MCP-1). In contrast, there is virtually no monocyte recruitment after injury in normal rabbits [66], the difference appearing

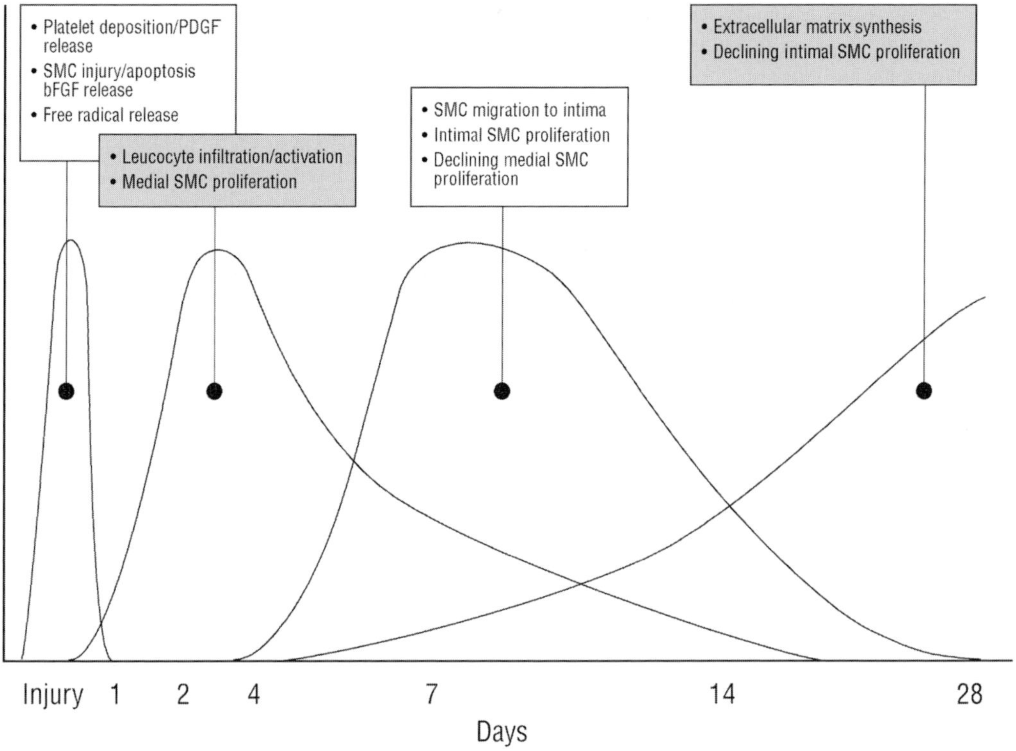

Fig. 12.1. Sequence of events leading to intimal hyperplasia after arterial injury.

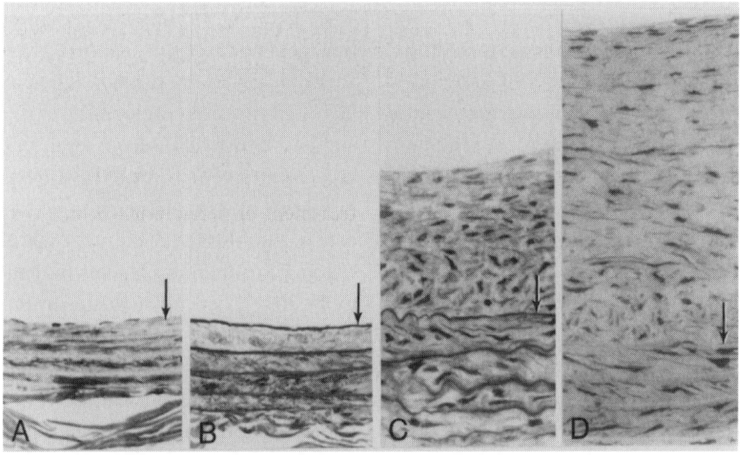

Fig. 12.2. Histologic cross-sections of injured rat carotid arteries: (a) normal vessel. Note the single layer of endothelium in the intima; (b) denuded vessel at two days. Note the loss of endothelium; (c) denuded vessel at two weeks. Intima is now markedly thickened due to smooth muscle migration and proliferation; and (d) denuded vessel at 12 weeks. Further intimal thickening has occurred. Internal elastic lamina indicated by an arrow. Lumen is at the top. (By permission Nature Publishing Group [36].)

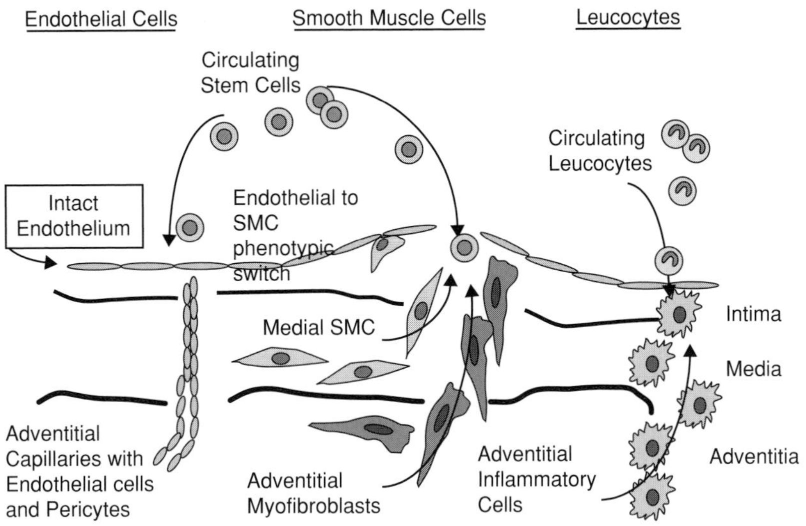

Fig. 12.3. Possible sources of intimal cells after arterial injury.

to be that MCP-1 induction is only transient in this case. However, in this latter case, blockade of neutrophil recruitment using an antibody to the β2 integrin, Mac1, inhibited medial SMC proliferation and intimal hyperplasia [66]. Further evidence for the role of leucocytes in intimal hyperplasia is that Mac1 knock-out mice develop smaller lesions after vascular injury [67].

There are differences in the absolute level of hyperplasia between species [39], and even between strains of mouse [4] and rat [68]. Differences in the thrombotic response [39] as well as differences in rates of recovery of the endothelium [69] may explain some of the variability, although the genetic basis of these differences has not yet been elucidated.

BIOCHEMICAL EVENTS DURING RESTENOSIS

Growth factors/cytokines

Activated platelets and SMCs release a number of growth factors after arterial injury, including platelet-derived growth factor (PDGF), basic fibroblast growth factor (bFGF), transforming growth factor-β (TGFβ), TGFα, platelet-derived endothelial cell growth factor, interleukin-1 (IL-1) and tumor necrosis factor (TNF) [70]. In addition, endothelial cells and macrophages, two other cells present in atherosclerotic vessels, can secrete vascular endothelial growth factor (VEGF), macrophage colony stimulating factor (MCSF) and granulocyte macrophage colony stimulating factor (GMCSF) [70]. Many of these factors have been shown to play some role in intimal hyperplasia after arterial injury (Table 12.1). However, we will focus on only three of these.

Platelet-derived growth factor plays a major role in the migration of SMCs [71; 72], while playing a minor role in SMC proliferation [23]. The β, but not the α, isoform of the PDGF receptor mediates intimal hyperplasia in non-human primates [73; 74]. This, in turn, suggests a role for the PDGF isoforms B and D [75; 76], and possibly C [77]. However, there is also evidence for a role of PDGF-AA and, therefore, PDGF receptor α in intimal hyperplasia in the rat [78]. Of interest, concomitant treatment of non-human primates with blocking antibodies to both PDGF receptor isoforms caused intimal regression in polytetrafluroethylene grafts, while treatment with either alone did not [79]. At present there is no evidence that PDGF plays a role in arterial remodelling.

Basic fibroblast growth factor stimulates medial SMC proliferation [80] and migration [81] to the intima in the injured rat carotid. However, bFGF plays no role in the proliferation of intimal SMCs [82], and the intimal hyperplastic response in bFGF knock-out mice is normal [83]. With regard to a possible role in remodelling, a blocking antibody to bFGF inhibits negative remodelling in the mouse carotid tie-off model [84],

Table 12.1. *Stimulatory factors for intimal hyperplasia after arterial injury*

Factor	Function	Reference
PDGF	Increases SMC migration and proliferation	23, 71
bFGF	Increases SMC migration and proliferation	23, 157
TGFβ	Increases SMC proliferation, EMC production	87, 88
EGF receptor agonist (EGF?)	Increases SMC proliferation	158
Insulin	Increases SMC migration and proliferation	159
IGF-1	Increases SMC proliferation	160, 161
TNFα	Increases MCP-1 expression	162
IL-1β	ND	163
Endothelin via ET-A receptor	ND	164, 165
Angiotensin II/AT2 receptor	Increases SMC proliferation, inhibits apoptosis	166
Thrombin	ND	167, 168
Factor Xa	Increases SMC proliferation	169
Tissue factor	Increases thrombus formation, SMC migration	170
Discoidin domain receptor-1	Mediates SMC migration, proliferation, MMP production	135
Thrombospondin-1	Inhibits endothelial cell healing	171
Alpha 1A-adrenoceptor agonist	ND	172

ND = not determined *in vivo*; EGF = epidermal growth factor; IGF-1 = insulin-like growth factor-1; ET-A = endothelin-A type receptor; TNF = tumour necrosis factor; IL-1 = interleukin-1; AT2 = angiotensin type 2 receptor.

and expression of bFGF correlates with positive remodelling caused by increased blood flow [85]. Finally, blocking both bFGF and PDGF with antibodies results in an additive inhibition of intimal hyperplasia [86].

Although infusion of TGFβ stimulates medial SMC proliferation [87] and antibody blockade slightly inhibits intimal hyperplasia [88], the more striking effect of blocking the action of TGFβ is on remodelling and ECM production. Blockade of TGFβ inhibited negative remodelling, the transition of adventitial fibroblasts to myofibroblasts, and the deposition of collagen and versican [88; 89].

Interactions among growth factors after injury are a significant though largely unexplored aspect of restenosis. For example, TGFβ can synergistically augment the mitogenic action of PDGF and bFGF [90]. In addition, IL-1β augments the proliferative effect of PDGF-BB on SMC by inhibiting expression of p21 and p27 [91], but inhibits PDGF-BB mediated SMC migration [92]. Platelet-derived growth factor also increases IL-1β binding to SMC [93]. Such interactions may augment hyperplasia in areas of inflammation (such as near stent struts) by slowing SMC movement and increasing proliferation.

Inhibitors

Numerous factors can act as inhibitors of intimal hyperplasia (Table 12.2). For example, nitric oxide (NO) can inhibit SMC migration and proliferation after arterial injury [94], and partially mediates the inhibitory effect of IL-1β on migration [95]. Heparin and heparan sulphate proteoglycans can inhibit SMC proliferation and migration [44; 96].

Coagulation cascade/fibrinolytic path

A central stimulant for thrombus formation after injury is tissue factor [19]. In a double injury model in rabbits, Courtman *et al.* found that inhibition of tissue factor prevented negative remodelling [97]. In recent years a intracellular signalling role for tissue factor has become apparent, further adding to its role after injury [98]. Thrombin [99] and factor Xa [100] can stimulate SMC

Table 12.2. *Inhibitory factors for intimal hyperplasia after arterial injury*

Factor	Function	Reference
Interferon-γ	Inhibits SMC proliferation	173
Hepatocyte growth factor	Increases endothelial cell coverage	174
Adiponectin	Inhibits SMC proliferation and migration	175
Interleukin 10	Decreases SMC proliferation and monocyte infiltration	176
Adrenomedullin	ND	177
Met-enkephalin (opioid growth factor)	Inhibits SMC proliferation	178
Somatostatin	Inhibits SMC migration	179, 180
Endothelin via ET-B receptor	Increases NO	181
Tissue Inhibitor of metalloproteinases-1	Inhibits SMC migration	182
Tissue Inhibitor of metalloproteinases-2	Inhibits SMC migration	183, 184
Tissue Inhibitor of metalloproteinases-3	Increases SMC apoptosis	185
Heparin/heparan sulphates	Inhibits SMC proliferation and migration	96, 186
NO	Inhibits SMC proliferation and migration	94, 187
ApoE	Inhibits SMC proliferation	188
estrogens	Inhibits SMC proliferation	189, 190

ND = not determined *in vivo*.

growth directly as well as indirectly through coagulation and platelet activation.

Balloon injury causes levels of the plasminogen activators, urokinase and tissue-type plasminogen activator, to increase in SMCs [101]. The plasminogen activators, in turn, proteolytically activate plasmin. The persistence of fibrin in the media after arterial injury in plasminogen knock-out mice [102] indicates the major role of plasmin in fibrinolysis. Several lines of evidence also indicate that urokinase is required for SMC migration through the vascular wall [103; 104] and thrombus [105]. In addition, the plasma urokinase concentration is also a predictor of restenosis [106].

Matrix metalloproteinases

Arterial injury in several animals [107; 108; 109], including the non-human primate [104], induces the production of several matrix metalloproteinases (MMPs). MMP9 is induced within hours and falls to baseline within a week, while MMP2 activation occurs within days. There are little data on the effect of angioplasty or other interventions on the expression of MMPs in humans. Most data come from tissue obtained months to years after intervention and these suggest decreased expression of MMPs compared to primary lesions [110; 111]. However, these tissues are mostly from failed interventions. With increasing time the restenotic tissue resembles advanced atherosclerosis and, thus, contains cells that express MMPs [110]. Blockade of MMPs with synthetic drugs or natural inhibitors reduces SMC migration from the arterial media in animals [43; 112; 112; 113]. This effect on SMC migration in the rat carotid injury model leads to a short term reduction in intimal hyperplasia [43; 112]. Small molecule MMP inhibitors have been shown to inhibit stent intimal hyperplasia in rabbits [114], but not in porcine coronary arteries [115]. In the later case the MMP inhibitor prevented negative arterial remodelling instead. In contrast, a MMP inhibitor prevented neither intimal hyperplasia nor negative arterial remodelling after angioplasty or stenting in cholesterol-fed, non-human primates [116]. These differences may result from differences between species, in the inhibitory profile of the specific inhibitor used or the type of arterial lesion existing before treatment.

Gene polymorphisms in MMP3 and MMP9 appear to play a role in atherogenesis, but only the MMP3 5A/6A polymorphism plays a role in restenosis [117; 118; 119]. Interestingly, this association with restenosis is only true for angioplasty and not stenting [118; 120]. The MMP3 promoter with the 6A allele, which is protective in both the progression of atherosclerosis and restenosis, has less activity than the promoter with the 5A allele [117]. The simplest explanation that MMP3 is needed to cause negative arterial remodelling is complicated by the observation that immunostaining for MMP3 was highest in positively remodelled arterial segments compared with negatively or intermediately remodelled segments [121].

The mechanism by which MMPs may mediate negative remodelling is not certain. For example, given that hydroximate-based MMP inhibitors can inhibit mitogen activated protein (MAP) kinase signalling [122] and collagen synthesis [123], and collagen synthesis inhibitors can inhibit SMC migration [124], the mechanism for these effects on restenosis goes beyond simply cleaving the ECM proteins [125].

The process of negative remodelling after angioplasty has been modelled *in vitro*. Smooth muscle cells embedded in collagen gel rafts cause the gels to contract slowly. Although contraction of collagen gels by skin fibroblasts is inhibited by a MMP inhibitor (marimastat) [126], a similar broad spectrum MMP inhibitor (batimastat) failed to inhibit non-human primate SMC mediated collagen gel contraction [116; Kenagy, unpublished data]. Interestingly, MMP9 knock-out SMCs have an impaired ability to contract collagen gels [17].

Extracellular matrix/receptors

While SMC proliferation decreases dramatically by two weeks in both the media and intima of the injured rat carotid artery, intimal hyperplasia continues as the result of ECM accumulation. The intimal area more than doubles between two and eight weeks, and the stable neointima is about 20% SMC and 80% ECM [127]. The accumulation of collagen occurs even as collagen synthesis is decreasing [128], presumably because degradation by MMPs is decreasing. Extracellular matrix factors induced by angioplasty [129] and stenting [130] include versican, perlecan, biglycan, elastin, hyaluronan and type I collagen. Biglycan and hyaluronan are also highly expressed in restenotic tissue in comparison with primary lesions [129; 131; 132; 133].

The list of cellular receptors for ECM components by which SMCs might directly act to remodel the artery includes the integrins, discoidin domain receptors (DDR) and CD44, all of which are induced after vascular injury [134; 135; 136]. The family of integrins provides the classic example of a binding partner, which is able to mediate subcellular signalling [137]. Smooth muscle cell mediated collagen gel contraction *in vitro is* dependent on β1 integrin [138]. Blockade of α vβ 3 integrin inhibited intimal hyperplasia [139; 140] without an effect on arterial remodelling. DDR1 has been shown to be required for SMC migration and MMP production [141], and CD44 mediates the stimulatory effect of hyaluronate on SMC mediated collagen gel contraction [142]. However, in all these cases a clear role in remodelling *in vivo* has not been established.

STRATEGIES TO PREVENT RESTENOSIS

Strategies to prevent restenosis will be only mentioned briefly, because this topic is covered in detail in Chapter 13. The most promising at this time is drug eluting stents, at least for those situations in which stents can be utilized successfully [143]. For example, sirolimus (rapamyacin) eluting stents show a clear benefit six months after stent placement [144], and in a small cohort no lesion formation or luminal narrowing was seen after two years [145]. Brachytherapy (radiation treatment) has shown much success, but exuberant hyperplasia at the ends of the stents or injured angioplasty zone can occur when radiation is not delivered in these areas (edge effect or 'candy wrapper') [146]. Gene therapy continues to hold promise with numerous promising candidates, but transfer efficiency remains the biggest challenge [147].

PREVENTION VS. REVERSAL OF RESTENOSIS

To date the pharmacological strategies employed for restenosis have been to prevent intimal hyperplasia. This means treatment of all patients, even though less than one-third of all vascular interventions fail. Another strategy is to develop the ability to screen for those patients at high risk or to develop a treatment that could reverse the restenotic process. Observations of an IL-1 receptor antagonist polymorphism [148] and genomic instability of TGFβ receptor II in SMCs of restenotic patients [149], suggest that screening may be possible in the future.

The possibility of reversing the restenotic process comes from the observation that intima formation in response to stents increases for about three months, but starts regressing spontaneously after six months [150; 151]. The mechanism of this spontaneous regression is unknown, but a model of graft intimal regression in non-human primates offers a promising direction of inquiry. In this model aorto-iliac, polytetrafluorethylene (PTFE) grafts are allowed to heal under normal shear stress. Shear stress is then switched from normal to high by constructing a downstream, arterio-venous fistula (AVF), which causes atrophy of the pre-existing intima [152]. This relationship between intimal thickness and wall shear stress has also been demonstrated in stented human coronary arteries [153]. Increased shear stress is associated with decreased SMC proliferation, increased SMC death [154] and increased proteolytic activity [155] as the pre-established PTFE graft intima atrophies. DNA microarray analysis of the high shear stress graft intima has revealed that over 500 out of ~30 000 genes or expressed sequence tags (ESTs) are differentially regulated compared to the normal shear intima [156]. These data should lead to drug candidates that may be useful for reversing stenosis in those situations where intimal hyperplasia is the primary cause.

REFERENCES

1. J. M. Ahmed, G. S. Mintz, N. J. Weissman *et al.*, Mechanism of lumen enlargement during intracoronary stent implantation – an intravascular ultrasound study. *Circulation*, **102** (2000), 7–10.
2. G. S. Mintz, A. D. Pichard, K. M. Kent *et al.*, Axial plaque redistribution as a mechanism of percutaneous transluminal coronary angioplasty. *American Journal of Cardiology*, **77** (1996), 427–30.
3. E. Allaire & A. W. Clowes. The intimal hyperplastic response. *Annals of Thoracic Surgery*, **64** (1997), S38–S46.
4. D. G. Kuhel, B. H. Zhu, D. P. Witte & D. Y. Hui, Distinction in genetic determinants for injury-induced neointimal hyperplasia and diet-induced atherosclerosis in inbred mice. *Arteriosclerosis, Thrombosis and Vascular Biology*, **22** (2002), 955–60.
5. P. Libby, Inflammation in atherosclerosis. *Nature*, **420** (2002), 868–74.
6. M. R. Bennett, & M. O'Sullivan, Mechanisms of angioplasty and stent restenosis: implications for design of rational therapy. *Pharmacology and Therapeutics*, **91** (2001), 149–66.
7. M. Nobuyoshi, T. Kimura, H. Nosaka *et al.*, Restenosis after successful percutaneous trans-luminal coronary angioplasty – serial angiographic follow-up of 229 patients. *Journal of the American College of Cardiology*, **12** (1998), 616–23.
8. M. Haude, R. Erbel, H. Issa & J. Meyer, Quantitative-analysis of elastic recoil after balloon angioplasty and after intracoronary implantation of balloon-expandable Palmaz-Schatz stents. *Journal of the American College of Cardiology*, **21** (1993), 26–34.
9. S. Glagov, E. Weisenberg, C. K. Zarins, R. Stankunavicius & G. J. Kolettis, Compensatory enlargement of human atherosclerotic coronary arteries. *New England Journal of Medicine*, **316** (1987), 1371–407.
10. S. Kiechl, J. Willeit & S. G. Bruneck, The natural course of atherosclerosis – part II: vascular remodeling. *Arteriosclerosis, Thrombosis and Vascular Biology*, **19** (1999), 1491–8.
11. T. Kimura, S. Kaburagi, T. Tamura *et al.*, Remodeling of human coronary arteries undergoing coronary angioplasty or atherectomy. *Circulation*, **96** (1997), 475–83.
12. H. R. Andersen, M. Mong, Thorwest & E. Falk, Remodeling rather than neointimal formation explains luminal narrowing after deep vessel wall injury – insights from a porcine coronary (re)stenosis model. *Circulation*, **93** (1996), 1716–24.
13. M. J. Post, C. Borst & R. E. Kuntz, The relative importance of arterial remodeling compared with intimal hyperplasia in lumen renarrowing after balloon angioplasty: a study in the normal rabbit and the hypercholesterolemic Yucatan micropig. *Circulation*, **89** (1994), 2816–21.
14. R. L. Geary, J. K. Williams, D. Golden *et al.*, Time course of cellular proliferation, intimal hyperplasia, and remodeling following angioplasty in monkeys with established atherosclerosis – a nonhuman primate model of restenosis. *Arteriosclerosis, Thrombosis and Vascular Biology*, **16** (1996), 34–43.

15. G. S. Mintz, J. J. Popma, A. D. Pichard *et al.*, Arterial remodeling after coronary angioplasty – a serial intravascular ultrasound study. *Circulation*, **94** (1996), 35–43.
16. H. Mudra, E. Regar, V. Klauss *et al.*, Serial follow-up after optimized ultrasound-guided deployment of Palmaz-Schatz stents – in-stent neointimal proliferation without significant reference segment response. *Circulation*, **95** (1997), 363–70.
17. Z. S. Galis, C. Johnson, D. Godin *et al.*, Targeted disruption of the matrix metalloproteinase-9 gene impairs smooth muscle cell migration arterial remodeling and geometrical. *Circulation Research*, **91** (2002), 852–9.
18. E. Ivan, J. J. Khatri, C. Johnson *et al.*, Expansive arterial remodeling is associated with increased neointimal macrophage foam cell content – the murine model of macrophage-rich carotid artery lesions. *Circulation*, **105** (2002), 2686–91.
19. C. M. Speidel, P. R. Eisenberg, W. Ruf, T. S. Edgington & D. R. Abendschein, Tissue factor mediates prolonged procoagulant activity on the luminal surface of balloon-injured aortas in rabbits. *Circulation*, **92** (1995), 3323–30.
20. D. P. Faxon, T. A. Sanborn, C. C. Haudenschild & T. J. Ryan, Effect of antiplatelet therapy on restenosis after experimental angioplasty. *American Journal of Cardiology*, **53** (1984), 72C–6C.
21. J. Fingerle, R. Johnson, A. W. Clowes, M. W. Majesky & M. A. Reidy, Role of platelets in smooth muscle cell proliferation and migration after vascular injury in rat carotid artery. *Proceedings of the National Academy of Sciences of the USA*, **86** (1989), 8412–6.
22. L. A. Harker, Role of platelets and thrombosis in mechanisms of acute occlusion and restenosis after angioplasty. *American Journal of Cardiology*, **60** (1987), B20–8.
23. C. D. Lewis, N. E. Olson, E. W. Raines, M. A. Reidy & C. L. Jackson, Modulation of smooth muscle proliferation in rat carotid artery by platelet-derived mediators and fibroblast growth factor-2. *Platelets*, **12** (2001), 352–8.
24. P. Libby & D. I. Simon, Inflammation and thrombosis – the clot thickens. *Circulation*, **103** (2001), 1718–20.
25. T. G. Diacovo, S. J. Roth, J. M. Buccola, D. F. Bainton & T. A. Springer, Neutrophil rolling, arrest, and transmigration across activated, surface-adherent platelets via sequential action of P-selectin and the beta(2)-integrin CD11b/CD18. *Blood*, **88** (1996), 146–57.
26. M. D. Rekhter, E. O'Brien, N. Shah *et al.*, The importance of thrombus organization and stellate cell phenotype in collagen I gene expression in human, coronary atherosclerotic and restenotic lesions. *Cardiovascular Research*, **32** (1996), 496–502.
27. K. Schafer, S. Konstantinides, C. Riedel *et al.*, Different mechanisms of increased luminal stenosis after arterial injury in mice deficient for urokinase- or tissue-type plasminogen activator. *Circulation*, **106** (2002), 1847–52.
28. C. Indolfi, D. Torella, C. Coppola *et al.*, Rat carotid artery dilation by PTCA balloon catheter induces neointima formation in presence of IEL rupture. *American Journal of Heart and Circulatory Physiology*, **283** (2002), H760–7.
29. W. Kerwin, A. Hooker, M. Spilker *et al.*, Quantitative magnetic resonance imaging analysis of neovasculature volume in carotid atherosclerotic plaque. *Circulation*, **107** (2003), 851–6.
30. C. Yuan, L. M. Mitsumori, M. S. Ferguson *et al.*, *In vivo* accuracy of multispectral magnetic resonance imaging for identifying lipid-rich necrotic cores and intraplaque hemorrhage in advanced human carotid plaques. *Circulation*, **104** (2001), 2051–6.
31. H. Perlman, L. Maillard, K. Krasinski & K. Walsh, Evidence for the rapid onset of apoptosis in medial smooth muscle cells after balloon injury. *Circulation*, **95** (1997), 981–7.
32. E. Rodriguez, E. H. Lambert, M. G. Magno & J. D. Mannion, Contractile smooth muscle cell apoptosis early after saphenous vein grafting. *Annals of Thoracic Surgery*, **70** (2000), 1145–52.
33. M. Kearney, A. Pieczek, L. Haley *et al.*, Histopathology of in-stent restenosis in patients with peripheral artery disease. *Circulation*, **95** (1997), 1998–2002.
34. M. Kollum, S. Kaiser, R. Kinscherf *et al.*, Apoptosis after stent implantation compared with balloon angioplasty in rabbits – role of macrophages. *Arteriosclerosis, Thrombosis and Vascular Biology*, **17** (1997), 2383–8.
35. G. Bauriedel, S. Schluckebier, R. Hutter *et al.*, Apoptosis in restenosis versus stable-angina atherosclerosis – implications for the pathogenesis of restenosis. *Arteriosclerosis, Thrombosis and Vascular Biology*, **18** (1998), 1132–9.
36. A. W. Clowes, M. A. Reidy & M. M. Clowes, Kinetics of cellular proliferation after arterial injury. I. Smooth

muscle growth in the absence of endothelium. *Laboratory Investigation*, **49** (1983), 327–33.

37. R. S. More, G. Rutty, M. J. Underwood, M. J. Brack & A. H. Gershlick, Assessment of myointimal cellular kinetics in a model of angioplasty by means of proliferating cell nuclear antigen expression. *American Heart Journal*, **128** (1994), 681–6.
38. R. D. Kenagy, S. Vergel, E. Mattsson *et al.*, The role of plasminogen, plasminogen activators, and matrix metalloproteinases in primate arterial smooth muscle cell migration. *Arteriosclerosis, Thrombosis and Vascular Biology*, **16** (1996), 1373–82.
39. R. S. Schwartz, Neointima and arterial injury: dogs, rats, pigs, and more. *Laboratory Investigation*, **71** (1994), 789–91.
40. A. Farb, D. K. Weber, F. D. Kolodgie, A. P. Burke & R. Virmani, Morphological predictors of restenosis after coronary stenting in humans. *Circulation*, **105** (2002), 2974–80.
41. A. W. Clowes & S. M. Schwartz, Significance of quiescent smooth muscle migration in the injured rat carotid artery. *Circulation Research*, **56** (1985), 139–45.
42. S. M. Schwartz, Smooth muscle migration in atherosclerosis and restenosis. *Journal of Clinical Investigation*, **100** (1997), S87–9.
43. N. Zempo, N. Koyama, R. D. Kenagy, H. J. Lea & A. W. Clowes, Regulation of vascular smooth muscle cell migration and proliferation *in vitro* and in injured rat arteries by a synthetic matrix metalloproteinase inhibitor. *Arteriosclerosis, Thrombosis and Vascular Biology*, **16** (1996), 28–33.
44. A. W. Clowes & M. M. Clowes, Kinetics of cellular proliferation after arterial injury. II. Inhibition of smooth muscle growth by heparin. *Laboratory Investigation*, **52** (1985), 611–6.
45. G. H. Li, S. J. Chen, S. Oparil, Y. F. Chen & J. A. Thompson, Direct *in vivo* evidence demonstrating neointimal migration of adventitial fibroblasts after balloon injury of rat carotid arteries. *Circulation*, **101** (2000), 1362–5.
46. N. A. Scott, G. D. Cipolla, C. E. Ross *et al.*, Identification of a potential role for the adventitia in vascular lesion formation after balloon overstretch injury of porcine coronary arteries. *Circulation*, **93** (1996), 2178–87.
47. E. Faggin, M. Puato, L. Zardo *et al.*, Smooth muscle-specific SM22 protein is expressed in the adventitial cells of balloon-injured rabbit carotid artery. *Arteriosclerosis, Thrombosis and Vascular Biology*, **19** (1999), 1393–404.
48. S. Sartore, A. Chiavegato, E. Faggin *et al.*, Contribution of adventitial fibroblasts to neointima formation and vascular remodeling – from innocent bystander to active participant. *Circulation Research*, **89** (2001), 1111–21.
49. T. Christen, V. Verin, M. L. Bochaton-Piallat *et al.*, Mechanisms of neointima formation and remodeling in the porcine coronary artery. *Circulation*, **103** (2001), 882–8.
50. C. I. Han, G. R. Campbell & J. H. Campbell, Circulating bone marrow cells can contribute to neointimal formation. *Journal of Vascular Research*, **38** (2001), 113–9.
51. P. Religa, K. Bojakowski, M. Maksymowicz *et al.*, Smooth-muscle progenitor cells of bone marrow origin contribute to the development of neointimal thickenings in rat aortic allografts and injured rat carotid arteries. *Transplantation*, **74** (2002), 1310–5.
52. K. Shimizu & R. N. Mitchell, Stem cell origins of intimal cells in graft arterial disease. *Current Atherosclerosis Reports*, **5** (2003), 230–7.
53. M. G. Frid, V. A. Kale & K. R. Stenmark, Mature vascular endothelium can give rise to smooth muscle cells via endothelial-mesenchymal transdifferentiation: *in vitro* analysis. *Circulation Research*, **90** (2002), 1189–96.
54. E. R. O'Brien, C. E. Alpers, D. K. Stewart *et al.*, Proliferation in primary and restenotic coronary atherectomy tissue: implications for antiproliferative therapy. *Circulation Research*, **73** (1993), 223–31.
55. P. R. Moreno, I. F. Palacios, M. N. Leon *et al.*, Histopathologic comparison of human coronary instent and post-balloon angioplasty restenotic tissue. *American Journal of Cardiology*, **84** (1999), 462–6.
56. E. R. O'Brien, S. Urieli-Shoval, M. R. Garvin *et al.*, Replication in restenotic atherectomy tissue. *Atherosclerosis*, **152** (2000), 117–26.
57. H. Koyama & M. A. Reidy, Reinjury of arterial lesions induces intimal smooth muscle cell replication that is not controlled by fibroblast growth factor 2. *Circulation Research*, **80** (1997), 408–17.
58. H. Koyama & M. A. Reidy, Expression of extracellular matrix proteins accompanies lesion growth in a model of intimal reinjury. *Circulation Research*, **82** (1998), 988–95.
59. F. G. P. Welt & C. Rogers, Inflammation and restenosis in the stent era. *Arteriosclerosis, Thrombosis and Vascular Biology*, **22** (2002), 1769–76.

60. P. R. Moreno, V. H. Bernardi, J. López-Cuéllar *et al.*, Macrophage infiltration predicts restenosis after coronary intervention in patients with unstable angina. *Circulation*, **94** (1996), 3098–102.
61. M. Schillinger, M. Exner, W. Mlekusch *et al.*, Vascular inflammation and percutaneous transluminal angioplasty of the femoropopliteal artery: association with restenosis. *Radiology*, **225** (2002), 21–6.
62. S. S. Smyth, E. D. Reis, W. Zhang *et al.*, Beta(3)-integrin-deficient mice but not P-selectin-deficient mice develop intimal hyperplasia after vascular injury: correlation with leukocyte recruitment to adherent platelets 1 hour after injury. *Circulation*, **103** (2001), 2501–7.
63. H. Tanaka, G. K. Sukhova, S. J. Swanson *et al.*, Sustained activation of vascular cells and leukocytes in the rabbit aorta after balloon injury. *Circulation*, **88** (1993), 1788–803.
64. M. Usui, K. Egashira, K. Ohtani *et al.*, Anti-monocyte chemoattractant protein-1 gene therapy inhibits restenotic changes (neointimal hyperplasia) after balloon injury in rats and monkeys. *FASEB Journal*, **16** (2002), 1838–40.
65. E. Mori, K. Komori, T. Yamaoka *et al.*, Essential role of monocyte chemoattractant protein-1 in development of restenotic changes (neointimal hyperplasia and constrictive remodeling) after balloon angioplasty in hypercholesterolemic rabbits. *Circulation*, **105** (2002), 2905–10.
66. F. G. P. Welt, E. R. Edelman, D. I. Simon & C. Rogers, Neutrophil, not macrophage, infiltration precedes neointimal thickening in balloon-injured arteries. *Arteriosclerosis, Thrombosis and Vascular Biology*, **20** (2000), 2553–8.
67. D. I. Simon, Z. Dhen, P. Seifert *et al.*, Decreased neointimal formation in Mac-1(-/-) mice reveals a role for inflammation in vascular repair after angioplasty. *Journal of Clinical Investigation*, **105** (2000), 293–300.
68. S. Assadnia, J. P. Rapp, A. L. Nestor *et al.*, Strain differences in neointimal hyperplasia in the rat. *Circulation Research*, **84** (1999), 1252–7.
69. D. Du Toit, E. Aavik, E. Taskinen *et al.*, Structure of carotid artery in baboon and rat and differences in their response to endothelial denudation angioplasty. *Annals of Medicine*, **33** (2001), 63–78.
70. R. Ross, The pathogenesis of atherosclerosis: a perspective for the 1990s. *Nature*, **362** (1993), 801–9.
71. C. L. Jackson, E. W. Raines, R. Ross & M. A. Reidy, Role of endogenous platelet-derived growth factor in arterial smooth muscle cell migration after balloon catheter injury. *Arteriosclerosis and Thrombosis*, **13** (1993), 1218–26.
72. A. Jawien, D. F. Bowen-Pope, V. Lindner, S. M. Schwartz & A. W. Clowes, Platelet-derived growth factor promotes smooth muscle migration and intimal thickening in a rat model of balloon angioplasty. *Journal of Clinical Investigation*, **89** (1992), 507–11.
73. N. A. Giese, M. M. H. Marijianowski, O. McCook *et al.*, The role of alpha and beta platelet-derived growth factor receptor in the vascular response to injury in nonhuman primates. *Arteriosclerosis, Thrombosis and Vascular Biology*, **19** (1999), 900–9.
74. M. G. Davies, E. L. Owens, D. P. Mason *et al.*, Effect of platelet-derived growth factor receptor-α and -β blockade on flow-induced neointimal formation in endothelialized baboon vascular grafts. *Circulation Research*, **86** (2000), 779–86.
75. C. E. Hart, J. W. Forstrom, J. D. Kelly *et al.*, Two classes of PDGF receptor recognize different isoforms of PDGF. *Science*, **240** (1988), 1529–31.
76. E. Bergsten, M. Uutela, X. Li *et al.*, PDGF-D is a specific, protease-activated ligand for the PDGF beta-receptor. *Nature Cell Biology*, **3** (2001), 512–6.
77. D. G. Gilbertson, M. E. Duff, J. W. West *et al.*, Platelet-derived growth factor C (PDGF-C), a novel growth factor that binds to PDGF alpha and beta receptor. *Journal of Biological Chemistry*, **276** (2001), 27406–14.
78. M. Kotani, N. Fukuda, H. Ando *et al.*, Chimeric DNA-RNA hammerhead ribozyme targeting PDGF A-chain mRNA specifically inhibits neointima formation in rat carotid artery after balloon injury. *Cardiovascular Research*, **57** (2003), 265–76.
79. M. J. Englesbe, S. Hawkins, P. C. Hsieh, *et al.*, Concomitant blockade of platelet-derived growth factor receptors -α and -β induces intimal atrophy in baboon PTFE grafts. *Journal of Vascular Surgery*, **39**(2) (2004), 440–6.
80. V. Lindner & M. A. Reidy, Proliferation of smooth muscle cells after vascular injury is inhibited by an antibody against basic fibroblast growth factor. *Proceedings of the National Academy of Sciences of the USA*, **88** (1991), 3739–43.
81. C. L. Jackson & M. A. Reidy, Basic fibroblast growth factor: its role in the control of smooth muscle cell

migration. *American Journal of Pathology*, **143** (1993), 1024–31.

82. N. E. Olson, S. Chao, V. Lindner & M. A. Reidy, Intimal smooth muscle cell proliferation after balloon catheter injury: the role of basic fibroblast growth factor. *American Journal of Pathology*, **140** (1992), 1017–23.
83. M. Zhou, R. L. Sutliffe, R. J. Paul *et al.*, Fibroblast growth factor 2 control of vascular tone. *Nature Medicine*, **4** (1998), 201–7.
84. S. R. Bryant, R. J. Bjercke, D. A. Erichsen, A. Rege & V. Lindner, Vascular remodeling in response to altered blood flow is mediated by fibroblast growth factor-2. *Circulation Research*, **84** (1999), 323–8.
85. T. M. Singh, K. Y. Abe, T. Sasaki, Y. J. Zhuang, H. Masuda, C. K. Zarins, Basic fibroblast growth factor expression precedes flow-induced arterial enlargement. *Journal of Surgical Research*, **77** (1998), 165–73.
86. C. Rutherford, W. Martin, M. Salame *et al.*, Substantial inhibition of neo-intimal response to balloon injury in the rat carotid artery using a combination of antibodies to platelet-derived growth factor-BB and basic fibroblast growth factor. *Atherosclerosis*, **130** (1997), 45–51.
87. M. W. Majesky, V. Lindner, D. R. Twardzik, S. M. Schwartz & M. A. Reidy, Production of transforming growth factor β_1 during repair of arterial injury. *Journal of Clinical Investigation*, **88** (1991), 904–10.
88. Y. G. Wolf, L. M. Rasmussen & E. Ruoslahti, Antibodies against transforming growth factor-β1 suppress intimal hyperplasia in a rat model. *Journal of Clinical Investigation*, **93** (1994), 1172–8.
89. J. D. Smith, S. R. Bryant, L. L. Couper *et al.*, Soluble transforming growth factor-β type II receptor inhibits negative remodeling, fibroblast transdifferentiation, and intimal lesion formation but not endothelial growth. *Circulation Research*, **84** (1999), 1212–22.
90. Y. Ko, H. Stiebler, G. Nickenig *et al.*, Synergistic action of angiotensin II, insulin-like growth factor-I, and transforming growth factor-β on platelet-derived growth factor-BB, basic fibroblastic growth factor, and epidermal growth factor-induced DNA synthesis in vascular smooth muscle cells. *American Journal of Hypertension*, **6** (1993), 496–9.
91. T. J. Nathe, J. Deou, B. Walsh *et al.*, Interleukin-1β inhibits expression of p21(WAF1/CIP1) and p27(KIP1) and enhances proliferation in response to platelet-derived growth factor-BB in smooth muscle cells. *Arteriosclerosis, Thrombosis and Vascular Biology*, **22** (2002), 1293–8.
92. M. J. Englesbe, J. Deou, B. D. Bourns, A. W. Clowes & G. Daum, Interleukin-1β inhibits PDGF-BB induced migration by cooperating with PDGF-BB to induce cyclo-oxygenase-2 expression in baboon aortic smooth muscle cells. *Journal of Vascular Surgery*, **39** (5) (2004), 1091–6.
93. S. Valles, C. J. Caunt, M. H. Walker & E. E. Qwarnstrom, PDGF enhancement of IL-1 receptor levels in smooth muscle cells involves induction of an attachment-regulated, heparan sulfate binding site (IL-1RIII). *Laboratory Investigation*, **82** (2002), 855–62.
94. L. Chen, G. Daum, R. Forough *et al.*, Overexpression of human endothelial nitric oxide synthase in rat vascular smooth muscle cells and in balloon-injured carotid artery. *Circulation Research*, **82** (1998), 862–70.
95. R. D. Kenagy & A. W. Clowes, Blockade of smooth muscle cell migration and proliferation in baboon aortic explants by interleukin-1β and tumor necrosis factor-α is nitric oxide-dependent and nitric oxide-independent. *Journal of Vascular Research*, **37** (2000), 381– 9.
96. A. W. Clowes & M. M. Clowes, Kinetics of cellular proliferation after arterial injury. IV. Heparin inhibits rat smooth muscle mitogenesis and migration. *Circulation Research*, **58** (1986), 839–45.
97. D. W. Courtman, S. M. Schwartz & C. E. Hart, Sequential injury of the rabbit abdominal aorta induces intramural coagulation and luminal narrowing independent of intimal mass – extrinsic pathway inhibition eliminates luminal narrowing. *Circulation Research*, **82** (1998), 996–1006.
98. H. H.Versteeg, M. P. Peppelenbosch & C. A. Spek, The pleiotropic effects of tissue factor: a possible role for factor VIIa-induced intracellular signalling? *Thrombosis and Haemostasis*, **86** (2001), 1353–9.
99. S. R. Coughlin, Thrombin signalling and protease-activated receptors. *Nature*, **407** (2000), 258–64.
100. F. N. Ko, Y. C. Yang, S. C. Huang & J. T. Ou, Coagulation factor Xa stimulates platelet-derived growth factor release and mitogenesis in cultured vascular smooth muscle cells of rat. *Journal of Clinical Investigation*, **98** (1996), 1493–501.
101. A. W. Clowes, M. M. Clowes, Y. P. T. Au, M. A. Reidy & D. Belin, Smooth muscle cells express urokinase during mitogenesis and tissue-type plasminogen activator during migration in injured rat carotid artery. *Circulation Research*, **67** (1990), 61–7.

102. S. J. Busuttil, C. Drumm, V. A. Ploplis & E. F. Plow, Endoluminal arterial injury in plasminogen-deficient mice. *Journal of Surgical Research*, **91** (2000) 159–64.
103. P. Carmeliet, L. Moons, J. M. Herbert *et al.*, Urokinase but not tissue plasminogen activator mediates arterial neointima formation in mice. *Circulation Research*, **81** (1997), 829–39.
104. R. D. Kenagy, S. Vergel, E. Mattsson *et al.*, The role of plasminogen, plasminogen activators, and matrix metalloproteinases in primate arterial smooth muscle cell migration. *Arteriosclerosis, Thrombosis and Vascular Biology*, **16** (1996), 1373–82.
105. K. Schäfer, S. Konstantinides, C. Riedel *et al.*, Different mechanisms of increased luminal stenosis after arterial injury in mice deficient for urokinase- or tissue-type plasminogen activator. *Circulation*, **106** (2002), 1847–52.
106. B. H. Strauss, H. K. Lau, K. A. Bowman *et al.*, Plasma urokinase antigen and plasminogen activator inhibitor-1 antigen levels predict angiographic coronary restenosis. *Circulation*, **100** (1999), 1616–22.
107. N. Zempo, R. D. Kenagy, Y. P. T. Au *et al.*, Matrix metalloproteinases of vascular wall cells are increased in balloon-injured rat carotid artery. *Journal of Vascular Surgery*, **20** (1994), 209–17.
108. H. Wang & J. A. Keiser, Expression of membrane-type matrix metalloproteinase in rabbit neointimal tissue and its correlation with matrix-metalloproteinase-2 activation. *Journal of Vascular Research*, **35** (1998), 45–54.
109. P. Carmeliet, L. Moons, M. Dewerchin *et al.*, Receptor-independent role of urokinase-type plasminogen activator in pericellular plasmin and matrix metalloproteinase proteolysis during vascular wound healing in mice. *Journal of Cell Biology*, **140**(1) (1998), 233–45.
110. S. T. Nikkari, R. L. Geary, T. Hatsukami *et al.*, Expression of collagen, interstitial collagenase, and tissue inhibitor of metalloproteinases-1 in restenosis after carotid endarterectomy. *American Journal of Pathology*, **148** (1996), 777–83.
111. S. C. Tyagi, L. Meyer, R. A. Schmaltz, H. K. Reddy & D. J. Voelker, Proteinases and restenosis in the human coronary artery: extracellular matrix production exceeds the expression of proteolytic activity. *Atherosclerosis*, **116** (1995), 43–57.
112. R. Forough, N. Koyama, D. Hasenstab *et al.*, Overexpression of tissue inhibitor of matrix metalloproteinase-1 inhibits vascular smooth muscle cell functions *in vitro* and *in vivo*. *Circulation Research*, **79** (1996), 812–20.
113. R. D. Kenagy, C. E. Hart, W. G. Stetler-Stevenson & A. W. Clowes, Primate smooth muscle cell migration from aortic explants is mediated by endogenous platelet-derived growth factor and basic fibroblast growth factor acting through matrix metalloproteinases 2 and 9. *Circulation*, **96** (1997), 3555–60.
114. C. Li, W. J. Cantor, N. Nili *et al.*, Arterial repair after stenting and the effects of GM6001, a matrix metalloproteinase inhibitor. *Journal of the American College of Cardiology*, **39** (2002), 1852–8.
115. B. J. G. L. De Smet, D. De Kleijn, R. Hanemaaijer *et al.*, Metalloproteinase inhibition reduces constrictive arterial remodeling after balloon angioplasty – a study in the atherosclerotic Yucatan micropig. *Circulation*, **101** (2000), 2962–7.
116. G. S. Cherr, S. J. Motew, J. A. Travis *et al.*, Metalloproteinase inhibition and the response to angioplasty and stenting in atherosclerotic primates. *Arteriosclerosis, Thrombosis and Vascular Biology*, **22** (2002), 161–6.
117. S. Ye, P. Eriksson, A. Hamsten *et al.*, Progression of coronary atherosclerosis is associated with a common genetic variant of the human stromelysin-1 promoter which results in reduced gene expression. *Journal of Biological Chemistry*, **271** (1996), 13055–60.
118. J. S. Kim, H. Y. Park, J. H. Kwon *et al.*, The roles of stromelysin-1 and the gelatinase B gene polymorphism in stable angina. *Yonsei Medical Journal*, **43** (2002), 473–81.
119. H. J. Cho, I. H. Chae, K. W. Park *et al.*, Functional polymorphism in the promoter region of the gelatinase B gene in relation to coronary artery disease and restenosis after percutaneous coronary intervention. *Journal of Human Genetics*, **47** (2002), 88–91.
120. S. Humphries, C. Bauters, A. Meirhaeghe *et al.*, The 5A6A polymorphism in the promoter of the stromelysin-1 (MMP3) gene as a risk factor for restenosis. *European Journal*, **23** (2002), 721–5.
121. P. Schoenhagen, D. G. Vince, K. M. Ziada *et al.*, Relation of matrix-metalloproteinase 3 found in coronary lesion samples retrieved by directional coronary atherectomy to intravascular ultrasound observations on coronary remodeling. *American Journal of Cardiology*, **89** (2002), 1354–9.
122. C. Lovdahl, J. Thyberg, A. Hultgardh-Nilsson, The synthetic metalloproteinase inhibitor batimastat

suppresses injury-induced phosphorylation of MAP kinase ERK1/ERK2 and phenotypic modification of arterial smooth muscle cells *in vitro*. *Journal of Vascular Research*, **37** (2000), 345–54.

123. B. H. Strauss, R. Robinson, W. B. Batchelor *et al.*, *In vivo* collagen turnover following experimental balloon angioplasty injury and the role of matrix metalloproteinases. *Circulation Research*, **79** (1996), 541–50.
124. E. F. Rocnik, B. M. C. Chan, J. G. Pickering, Evidence for a role of collagen synthesis in arterial smooth muscle cell migration. *Journal of Clinical Investigation*, **101** (1998), 1889–98.
125. W. C. Parks, Who are the proteolytic culprits in vascular disease? *Journal of Clinical Investigation*, **104** (1999), 1167–8.
126. K. A. Scott, E. J. Wood & E. H. Karran, A matrix metalloproteinase inhibitor which prevents fibroblast-mediated collagen lattice contraction. *FEBS Letters*, **441** (1998), 137–40.
127. A. W. Clowes, M. A. Reidy & M. M. Clowes Mechanisms of stenosis after arterial injury. *Laboratory Investigation*, **49** (1983), 208–15.
128. B. H. Strauss, R. J. Chisholm, F. W. Keeley, Extracellular matrix remodeling after balloon angioplasty injury in a rabbit model of restenosis. *Circulation Research*, **75** (1994), 650–8.
129. S. T. Nikkari, H. T. Järveläinen, T. N. Wight, M. Ferguson & A. W. Clowes, Smooth muscle cell expression of extracellular matrix genes after arterial injury. *American Journal of Pathology*, **144** (1994), 1348–56.
130. I. M. Chung, H. K. Gold, S. M. Schwartz *et al.*, Enhanced extracellular matrix accumulation in restenosis of coronary arteries after stent deployment. *Journal of the American Journal of Cardiology*, **40** (2002), 2072–81.
131. R. Riessen, J. M. Isner, E. Blessing *et al.*, Regional differences in the distribution of the proteoglycans biglycan and decorin in the extracellular matrix of atherosclerotic and restenotic human coronary arteries. *American Journal of Pathology*, **144** (1994), 962–74.
132. R. Riessen, T. N. Wight, C. Pastore, C. Henley & J. M. Isner, Distribution of hyaluronan during extracellular matrix remodeling in human restenotic arteries and balloon-injured aat carotid arteries. *Circulation*, **93** (1996), 1141–7.
133. C. Glover, X. L. Ma, Y. X. Chen *et al.*, Human in-stent restenosis tissue obtained by means of coronary atherectomy consists of an abundant proteoglycan matrix with a paucity of cell proliferation. *American Heart Journal*, **144** (2002), 702–9.
134. P. J. Gotwals, G. Chi-Rosso, V. Lindner *et al.*, The α 1β 1 integrin is expressed during neointima formation in rat arteries and mediates collagen matrix reorganization. *Journal of Clinical Investigation*, **97** (2001), 2469–77.
135. G. Hou, W. Vogel, M. P. Bendeck, The discoidin domain receptor tyrosine kinase DDR1 in arterial wound repair. *Journal of Clinical Investigation*, **107** 2001, 727–35.
136. M. Jain, Q. He, W. S. Lee *et al.*, Role of CD44 in the reaction of vascular smooth muscle cells to arterial wall injury. *Journal of Clinical Investigation*, **97** (1996), 596–603.
137. F. G. Giancotti & E. Ruoslahti, Integrin signaling. *Science*, **285** (1999), 1028–32.
138. R. T. Lee, F. Berditchevski, G. C. Cheng & M. E. Hemler, Integrin-mediated collagen matrix reorganization by cultured human vascular smooth muscle cells. *Circulation Research*, **76** (1995), 209–14.
139. S. S. Srivatsa, L. A. Fitzpatrick, P. W. Tsao *et al.*, Selective α vβ 3 integrin blockade potently limits neointimal hyperplasia and lumen stenosis following deep coronary arterial stent injury: evidence for the functional importance of integrin α vβ 3 and osteopontin expression during neointima formation. *Cardiovascular Research*, **36** (1997), 408–28.
140. E. T. Choi, L. Engel, A. D. Callow *et al.*, Inhibition of neointimal hyperplasia by blocking α vβ 3 integrin with a small peptide antagonist G*penGRGDSPCA*. *Journal of Vascular Surgery*, **19** (1994), 125–34.
141. G. P. Hou, W. F. Vogel & M. P. Bendeck, Tyrosine kinase activity of discoidin domain receptor 1 is necessary for smooth muscle cell migration and matrix metalloproteinase expression. *Circulation Research*, **90** (2002), 1147–9.
142. J. A. Travis, M. G. Hughes, J. M. Wong, W. D. Wagner & R. L. Geary, Hyaluronan enhances contraction of collagen by smooth muscle cells and adventitial fibroblasts – role of CD44 and implications for constrictive remodeling. *Circulation Research*, **88** (2001), 77–83.
143. R. Fattori & T. Piva, Drug-eluting stents in vascular intervention. *Lancet*, **361** (2003), 247–9.

144. P. W. Serruys, M. Degertekin, K. Tanabe *et al.*, Intravascular ultrasound findings in the multicenter, randomized, double-blind RAVEL (RAndomized study with the sirolimus-eluting VElocity balloon-expandable stent in the treatment of patients with *de novo* native coronary artery Lesions) trial. *Circulation*, **106** (2002), 798–803.
145. J. E. Sousa, M. A. Costa, A. G. Sousa *et al.*, Two-year angiographic and intravascular ultrasound follow-up after implantation of sirolimus-eluting stents in human coronary arteries. *Circulation*, **107** (2003), 381–3.
146. P. Nguyen-Ho, G. L. Kaluza, P. T. Zymek & A. E. Raizner, Intracoronary brachytherapy. *Catheterization and Cardiovascular Interventions*, **56** (2002), 281–8.
147. J. Rutanen, H. Puhakka & S. Yla-Herttuala, Post-intervention vessel remodeling. *Gene Therapy*, **9** (2002), 1487–91.
148. S. E. Francis, N. J. Camp, A. J. Burton *et al.*, Interleukin 1 receptor antagonist gene polymorphism and restenosis after coronary angioplasty. *Heart*, **86** (2001), 336–40.
149. T. A. McCaffrey, B. H. Du, S. Consigli *et al.*, Genomic instability in the type II TGF-β 1 receptor gene in atherosclerotic and restenotic vascular cells. *Journal of Clinical Investigation*, **100** (1997), 2182–8.
150. M. Asakura, Y. Ueda, S. Nanto *et al.*, Remodeling of in-stent neointima, which became thinner and transparent over 3 years – Serial angiographic and angioscopic follow-up. *Circulation*, **97** (1998), 2003–6.
151. N. Kuroda, Y. Kobayashi, M. Nameki *et al.*, Intimal hyperplasia regression from 6 to 12 months after stenting. *American Journal of Cardiology*, **89** (2002), 869–72.
152. E. J. R. Mattsson, T. R. Kohler, S. M. Vergel & A. W. Clowes, Increased blood flow induces regression of intimal hyperplasia. *Arteriosclerosis, Thrombosis and Vascular Biology*, **17** (1997), 2245–9.
153. J. J. Wentzel, R. Krams, J. C. H. Schuurbiers *et al.*, Relationship between neointimal thickness and shear stress after wallstent implantation in human coronary arteries. *Circulation*, **103** (2001), 1740–5.
154. S. A. Berceli, M. G. Davies, R. D. Kenagy & A. W. Clowes, Flow-induced neointimal regression in baboon polytetrafluoroethylene grafts is associated with decreased cell proliferation and increased apoptosis. *Journal of Vascular Surgery*, **36** (2002), 1248–55.
155. R. D. Kenagy, J. W. Fischer, M. G. Davies *et al.*, Increased plasmin and serine proteinase activity during flow-induced intimal atrophy in baboon PTFE grafts. *Arteriosclerosis, Thrombosis and Vascular Biology*, **22** (2002), 400–4.
156. P. C. H. Hsieh, RjD. Kenagy, E. R. Mulvihill *et al.*, BMP4: potential regulator of shear stress-induced graft neointimal atrophy. *Journal of Vascular Surgery*, **43** (2006), 150–8.
157. C. L. Jackson & M. A. Reidy, Basic fibroblast growth factor: its role in the control of smooth muscle cell migration. *American Journal of Pathology*, **143** (1993), 1024–31.
158. B. M. C. Chan, A. Kalmes, S. Hawkins, G. Daum & A. W. Clowes, Blockade of the edidermal growth factor receptor decreases intimal hyperplasia in balloon-injured rat carotid artery. *Journal of Vascular Surgery*, **37** (3) (2003), 644–9.
159. C. Indolfi, D. Torella, L. Cavuto *et al.*, Effects of balloon injury on neointimal hyperplasia in streptozotocin-induced diabetes and in hyperinsulinemic nondiabetic pancreatic islet-transplanted rats. *Circulation*, **103** (2001), 2980–6.
160. P. Hayry, M. Myllarniemi, E. Aavik *et al.*, Stabile D-peptide analog of insulin-like growth factor-1 inhibits smooth muscle cell proliferation after carotid ballooning injury in the rat. *FASEB Journal*, **9** (1995), 1336–44.
161. B. H. Zhu, G. S. Zhao, D. P. Witte, D. Y. Hui & J. A. Fagin, Targeted overexpression of IGF-I in smooth muscle cells of transgenic mice enhances neointimal formation through increased proliferation and cell migration after intraarterial injury. *Endocrinology*, **142** (2001), 3598–606.
162. M. A. Zimmerman, C. H. Selzman, L. L. Reznikov *et al.*, Lack of TNF-alpha attenuates intimal hyperplasia after mouse carotid artery injury. *American Journal of Physiology – Regulatory, Integrative and Comparative Physiology*, **283** (2002), R505–12.
163. J. E. Rectenwald, L. L. Moldawer, T. S. Huber, J. M. Seeger & C. K. Ozaki, Direct evidence for cytokine involvement in neointimal hyperplasia. *Circulation*, **102** (2000), 1697–702.
164. W. R. Huckle, M. D. Drag, W. R. Acker *et al.*, Effects of L-749,329, an ET(A)/ET(B) endothelin receptor antagonist, in a porcine coronary artery injury model of vascular restenosis. *Circulation*, **103** (2001), 1899–905.
165. C. J. McKenna, S. E. Burke, T. J. Opgenorth *et al.*, Selective ET(A) receptor antagonism reduces neointimal hyperplasia in a porcine coronary stent model. *Circulation*, **97** (1998), 2551–6.

166. J. Lemay, P. Hamet & D. DeBlois, Losartan-induced apoptosis as a novel mechanism for the prevention of vascular lesion formation after injury. *Journal of the Renin-Angiotensin-Aldosterone System*, **1** (2000), 46–50.
167. R. Gallo, A. Padurean, V. Toschi, J. Bichler & J. T. Fallon, Prolonged thrombin inhibition reduces restenosis after balloon angioplasty in porcine coronary arteries. *Circulation*, **97** (1998), 588.
168. C. Gerdes, V. Faber-Steinfeld, Ö Yalkinoglu & S. Wohlfeil, Comparison of the effects of the thrombin inhibitor r-hirudin in four animal models of neointima formation after arterial injury. *Arteriosclerosis, Thrombosis and Vascular Biology*, **16** (1996), 1306–11.
169. J. Herbert, F. Bono, J. Herault *et al.*, Effector protease receptor 1 mediates the mitogenic activity of factor Xa for vascular smooth muscle cells *in vitro* and *in vivo*. *Journal of Clinical Investigation*, **101** (1998), 993–1000.
170. M. Roqué, E. D. Reis, V. Fuster *et al.*, Inhibition of tissue factor reduces thrombus formation and intimal hyperplasia after porcine coronary angioplasty. *Journal of the American College of Cardiology*, **36** (2000), 2303–10.
171. D. Chen, T. Asahara, K. Krasinski *et al.*, Antibody blockade of thrombospondin accelerates reendothelialization and reduces neointima formation in balloon-injured rat carotid artery. *Circulation*, **100** (1999), 849–54.
172. J. C. Teeters, C. Erami, H. Zhang & J. E. Faber, Systemic α 1A-adrenoceptor antagonist inhibits neointimal growth after balloon injury of rat carotid artery. *American Journal of Heart and Circulatory Physiology*, **284** (2003), H385–92.
173. G. K. Hansson, L. Jonasson, J. Holm, M. M. Clowes & A. W. Clowes, Gamma interferon regulates vascular smooth muscle proliferation and Ia expression *in vitro* and *in vivo*. *Circulation Research*, **63** (1988), 712–9.
174. K. Hayashi, S. Nakamura, R. Morishita *et al.*, *In vivo* transfer of human hepatocyte growth factor gene accelerates re-endothelialization and inhibits neointimal formation after balloon injury in rat model. *Gene Therapy*, **7** (2000), 1664–71.
175. M. Matsuda, I. Shimomura, M. Sata *et al.*, Role of adiponectin in preventing vascular stenosis. The missing link of adipo-vascular axis. *Journal of Biological Chemistry*, **277** (2002), 37487–91.
176. L. J. Feldman, L. Aguirre, M. Ziol *et al.*, Interleukin-10 inhibits intimal hyperplasia after angioplasty or stent implantation in hypercholesterolemic rabbits. *Circulation*, **101** (2000), 908–16.
177. K. Shimizu, H. Tanaka, M. Sunamori, F. Marumo & M. Shichiri, Adrenomedullin receptor antagonism by calcitonin gene-related peptide(8–37) inhibits carotid artery neointimal hyperplasia after balloon injury. *Circulation Research*, **85** (1999), 1199–205.
178. I. S. Zagon, F. M. Essis, Jr., M. F. Verderame *et al.*, Opioid growth factor inhibits intimal hyperplasia in balloon-injured rat carotid artery. *Journal of Vascular Surgery*, **37** (2003), 636–43.
179. E. Aavik, N. M. Luoto, L. Petrov *et al.*, Elimination of vascular fibrointimal hyperplasia by somatostatin receptor 1.4 selective agonist. *FASEB Journal*, **16** (2002), NIL202–23.
180. J. T. Light, J. A. Bellan, I. L. Chen *et al.*, Angiopeptin enhances acetylcholine-induced relaxation and inhibits intimal hyperplasia after vascular injury. *American Journal of Heart and Circulatory Physiology*, **265** (1993), H1265–74.
181. N. Murakoshi, T. Miyauchi, Y. Kakinuma *et al.*, Vascular endothelin-B receptor system *in vivo* plays a favorable inhibitory, role in vascular remodeling after injury revealed by endothelin-B receptor-knockout mice. *Circulation*, **106** (2002), 1991–8.
182. R. Forough, N. Koyama, D. Hasenstab *et al.*, Overexpression of tissue inhibitor of matrix metalloproteinase-1 inhibits vascular smooth muscle cell functions *in vitro* and *in vivo*. *Circulation Research*, **79** (1996), 812–20.
183. Y. H. Hu, A. H. Baker, Y. P. Zou, A. C. Newby & Q. B. Xu, Local gene transfer of tissue inhibitor of metalloproteinase-2 influences vein graft remodeling in a mouse model. *Arteriosclerosis, Thrombosis and Vascular Biology*, **21** (2001), 1275–80.
184. L. Cheng, G. Mantile, R. Pauly *et al.*, Adenovirus-mediated gene transfer of the human tissue inhibitor of metalloproteinase-2 blocks vascular smooth muscle cell invasiveness *in vitro* and modulates neointimal development *in vivo*. *Circulation*, **98** (1998), 2195–201.
185. S. J. George, C. T. Lloyd, G. D. Angelini, A. C. Newby & A. H. Baker, Inhibition of late vein graft neointima formation in human and porcine models by adenovirus-mediated overexpression of tissue inhibitor of metalloproteinase-3. *Circulation*, **101** (2000), 296–304.

186. M. A. Nugent, H. M. Nugent, R. V. Iozzo, K. Sanchack & E. R. Edelman, Perlecan is required to inhibit thrombosis after deep vascular injury and contributes to endothelial cell-mediated inhibition of intimal hyperplasia. *Proceedings of the National Academy of Sciences of the USA*, **97** (2000), 6722–7.
187. T. Le Tourneau, E. Van Belle, D. Corseaux *et al.*, Role of nitric oxide in restenosis after experimental balloon angioplasty in the hypercholesterolemic rabbit: effects on neointimal hyperplasia and vascular remodeling. *Journal of the American College of Cardiology*, **33** (1999), 876–82.
188. B. Zhu, D. G. Kuhel, D. P. Witte & D. Y. Hui, Apolipoprotein E inhibits neointimal hyperplasia after arterial injury in mice. *American Journal of Pathology*, **157** (2000), 1839–48.
189. M. L. Foegh, S. Asotra, M. H. Howell & P. W. Ramwell, Estradiol inhibition of arterial neointimal hyperplasia after balloon injury. *Journal of Vascular Surgery*, **19** (1994), 722–6.
190. T. R. Sullivan, Jr., R. H. Karas, M. Aronovitz *et al.*, Estrogen inhibits the response-to-injury in a mouse carotid artery model. *Journal of Clinical Investigation*, **96** (1995), 2482–8.

13 • Restenosis: treatment options current and future

JOHN BINGLEY, JULIE CAMPBELL, GORDON CAMPBELL AND PHILIP WALKER

INTRODUCTION

As we approach the second century of modern vascular surgical practice, one hundred years after Alexis Carrel's pioneering work on arterial and graft anastomoses, the narrowing, or restenosis, of arteries and grafts after intervention to improve blood flow continues to provide vascular surgeons with technical challenges and difficult management decisions [1]. The recent rise in coronary and peripheral endoluminal interventions has forced intense research into the mechanisms and prevention of restenosis because of higher restenosis rates compared with traditional revascularization techniques. This is nowhere more evident than in coronary artery angioplasty and stenting. The substantial body of recent research on restenosis reflects the active interest in causes and treatments of restenosis from the perspective of the interventionalist. This chapter focuses on human data, where at all possible, since it is written with the clinician in mind. Where human data is lacking, *in vivo* experimental evidence is relied upon.

Recent clinical trials of restenosis treatments have been performed predominantly by cardiologists and interventional radiologists. While this is for the most part admirable and has led to the advancement of our understanding of mechanisms in restenosis, there are some aspects of restenosis in the peripheral vascular tree that are not well represented in recent restenosis research. Understanding the mechanisms contributing to restenosis, and methods of prevention, is a priority for every vascular surgeon.

CAUSES OF VESSEL NARROWING AFTER VASCULAR SURGERY (SEE CHAPTER 12)

Restenosis is the narrowing of a conduit after an intervention to improve flow through it. There are several reasons for vessel narrowing after intervention (Table 13.1). Conceptually the causes for renarrowing after intervention can be divided into three major categories based on their time of onset. It needs to be acknowledged that this division is a simplification since early restenoses undoubtedly contribute to intermediate restenoses [2; 3], and quite probably both then contribute to the slow development of atheroma [4].

Early onset narrowing

Early onset narrowing, around the time of intervention and the subsequent few days, is largely within the control of the surgeon. From time to time stenoses are fashioned unintentionally through the failure of accurate technique in suturing, or failure to relieve stenosis adequately with angioplasty. Other early closures relate to procedural errors leaving intimal flaps and dissections, poor tunnelling of conduit leaving kinking, twists or compression, and even zealous wound closure with external compression [5; 6]. All these represent narrowing rather than true renarrowing.

Acute thrombosis related to platelet and thrombus deposition on the injured arterial wall or graft material are to a degree unpreventable, since all operated arterial and venous surfaces, as well as graft surfaces, will rapidly develop a lining of fibrin and platelets [7; 8]. The use of platelet inhibitors (aspirin, clopidogrel, dextrans, antiplatelet antibodies) before and during surgery or angioplasty, as well as the use of heparin during surgery, may reduce the degree of early thrombus formation [9; 10; 11]. In addition, maintenance of high flow through the graft or operative site by the provision of an adequate systolic blood pressure can reduce the degree of thrombosis [10].

Intermediate onset narrowing

Intermediate onset narrowing occurring six weeks to several years after injury is what most surgeons refer to as restenosis. It is due to two processes. Neointimal

Table 13.1. *Causes of luminal narrowing after surgery/angioplasty categories by time of onset*

Early onset: acute closure (minutes to days)
1. failure to produce sufficient lumen diameter (poor suturing or angioplasty failure)
2. acute thrombosis
3. dissection
4. intimal flap
5. spasm/elastic recoil
6. external compression
7. graft twist or kink
8. retained valve cusp (*in situ* bypass)
9. low flow

Intermediate onset: *restenosis* (weeks to months to years)
1. neointimal hyperplasia
   a. cellular mass (smooth muscle cell, macrophage, ?stem cell)
   b. extracellular matrix
2. vessel wall remodelling
   a. adventitial and medial reaction (wound healing)
   b. shear stress
   c. low flow

Late onset: (several years)
1. neointimal hyperplasia
2. vessel wall remodelling
3. atheroma

hyperplasia describes the development within the innermost layer of the injured artery, vein or conduit of a cell and extracellular matrix mass that may encroach on the lumen. Medial smooth muscle cells (SMCs), analogous to wound fibroblasts, undergo a change in their phenotype with injury after which they are free to migrate to, and proliferate within, the intima and subintima [12; 13]. Recently, the possibility of circulating cells, including stem cells, contributing to the cell population of the neointima has been raised and remains the subject of intense investigation [12]. Smooth muscle cell precursor cells have been identified in the buffy coat of human blood, differentiating as SMCs in cell culture [14]. Smooth muscle cell changes are associated initially with the degradation of existing arterial matrix structures through the action of matrix metalloproteinases and endoglycosidases that alter the environment of the cell, freeing it from its previously secure footing [15; 16]. Once the SMC has entered the intimal area it produces a new extracellular matrix that matures (and alters in composition) with time [17; 18]. The changes in SMC phenotype and its environment are accompanied by a complex change in genetic expression [19]. Incorporated into this neointima may be a thrombus present from the time of surgery. The thrombus itself is a powerful trigger for neointimal formation.

The appreciation that the neointima is not the only process contributing to a narrowed lumen after successful vascular intervention has occurred only recently [20]. With the introduction of the arterial stent (primarily an intervention to rescue the artery from acute closure due to dissection or recoil) came the realization that all layers of the arterial wall changed with injury. The stented artery, despite developing a profuse neointimal hyperplasia, may remain more widely patent than when angioplastied only. Remodelling refers to these changes in structure and geometry of the vessel wall with disease progression. A reduction in overall vessel diameter, when it does happen, probably occurs through the action of SMCs and matrix-degrading enzymes in the media, as well as myofibroblasts in the adventitia [18; 21; 22; 23], and is analogous to healing wound contraction. However, some arteries increase in circumference, while others stay the same or decrease. The relative contributions of the neointima and remodelling to luminal diameter are thus variable, and to some degree unpredictable [20].

Late onset narrowing

Atheroma can occur in endarterectomized arteries, vein grafts and synthetic grafts but takes several years to develop [24; 25]. Moreover, atheroma is an active disease in many patients with peripheral vascular disease, and while the treated area may remain atheroma-free complicated atheroma upstream and downstream can advance and create flow limitations that then threaten the graft or stent [4].

PREVENTING RESTENOSIS

A simple problem, a simple solution?

The evolution of treatments for restenosis reflects the evolution of the recent science of vascular biology and is best understood in its historical context. The science has not always preceded, nor predicted, the treatment successes. For instance, the success of the stent in preventing restenosis led to a fundamental change in our understanding of restenosis, which until that time had focused on the neointima. This chapter will attempt to place the treatments for restenosis – both the successes and the failures – in a historical perspective to allow a better appreciation of the manner in which science and clinical management progresses.

Research into restenosis has revealed a complex biology behind an apparently simple problem, but this only developed over time as techniques for investigation became available. Prior to the 1980s most restenosis prevention in cardiac and vascular surgery conceptually involved bypass grafts and haemodynamics. It has already been pointed out that restenosis is less in most peripheral arterial grafts than in angioplastied arteries. Gruntzig *et al.* [26] in refining percutaneous coronary angioplasty for practical use, found restenosis the major stumbling block to a new and safer coronary artery intervention. Subsequently, most recent restenosis research has focused on the prevention after angioplasty injury.

Systemic treatments for restenosis

The first recent wave of anti-restenosis treatments began with the coronary angioplasty revolution of the 1980s that produced restenosis rates after coronary balloon angioplasty rarely lower than 40% [27]. The pathogenesis of restenosis was not well understood, based on the results of cell culture experiments and some animal models, as well as small studies on fragments of human tissue excised via atherectomy or at autopsy [28]. Indeed, the occurrence of restenosis after angioplasty inspired a generation of vascular biologists and clinicians to probe deeply into the processes involved, in a way restenosis in vascular grafts had failed to do for the preceding generation of cardiac and vascular surgeons. Restenosis of vascular grafts has become appreciated more recently with the advent of Duplex scanning surveillance which uncovered previously unrecognized graft narrowings [4].

In cell culture, a variety of therapeutic agents was shown to inhibit SMC proliferation, prevent SMC phenotype change that accompanies neointimal formation and promote or prevent SMC matrix formation. When trialled in rat, rabbit, pig and primate models of restenosis, systemically delivered treatments were shown to be effective in 'treating' restenosis compared with controls [29].

Many of these pharmacological therapies were cardiovascular and anti-inflammatory drugs already in clinical use and shown to be relatively safe in humans. In some cases their use can best be explained by naïve optimism on the part of the treating physician. Other drugs were novel agents not previously used in cardiovascular medicine. Despite excellent laboratory and animal data, none was effective in human trials in preventing restenosis after angioplasty of the coronary arteries [29]. Nor were these drugs shown to be effective in preventing restenosis in bypass grafts or after peripheral angioplasty.

Despite this failure, trials of systemic treatments still occur. The PRESTO trial of 11 500 patients given the anti-allergic drug tranilast after angioplasty, which had shown success in preventing coronary restenosis after angioplasty and stenting in small Japanese trials [30], has been very recently concluded. Predictably the authors reported failure of tranilast to prevent restenosis after angioplasty compared with the placebo [31]. Unfortunately this is unlikely to be the last trial of a systemic agent to prevent restenosis.

This simple problem of arterial narrowing after injury did not have a simple solution, with research revealing an increasingly complex biology. However, this period of intense research and failed systemic therapy to prevent restenosis was not all loss and no gain. Balloon-injury animal models provided us with an extraordinary depth of understanding of the complexity of the response-to-injury process in the artery, evidenced in the preceding chapter. Moreover, balloon-injured artery models were also being used to investigate atherogenesis, based on the response-to-injury hypothesis of Ross, in which an injured endothelium is seen as the important pathogenic event [32].

Arterial injury research stimulated the discovery of growth factors and cytokines, led by Ross, with the discovery of platelet-derived growth factor (PDGF). Soon following were discoveries of fibroblast growth factor (FGF), transforming growth factors (TGF), other growth factors, leukaemia inhibitory factor (LIF), the interleukins and others [1; 33; 34; 35]. The findings of restenosis research had implications for wound healing biology and treatment in general.

FAILURE OF SYSTEMIC THERAPY FOR RESTENOSIS PREVENTION

There are several possible reasons for this failure of a standard pharmacological approach to prevent restenosis. Firstly, there are limitations to the use of a therapeutic agent imposed by the agents' own toxicity. Secondly, the animal models of arterial injury only approximated the human situation in part. Thirdly, advances in interventional cardiology coincided with major discoveries in biomedical sciences, including the revolution in genetics, which provided a newer and better targeted range of intervention strategies. And finally, the understanding of the fundamental process of restenosis was incomplete or inaccurate.

Systemic toxicity, topical delivery

Firstly, systemic therapies are limited by the toxic threshold of the agent in question. Heparin provides an excellent example of this problem. Clowes and Karnovsky showed heparin to be inhibitory to SMC proliferation and migration *in vitro*, and reduced neointimal formation *in vivo* [21]. A number of animal experiment publications followed showing that heparin, low molecular weight heparin, heparan sulphates and heparin-like analogues impressively reduced neointimal formation [21; 36; 37; 38]. Almost all clinical angioplasty procedures use heparin in one or other form for anticoagulation. However, in clinical trials, heparin failed to reduce restenosis rates after coronary angioplasty and in one instance the trial was ceased because of an apparent increase in restenosis compared with placebo [39; 40; 41]. Edelman and Karnovsky [42] then showed elegantly the delivery of heparin in divided daily doses (in the manner typically used in clinical work) did indeed promote neointimal formation in animal experiments, compared with the constant delivery of heparin either through infusion pumps or by peri-adventitial delivery which reduced neointimal formation. In hindsight, low concentrations of heparins were noted to promote SMC proliferation *in vitro* [17]. The continuous delivery of high-dose heparin in clinic was limited, however, by the risk of associated bleeding.

The antiproliferative and anticoagulant effects of heparin are independent properties of the heparin molecule [43]. Advances in carbohydrate chemistry and drug designs have allowed modified heparins to be synthesized with the antiproliferative properties of heparin but without the anticoagulant side effects. Despite this, heparins and their derivatives to date have failed to prevent restenosis in humans after angioplasty.

One solution to this problem of systemic toxicity is to deliver the drug topically. Two routes of drug application to the arterial media are available. Either the drug can be absorbed, or delivered, from the luminal side, or it can be delivered from the outside of the artery, the adventitial side. Modified angioplasty balloons were designed to deliver concentrated therapeutic agents to the site of angioplasty. Some 'sweated' their drug onto the injured luminal surface, or injected the therapeutic agent at pressure into the arterial media [44]. Other balloons bathe the angioplasty site in the agent using a double balloon device [45] (Figure 13.1). Still others deliver drug in a gel coating designed to stick to the angioplasty site [46]. These various techniques are troubled by washout, and limited residency of the drug at the luminal surface and in the arterial media [45]. Pressurized injection into the arterial media further created dissection with acute narrowing [47]. Furthermore, delivery balloons can dislodge stents from their optimum positioning [48]. Currently, agents delivered by modified balloons fail to prevent restenosis more effectively than angioplasty alone.

Grafts and stents (see later) have been modified with the intention of limiting restenosis. Synthetic grafts have been seeded with endothelial cells in an attempt to have them totally re-endothelialize, and thus (in theory) to have lower thrombogenicity and less restenosis. The failure of this technique to reduce thrombosis and restenosis in humans may be largely due to the difficulty in having the endothelial cells remain attached to the graft [49]. However, even an intact endothelium is not necessarily a benign endothelium, and activated endothelial cells promote cell and platelet adhesion, which are early events in neointimal formation [32; 50].

While drug delivery via the peri-adventitial route is effective in animal models of restenosis [17; 42; 51; 52; 53], access to the peri-adventitia is limited for the interventional cardiologist. In peripheral vascular surgery, the surgeon has ready access to the peri-adventitial space as a site for therapeutic deposition. Failure to adopt it as a therapeutic choice may reflect the extent to which restenosis research has been driven recently by angioplasty interventionists, rather than a failure of concept.

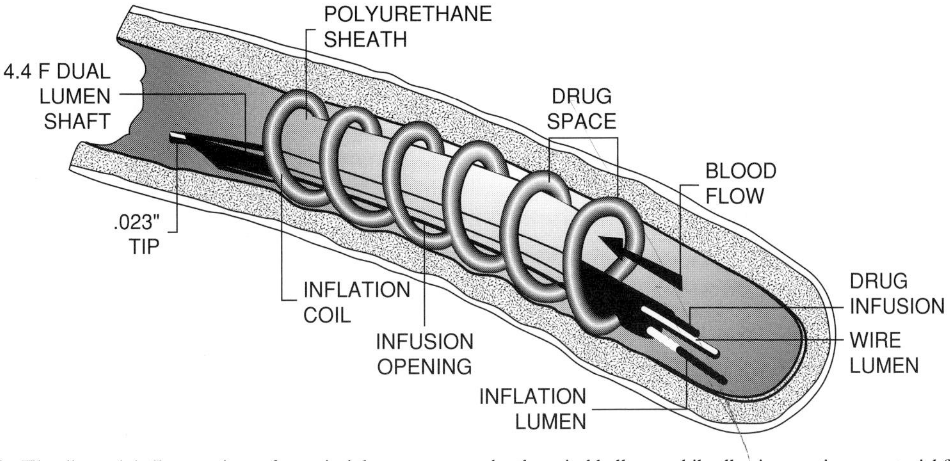

Fig. 13.1. The dispatch balloon catheter for topical drug delivery to the arterial wall. Therapeutic agent is delivered via a separate channel to bathe the arterial wall within an area limited by the spiral balloon, while allowing continuous arterial flow through the central channel [45].

Animal models

A second reason for the failure of standard systemic therapy to prevent restenosis lies in the animal models and the way in which they are utilized. Beyond doubt, arterial injury models have assisted enormously in exploring the biology of the injured artery and early neointima. Doubt arises, however, as to whether there is analogous pathobiology between the acutely injured (previously normal) animal artery and the angioplastied, stenotic, atheromatous human artery [28]. Double injury models were devised where angioplasty was performed on a previously injured artery. Still, these are relatively acute arterial models, not models of the timescales seen in clinically advanced, complicated atheroma. The relevance of angioplasty models to clinical outcomes continues to be controversial.

The failure of systemic therapies to prevent human restenosis after angioplasty as they did in animal models may also be explained by a comparison of the pathology being measured in these models. The focus of the earlier period of restenosis research was neointimal formation as the culpable lesion, with the central role attributed to SMC migration and proliferation, as well as matrix production. One assumption of the arterial injury models was that if the neointima could be prevented from developing at the time of injury, neointima would not subsequently develop. Hence markers of SMC proliferation (BrdU, tritiated thymidine, etc), SMC phenotypic state (e.g. actin and myosin subtype expression, ultrastructural markers), matrix production (collagen and metalloprotease assays) and the volume of neointima produced (neointimal cross-sectional area, intima-media ratio) were measured [54; 55; 56; 57; 58]. By and large these measures were performed in cell culture or at very early timepoints after injury and rarely carried beyond two to four weeks. In contrast, clinical results were being expressed in terms of six month restenosis rates, with assessment of the lumen measured by angiography rather than the neointima measured by histology. Very few animal studies of balloon-injured arteries took measurements out as long as six months.

Campbell *et al.* and others have recently shown the contribution of cells from the circulation (bone marrow stem cells) to the neointima in a mouse model [12]. These data open up the possibility that the genesis of neointimal formation may be distant from the focal response at the time of angioplasty in both time and cell origin. Human data for stem cell contribution to the restenosing arterial injury remain to be determined.

Genetic manipulation

A third explanation for why systemic therapy fails to prevent restenosis after angioplasty in humans is that the target of pharmacological therapies was not the best target possible. The angioplasty revolution coincided with a major advance in biomedical research in the polymerase chain reaction and automated gene sequencing.

The genetic code, now held as the vital source of all cell activities and responses, is considered a better site for manipulation of responses to arterial injury.

This approach reflected, and still reflects, the general movement away from protein-based towards gene-based concepts of pathology, made possible by the new tools for genetic investigation. The genetic changes that occurred with angioplasty were identified in animal models of injury and techniques for manipulating these genes were developed. Not only the downstream products of the genetic code (proteins), but also the genetic steps necessary for the entrance to the cell cycle were manipulated to interrupt the fundamental steps involved in cell migration and replication, without which the SMC and other cells cannot migrate to and proliferate within the neointima [59]. It is important to understand that the pharmacopoeia previously used already had tools for this manipulation and that this new approach reflected a new tool rather than a new concept in restenosis therapy: i.e. the neointima remained supreme as the cause for restenosis.

Manipulation of the genetic code can occur at several levels. Transcription of the DNA into RNA can be modified through direct insertion of genomic material upstream of the gene target in question, or by alteration of the gene itself to produce an abnormal or dysfunctional protein product. This usually requires transfer of genetic material into the genome by deliberate viral infection or *transfection*. Targets for this form of genetic manipulation included the many protein products and their receptors already targeted unsuccessfully through pharmacology, as well as novel targets such as genes to promote cell death (apoptosis) and inhibit cell cycle entry (oncogene and promotor genes).

The protein product produced by RNA through translation was also targeted, requiring a slightly less precise delivery, since the treatment only needs to enter the cytoplasm rather than the nucleus and thence the appropriate place in the genome. Antisense olignucleotides, short sequences of 12–20 or more nucleotides designed highly specifically against the known genetic sequence of the chosen target, were introduced into the cell by electroporation (electric current-induced holes in the bilipid envelope) or incorporated into lysosomes. The use of oligonucleotides to manipulate the biology of SMCs and other cells *in vitro*, and to limit neointimal formation *in vivo* was readily demonstrated [60; 61]. Of concern for the stated high specificity of these genetic tools were studies that demonstrated antisense (exactly opposite sequences) and *nonsense* (scrambled combinations of the same nucleotides as used in the antisense sequences) oligonucleotides were equally as effective in preventing the changes in biology, dependent only on four continuous guanosine residues [62]. This suggested that the presumed highly specific tools were acting in a less specific manner, perhaps through enzyme inhibition or other mechanisms.

Demonstrated initially in cell culture, transfer of the genetic treatment into the genome was able to reduce proliferation of the cells of the neointima, especially the SMCs [63]. *In vivo* transfection is more difficult, but continued refinements to the genetic agent [64] and to delivery techniques, including the use of infusion balloons [60; 61], injury-targeted retroviruses [65] and stents [66], allowed adequate transfection rates, with a significant reduction in neointimal formation in animal models of injury. Currently, several genetic treatments are undergoing clinical trials for a variety of cardiovascular and other conditions. However, to date none is effective in restenosis prevention after angioplasty and bypass grafting in humans [67]. Concerns for genetic therapies, with the potential for targeted gene therapy to act in ectopic sites [68], remain speculative.

Remodelling

The use of systemic and genetic agents fails to fulfil in humans the promise shown in animal experiments for all the above reasons, and one more. Neointimal formation is not the only process that leads to arterial restenosis after injury. The changes in the overall arterial dimensions after injury make a major contribution to the final dimension of the arterial lumen. This concept was not new in arterial pathology. Glagov *et al.* showed that the artery can enlarge to accommodate the developing atheromatous lesion without lumen narrowing [69]. In peripheral bypass surgery, bigger arteries develop less restenosis, patched carotid endarterectomies develop less restenosis and the use of bigger diameter infrainguinal grafts provides a better patency rate in the follow-up, suggesting overall vessel dimension is an important contributor to luminal narrowing.

In the clinic, the overall vessel dimension changes had gone unnoticed for a simple reason. Restenosis is measured in the follow-up angiogram by luminal measurements. Angiography training teaches that the 'lumenogram' demonstrates only the flow channel and the vessel wall (remodelled, aneurysmal, lined with thrombus) is not displayed. This became apparent with the introduction of intravascular ultrasound (IVUS) to clinical practice, since IVUS readily measures not only the flow channel but also the dimensions of the various layers of the arterial wall. In the laboratory, the new science of post-angioplasty restenosis had focused on the neointima, spurred on by newer tools such as genetic sequencing and manipulation that allowed even finer micromolecular understanding and intervention.

The introduction of the arterial stent helped complete this incomplete understanding of restenosis pathogenesis. Arterial stents were introduced to maintain the early angioplasty gain and for the prevention of early vessel closure, as well as for the prevention of restenosis. They overcome spasm or recoil, as well as controlling the dissection produced by the angioplasty balloon. In the coronary arteries, this early vessel closure was as high as 10%. Trialled initially in dogs and rabbits, stents were first reported in human trials in 1987 in the coronary and iliac arteries [70].

Arterial stenting immediately gained popularity in clinical work. In the iliac arteries, this was well justified, with excellent patency rates of up to five years. The first randomized controlled trial for the prevention of restenosis using stents against balloon angioplasty alone was reported in 1994 [71]. Whereas iliac stents were patent above 60% up to five years, coronary stents continued to be troubled by unacceptably high restenosis rates (TASC pS108). While the coronary stent reduced the restenosis rate compared with angioplasty alone, the six month >50% luminal diameter restenosis rate rarely fell below 30%.

Risks for in-stent restenosis are patients with acute ischaemic syndromes, diabetes, renal failure, multiple or longer lesions, occluded vessels and vessels of a smaller calibre [72; 73]. Treating in-stent restenosis became, and remains, a growth industry of its own. Attempts to aggressively clean the stent of microparticles resident from manufacture to prevent foreign body reactions [74] and to avoid over-expansion or over-sizing of the stents had no demonstrable clinical benefit in restenosis prevention.

Devices to remove the neointimal hyperplasia from the lumen of the stenosed stent have been developed, including atherectomy devices (e.g. rotablator) that core out the disease, cutting balloons that slice it out, lasers that vaporize it out, further angioplasty and stents-in-stents to push it out, and ultrasound probes that pulverize it out [75]. Each device has its champions and ongoing arguments as to which is technically better [76]. While technically adequate in the short term, these devices provide at best unpredictable longer term success. All were developed to treat post-angioplasty restenosis alone and found a new use with the introduction of stents [77]. The failure of these approaches to solve the problem once and for all, often requiring multiple procedures for recurring restenosis, had these patients occasionally referred to the cardiac or vascular surgeon for stent removal or bypass.

It is the prevention of remodelling and early spasm and dissection, as well as later remodelling, not neointimal formation, which the arterial stent most readily attends. Autopsy specimens and animal work demonstrate the stent itself excites a profuse neointima. Scientific data have now demonstrated that vascular remodelling, not the neointima, was the primary source of restenosis. Ironically, the continued problem of in-stent restenosis was basically a problem of profuse neointimal formation.

The science of neointimal formation and prevention, studied in depth over two decades, showed its benefits. It was known that systemic therapies failed to prevent the neointima forming, and focal delivery of treatment was required to maximize the effect and yet avoid systemic side effects. Treatments for in-stent restenosis thus focus on the site of injury itself. Delivery of drug incorporated into the surface of the stent, and radiation (brachytherapy) to the angioplastied and stented artery, together produced the first real advances in in-stent restenosis prevention.

Brachytherapy

Radiation forms of β-emission (electron) and γ-emission (high-energy electromagnetic irradiation) are the basis for brachytherapy. Energy from these particles ionizes molecules within the irradiated tissue, causing irreparable damage to the cell and its genome. Radiation thus inhibits the neointimal response to injury by effectively killing the cell, or at best preventing its proliferation. Measured per unit of tissue, the energy imparted is labelled as a *Gray* (Gy). Typical dosages for peripheral brachytherapy in restenosis prevention are 12–23 Gy and these can require 20–30 minutes exposure ('dwell time') for delivery. Dosage is optimized to deliver sufficient therapy to a depth of 20 mm from the luminal surface. The penetration through tissue is higher for γ-than β-emitters, and the use of γ-emitters requires more careful shielding and handling. β-emitters, with greater loss of energy to the surrounding tissues, and higher energy dose per emission, are ideally suited to close irradiation of tissues. The radiation affects both neointimal formation and vascular remodelling [78], and thus in theory covers both the major contributors to restenosis.

Radiation can be delivered to the angioplastied stented arterial stenosis from an external source, from within the lumen or from the stent itself. All three approaches have found enthusiasts for their use. All three techniques have problems of their own. External beam brachytherapy is non-invasive but has the greatest potential for collateral tissue damage. Delivery from within the lumen requires a catheter-based delivery. This can be in the form of a guide-wire (typically Ir-192), a balloon filled with gas (Xe-133) [79] or liquid (Re-188) [80], or a centring catheter system (e.g. PARIS catheter, Guidant, Santa Clara, California) [81]. Centring the radiation source ensures an even dose of irradiation to the entire wall exposed, since tissue penetration is proportional to distance from the source. This is particularly a problem in curved arteries, those with heavy calcification and where angioplasty has failed to totally relieve the stenosis. Stent-based radiation (e.g. P-32, Re-186) in theory provides the greatest accuracy in delivery, however, current techniques and stent design ensure only irregular dose delivery in the region of the stent [82; 83].

Clinical trials of brachytherapy for coronary and peripheral restenosis prevention following angioplasty alone or with stenting have shown promise compared with the controls. This is in marked contrast with almost all previous clinical trials in post-angioplasty restenosis, and deserves recognition and praise after two decades of therapeutic failures in preventing neointimal formation in humans. These trials have been concentrated in the coronary sphere [84; 85; 86; 87], where benefit in event-free survival and reduced target vessel revascularization have been shown [88]. For example, the START trial, using 90Sr/90Y beta-source for treatment of in-stent restenosis with doses of 18–23 Gy adjusted for vessel size, recorded death, myocardial infarction and target-vessel revascularization in 28.7% placebo patients compared with 19.1% irradiated patients ($P = 0.024$) at eight months. On angiography at eight-months, restenosis was significantly reduced from 45.2% in the placebo group to 28.8% in irradiated patients [89]. Single centre studies are demonstrating that these benefits are durable up to five years [90].

Some high-risk groups for in-stent restenosis were beneficiaries of brachytherapy. Brachytherapy reduces six month in-stent restenosis in coronary arteries, target vessel revascularization and coronary events in diabetics to a rate similar to that in non-diabetics [91; 92]. Patients with chronic renal failure have similar rates of restenosis and revascularizations as non-renal failure patients, although with higher six month mortality rates (7.2% vs. 1.9%, respectively) [91].

Notable in these series are the sub-groups for whom brachytherapy was less successful, including those lesions greater than 20 mm. This is relevant to the treatment of lesions of the superficial femoral artery especially, since trials to date show a mean lesion lengths of 8–18 cm. Most involve angioplasty alone [93; 94; 95] while, few treatments include in-stent restenotic lesions [96]. Minar *et al.* randomized 113 patients to either PTA and Ir-192 brachytherapy of femoro-popliteal segments or PTA alone [94]. Six month restenosis rates on Duplex US were 28% in the brachytherapy group compared with 53% in the PTA alone group, and 12 month patency rates were 63% vs. 35%, respectively. The study shows while brachytherapy improves the results of PTA alone in the femoro-popliteal segment, it fails to make PTA a comparable procedure for vein, or even synthetic, bypass grafting. Hagennars *et al.* published a small randomized trial, showing a reduction in restenosis in angioplastied femoro-popliteal segments at six months after Ir-192 brachytherapy. With an incomplete follow-up, and small numbers, the study is methodologically flawed. Awaited are the results of the PARIS (Peripheral Artery Radiation Investigational Study) trial, the first prospective placebo-controlled, multicentre, randomized trial of brachytherapy in lower limb angioplasty. Delivery of radiation is transluminally via centring catheter systems using Ir-192. The feasability trial demonstrated angiographic restenosis of 17.2% at six months and clinical restenosis of 13% at 12 months [81]. These results are more promising than previously published results, but require longer term confirmation.

The use of angioplasty and stenting in saphenous vein grafts (SVG) is controversial, as is the use of brachytherapy. Retrospective analysis of the WRIST and SVGWRIST data show similar benefits in SVG and native vessel in-stent restenosis rates at six months after Ir-192 brachytherapy [97]. A recent small prospective series showed a benefit in reducing in-stent restenosis by Ir-192 brachytherapy after successful treatment of the restenosis through one or a combination of angioplasty, atherectomy or stent-in-stent placement. With a six month restenosis rate of 21% in the irradiated group compared with 44% in the placebo group ($P = 0.005$) the benefits compared with re-do cardiac surgery may be substantial. In peripheral bypass, the relative ease of surveillance with Duplex and ease of vein patch angioplasty for developing stenoses [4], makes open surgery for graft stenosis a low risk and desirable option in comparison with angioplasty and brachytherapy.

Despite clinical success in limiting restenosis after angioplasty, there are several problems with post-angioplasty brachytherapy. Late thrombosis, perhaps from a failure of adequate luminal healing after irradiation, has required the longer term use of antiplatelet agents (aspirin and clopidogrel). In femoro-popliteal segments thromboses occur despite the addition of clopidogrel and aspirin in stented segments [96; 98]. Edge-effect, either due to inadequate irradiation of the angioplastied and stented region, or from geographic miss with irradiation beyond the injured region, is seen in a 'candy-wrapper' appearance on angiogram [99]. This leaves tight stenoses at the ends of the stent. 'Hot-' and 'cold-ended' stents were developed to combat the edge-effect, covering both possible pathogeneses by increasing or decreasing the radiation dose incorporated into the radioactive stent. 'Cold-end' stents fail to reduce restenosis, moving the site of maximal restenosis from the stent end to the junction between the radiation and non-radiation zones [100].

Concern about the use of irradiation to reduce neointimal formation after angioplasty is founded on the knowledge that radiation is itself a source for arterial stenosis seen by vascular surgeons many years after therapy. Radiation injury of arteries has been known since the end of the nineteenth century and its induction of accelerated atherosclerosis known since the 1940s. The use of deep x-ray therapy for head and neck squamous cell carcinoma produces carotid atheroma years from the time of therapy [101]. Catheter-delivered radiation in clinical doses is shown in animal models to produce acute vasculitis 20–30 mm beyond the target vessel in both the coronary and iliac arteries of pigs [102]. Persistent dissections six months after PTA in irradiated groups compared with controls also raise concerns about vessel healing [78]. The effect of radiation, with its potential to cause problems many years after therapy, makes the long term role for brachytherapy uncertain.

Drug-eluting stents

A second recent approach to preventing restenosis after angioplasty, slightly lagging in time behind brachytherapy, combined the use of stents (to overcome vascular remodelling) and topical therapy (to reduce the profuse neointima produced by the presence of the stent). The incorporation of pharmaceutical agents into the stent structure itself, from where the drug diffuses out over time to limit neointimal formation – the 'drug-eluting stent' – has recently excited great interest. The intense work on systemic therapeutics from the 1980s and early 1990s already showed many pharmacological agents could reduce the neointimal response to injury in animal models, and stent manufacturers had a cupboard full of potentially therapeutic drugs to choose from.

Several drug-eluting stents show benefit in human and animal models in the prevention of restenosis after angioplasty (Table 13.2). For reasons mentioned above, the animal results must be treated with caution. Human data for coronary-placed drug-eluting stents, however, is emerging and is impressive. The Cypher stent (Cordis), which incorporates sirolimus into a standard coronary stent (Figure 13.2), has been tested in two prospective trials of in-stent restenosis prevention [103; 104]. The former, a pilot study in 45 patients using stents that were fast-eluting (>80% release of sirolimus under 14 days) or slow-eluting (>80% release under 28 days), demonstrated a remarkable 0% restenosis rate at 12 months, but lacked a control group. The latter study of 238 patients randomized to either a naked stent or slow-eluting sirolimus stent demonstrated a six month 0% restenosis in the sirolimus stent group compared with 26.6% in the naked stent group. At a one year follow-up the rate of major cardiac events was 5.8% in the sirolimus stent group and 28.8% in the naked stent group.

Not all drug-eluting stents may be equal, however. First reports of human trials with a QP2 (paclitaxel derivative) coated coronary stent showed 8 of 13 patients (61.5%) with restenosis at 12 months, despite only 13% restenosis at six months [105]. Variations in the efficacy

Table 13.2. *Drug-eluting stents in human or animal research models*

Drug	Stent	Animal model	% Restenosis	Timepoint	Reference
Sirolimus	Bx Velocity	Human	0	24 months	133
QP2 (paclitaxel derivative)		Human	61.5%	12 months	105
Heparin	JoStent	Human	33%	6 months	135
Paclitaxel	Gianturco-Roubin II	Porcine coronary	27%	4 weeks	134
Iloprost/hirudin	Palmaz-Schatz	Porcine and Ovine	55%	4 weeks	131
Dexamethasone	Tantalum wire	Porcine	No reduction compared with controls	4 weeks	44
Batimastat (MMP inhibitor)	Matrix LO	Rabbit	NA	4 weeks	www.britbio.co.uk/bbstent.htm
Angiopeptin	BioDivYsio	Porcine	No reduction compared with controls	4 weeks	132

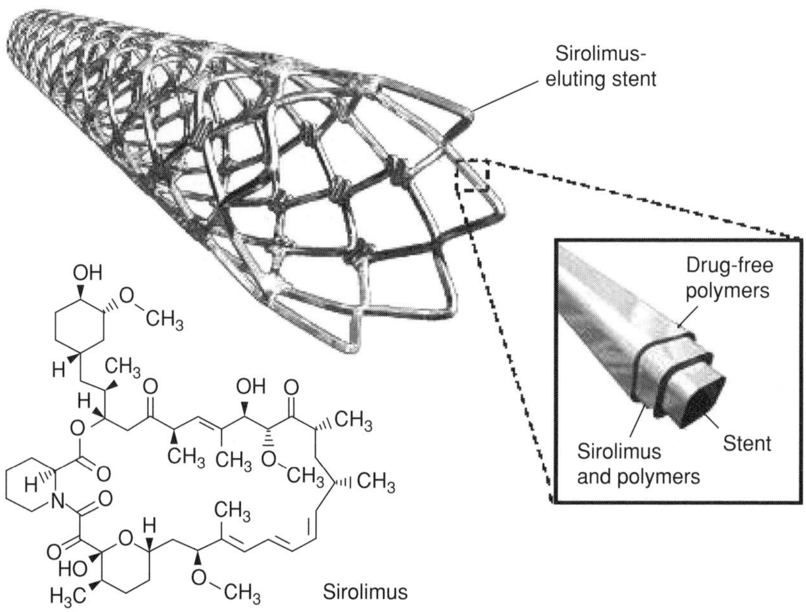

Fig. 13.2. The cypher stent (Johnson and Johnson, New Jersey). Sirolimus (rapamycin) is incorporated into a polymer layer coating the stent. This is then covered by a further polymer coating allowing slow elution of the drug over approximately 28 days.

of each system will depend not only on the therapeutic agent, but also the polymer or other coating used for controlled release of the drug [106]. Each drug-eluting stent will require empirical in-human testing to properly ascertain its ability to prevent restenosis.

Clearly the advantage of the drug-eluting stents over catheter or external (but not stent-based) brachytherapy is the lack of a second procedure, or prolonged primary procedure, to prevent restenosis. The introduction of the drug-eluting stents may well significantly reduce the degree of restenosis in the coronary artery, although larger trials will be welcome. But are they the salvation of peripheral arterial restenoses? In the peripheral vasculature the stent faces external pressures (in the adductor canal or under the inguinal ligament, or the cubital fossa at the end of the polytetrafluorethylene (PTFE) dialysis loop, for example) not present in the coronary artery. These sites are potentially problematic for stenting, since the external pressures remodel the stent, leaving it buckled or with broken struts [107; 108]. Also, the stenotic segments are longer in the peripheries and angioplastied lengths are measured in centimetres not millimetres. One early report of sirolimus-eluting SMART stents in the femoro-popliteal segment, with 18 patients in each group, showed no significant difference in percentage diameter reduction compared with naked stents (22.6% vs. 30.9%, respectively) at six months [108], suggesting that results from coronary arteries cannot easily be translated to the peripheral vasculature.

Covered stents and stent-grafts

Another approach to preventing restenosis in femoro-popliteal segments after angioplasty and stenting is to cover the stent with a graft material to inhibit ingrowth of neointimal genesis cells from the arterial wall (Figure 13.3). Perhaps the new evidence for circulating cells as potential precursors of neointimal formation has relevance here, for covered stent trials for treatment of stenosis have failed to show long term benefit to date [109; 110]. A cohort of 30 patients undergoing dacron-covered stenting of femoro-popliteal segments had 23% primary patency rates at two years, and 17% at three and four years [111]. Further, the patients were all given oral anticoagulation and despite this 17% suffered acute thrombosis in the first 24 hours. Also, more than half of the patients experienced pain in the stent-grafted segment for a mean of five days beyond placement. Better

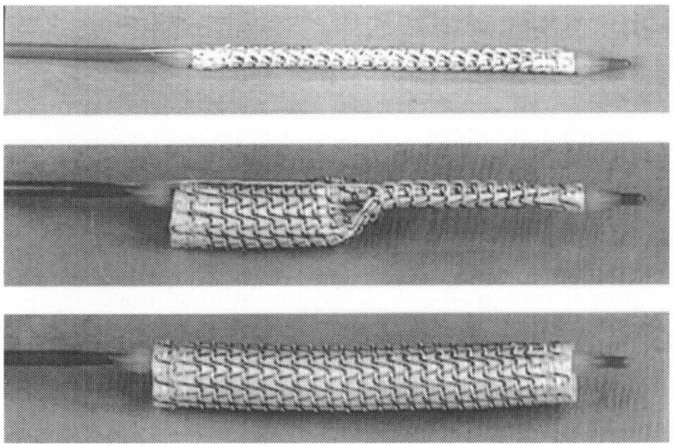

Fig. 13.3. The Hemobahn endoprosthesis (W. Gone and Associates, Flagstaff, Arizona) is a self-expanding endoluminal prosthesis. The prosthesis is composed of an ultra thin (100 μm wall thickness, 30 μm internodal distance) expanded polytetrafluoroethylene graft on the luminal surface attached to self-expanding nitinol (nickel-titanium) stent.

results have been reported with PTFE-covered stents (73% primary patency at one year) although the follow-up period was shorter than for the dacron-covered grafts [112].

Novel and future methods for the prevention and treatment of in-stent restenosis

Novel methods for the prevention of restenosis after angioplasty alone or within stents abound. We include here reference to systemic therapeutic agents that have animal but no human evidence for preventing restenosis, although they may not bear fruit in clinical medicine. Photodynamic therapy, using an agent activated by light spectrum electromagnetic radiation, reduces restenosis in animal experiments following angioplasty. Sonodynamic therapy, using externally applied ultrasound energy after intravenous administration of a chlorin derivative 'sensitizer' showed reduced in-stent restenosis in rabbit iliac arteries compared with controls [113]. Similar use of ultrasound from an intravascular-positioned probe 'decelerates' neointimal formation in a porcine femoral artery stent model [114]. Magnetized balloon expandable stents showed reduced neointimal formation compared with standard Palmaz stents in a dog coronary model [115]. Pre-treatment of the angioplastied site with low-power red laser light reduced in-stent restenosis in a porcine coronary model [116].

Open surgical considerations in restenosis prevention and treatment

The potential for angioplasty to extend the treatment of peripheral vascular disease was recognized early in the development of the procedure [117]. Bypass surgery suffers less frequently from restenosis, yet it does occur and requires treatment. Surveillance of femoropopliteal vein grafts, with treatment of stenoses before grafts occlude, is beneficial in indicating the need for intervention to treat a restenotic segment [2]. Erickson *et al.*, using Duplex surveillance follow-up of 556 *in situ* vein grafts that performed overwhelmingly for critical ischaemia (93%), found a stenosis within a femoropopliteal bypass vein graft can occur at any time within the life of the graft, with mean time to detection of stenosis at 12 months after initial surgery [4]. Some 30% of grafts required one or more interventions over the lifetime of the graft, with 18% of abnormalities detected more than two years after initial surgery. Threats to graft patency were low flow states and >75% stenoses.

Treatment of peripheral arterial and fistula restenoses has until recently been the domain of traditional vascular surgery. Open surgery employing endarterectomy and patch angioplasty or bypass for symptomatic or high grade restenotic lesions can be achieved with acceptably low morbidity and mortality [24]. Endarterectomy and patch angioplasty are deliberate attempts by the surgeon to remodel the vessel, changing its overall dimensions. So too is choice of conduit size. A larger (>6 mm) conduit retains a higher patency than a narrower one in the infrainguinal bypass procedure [118]. Bypass surgery, while not strictly a treatment for restenosis in that it does not relieve the narrowed vessel, is nevertheless a useful technique for providing an alternative conduit for improving distal perfusion. Bypass has several considerations of its own in restenosis prevention. The handling of the vein used for bypass, including aggressive inflation, or multiple dilatations and thrombectomies, influences platelet deposition and the healing of the vein as it arterializes on exposure to systemic pressure [7]. Imperfect valvulotomy for *in situ* bypass is strictly a stenosis rather than restenosis and thus a cause of early graft failure, as well as a potential stimulus for later restenosis.

Haemodynamic forces are considered important contributors to restenosis through both neointimal hyperplasia formation and vascular remodelling. The influences of sheer stress gradients on neointimal formation and post-stenotic dilatation are evidence for this [16; 119; 120]. Indirect human evidence of haemodynamic contributions may be found in the higher rate of graft failure with low flow states and poor run off [4]. Wentzel *et al.* [121] demonstrated the relationship between shear stress and neointimal hyperplasia in human coronary stents using a combination of angiography and intravascular ultrasound (ANGUS). In patients without hypercholesterolaemia, there was a direct relationship between neointimal thickness and low shear stress within the stent. Within the curved course of the coronary stents, maximum neointimal thickness was found on the inner curve of the stent, where shear stress was lowest.

How shear stress can be influenced in the peripheral vasculature to prevent restenosis is at best speculative. The size, shape and angle of bypass anastomoses may influence the development of subsequent neointimal hyperplasia [122]. Computer modelling for reducing sheer stresses and sheer stress gradients indicates an optimum design for end-to-side anastomoses. Characteristics of the optimum design include a low (10–15°) incidence angle relative to the long axis of the artery, a ratio of graft to native vessel diameter of 1.6:1 and a long tapering narrow toe. This design demonstrated minimal shear stress gradients at resting and exercise flow rates, compared with both a standard (45° incidence angle) end-to-side anastomoses and anastomosis modified with a Taylor patch [123] (Figure 13.4). For this there remains only conceptual and animal proof, not human data. Improving flow through a treated segment of artery also depends on ensuring adequate inflow and outflow. Upstream stenoses are usually treated first, and the problem thus becomes one of improving the flow through the distal vascular bed.

Reducing the resistance of the distal vascular bed is no easy matter, since ischaemia is itself a powerful vasodilator and promoter of angiogenesis. While fashioning an arterio-venous fistula beyond a bypass graft may maintain the graft patency it does not improve distal perfusion or limb survival. Promotion of angiogenesis through growth factor stimulation within the run off territory might assist this.

Compliance matching of synthetic and native vessels may also reduce restenosis rates. Mismatch of compliance between the PTFE and vein at the venous end of a dialysis fistulae, as well as external compression in the cubital fossa, are likely to be causes for the persisting

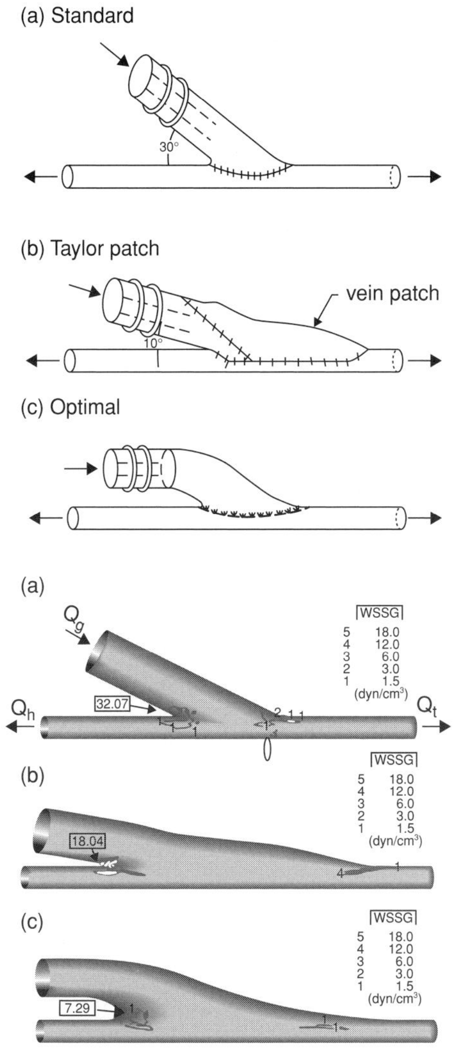

Fig. 13.4. Anastomotic design to reduce shear stress gradient[123].

problem of arterio-venous fistula stenosis. Similar compliance mismatches are seen in coronary stents [121]. Angioplasty and stenting are uniformly bad treatments for this problem, with superior results achieved through patch angioplasty or re-siting the distal anastomosis. The compliance match of artery and vein is far superior to that of dacron or PTFE [124]. Future conduit design will incorporate this feature. Compliance matched stents are planned for clinical testing in the near future [125].

Restenosis following carotid endarterectomy occurs in approximately 10% of cases; however, less than 2% require intervention over a 20 year follow-up ([24] Gagne). The rate is lower in men and patients whose arteries are closed with a patch [24]. There is continued debate about the protective effects of PTFE, polyurethane, bovine pericardial, vein or dacron as the ideal patch material to prevent restenosis [24; 126; 127]. One major problem with open re-operation in the neck is injury to the cranial nerves X and XII, and other structures incorporated in scarred tissue. Similar problems exist for irradiated necks. Carotid stenting, with the attendant problems associated with coronary stenting, has been offered recently as an alternative therapy. Controversy remains as to the restenosis rates with primary and secondary carotid stenting. Treatments for this are discussed above.

Finally, the vascular surgeon has available the adventitial surface of the vessel for delivery of anti-restenotic therapy at the site of anastomosis or endarterectomy. This provides an alternative site for topical drug delivery. It has been shown to be useful in animal models for reducing neointimal hyperplasia after angioplasty and in vein grafts [37; 128; 129; 130] but remains untested to any degree in humans. However, as with any other local treatment that aims to limit neointimal hyperplasia, if it is uncoupled from treatment to overcome the effects of vascular remodelling it is unlikely to be successful. Fortunately, a number of open vascular techniques, as indicated, do improve vessel dimensions. The possibilities for this avenue of therapy remain to be explored.

CONCLUSIONS

Angioplasty and stenting are associated with higher rates of restenosis than traditional open surgery. Combining the two major pathological processes involved – **neointimal hyperplasia** and **vascular remodelling** – with concepts of special importance in the peripheral vasculature, allows the vascular surgeon a range of options in preventing and treating restenosis. Therapies that aim primarily to prevent one pathological process without considering the other are unlikely to succeed in long term restenosis prevention. Consideration of this should be made when planning new clinical treatments for restenosis prevention based on positive animal data. Traditional treatments of restenosis including patch angioplasty, endarterectomy and bypass (which skirts the issue rather than treating it) are practical and useful and – even in the current age of endoluminal technology – frequently necessary. Future methods to limit restenosis may encompass new conduit and anastomotic design, targeted drug delivery, genetic therapies and improving resistance patterns in the distal vascular bed. With the spectacular failure of many promising therapies in restenosis prevention treatment, a new treatment can only be deemed a success when shown effective in well-designed prospective studies in humans.

REFERENCES

1. R. B. Rutherford, Basic vascular surgical techniques. In *Vascular Surgery*, 5th edn, ed. R. B. Rutherford. (Philadelphia: W. B. Saunders, 2000), pp. 476–7.
2. M. M. Idu, J. D. Blankenstein, P. de Gier, E. Truyen & J. Buth, Impact of a color-flow duplex surveillance program on infrainguinal vein graft patency: a five-year experience. *Journal of Vascular Surgery*, **17**(1) (1993), 42–53.
3. T. Igawa, Y. Nagamura, Y. Ozeki, H. Itoh & F. Unemi, Stenosis enhances role of platelets in growth of regional thrombus and intimal wall thickening in rat carotid arteries. *Circulation Research*, **77**(2) (1995), 310–6.
4. C. A. Erickson, J. B. Towne, G. R. Seabrook, J. A. Freischlag & R. A. Cambria, Ongoing vascular laboratory surveillance is essential to maximize long-term *in situ* saphenous vein bypass patency. *Journal of Vascular Surgery*, **23**(1) (1996), 18–27.
5. J. L. Mills, R. M. Fujitani & S. M. Taylor, Contribution of routine intraoperative completion arteriography to early infrainguinal bypass patency. *American Journal of Surgery*, **164**(5) (1992), 506–11.
6. D. B. Walsh, Technical adequacy and graft thrombosis. In *Vascular Surgery*, 5th edn, ed. R. B. Rutherford. (Philadelphia: W. B. Saunders, 2000), pp. 708–26.
7. T. G. Nielsen, B. Hesse, M. W. Boehme & T. V. Schroeder, Intraoperative endothelial damage is associated with increased risk of stenoses in infrainguinal vein grafts. *European Journal of Vascular and Endovascular Surgery*, **21**(6) (2001), 513–9.
8. T. W. Wakefield, B. L. Shulkin, E. P. Fellows *et al.*, Platelet reactivity in human aortic grafts: a prospective, randomized midterm study of platelet adherence and release products in Dacron and polytetrafluoroethylene conduits. *Journal of Vascular Surgery*, **9**(2) (1989), 234–43.
9. L. A. Harker, Clinical trials evaluating platelet-modifying drugs in patients with atherosclerotic cardiovascular disease and thrombosis. *Circulation*, **73**(2) (1986), 206–23.
10. B. L. Johnson, D. F. Bandyk, M. R. Back, A. J. Avino & S. M. Roth, Intraoperative duplex monitoring of infrainguinal vein bypass procedures. *Journal of Vascular Surgery*, **31**(4) (2000), 678–90.
11. J. P. Zidar, Rationale for low-molecular weight heparin in coronary stenting. *American Heart Journal*, **134**(5) (1997), S81–7.
12. J. H. Campbell, C. L. Han & G. R. Campbell, Neointimal formation by circulating bone marrow cells. *Annals of the New York Academy of Sciences*, **947** (2001), 18–25.
13. J. S. Forrester, M. Fishbein, R. Helfant & J. Fagin, A paradigm for restenosis based on cell biology: clues for the development of new preventive therapies. *Journal of the American College of Cardiology*, **17**(3) (1991), 758–69.
14. D. Simper, P. G. Stalboerger, C. J. Panetta, S. Wang & N. M. Caplice, Smooth muscle progenitor cells in human blood. *Circulation*, **106**(10) (2002), 1199–204.
15. D. P. Faxon, W. Coats & J. Currier, Remodeling of the coronary artery after vascular injury. *Progress in Cardiovascular Diseases*, **40**(2) (1997), 129–40.
16. E. J. Mattsson, T. R. Kohler, S. M. Vergel & A. W. Clowes, Increased blood flow induces regression of intimal hyperplasia. *Arteriosclerosis, Thrombosis and Vascular Biology*, **17**(10) (1997), 2245–9.
17. J. A. Bingley, I. P. Hayward, J. H. Campbell & G. R. Campbell, Arterial heparan sulfate proteoglycans inhibit vascular smooth muscle cell proliferation and phenotype change *in vitro* and neointimal formation *in vivo*. *Journal of Vascular Surgery*, **28**(2) (1998), 308–18.
18. R. L. Geary, S. T. Nikkari, W. D. Wagner *et al.*, Wound healing: a paradigm for lumen narrowing after arterial reconstruction. *Journal of Vascular Surgery*, **27**(1) (1998), 96–108.
19. A. C. Newby & A. H. Baker, Targets for gene therapy of vein grafts. *Current Opinion in Cardiology*, **14**(6) (1999), 489–94.
20. D. P. Faxon, Predicting restenosis: bigger is better but not best. *Circulation*, **101**(9) (2000), 946–7.
21. A. W. Clowes & M. J. Karnowsky, Suppression by heparin of smooth muscle cell proliferation in injured arteries. *Nature*, **265**(5595) (1977), 625–6.

22. M. R. Ward, P. S. Tsao, A. Agrotis *et al.*, Low blood flow after angioplasty augments mechanisms of restenosis: inward vessel remodeling, cell migration, and activity of genes regulating migration. *Arteriosclerosis, Thrombosis and Vascular Biology*, **21**(2) (2001), 208–13.
23. J. Wilcox, E. Okamoto, K. Nakahara & J. Vinten-Johansen, Perivascular responses after angioplasty which may contribute postangioplasty restenosis: a role for circulating myofibroblast precursors. *Annals of the New York Academy of Sciences*, **947** (2001), 68–90.
24. J. P. Archie, Jr., Reoperations for carotid artery stenosis: role of primary and secondary reconstructions. *Journal of Vascular Surgery*, **33**(3) (2001), 495–503.
25. T. Reifsnyder, J. B. Towne, G. R. Seabrook, J. F. Blari & D. F. Bandyk, Biological characteristics of long-term autogenous vein grafts: a dynamic evolution. *Journal of Vascular Surgery*, **17** (1993), 207–17.
26. A. R. Gruntzig, A. Senning, W. E. Siegenthaler, Nonoperative dilatation of coronary-artery stenosis: percutaneous transluminal coronary angioplasty. *New England Journal of Medicine*, **301**(2) (1979), 61–8.
27. P. W. Serruys, H. E. Luijten, K. J. Beatt *et al.*, Incidence of restenosis after successful coronary angioplasty: a time-related phenomenon. *Circulation*, **77**(2) (1988), 361–71.
28. C. Glover & E. R. O'Brien, Pathophysiological insights from studies of retrieved coronary atherectomy tissue. *Seminars in Interventional Cardiology*, **5**(4) (2000), 167–73.
29. J. P. R. Herrman, W. R. M. Hermans, J. Vos & P. W. Serruys, Pharmacological approaches to the prevention of restenosis following angioplasty. *Drugs*, **46**(1) (1993), 18–52.
30. H. Tamai, K. Katoh, T. Yamaguchi *et al.*, The impact of tranilast on restenosis after coronary angioplasty: the Second Tranilast Restenosis Following Angioplasty Trial (TREAT-2). *American Heart Journal*, **143**(3) (2002), 506–13.
31. D. R. Holmes, Jr., M. Savage, J. M. LaBlanche *et al.*, Results of Prevention of REStenosis with Tranilast and its Outcomes (PRESTO) trial. *Circulation*, **106**(10) (2002), 1243–50.
32. R. Ross The pathogenesis of atherosclerosis: a perspective for the 1990s. *Nature*, **362**(6423) (1993), 801–9.
33. V. Lindner, Role of basic fibroblast growth factor and platelet-derived growth factor (B-chain) in neointima formation after arterial injury. *Zeitschrift fur Kardiologie*, **84** (Suppl 4) (1995), 137–44.
34. C. S. Moran, J. H. Campbell & G. R. Campbell, Induction of smooth muscle cell nitric oxide synthase by human leukaemia inhibitory factor: effects *in vitro* and *in vivo*. *Journal of Vascular Research*, **34**(5) (1997), 378–85.
35. E. G. Nabel, L. Shum, V. J. Pompili *et al.*, Direct transfer of transforming growth factor beta 1 gene into arteries stimulates fibrocellular hyperplasia. *Proceedings of the National Academy of Sciences of the USA*, **90**(22) (1993), 10759–63.
36. J. W. Currier, T. K. Pow, C. C. Haudenschild, A. C. Minihan & D. P. Faxon, Low molecular weight heparin (enoxaparin) reduces restenosis after iliac angioplasty in the hypercholesterolemic rabbit. *Journal of the American College of Cardiology* **17**(6) (Suppl B) (1991), 118B–25B.
37. J. A. Bingley, J. H. Campbell, I. P. Hayward & G. R. Campbell, Inhibition of neointimal formation by natural heparan sulphate proteoglycans of the arterial wall. *Annals of the New York Academy of Sciences*, **811** (1997), 238–44.
38. H. C. Herrmann, S. S. Okada, E. Hozakowska *et al.*, Inhibition of smooth muscle cell proliferation and experimental angioplasty restenosis by beta-cyclodextrin tetradecasulfate. *Arteriosclerosis and Thrombosis*, **13**(6) (1993), 924–31.
39. S. G. Ellis, G. S. Roubin, J. Wilentz, J. S. Douglas, Jr. & S. B. King, 3rd, Effect of 18- to 24-hour heparin administration for prevention of restenosis after uncomplicated coronary angioplasty. *American Heart Journal*, **117**(4) (1989), 777–82.
40. D. P. Faxon, T. E. Spiro, S. Minor *et al.*, Low molecular weight heparin in prevention of restenosis after angioplasty. Results of Enoxaparin Restenosis (ERA) Trial. *Circulation*, **90**(2) (1994), 908–14.
41. K. G. Lehmann, R. J. Doria, J. M. Feuer, J. X. Hall & D. T. Hoang, Paradoxical increase in restenosis rate with chronic heparin use. *Journal of the American College of Cardiology*, **17** (1991), 181A.
42. E. R. Edelman & M. J. Karnovsky, Contrasting effects of the intermittent and continuous administration of heparin in experimental restenosis. *Circulation*, **89**(2) (1994), 770–6.
43. S. Uhlrich, O. Lagente, J. Choay, Y. Courtois & M. Lenfant, Structural activity relationship in heparin: stimulation of non-vascular cells by a synthetic heparin pentasaccharide in cooperation with human acidic

fibroblast growth factors. *Biochemical and Biophysical Research Communication*, **139**(2) (1986), 728–32.
44. A. M. Lincoff, E. J. Topol & S. G. Ellis, Local drug delivery for the prevention of restenosis. *Circulation*, **90**(4) (1994), 2070–84.
45. R. L. Wilensky, K. L. March, I. Gradus-Pizlo, A. J. Spaedy & D. R. Hathaway, Methods and devices for local drug delivery in coronary and peripheral arteries. *Trends in Cardiovascular Medicine*, **3** (1993) 163–70.
46. R. L. Wilensky, K. L. March, I. Gradus-Pizlo, D. S. Schauwecker & D. R. Hatheway, Enhanced localization and retention of microparticles following intramural delivery into atherosclerotic arteries using a new delivery catheter. *Journal of the American College of Cardiology*, **21**(2) (1993), 185A.
47. T. K. Nasser, R. L. Wilensky, K. Mehdi, K. L. March, Microparticle deposition in periarterial microvasculature and intramural dissections after porous balloon delivery into atherosclerotic vessels: quantitation and localization by confocal scanning laser microscopy. *American Heart Journal*, **131**(5) (1996), 892–8.
48. A. Baumbach, M. Oberhoff, C. Herdeg *et al.*, Local delivery of a low molecular weight heparin following stent implantation in the pig coronary artery. *Basic Research in Cardiology*, **95**(3) (2000), 173–8.
49. M. Herring, J. Smith, M. Dalsing *et al.*, Endothelial seeding of polytetrafluoroethylene femoral popliteal bypasses: the failure of low-density seeding to improve patency. *Journal of Vascular Surgery*, **20**(4) (1994), 650–5.
50. N. Jensen, B. Lindblad & D. Bergqvist, Endothelial cell seeded dacron aortobifurcated grafts: platelet deposition and long-term follow-up. *Journal of Cardiovascular Surgery*, **35**(5) (1994), 425–9.
51. M. Simons, E. R. Edelman, J. DeKeyser, R. Langer & R. Rosenberg, Antisense c-myb oligonucleotides inhibit arterial smooth muscle cell accumulation *in vivo*. *Nature*, **359** (1992), 67–70.
52. A. E. Villa, L. A. Guzman, W. Chen *et al.*, Local delivery of dexamethasone for prevention of neointimal proliferation in a rat model of balloon angioplasty. *Journal of Clinical Investigation*, **93**(3) (1994) 1243–9.
53. T. Okada, D. H. Bark & M. R. Mayberg, Localized release of perivascular heparin inhibits intimal proliferation after endothelial injury without systemic anticoagulation. *Neurosurgery*, **25**(6) (1989), 892–8.
54. S. M. London & M. R. Mayberg, Kinetics of bromodeoxyuridine uptake by smooth muscle cells after arterial injury. *Journal of Vascular Research*, **31**(5) (1994), 247–55.
55. M. P. Bendeck, N. Zempo, A. W. Clowes, R. E. Galardy & M. A. Reidy, Smooth muscle cell migration and matrix metalloproteinase expression after arterial injury in the rat. *Circulation Research*, **75**(3) (1994), 539–45.
56. N. Zempo, R. D. Kenagy, Y. P. Au *et al.*, Matrix metalloproteinases of vascular wall cells are increased in balloon-injured rat carotid artery. *Journal of Vascular Surgery*, **20**(2) (1994), 209–17.
57. E. W. Koo & A. I. Gotlieb, Neointimal formation in the porcine aortic organ culture. I. Cellular dynamics over 1 month. *Laboratory Investigation*, **64**(6) (1991), 743–53.
58. H. Hanke, T. Strohschneider, M. Oberhoff, E. Betz & K. R. Karsch, Time course of smooth muscle cell proliferation in the intima and media of arteries following experimental angioplasty. *Circulation Research*, **67**(3) (1990), 651–9.
59. D. W. Muller, The role of proto-oncogenes in coronary restenosis. *Progress in Cardiovascular Diseases*, **40**(2) (1997), 117–28.
60. A. B. Buchwald, A. H. Wagner, C. Webel & M. Hecker, Decoy oligodeoxynucleotide against activator protein-1 reduces neointimal proliferation after coronary angioplasty in hypercholesterolemic minipigs. *Journal of the American College of Cardiology*, **39**(4) (2002), 732–8.
61. N. N. Kipshidze, H. S. Kim, P. Iversen *et al.*, Intramural coronary delivery of advanced antisense oligonucleotides reduces neointimal formation in the porcine stent restenosis model. *Journal of the American College of Cardiology*, **39**(10) (2002), 1686–91.
62. T. L. Burgess, E. F. Fisher, S. L. Ross *et al.*, The antiproliferative activity of c-myb and c-myc antisense oligonucleotides in smooth muscle cells is caused by a nonantisense mechanism. *Proceedings of the National Academy of Sciences of the USA*, **92**(9) (1995), 4051–5.
63. S. Ribault, P. Neuville, A. Mechine-Neuville *et al.*, Chimeric smooth muscle-specific enhancer/promoters: valuable tools for adenovirus-mediated cardiovascular gene therapy. *Circulation Research*, **88**(5) (2001), 468–75.
64. J. G. Pickering, J. M. Isner, C. M. Ford *et al.*, Processing of chimeric antisense oligonucleotides by human vascular smooth muscle cells and human atherosclerotic plaque. Implications for antisense therapy of restenosis after angioplasty. *Circulation*, **93**(4) (1996), 772–80.
65. E. M. Gordon, N. L. Zhu, M. Forney Prescott *et al.*, Lesion-targeted injectable vectors for vascular restenosis. *Human Gene Therapy*, **12**(10) (2001), 1277–87.

66. B. D. Klugherz, C. Song, S. DeFelice *et al.*, Gene delivery to pig coronary arteries from stents carrying antibody-tethered adenovirus. *Human Gene Therapy*, **13**(3) (2002), 443–54.
67. M. J. Kutryk, D. P. Foley, M. van den Brand *et al.*, ITALICS Trial. Local intracoronary administration of antisense oligonucleotide against c-myc for the prevention of in-stent restenosis: results of the randomized investigation by the Thoraxcenter of antisense DNA using local delivery and IVUS after coronary stenting (ITALICS) trial. *Journal of the American College of Cardiology*, **39**(2) (2002), 281–7.
68. M. O. Hiltunen, M. P. Turunen, A. M. Turunen *et al.*, Biodistribution of adenoviral vector to nontarget tissues after local *in vivo* gene transfer to arterial wall using intravascular and periadventitial gene delivery methods. *FASEB Journal*, **14**(14) (2000), 2230–6.
69. S. Glagov, E. Weisenberg, C. K. Zarins, R. Stankunavicius & G. J. Kolettis, Compensatory enlargement of human atherosclerotic coronary arteries. *New England Journal of Medicine*, **316** (1987), 1371–5.
70. U. Sigwart, J. Puel, V. Mirkovitch, F. Joffre & L. Kappenberger, Intravascular stents to prevent occlusion and restenosis after transluminal angioplasty. *New England Journal of Medicine*, **316**(12) (1987), 701–6.
71. D. L. Fischman, M. B. Leon, D. S. Baim *et al.*, A randomized comparison of coronary-stent placement and balloon angioplasty in the treatment of coronary artery disease. Stent Restenosis Study Investigators. *New England Journal of Medicine*, **331**(8) (1994), 496–501.
72. R. W. Asinger, T. D. Henry, C. A. Herzog, P. R. Paulsen & R. L. Kane, Clinical outcomes of PTCA in chronic renal failure: a case-control study for comorbid features and evaluation of dialysis dependence. *Journal of Invasive Cardiology*, **13**(1) (2001), 21–8.
73. G. N. Levine, A. K. Jacobs, G. P. Keeler *et al.*, Impact of diabetes mellitus on percutaneous revascularization (CAVEAT-I). CAVEAT-I Investigators. Coronary Angioplasty Versus Excisional Atherectomy Trial. *American Journal of Cardiology*, **79**(6) (1997), 748–55.
74. A. Bayes-Genis, A. R. Camrud, M. Jorgenson *et al.*, Pressure rinsing of coronary stents immediately before implantation reduces inflammation and neointimal hyperplasia. *Journal of the American College of Cardiology*, **38**(2) (2001), 562–8.
75. S. Reith, P. W. Radke, O. Volk, J. vom Dahl & H. G. Klues, The place of rotablator for treatment of in-stent restenosis. *Seminars in Interventional Cardiology*, **5**(4) (2000), 199–208.
76. P. Braun, E. Stroh & K. W. Heinrich, Rotablator versus cutting balloon for the treatment of long in-stent restenoses. *Journal of Invasive Cardiology*, **14**(6) (2002), 291–6.
77. M. Adamian, A. Colombo, C. Briguori *et al.*, Cutting balloon angioplasty for the treatment of in-stent restenosis: a matched comparison with rotational atherectomy, additional stent implantation and balloon angioplasty. *Journal of the American College of Cardiology*, **38**(3) (2001), 672–9.
78. T. Hagenaars, I. F. Po, M. R. van Sambeek *et al.*, Gamma radiation induces positive vascular remodeling after balloon angioplasty: a prospective, randomized intravascular ultrasound scan study. *Journal of Vascular Surgery*, **36**(2) (2002), 318–24.
79. M. Apple, R. Waksman, R. C. Chan *et al.*, Radioactive 133-Xenon gas-filled balloon to prevent restenosis: dosimetry, efficacy, and safety considerations. *Circulation*, **106**(6) (2002), 725–9.
80. P. K. Coussement, P. Stella, H. Vanbilloen *et al.*, Intracoronary beta-radiation of *de novo* coronary lesions using a (186)Re liquid-filled balloon system: six-month results from a clinical feasibility study. *Catheterization and Cardiovascular Interventions*, **55**(1) (2002), 28–36.
81. R. Waksman, J. R. Laird, C. T. Jurkovitz *et al.*, Peripheral Artery Radiation Investigational Study (PARIS) Investigators. Intravascular radiation therapy after balloon angioplasty of narrowed femoropopliteal arteries to prevent restenosis: results of the PARIS feasibility clinical trial. *Journal of Vascular and Interventional Radiology*, **12**(8) (2001), 915–21.
82. A. N. Sidawy, J. M. Weiswasser & R. Waksman, Peripheral vascular brachytherapy. *Journal of Vascular Surgery*, **35**(5) (2002), 1041–7.
83. G. Tepe, L. M. Dinkelborg, U. Brehme *et al.*, Prophylaxis of restenosis with (186)re-labeled stents in a rabbit model. *Circulation*, **104**(4) (2001), 480–5.
84. A. E. Raizner, S. N. Oesterle, R. Waksman *et al.*, Inhibition of restenosis with beta-emitting radiotherapy: report of the Proliferation Reduction with Vascular Energy Trial (PREVENT). *Circulation*, **102** (2000), 951–8.
85. V. Verin, Y. Popowski, B. de Bruyne *et al.*, Endoluminal beta-radiation therapy for the prevention of coronary

restenosis after balloon angioplasty. The Dose-Finding Study Group. *New England Journal of Medicine*, **344** (2001), 243–9.

86. P. S. Teirstein, V. Massullo, S. Jani *et al.*, Catheter-based radiotherapy to inhibit restenosis after coronary stenting. *New England Journal of Medicine*, **336** (1997), 1697–703.
87. S. Malhotra & P. S. Teirstein, The SCRIPPS trial: catheter-based radiotherapy to inhibit coronary restenosis. *Journal of Invasive Cardiology*, **12** (2000), 330–2.
88. J. J. Popma, M. Suntharalingam, A. J. Lansky, Stents And Radiation Therapy (START) Investigators. Randomized trial of 90Sr/90Y beta-radiation versus placebo control for treatment of in-stent restenosis *Circulation*, **106**(9) (2002), 1090–6.
89. M. Suntharalingam, W. Laskey, A. J. Lansky *et al.*, Clinical and angiographic outcomes after use of 90Strontium/90Yttrium beta radiation for the treatment of in-stent restenosis: results from the Stents and Radiation Therapy 40 (START 40) registry. *International Journal of Radiation Oncology, Biology, Physics*, **52**(4) (2002), 1075–82.
90. M. A. Grise, V. Massullo, S. Jani *et al.*, Five-year clinical follow-up after intracoronary radiation: results of a randomized clinical trial. *Circulation*, **105**(23) (2002), 2737–40.
91. L. Gruberg, R. Waksman, A. E. Ajani *et al.*, The effect of intracoronary radiation for the treatment of recurrent in-stent restenosis in patients with diabetes mellitus. *Journal of the American College of Cardiology*, **39**(12) (2002), 1930–6.
92. J. W. Moses, I. Moussa, M. B. Leon *et al.*, Effect of catheter-based iridium-192 gamma brachytherapy on the added risk of restenosis from diabetes mellitus after intervention for in-stent restenosis (subanalysis of the GAMMA I Randomized Trial). *American Journal of Cardiology*, **90**(3) (2002), 243–7.
93. K. Krueger, P. Landwehr, M. Bendel *et al.*, Endovascular gamma irradiation of femoropopliteal *de novo* stenoses immediately after PTA: interim results of prospective randomized controlled trial. *Radiology*, **224**(2) (2002), 519–28.
94. E. Minar, B. Pokrajac, R. Ahmadi *et al.*, Brachytherapy for prophylaxis of restenosis after long-segment femoropopliteal angioplasty: pilot study. *Radiology*, **208** (1998), 173–9.
95. D. Liermann, J. Kirchner, R. Bauernsachs, B. Schopohl & H. D. Bottcher, Brachytherapy with iridium-192 HDR to prevent from restenosis in peripheral arteries. An update. **23** (1998), 394–400.
96. R. M. Wolfram, B. Pokrajac, R. Ahmadi *et al.*, Endovascular brachytherapy for prophylaxis against restenosis after long-segment femoropopliteal placement of stents: initial results. *Radiology*, **220**(3) (2001), 724–9.
97. M. T. Castagna, G. S. Mintz, R. Waksman *et al.*, Comparative efficacy of gamma-irradiation for treatment of in-stent restenosis in saphenous vein graft versus native coronary artery in-stent restenosis: an intravascular ultrasound study. *Circulation*, **104**(25) (2001), 3020–2.
98. W. J. Hofmann, M. Kopp, B. Kofler *et al.*, Preliminary observations on the need for control angiography after peripheral endovascular brachytherapy using a centering balloon. *Journal of Endovascular Therapy*, **9**(2) (2002), 241–5.
99. G. Sianos, I. P. Kay, M. A. Costa *et al.*, Geographical miss during catheter-based intracoronary beta-radiation: incidence and implications in the BRIE study. Beta-Radiation In Europe. *Journal of the American College of Cardiology*, **38**(2) (2001), 415–20.
100. A. J. Wardeh, R. Albiero, I. P. Kay *et al.*, Angiographical follow-up after radioactive 'cold ends' stent implantation: a multicenter trial. *Circulation*, **105**(5) (2002), 550–3.
101. B. J. Carmody, S. Arora, R. Avena *et al.*, Accelerated carotid artery disease after high-dose head and neck radiotherapy: is there a role for routine carotid duplex surveillance? *Journal of Vascular Surgery*, **30**(6) (1999), 1045–51.
102. L. F. Fajardo L.-G., S. D. Prionas, G. L. Kaluza & A. E. Raizner, Acute vasculitis after endovascular brachytherapy. *International Journal of Radiation Oncology, Biology, Physics*, **53**(3) (2002), 714–9.
103. M. C. Morice, P. W. Serruys, J. E. Sousa *et al.*, RAVEL study group. Randomized study with the sirolimus-coated bx velocity balloon-expandable stent in the treatment of patients with *de novo* native coronary artery lesions. A randomized comparison of a sirolimus-eluting stent with a standard stent for coronary revascularization. *New England Journal of Medicine*, **346**(23) (2002), 1773–80.
104. J. E. Sousa, M. A. Costa, A. C. Abizaid *et al.*, Sustained suppression of neointimal proliferation by sirolimus-eluting stents: one-year angiographic and intravascular ultrasound follow-up. *Circulation*, **104**(17) (2001), 2007–11.

105. F. Liistro, G. Stankovic, C. Di Mario *et al.*, First clinical experience with a paclitaxel derivate-eluting polymer stent system implantation for in-stent restenosis: immediate and long-term clinical and angiographic outcome. *Circulation*, **105**(16) (2002), 1883–6.
106. A. Farb, P. F. Heller, S. Shroff *et al.*, Pathological analysis of local delivery of paclitaxel via a polymer-coated stent. *Circulation*, **104**(4) (2001), 473–9.
107. K. Rosenfield, R. Schainfeld, A. Pieczek, L. Haley & J. M. Isner, Restenosis of endovascular stents from stent compression. *Journal of the American College of Cardiology*, **29**(2) (1997), 328–38.
108. S. H. Duda, B. Pusich, G. Richter *et al.*, Sirolimus-eluting stents for the treatment of obstructive superficial femoral artery disease: six-month results. *Circulation*, **106**(12) (2002), 1505–9.
109. P. B. Sick, O. Brosteanu, J. Niebauer, C. Hehrlein, G. Schuler, Neointima formation after stent implantation in an experimental model of restenosis: polytetrafluoroethylene-covered versus uncovered stainless steel stents. *Heart Disease*, **4**(1) (2002), 18–25.
110. P. B. Lundquist, B. Kalin, P. Olofsson & J. Swedenborg, Endovascular treatment of atherosclerotic lower limb lesions using a PTFE-collared stent-graft. *Journal of Endovascular Therapy*, **7**(3) (2000), 221–6.
111. R. Ahmadi, M. Schillinger, T. Maca & E. Minar, Femoropopliteal arteries: immediate and long-term results with a dacron-covered stent-graft. *Radiology*, **223**(2) (2002), 345–50.
112. G. Bauermeister, Endovascular stent-grafting in the treatment of superficial femoral artery occlusive disease. *Journal of Endovascular Therapy*, **8**(3) (2001), 315–20.
113. K. Arakawa, K. Hagisawa, H. Kusano *et al.*, Sonodynamic therapy decreased neointimal hyperplasia after stenting in the rabbit iliac artery. *Circulation*, **105**(2) (2002), 149–51.
114. P. J. Fitzgerald, A. Takagi, M. P. Moore *et al.*, Intravascular sonotherapy decreases neointimal hyperplasia after stent implantation in swine. *Circulation*, **103**(14) (2001), 1828–31.
115. A. Lu, G. Jia, G. Gao & X. Wang, The effect of magnetic stent on coronary restenosis after percutaneous transluminal coronary angioplasty in dogs. *Chinese Medical Journal*, **114**(8) (2001), 821–3.
116. I. K. De Scheerder, K. Wang, X. R. Zhou *et al.*, Optimal dosing of intravascular low-power red laser light as an adjunct to coronary stent implantation: insights from a porcine coronary stent model. *Journal of Clinical Laser Medicine and Surgery*, **19**(5) (2001), 261–5.
117. C. K. Zarins, C. T. Lu, A. E. McDonnell & W. M. Whitehouse, Jr., Limb salvage by percutaneous transluminal recanalization of the occluded superficial femoral artery. *Surgery*, **87**(6) (1980), 701–8.
118. W. M. Abbott, R. M. Green, T. Matsumoto *et al.*, Prosthetic above-knee femoropopliteal bypass grafting: results of a multicenter randomized prospective trial. Above-Knee Femoropopliteal Study Group. *Journal of Vascular Surgery*, **25**(1) (1997), 19–28.
119. A. Dardik, A. Liu & B. J. Ballermann, Chronic *in vitro* shear stress stimulates endothelial cell retention on prosthetic vascular grafts and reduces subsequent in vivo neointimal thickness. *Journal of Vascular Surgery*, **29**(1) (1999), 157–67.
120. M. H. Wu, Y. Kouchi, Y. Onuki *et al.*, Effect of differential shear stress on platelet aggregation, surface thrombosis, and endothelialization of bilateral carotid-femoral grafts in the dog. *Journal of Vascular Surgery*, **22**(4) (1995), 382–92.
121. J. J. Wentzel, D. M. Whelan, W. J. van der Giessen *et al.*, Coronary stent implantation changes 3-D vessel geometry and 3-D shear stress distribution. *Journal of Biomechanics*, **33**(10) (2000), 1287–95.
122. C. Kleinstreuer, S. Hyun, J. R. Buchanan, Jr. *et al.*, Hemodynamic parameters and early intimal thickening in branching blood vessels. *Critical Reviews in Biomedical Engineering*, **29**(1) (2001), 1–64.
123. M. Lei, J. P. Archie & C. Kleinstreuer, Computational design of a bypass graft that minimizes wall shear stress gradients in the region of the distal anastomosis. *Journal of Vascular Surgery*, **25**(4) (1997), 637–46.
124. D. A. Summer, Essential haemodynamic principles. In *Vascular Surgery*, 5th edn, ed. R. B. Rutherford. (New York: W. B. Saunders, 2000), pp. 91–2.
125. J. L. Berry, E. Manoach, C. Mekkaoui *et al.*, Hemodynamics and wall mechanics of a compliance matching stent: *in vitro* and *in vivo* analysis. *Journal of Vascular and Interventional Radiology*, **13**(1) (2002), 97–105.
126. P. J. O'Hara, N. R. Hertzer, E. J. Mascha *et al.*, A prospective, randomized study of saphenous vein patching versus synthetic patching during carotid endarterectomy. *Journal of Vascular Surgery*, **35**(2) (2002), 324–32.

127. V. Trisal, T. Paulson, S. S. Hans & V. Mittal, Carotid artery restenosis: an ongoing disease process. *American Surgeon*, **68**(3) (2002), 275–80.
128. K. J. Airenne, M. O. Hiltunen, M. P. Turunen *et al.*, Baculovirus-mediated periadventitial gene transfer to rabbit carotid artery. *Gene Therapy*, **7**(17) (2000), 1499–504.
129. R. Brauner, H. Laks, D. C. Drinkwater *et al.*, Controlled periadventitial administration of verapamil inhibits neointimal smooth muscle cell proliferation and ameliorates vasomotor abnormalities in experimental vein bypass grafts. *Journal of Thoracic and Cardiovascular Surgery*, **114**(1) (1997), 53–63.
130. G. J. Toes, E. S. Barnathan, H. Liu, Inhibition of vein graft intimal and medial thickening by periadventitial application of a sulfated carbohydrate polymer. *Journal of Vascular Surgery*, **23**(4) (1996), 650–6.
131. E. Alt, I. Haehnel, C. Beilharz *et al.*, Inhibition of neointima formation after experimental coronary artery stenting: a new biodegradable stent coating releasing hirudin and the prostacyclin analogue iloprost. *Circulation*, **101**(12) (2000), 1453–8.
132. J. Armstrong, J. Gunn, N. Arnold *et al.*, Angiopeptin-eluting stents: observations in human vessels and pig coronary arteries. *Journal of Invasive Cardiology*, **14**(5) (2002), 230–8.
133. M. Degertekin, P. W. Serruys, D. P. Foley *et al.*, Persistent inhibition of neointimal hyperplasia after sirolimus-eluting stent implantation: long-term (up to 2 years) clinical, angiographic, and intravascular ultrasound follow-up. *Circulation*, **106**(13) (2002), 1610–3.
134. M. K. Hong, R. Kornowski, O. Bramwell, A. O. Ragheb & M. B. Leon, Paclitaxel-coated Gianturco-Roubin II (GR II) stents reduce neointimal hyperplasia in a porcine coronary in-stent restenosis model. *Coronary Artery Disease*, **12**(6) (2001), 513–5.
135. J. Wohrle, E. Al-Khayer, U. Grotzinger *et al.*, Comparison of the heparin coated vs. the uncoated Jostent – no influence on restenosis or clinical outcome. *European Heart Journal*, **22**(19) (2001), 1808–16.

14 • Pathogenesis of abdominal aortic aneurysms – a review

JOHN EVANS AND MATTHEW M. THOMPSON

INTRODUCTION

In recent years, the pathophysiology of abdominal aortic aneurysms (AAAs) has become better understood. Whilst it is accepted that the biomechanical effects of hypertension and increased physical forces do have a role to play, there is now increasing interest in the biochemical and cellular events occurring within the aortic wall. It has been recognized that a greater understanding of these events may well explain why aneurysms rupture at different sizes in different individuals, despite risk factors remaining the same. In addition, it is hoped that an understanding of these events may lead to new strategies for medical treatment of aneurysms.

The fundamentals of research into aneurysm pathogenesis can be divided into these areas:

- Epidemiology
- Histology
- Biomechanical effects of blood flow within the aorta
- Genetics
- Abnormal proteolysis
- Inflammation and the immune response, and more recently
- Oxidative stress

By necessity, there is much overlap between these areas, but for the purposes of this review, each will be considered separately.

EPIDEMIOLOGY

One of the first steps in studying a disease process is to examine the epidemiology. The identification of disease associations is never sufficient to prove causality, but will at least provide a scientifically sound basis for further study. Associations may be both positive and negative, and some remain unclear. Proven associations with abdominal aortic aneurysms may be divided into eight areas:

(1) Family history
(2) Smoking
(3) Gender
(4) Age
(5) Lipids
(6) Blood pressure
(7) Race
(8) Diabetes

Family history

Familial studies may well help to identify whether there is a genetic component to the disease pathogenesis. Family studies into AAA began in earnest in 1977, when Clifton first reported a family of three brothers, all of whom underwent surgery for AAA [1]. By 1984, Tilson and Seashore had a series of 50 families in whom the incidence of AAA was too high to be explained by random chance [40]. In 1989, Bengtsson *et al.* published the results of a trial which screened siblings of patients with known AAA [2]. Of 87 patients who accepted the invitation for screening, ten brothers (29%) and three sisters (6%) were found to have dilatation of the aorta, a much higher prevalence than in the general population. Bengtsson *et al.*, have also looked at the prevalence of AAA in the offspring of patients dying from ruptured AAA, and in that study eight out of 39 sons (20.5%) were found to be affected. The more recent study of Salo *et al.* [3] showed that having an affected sibling increased the relative risk by 4.33 times, such that the prevalence in male siblings over 60 was as high as 18%. This risk factor was independent of the sex or age of the proband.

Smoking

Smoking has been clearly and irrefutably associated with both AAA and atherosclerosis in numerous studies. Wilmink *et al.* reported a case-control study including 447 individuals and concluded that smoking increased

Table 14.1. *Risk factors associated with aneurysm development in published studies*

	Risk factor										
Study	M	F	Smoking	Age	FH	C	Chol	LDL	HDL	DM	BP↑
Lederle [13]	↑	↓	↑	↑	↑	↑	↑			↓	↑
Tornwall [12]			↑	↑			↑		↓		↑*
Singh [109]	↑	↓	↑						↓		↑ #
Pleumeekers [112]	↑	↓	↑	↑			↑				
Blanchard [11]	↑	↓	↑	↑			↔	↔	↔	↓	↑*
Vardulaki [6]	↑	↓	↑	↑							↑
Bengtsson [14]	↑	↓	↔	↔	↑						↔
Salo [3]	↑	↓		↑	↑						

M = Male sex; F = Female sex; FH = Positive family history; C = Caucasian race; Chol = Raised plasma cholesterol; LDL = Low-density lipoprotein; HDL = High density lipoprotein; DM = Diabetes mellitus; BP↑ = Hypertension; * Indicates studies in which both an increase in systolic and diastolic hypertension were found to be independent risk factors; # = Studies in which taking medication for hypertension was more significant than hypertension itself.

the relative risk by 7.6 times [4]. Moreover, even ex-smokers had a three-fold increase in risk. Duration of smoking was important, with each year of smoking increasing the relative risk of AAA by 4%. The amount smoked was not shown to influence the prevalence of AAA and after stopping smoking the risk declined only very gradually. Interestingly, smoking gave a higher relative risk of small rather than large aneurysms. The amount smoked was estimated by the level of plasma cotinine, a metabolite of nicotine. This was higher in patients with small AAAs. Perhaps unexpectedly, the levels of cotinine did not differ between patients with stable or expanding aneurysms. These findings suggest that smoking is a risk factor for aneurysm initiation rather than expansion.

This contrasts markedly with the report of MacSweeney *et al.* [5], which followed 43 patients with small aneurysms for three years and assessed the size of their aneurysms with serial ultrasound scans. Growth rates in patients who did not smoke averaged 0.9 mm per year compared to 1.6 mm per year in smokers ($p = 0.038$). These higher growth rates correlated significantly with serum cotinine levels. The results of Valdulaki *et al.* [6] also contrast with those of Wilmink – in this study the level of exposure to cigarette smoke was found to be more significant than the duration of smoking.

As yet, nobody has proven a causative link between smoking and AAA formation, but one paper looking at the effect of cigarette smoking on fluid extracted from iatrogenic skin blisters provides a possible theory [7]. In this study, blister fluid from the skin of smokers showed lower rates of collagen synthesis, lower levels of tissue inhibitor of metalloproteinase-1 (TIMP-1) and higher levels of matrix metalloproteinase 8 (MMP8).

Gender and age

In common with atherosclerotic disease, males have consistently been shown to be affected more than females [8; 9; 10]. Similarly, the age is a well-recognized risk factor, the incidence increasing with age. Papers dealing with these factors are summarized in Table 14.1.

Plasma lipid levels

There is a more complicated relationship between plasma lipid levels and the risk of AAA. Blanchard *et al.* failed to show any correlation between cholesterol levels, low-density lipoprotein (LDL) or high-density lipoprotein (HDL) and aneurysm risk [11]. Tornwall, however, showed an increased risk in patients whose plasma cholesterol was high and a protective effect was seen in patients whose serum HDL was high [12]. Also,

Singh *et al.* showed that low serum HDL gave an increased risk of AAA [109]. The work of Lederle with the American veterans also showed high cholesterol to be an independent risk factor [8; 13].

Blood pressure

There is some disagreement in the literature regarding the effect of hypertension on aneurysm risk. The American Veterans study [13] represented the largest of its type and showed hypertension to be an independent risk factor. Singh, however, only showed that taking medication for high blood pressure was a risk factor, whereas hypertension itself was significant in women [109]. Tornwall and Blanchard both showed both systolic and diastolic hypertension to be risks [11; 12]. A study of all men born in Malmo in the year 1914 failed to demonstrate hypertension as a risk factor at all [14].

Experimentally, AAAs artificially induced into hypertensive rats were found to grow larger than those in normotensives [15] and the dilatation correlated well with systolic pressure.

Race

Abdominal aortic aneurysm is predominantly a disease of Caucasians; indeed one recent study of familial AAAs identified 233 multiplex families in a multinational investigation and all of them were white [16]. Racial studies have predominantly come from America and have concentrated on the different prevalences in the Afro-American and Caucasian communities. Lederle *et al.* have shown a reduced risk in black people [13] and LaMorte *et al.* have shown a black:white odds ratio of 0.29 [17]. Whether or not this racial disparity is related to the distribution of diabetes is an interesting theory but remains unproven.

One English study has looked at the racial differences in patients presenting with aneurysms in Bradford, UK [18]. Over a seven year period, 233 AAAs were identified. Given the racial mix of the catchment area, 28 of these could have been expected to be in Asian patients. In reality, none were. Although assumptions made on this evidence alone would be fraught with difficulties given differing rates of racial uptake of healthcare facilities, it does provide some evidence that AAA is more common in people of Caucasian origin than Asians.

Diabetes

Diabetes is known to be a risk factor for atherosclerotic disease, but has been shown consistently to be protective against abdominal aneurysms (see Table 14.1) [11; 13; 17].

HISTOLOGY

Microscopic examination of the structure of the wall of AAAs and comparison with the normal structure of the aortic wall gave some of the earliest insights into the development of AAAs. The normal structure of the aortic wall consists of well-organized elastin lamellae held together in a collagen matrix. By contrast, aneurysms are characterized by a loss of elastin lamellae, changes in the elastin:collagen ratio and a marked inflammatory infiltrate. Zatina *et al.* demonstrated that loss of the normal lamellar architecture can lead to aneurysm formation, and Terpin and Roach showed a decrease in the number of aortic elastin layers in a group of lathyritic turkeys that were highly susceptible to aortic rupture [19; 20].

Inflammation is a feature of nearly all aneurysms and *in vitro* experiments by Anidjar *et al.* showed that the intensity of the inflammatory infiltrate correlated well with the size of the enlarging aneurysm [84]. A standardized scale of inflammatory response has been suggested, the Histological Inflammation Scale of Aneurysms. This categorized aneurysms into five groups:

(A) Mixed acute and chronic inflammation
(O) No inflammation
(1) Mild chronic inflammation
(2) Moderate chronic inflammation
(3) Severe chronic inflammation

The majority of aneurysms fell into group 1, whereas 5.4% fell into group 3, marking them out as 'inflammatory' aneurysms [21].

A study of mRNA levels in normal and aneurysmal aortic walls showed that there was an increase in the expression of mRNA coding for collagen I, but that mRNA coding for elastin was not increased. This may, in part, explain the changes seen in the elastin:collagen ratio in AAAs [22]. Whether or not the amount of elastin cross-linkages is relevant to AAA formation is a matter of some debate, but Ghandi *et al.* showed that an apparent decrease in elastin cross-linkage was only in proportion to the absolute decrease in elastin content [110]. Conversely, Minion argued that elastin actually increased in AAAs, but not to the same degree as collagen [23].

BIOMECHANICAL EFFECTS

It has long been known that aortic aneurysms occur mainly in the infrarenal aorta and as far back as 1967 it was suggested that this might be due to a reduction in the elastic lamellae in this region when compared with the thoracic aorta [24]. Zatina *et al.* investigated the role of the medial lamellar architecture in the formation of aneurysms in porcine thoracic aorta [19]. Two hypotheses were postulated as to why the human infrarenal aorta was particularly susceptible to aneurysm formation: firstly, that the blood supply to the vessel wall was less at this point than is seen in other areas of the aorta and, secondly, that the number of elastin lamellae was smaller than in other mammals of comparable size.

To test these hypotheses, the vasal blood flow of the porcine aortas was surgically ablated and the aortas were physically crushed to reduce the number of intact lamellae. The findings were revealing; whilst ligation of the vasa vasorum led to cell death in the medial compartment it did not lead to significant alterations in the extracellular matrix, nor to the formation of aneurysms in the two-month period of the follow-up. However, destruction of the elastic lamellae led to aneurysm formation in both ischaemic and non-ischaemic aortas, providing the number of intact lamellae fell beneath a critical threshold. The authors pointed out, however, that prolonged mural ischaemia may eventually lead to alterations in the matrix composition and so could not be discounted as a contributing factor.

Elastin supplies most of the expansile properties of the aorta, as well as contributing to tensile strength. Decreased elastin therefore leads to higher pressures, greater shearing forces and a weaker aortic wall. Combined with the fact that elastin concentration declines with age and is not replaced, this explains why the peak age incidence for AAAs is in the eighth decade [25; 26].

In 1991 Dobrin and Anidjar demonstrated that a reduction in elastin alone was sufficient to allow dilatation of the vessel in arteries cultured *in vitro*, and that loss of elastin alone caused the characteristic tortuosity seen in ectatic vessels [27]. However, loss of collagen from the vessels also led to dilatation and perhaps more significantly also caused the vessel to rupture in every case. This experiment utilized both canine carotid arteries and human iliac arteries *in vitro*, but considerable work has been done using a similar *in vivo* model [28].

In this model, healthy adult rats underwent laparotomy, at which point ligatures were placed around a section of the infrarenal aorta. Once the section was isolated, it was infused with elastase, which initiated the protein degradation. The elastase was then washed out and the circulation restored. This technique always led to aneurysm formation when pancreatic elastase was infused, but other agents have also been investigated [27].

Quantifying the extent to which biomechanical variables contribute to aneurysm formation has not been easy. Many experimental studies have suggested that hypertension should be a risk factor, notably those of Reilly and Tilson [15; 29]. However, there remains no consistent epidemiological data to support this hypothesis. Nevertheless, experimental models of aneurysmal disease have shown that hypertension can increase both the size of the aneurysm and the rate of rupture [30]. What is not clear is the mechanism by which hypertension can induce or support the formation of aneurysms. In one study, patients on beta-blocking medication had a reduced incidence of ruptured aneurysms and there has been considerable work undertaken to investigate the reasons for this [31; 32; 33].

Clinical experiments into the use of beta blockade to retard aneurysm growth were thus thought to be of utmost importance, and a multicentre, double-blinded, randomized and controlled trial was initiated. The results of this trial were reported in 2002 [34].

The Stanford group has developed a model to look at atherosclerosis in hypertension [35]. New Zealand white rabbits were fed an atherogenic diet for three weeks to initiate plaque formation. Dacron bands were then placed around the thoracic aorta to create a hypertensive segment proximal to the stenosis. That this area did indeed become hypertensive was confirmed by comparison to both operated controls with no dacron bands and to non-operated controls. In the banded group, the mean systolic pressure was 89 mm Hg $+/-3$ compared to 64 mm Hg $+/-4$ in the operated controls and 74 mm Hg $+/-3$ in the non-operated group. The main findings in this experiment were that when the hypertensive section of the aorta was analysed immunohistochemically and using epifluorescent microscopy, there was a dramatic increase in monocyte binding and the expression of endothelial vascular cell adhesion molecule 1

(VCAM 1). These were accompanied by increased intimal thickness and an accumulation of macrophages. A follow-up experiment looked at the same model of hypertension but this time added either a loose or firm wrap around the hypertensive segment [36]. This had the effect of preventing excessive wall motion when compared to the coarcted group with no wrap, leading to a level of wall motion similar to that seen in the non-coarcted aorta. Interestingly, despite the hypertension, the level of intimal thickening in the aortas in which excessive wall motion was inhibited was much less than that seen in the coarcted group without a wrap. These results suggest that it is the motion of the vessel wall that is a key factor and not purely the rise in blood pressure.

Another series of aortic banding experiments investigated the effects of coarctation on the nitric oxide system and will be dealt with in the section concerning oxidative stress [37; 38].

GENETICS

Aortic aneurysms share many of the same risk factors as atherosclerosis such as age, sex and smoking, and for this reason were considered to be a product of the same disease process. However, in the mid-1980s evidence began to accumulate to suggest that AAAs were more common in Caucasians than in Afro-Caribbeans, whilst the reverse is true of atherosclerosis [17; 39]. In addition, the fact that aneurysms tend to run in families was first documented in 1977 and since then several other observers have identified a familial component [1; 40; 41]. Proving a family link is not easy, and Collin has outlined some of the problems involved [42].

Questionnaires suffer three major drawbacks. Firstly, asking patients whether any of their relatives have aneurysms will only identify the incident cases, whereas the lifetime prevalence is at least three times the incidence. Secondly, due to the age of most AAA patients, it is possible that they may be separated from other members of their family and may be unaware of or have forgotten their families' medical histories. Thirdly, as AAA is a disease of old age, the relatives of the patient may simply be too young to have developed an aneurysm at the time of the questionnaire. Similarly, many patients with a propensity to develop aneurysms will die of other causes before the disease manifests itself. Nonetheless, telephone questionnaires have been undertaken. Verloes *et al.* performed a segregation analysis on data obtained from 324 probands, concluding that a single gene effect with dominant inheritance was the most likely explanation for the pattern of inheritance seen in their subjects.

Family screening studies have been conducted successfully using ultrasound, giving an average prevalence of 24% in first order male relatives compared with between 5%–10% in males with no affected relatives [2; 43; 44; 45; 46].

With this strong evidence that aneurysms were familial and not simply an advanced form of atherosclerosis, the search for genetic factors began in earnest.

The pattern of inheritance of possible candidate genes for aneurysmal disease has been investigated in an important recent paper. Kuivaniemi *et al.* led an international team that was able to identify 233 families with multiple affected members, every single family being Caucasian [16]. There was an average of 2.8 members of each family affected, although some had six or seven, and one family even had eight members affected. It was found that no single inheritance mode could explain the pattern of inheritance seen. Some 72% of cases could be explained by an autosomal recessive gene, whilst 25% could have been autosomal dominant. The remainder would have had to be an autosomal dominant with incomplete penetrance.

A variety of genes have been suggested as likely candidates. These include genes coding for the matrix proteins, proteolytic enzymes and their inhibitors, and two genes on chromosome 16 coding for the haptoglobin alpha chain and its neighbouring cholesterol-ester transfer protein [47].

Collagen is the major constituent of the extracellular matrix, particularly types I and III. Type III has been shown to be deficient in a group of patients with familial AAA [48] and a variation of the gene COL3A1 has been associated with the development of AAAs. Interestingly, the aneurysm wall in patients with this variant was found to be less elastic [49]. Kontusaari *et al.* investigated two families with mutations in this gene that developed aneurysms in a dominantly inherited manner [50]. In one of these families, collagen type III synthesis was severely impaired and they went on to develop a range of symptoms from AAA to full-blown Ehlers-Danlos syndrome. Conversely, by sequencing DNA from 50 unrelated patients with AAA, Tromp *et al.* showed that mutation in the gene coding for collagen type III was in fact a rare cause of AAAs [51].

An examination of the influence of differing collagen gene expression revealed some interesting results. Whereas mRNA for type I and type III collagen was increased in patients with aneurysms and in patients with aorto-occlusive disease, the actual concentration of collagen in aneurysmal aortas was reduced. This implies that far from varying rates of collagen synthesis causing aneurysm development, the real key is more likely to lie in different rates of collagen breakdown [52].

By contrast, Mesh *at al.* [22] sought to explain the different ratios of elastin:collagen in AAAs in terms of increased collagen synthesis rather than an increase in elastolysis. They showed that the expression of mRNA for type I collagen was indeed up-regulated in aneurysms and that the synthesis of elastin failed to increase accordingly. This effect is independent of age and the decrease in elastin may explain why AAAs develop in these patients.

The tissue inhibitors of metalloproteinases (TIMPs) are natural antagonists of the matrix metalloproteinases (MMPs). and one hypothesis suggests that aneurysm development may be a result of either a mutation in the genes coding for these molecules or a failure in expression. However, when Tilson *et al.* looked at the expression of TIMPs by fibroblasts from AAAs, they found these were all at normal levels. In addition, whilst a single-point mutation of the gene coding for TIMP-1 was found in two out of six patients, this did not affect the amino acid transcription [53].

The cathepsins are cysteine proteases with powerful elastolytic properties. They have been demonstrated in atherosclerotic plaques. Cultured smooth muscle cells secreted cathepsin-S when stimulated with interferon-γ or interleukin-1β [54]. In arterial smooth muscle cells they are naturally inhibited by cystatin C, for which a polymorphism has been identified in the signal peptide. In a study of 424 patients with AAAs, the growth rate of the aneurysm was significantly less in patients with the homozygous allele, AA. This suggests that the cathepsins have a role in aneurysm development [55].

Autoimmunity has been postulated as a possible cause of AAAs, and a study from Japan looked at the link between HLA haplotype and aneurysm prevalence [56]. They observed that the HLA-DR2(15) antigen was found in twice as many patients with AAA as without. Another Japanese case-control study aimed to investigate the relationship between mutation of the gene coding for platelet-activating factor acetylhydrolase (PAF-AH) and aneurysms. They found a significant increase in the mutant allele in patients with aneurysms than in the control group [57]. Another polymorphism that has been investigated consists of a single base pair deletion in the plasminogen activator inhibitor, PAI-1. The proportion of patients with the three genotypes (4G/4G, 4G/5G and 5G/5G) in the group with AAAs matched that of the general population. However, those with the heterozygous pattern displayed faster aneurysm growth than the homozygous 4G/4G, and the 5G/5G showed faster growth still ($p = 0.07$) [58].

Genetic variation in the haptoglobin gene and neighbouring cholesterol-ester transfer protein gene on the long arm of chromosome 16 were found to be increased in patients with AAAs when compared to healthy control subjects [59]. These genotypes were associated with an increased rate of aneurysm expansion and homogenates from the aortic walls of such patients also displayed increased proteolysis *in vitro*.

An exciting prospect for the future is the use of human gene array technology. One recent study was able to evaluate 265 different genes in a group of patients with either AAA, aorto-occlusive disease or neither [60]. Of the 265 genes studied, 11 showed significant differences when corrected and standardized. The results for these 11 genes are summarized in Table 14.2.

Table 14.2. *Differing gene expression in patients with abdominal aortic aneurysms (AAAs) or aorto-occlusive disease (AOD) when compared with control subjects*

Gene	AAA	AOD
Collagen type VI α 1	↓	
Glycoprotein III A	↓	
α -2 macroglobulin	↓	
MMP-9	↑	↑
Intercellular adhesion molecule-1	↑	↑
Interferon-β receptor	↑	↑
Laminin α-4		↑
Insulin-like growth factor-2 receptor		↑
Integrin α-5	↓	↓
Ephrin A5	↓	↓
Rho/rac guanine nuclear exchange factor	↓	↓

↑ = Increased gene expression seen.
↓ = Decreased gene expression.

ABNORMAL PROTEOLYSIS

The elastin:collagen ratio has consistently been shown to be reduced in AAAs when compared with normal aortas [61; 62; 63; 64], leading to loss of elasticity and weakening of the aneurysmal wall. This may not be simply due to increased elastin degradation, as Minion has shown that the total elastin content of the aneurysmal wall may actually increase, but that the corresponding increase in collagen is much greater [23]. Despite this evidence, there is little doubt that proteolysis plays an important role in aneurysm development [65]. Aneurysmal disease differs from stenotic disease by the intensity of proteolytic activity within the extracellular matrix. The established association with chronic lung disease supports the argument that elastolysis is a major contributory factor, and indeed this is an area in which there has been much research [66; 67; 68].

For some time, the cause of elastin degradation remained unknown, but even as early as 1980 Busuttil *et al.* described increased collagenase activity [69]. Vine and Powell in 1991 found a spectrum of collagenase activity in the aortic wall of both atherosclerotic and aneurysmal vessels ranging from 55–92 kDa [68]. Importantly, although the collagenase activity was limited, it increased dramatically when TIMPs were destroyed. Thompson *et al.* also described the increased expression of a 92 kDa gelatinase in AAAs when compared with both normal aortas and aorto-occlusive disease, and localized this to the area around infiltrating macrophages [67]. This gelatinase is part of a family of zinc-dependent proteolytic enzymes, the matrix metalloproteinases (MMPs), now known as MMP9. In the same year, Freestone *et al.* further elucidated the relative amounts of both MMP9 and MMP2 by a combination of gelatin zymography and immunoblotting [70]. This study demonstrated that the principal gelatinase in smaller aneurysms was MMP2, but that in larger aneurysms MMP9 predominated. McMillan *et al.* investigated mRNA levels for MMPs in AAAs and found that MMP9 was maximally expressed in moderate diameter (5–6.9 cm) rather than large (>7 cm) or small (<4 cm) aneurysms [111]. These findings suggested that whilst MMP9 was responsible for the rapid growth that was seen in this size of aneurysm, other enzymes were responsible for initiation and rupture.

Pyo *et al.*'s paper elegantly proves a link between MMP9 and aneurysm pathogenesis by looking at the effect of inhibiting it both pharmacologically and by targeted gene disruption [71]. Mice that were deficient in the MMP9 gene failed to develop aneurysms as their wild-type counterparts did when subjected to elastase perfusion of the aorta. Bone marrow transplants from each group to the other reversed the response to elastase infusion, demonstrating that the expression of MMP9 by inflammatory cells is crucial to aneurysm development.

Other MMPs have also been implicated in the development of AAAs [72; 73; 74], particularly MMP1 and MMP3. Vine and Powell also found immunoreactive MMP1 in extracts from AAAs [68]. and more recently the expression of MMP3, as measured by reverse transcriptase polymerase chain reaction (rt-PCR), was found to be elevated in AAAs when compared to aorto-occlusive disease [75].

Matrix metalloproteinase 13 is a recently described enzyme also known as collagenase-3 and its expression is tightly regulated. Mao *et al.* measured its concentrations in AAAs and atherosclerotic disease using rt-PCR and compared them to normal aortas taken from organ donors [76]. Whilst MMP13 was not expressed at all in normal tissue, it was found in atherosclerotic disease and in significantly higher concentrations in AAAs. Expression was localized to medial smooth muscle cells in the aortic tissue, and could also be detected in human vascular smooth muscle cells in culture.

Membrane type MMP1 (MT MMP1) is an activator of MMP2 and was found to be increased in aneurysmal aorta when compared to normal or atherosclerotic aorta. Membrane type MMP1 was localized to aortic smooth muscle cells and macrophages in aneurysmal tissue by immunohistochemical analysis. The ability to activate MMP2 was confirmed by the addition of radiolabelled pro-MMP2, and determination of the subsequent amount of radiolabelled active MMP2.

In vivo, the activity of MMPs is tightly controlled by their natural inhibitors, the TIMPs. In 2000, Olson demonstrated that TIMP-1 bound to both the monomeric and dimeric forms of MMP9, whereas TIMP-2 bound only to the active form [77]. Whilst it has been shown that the TIMPs are present in large quantities in AAAs, it has been suggested that it is an imbalance between MMPs and TIMPs that leads to the net increase in proteolysis seen [78; 79]. Knox *et al.* in particular showed that whilst the expression of

TIMPs was increased in both AAAs and aorto-occlusive disease when compared to normal aorta, the increase was not in proportion to that of MMPs [79]. Tamarina *et al.* also showed that the TIMP:MMP ratio was actually decreased in AAAs, despite an absolute increase in TIMP levels [80].

Whilst there has been considerable work published in the area of collagenases and other metalloproteinases in AAAs, less is known about the role of serine proteases. Elastases of approximately 20–30 kDa have been demonstrated in the inner aspect of the media in AAAs [81]. This elastase works best in the alkaline range, and is inhibited by α-1 anti-trypsin. The fact that it is also inhibited by phenylmethylsulphonyl fluoride (PMSF) confirms that it is indeed a serine protease.

Five distinct serine proteases have been separated by gel electrophoresis from aortic aneurysm tissue [82]. suggesting there is a spectrum of enzymes at work.

In addition to MMPs and serine proteases, there is also the cysteine protease group. These differ from serine proteases by the substitution of an Asn residue for an Asp in the catalytic triad. Cathepsins S and K are examples of this type of elastase and have been shown to be produced in abundance by smooth muscle cells in atheroma [54]. They are inhibited by cystatin C, the expression of which is governed by a polymorphism of its signal peptide. As discussed previously, patients in whom the cathepsins were not inhibited displayed faster growing aneurysms [55].

INFLAMMATION AND THE IMMUNE RESPONSE

Inflammation is a characteristic feature of all AAAs, not just those previously thought of as 'inflammatory aneurysms' [21; 63; 66; 83]. In 1992, Anidjar *et al.*, demonstrated that during the development of aneurysms using the rat model, the timing of the inflammatory infiltrate correlated well with aneurysm expansion [84]. Elastolysis continued well after the infusion of elastase was discontinued, suggesting the inflammatory infiltrate was capable of activating endogenous elastolysis [85]. Similarly, Freestone *et al.* showed that in enlarging AAAs there was a denser inflammatory infiltrate when compared to small aneurysms [70].

Another method of inducing aortic damage in an animal model is the application of calcium chloride to the outside of the aorta in rabbits [86]. In a series of experiments by Freestone *et al.* this caused both medial injury with calcification as well as endothelial damage, echoing the pattern seen in most aneurysms. Interestingly, in this model, inflammation induced by the addition of thioglycollate to healthy aortas had no effect, but significantly increased the rate of dilatation in aortas that had previously been damaged by calcium chloride. Inflammation by itself would therefore seem to be insufficient to induce aneurysms in healthy aortas, but hastens their development in those that are already damaged. In a related result, it was found that the instillation of pure elastase into the isolated infrarenal aorta was unable, by itself, to induce aneurysm formation, but required the addition of an agent such as thioglycollate to initiate an inflammatory response [87].

Koch *et al.* have developed a scale for the measurement of inflammation in AAAs that allows some degree of standardization between investigators [88]. By immunostaining individually for T cells, B cells, macrophages, T-helper and T-suppressor cells, a gradient of inflammatory infiltration was demonstrated. Unsurprisingly, the highest level was described in 'inflammatory' aneurysms, followed by normal AAAs, then aorto-occlusive disease and finally the normal aorta. These results also suggested an immune-mediated aetiology behind the development of AAAs.

Proinflammatory cytokines have been demonstrated in the aneurysmal wall. In 1994 Szekanecz *et al.* analysed conditioned medium in which human aortic aneurysmal explants had been cultured [89]. The levels of interleukin-6 and interferon-γ were found to be significantly elevated when compared with both atherosclerotic and normal control tissue, although there was no difference seen in interleukin-2 and interleukin-4. Using homogenates of aortic tissue, interleukin-1β (IL-1β) and tumour necrosis factor-α (TNFα) were also both shown to be raised [90]. Taking this one step further, the addition of TNFα and IL-1β increased the expression of intercellular adhesion molecule 1 in human aortic endothelial cells, partially explaining the recruitment of inflammatory cells into the aneurysm. Conversely, by blocking the leucocyte adhesion molecule CD18 using specific antibodies, the growth rate of experimental aneurysms was significantly slowed [91; 92]. Keen *et al.* also found that the addition of

IL-1β to vascular smooth muscle cell cultures resulted in a dose-dependent increase in the expression of collagenase [93].

Perhaps some of the best evidence that inflammation is crucial to aneurysm development can be seen in studies using indomethacin. In 1996 it was shown that indomethacin prevented the development of aneurysms in the rat/elastase infusion model [94] and that this was due at least in part to a reduction in MMP9. Three years later the same group went further to elucidate that the effect was manifested through cyclo-oxygenase 2 (COX-2) and not COX-1 [95]. Franklin *et al.* combined *in vitro* studies of the effects of indomethacin on aneurysm development with a clinical case-control study to look at the effects *in vivo* [96; 97; 98]. In the laboratory experiments, the secretion of inflammatory cytokines was inhibited, whilst the case-control study demonstrated slower aneurysm growth in patients taking non-steroidals.

Gregory *et al.* have also hypothesised that there may be an autoimmune basis for aneurysm development [99]. The identification of immunoglobulin G (IgG) within the aneurysmal aortic wall led to the search for a putative autoantigen. They identified a peptide belonging to the microfibril-associated glycoprotein family, MAGP-3. Further support for the autoimmune theory can be found in the relationship between AAA formation and the major histocompatibility locus, HLA-DR. Mutations at this locus are implicated in a variety of autoimmune disorders, notably rheumatoid arthritis. Tilson *et al.* showed that the frequency of mutations in the HLA-DR locus in African Americans were far more common than could be explained by chance. These findings were especially interesting due to the fact that AAAs are extremely rare in Afro-Caribbeans [100].

OXIDATIVE STRESS

The action of reactive oxygen species has been implicated in the aetiology of many disease processes [101; 102; 103]. In particular, the effect of oxidative stress on many aspects of vascular biology has come under intense scrutiny over the past few years [104; 105; 106; 107]. In order to demonstrate an improvement in endothelial function when oxidative stress was reduced, Higashi *et al.* investigated patients with and without renal artery stenosis [107]. Renal artery stenosis is known to activate the renin-angiotensin axis and thereby cause a global increase in oxidative stress. In this experiment, the degree of oxidative stress was measured in two ways. Firstly, by urinary excretion of 8-hydroxy 2-deoxyguanosine (8-OHdg), an oxidized base which is an indicator of the degree of oxidation of DNA, and, secondly, by the levels of serum malondialdehyde modified low density lipoprotein (mm-LDL), both of which are recognized indices of total body oxidative stress. Endothelial function was assessed by the administration of acetylcholine (ACh), which causes vasodilatation in healthy endothelium, and by the administration of isosorbide dinitrate, which causes vasodilatation independently of endothelial function. The degree of vasodilatation after each stimulus was measured using forearm plethysmography.

In the patients with renovascular hypertension, the response to ACh was reduced and there were higher levels of the markers of oxidative stress. Following renal arterial angioplasty, the serum mm-LDL and the urinary 8-OHdg dropped, and the degree of vasodilatation improved, thereby neatly demonstrating a link between systemic oxidative stress and vascular endothelial function.

Other products of oxidation, namely mildly oxidized LDL (MoxLDL), have been implicated in the process of atherosclerosis by activating platelet-derived growth factor beta-receptor (PGDFbR) in cultured vascular endothelial cells [106]. Reactive oxygen species were increased by up to 70% in bovine aortic endothelial cells cultured in high concentrations of glucose for two weeks. This also caused an increase in both the expression and activity of MMP9. The addition of antioxidants significantly reduced the activity of MMP9, whereas the addition of inhibitors of protein kinase C had no effect. These results suggest that the increased proteolytic activity seen in the extracellular matrix in patients with diabetes mellitus is due, at least in part, to the effects of oxidation, and may help to explain a link between aneurysm formation and oxidative stress.

A further series of aortic banding experiments have demonstrated that in areas of high pressure there is an up-regulation of endothelial nitric oxide synthase (eNOS) when compared with tissues downstream of the artificial coarctation [38]. Measuring nitrotyrosine in the same tissues gave some indication of the degree of nitric oxide breakdown and sequestration by reactive oxygen species. In the areas above the banding (heart, brain and thoracic aorta) the levels of nitrotyrosine were much higher than in areas not exposed to high pressures (distal aorta). The inactivation of nitric oxide due to oxidative damage in areas of high pressure is another indication of vascular endothelial dysfunction, which may contribute to the pathogenesis of aneurysms.

Combining the *in vitro* elastase perfusion rat model of Anidjar *et al.* with modern cDNA microassay analysis, Yajima *et al.* looked at the expression of 8799 genes in rats with induced aortic aneurysms, and compared them with genes expressed in rats that had undergone sham operations [108]. Using this technique they were able to identify over 200 genes whose expression had more than doubled in the aneurysm group. Significantly, this included many genes reflecting an increase in oxidative stress, notably heme oxygenase, inducible nitric oxide synthase (iNOS), 12-lipoxygenase and heart cytochrome C oxidase, subunit VIa. Conversely, antioxidant genes such as superoxide dismutase, reduced NAD-cytochrome b-5 reductase and glutathione S reductase were found to be down-regulated. These two complementary findings both point to oxidative stress playing a major role in AAA development.

FUTURE RESEARCH AREAS

Future research into the aneurysmal process is likely to make use of powerful analytic tools including gene chip technology and proteomics. The ultimate aim of understanding the pathogenesis of aneurysms is to target the process of expansion and rupture, and to inhibit these.

REFERENCES

1. M. A. Clifton, Familial abdominal aortic aneurysms. *British Journal of Surgery*, **64**(11) (1977), 765–6.
2. H. Bengtsson, O. Norrgard, K. A. Angquist *et al.*, Ultrasonographic screening of the abdominal aorta among siblings of patients with abdominal aortic aneurysms. *British Journal of Surgery*, **76**(6) (1989), 589–91.
3. J. A. Salo, S. Soisalon-Soininen, S. Bondestam & P. S. Mattila, Familial occurrence of abdominal aortic aneurysm. *Annals of Internal Medicine*, **130**(8) (1999), 637–42.
4. T. B. Wilmink, C. R. Quick & N. E. Day, The association between cigarette smoking and abdominal aortic aneurysms. *Journal of Vascular Surgery*, **30**(6) (1999), 1099–105.
5. S. T. MacSweeney, M. Ellis, P. C. Worrell, R. M. Greenhalgh & J. T. Powell, Smoking and growth rate of small abdominal aortic aneurysms. *Lancet*, **344**(8923) (1994), 651–2.
6. K. A. Vardulaki, N. M. Walker, N. E. Day *et al.*, Quantifying the risks of hypertension, age, sex and smoking in patients with abdominal aortic aneurysm. *British Journal of Surgery*, **87**(2) (2000), 195–200.
7. A. Knuutinen, N. Kokkonen, J. Risteli *et al.*, Smoking affects collagen synthesis and extracellular matrix turnover in human skin. *British Journal of Dermatology*, **146**(4) (2002), 588–94.
8. F. A. Lederle, G. R. Johnson & S. E. Wilson, Abdominal aortic aneurysm in women. *Journal of Vascular Surgery*, **34**(1) (2001), 122–6.
   CORPORATE NAME: Aneurysm Detection and Management Veterans Affairs Cooperative Study.
9. P. F. Lawrence, C. Gazak, L. Bhirangi *et al.*, The epidemiology of surgically repaired aneurysms in the United States. *Journal of Vascular Surgery*, **30**(4) (1999), 632–40.
10. W. M. Castleden & J. C. Mercer, Abdominal aortic aneurysms in Western Australia: descriptive epidemiology and patterns of rupture. *British Journal of Surgery*, **72**(2) (1985), 109–12.
11. J. F. Blanchard, H. K. Armenian & P. P. Friesen, Risk factors for abdominal aortic aneurysm: results of a case-control study. *American Journal of Epidemiology*, **151**(6) (2000), 575–83.
12. M. E. Tornwall, J. Virtamo, J. K. Haukka, D. Albanes & J. K. Huttunen, Life-style factors and risk for abdominal aortic aneurysm in a cohort of Finnish male smokers. *Epidemiology*, **12**(1) (2001), 94–100.
13. F. A. Lederle, G. R. Johnson, S. E. Wilson *et al.*, Prevalence and associations of abdominal aortic aneurysm detected through screening. Aneurysm Detection and Management (ADAM) Veterans Affairs Cooperative Study Group. *Annals of Internal Medicine*, **126**(6) (1997), 441–9.
14. H. Bengtsson, D. Bergqvist, O. Ekberg, L. Janzon, A population based screening of abdominal aortic aneurysms (AAA). *European Journal of Vascular Surgery*, **5**(1) (1991), 53–7.
15. S. Anidjar, M. Osborne-Pellegrin, M. Coutard, J. B. Michel, Arterial hypertension and aneurysmal dilatation. *Kidney International Supplement*, **37** (1992), S61–6.

16. H. Kuivaniemi, H. Shibamura, C. Arthur *et al.*, Familial abdominal aortic aneurysms: collection of 233 multiplex families. *Journal of Vascular Surgery*, **37**(2) (2003), 340–5.
17. W. W. LaMorte, T. E. Scott & J. O. Menzoian, Racial differences in the incidence of femoral bypass and abdominal aortic aneurysmectomy in Massachusetts: relationship to cardiovascular risk factors. *Journal of Vascular Surgery*, **21**(3) (1995), 422–31.
18. J. I. Spark, J. L. Baker, P. Vowden & D. Wilkinson, Epidemiology of abdominal aortic aneurysms in the Asian community. *British Journal of Surgery*, **88**(3) (2001), 382–4.
19. M. A. Zatina, C. K. Zarins, B. L. Gewertz & S. Glagov, Role of medial lamellar architecture in the pathogenesis of aortic aneurysms. *Journal of Vascular Surgery*, **1**(3) (1984), 442–8.
20. T. Terpin & M. R. Roach, A biophysical and histological analysis of factors that lead to aortic rupture in normal and lathyritic turkeys. *Canadian Journal of Physiology and Pharmacology*, **65**(3) (1987), 395–400.
21. A. Rijbroek, F. L. Moll, H. A. von Dijk, R. Meijer & J. W. Jansen, Inflammation of the abdominal aortic aneurysm wall. *European Journal of Vascular Surgery*, **8**(1) (1994), 41–6.
22. C. L. Mesh, B. T. Baxter, W. H. Pearce *et al.*, Collagen and elastin gene expression in aortic aneurysms. *Surgery*, **112**(2) (1992), 256–62.
23. D. J. Minion, V. A. Davis, P. A. Nejezchleb *et al.*, Elastin is increased in abdominal aortic aneurysms. *Journal of Surgical Research*, **57**(4) (1994), 443–6.
24. H. Wolinsky & S. A. Glagov, lamellar unit of aortic medial structure and function in mammals. *Circulation Research*, **20**(1) (1967), 99–111.
25. R. A. Scott, H. A. Ashton & D. N. Kay, Abdominal aortic aneurysm in 4237 screened patients: prevalence, development and management over 6 years. *British Journal of Surgery*, **78**(9) (1991), 1122–5.
26. J. Collin, Prevalence, development and management of acute aortic aneurysm. *British Journal of Surgery*, **79**(4) (1992), 372.
27. P. B. Dobrin & S. Anidjar, Pathophysiology of arterial aneurysms. *Archives de Maladies du Coeur et des Vaisseaux* **84**(3) (1991), 357–62.
28. S. Anidjar, J. L. Salzmann, D. Gentric *et al.*, Elastase-induced experimental aneurysms in rats. *Circulation*, **82**(3) (1990), 973–81.
29. J. M. Reilly & M. D. Tilson, Incidence and etiology of abdominal aortic aneurysms. *Surgical Clinics of North America*, **69**(4) (1989), 705–11.
30. M. A. Ricci, J. M. Slaiby, G. R. Gadowski *et al.*, Effects of hypertension and propranolol upon aneurysm expansion in the Anidjar/Dobrin aneurysm model. *Annals of the New York Academy of Sciences*, **800** (1996), 89–96.
31. S. D. Leach, A. L. Toole, H. Stern, R. W. DeNatale & M. D. Tilson, Effect of beta-adrenergic blockade on the growth rate of abdominal aortic aneurysms. *Achives of Surgery*, **123**(5) (1988), 606–9.
32. M. A. Ricci, D. B. Pilcher & R. McBride, Design of a trial to evaluate the effect of propranolol upon abdominal aortic aneurysm expansion. *Annals of the New York Academy of Sciences*, **800** (1996), 252–3.
33. G. R. Gadowski, D. B. Pilcher & M. A. Ricci, Abdominal aortic aneurysm expansion rate: effect of size and beta-adrenergic blockade. *Journal of Vascular Surgery*, **19**(4) (1994), 727–31.
34. Propanolol Aneurysm Trial Investigators, Propranolol for small abdominal aortic aneurysms: results of a randomized trial. *Journal of Vascular Surgery*, **35**(1) (2002), 72–9.
35. B. I. Tropea, P. Huie, J. P. Cooke *et al.*, Hypertension-enhanced monocyte adhesion in experimental atherosclerosis. *Journal of Vascular Surgery*, **23**(4) (1996), 596–605.
36. B. I. Tropea, S. P. Schwarzacher, A. Chang *et al.*, Reduction of aortic wall motion inhibits hypertension-mediated experimental atherosclerosis. *Arteriosclerosis, Thrombosis and Vascular Biology*, **20**(9) (2000), 2127–33.
37. C. H. Barton, Z. Ni & N. D. Vaziri, Effect of severe aortic banding above the renal arteries on nitric oxide synthase isotype expression. *Kidney International*, **59**(2) (2001), 654–61.
38. C. H. Barton, Z. Ni & N. D. Vaziri, Enhanced nitric oxide inactivation in aortic coarctation-induced hypertension. *Kidney International*, **60**(3) (2001), 1083–7.
39. J. V. Robbs, R. R. Human & P. Rajaruthnam, Operative treatment of nonspecific aortoarteritis (Takayasu's arteritis). *Journal of Vascular Surgery*, **3**(4) (1986), 605–16.
40. M. D. Tilson & M. R. Seashore, Fifty families with abdominal aortic aneurysms in two or more first-order

relatives. *American Journal of Surgery*, **147**(4) (1984), 551–3.
41. J. Collin & J. Walton, Is abdominal aortic aneurysm familial? *British Medical Journal*, **299**(6697) (1989), 493.
42. J. Collin The Oxford Screening Program for aortic aneurysm and screening first-order male siblings of probands with abdominal aortic aneurysm. *Annals of the New York Academy of Sciences*, **800** (1996), 36–43.
43. M. W. Webster, P. L. St. Jean, D. L. Steed, R. E. Ferrell & P. P. Majumder, Abdominal aortic aneurysm: results of a family study. *Journal of Vascular Surgery*, **13**(3) (1991), 366–72.
44. D. C. Adams, B. R. Tulloh, S. W. Galloway *et al.*, Familial abdominal aortic aneurysm: prevalence and implications for screening. *European Journal of Vascular Surgery*, **7**(6) (1993), 709–12.
45. P. Fitzgerald, D. Ramsbottom, P. Burke *et al.*, Abdominal aortic aneurysm in the Irish population: a familial screening study. *British Journal of Surgery*, **82**(4) (1995), 483–6.
46. P. A. Baird, A. D. Sadovnick, I. M. Yee, C. W. Cole & L. Cole, Sibling risks of abdominal aortic aneurysm. *Lancet*, **346**(8975) (1995), 601–4.
47. A. Verloes, N. Sakalihasan, R. Limet & L. Koulischer, Genetic aspects of abdominal aortic aneurysm. *Annals of the New York Academy of Sciences*, **800** (1996), 44–55.
48. S. Menashi, J. S. Campa, R. M. Greenhalgh & J. T. Powell, Collagen in abdominal aortic aneurysm: typing, content, and degradation. *Journal of Vascular Surgery*, **6**(6) (1987), 578–82.
49. J. T. Powell, J. Adamson, S. T. MacSweeney *et al.*, Genetic variants of collagen III and abdominal aortic aneurysm. *European Journal of Vascular Surgery*, **5**(2) (1991), 145–8.
50. S. Kontusaari, G. Tromp, H. Kuivaniemi, A. M. Romanic & D. J. Prockop, A mutation in the gene for type III procollagen (COL3A1) in a family with aortic aneurysms. *Journal of Clinical Investigation*, **86**(5) (1990), 1465–73.
51. G. Tromp, Y. Wu, D. J. Prockop *et al.*, Sequencing of cDNA from 50 unrelated patients reveals that mutations in the triple-helical domain of type III procollagen are an infrequent cause of aortic aneurysms. *Journal of Clinical Investigation*, **91**(6) (1993), 2539–45.
52. G. S. McGee, B. T. Baxter, V. P. Shively *et al.*, Aneurysm or occlusive disease – factors determining the clinical course of atherosclerosis of the infrarenal aorta. *Surgery* **110**(2) (1991), 370–6.
53. M. D. Tilson, J. M. Reilly, C. M. Brophy, E. L. Webster & T. R. Barnett, Expression and sequence of the gene for tissue inhibitor of metalloproteinases in patients with abdominal aortic aneurysms. *Journal of Vascular Surgery*, **18**(2) (1993), 266–70.
54. G. K. Sukhova, G. P. Shi, D. I. Simon, H. A. Chapman & P. Libby, Expression of the elastolytic cathepsins S and K in human atheroma and regulation of their production in smooth muscle cells. *Journal of Clinical Investigation*, **102**(3) (1998), 576–83.
55. P. Eriksson, K. G. Jones, L. C. Brown *et al.*, Genetic approach to the role of cysteine proteases in the expansion of abdominal aortic aneurysms. *British Journal of Surgery*, **91**(1) (2004), 86–9.
56. H. Hirose, M. Takagi, N. Miyagawa *et al.*, Genetic risk factor for abdominal aortic aneurysm: HLA-DR2(15), a Japanese study. *Journal of Vascular Surgery*, **27**(3) (1998), 500–3.
57. N. Unno, T. Nakamura, H. Mitsuoka *et al.*, Association of a G994 –>T missense mutation in the plasma platelet-activating factor acetylhydrolase gene with risk of abdominal aortic aneurysm. (In Japanese.) *Annals of Surgery*, **235**(2) (2002), 297–302.
58. K. Jones, J. Powell, L. Brown *et al.*, The influence of 4G/5G polymorphism in the plasminogen activator inhibitor-1 gene promoter on the incidence, growth and operative risk of abdominal aortic aneurysm. *European Journal of Vascular and Endovascular Surgery*, **23**(5) (2002), 421–5.
59. J. T. Powell, A. Bashir, S. Dawson *et al.*, Genetic variation on chromosome 16 is associated with abdominal aortic aneurysm. *Clinical Science (London)*, **78**(1) (1990), 13–6.
60. P. J. Armstrong, J. M. Johanning, W. C. Calton, Jr. *et al.*, Differential gene expression in human abdominal aorta: aneurysmal versus occlusive disease. *Journal of Vascular Surgery*, **35**(2) (2002), 346–55.
61. P. B. Dobrin, N. Baumgartner, S. Anidjar, G. Chejfec & R. Mrkvicka, Inflammatory aspects of experimental aneurysms. Effect of methylprednisolone and cyclosporine. *Annals of the New York Academy of Sciences*, **800** (1996), 74–88.
62. G. D. Treharne, J. R. Boyle, S. Goodall *et al.*, Marimastat inhibits elastin degradation and matrix metalloproteinase 2 activity in a model of aneurysm disease. *British Journal of Surgery*, **86**(8) (1999), 1053–8.
63. J. Satta, A. Laurila, P. Paakko *et al.*, Chronic inflammation and elastin degradation in abdominal

aortic aneurysm disease: an immunohistochemical and electron microscopic study. *European Journal of Vascular and Endovascular Surgery*, **15**(4) (1998), 313–9.
64. J. J. Grange, V. Davis & B. T. Baxter, Pathogenesis of abdominal aortic aneurysm: an update and look toward the future. *Cardiovascular Surgery*, **5**(3) (1997), 256–65.
65. S. Anidjar & E. Kieffer, Pathogenesis of acquired aneurysms of the abdominal aorta. *Annals of Vascular Surgery*, **6**(3) (1992), 298–305.
66. P. K. Shah, Inflammation, metalloproteinases, and increased proteolysis: an emerging pathophysiological paradigm in aortic aneurysm. *Circulation*, **96**(7) (1997), 2115–7.
67. R. W. Thompson, D. R. Holmes, R. A. Mertens *et al.*, Production and localization of 92-kilodalton gelatinase in abdominal aortic aneurysms. An elastolytic metalloproteinase expressed by aneurysm-infiltrating macrophages. *Journal of Clinical Investigation*, **96**(1) (1995), 318–26.
68. N. Vine & J. T. Powell, Metalloproteinases in degenerative aortic disease. *Clinical Science (London)*, **81**(2) (1991), 233–9.
69. R. W. Busuttil, A. M. Abou-Zamzam & H. I. Machleder, Collagenase activity of the human aorta. A comparison of patients with and without abdominal aortic aneurysms. *Archives of Surgery*, **115**(11) (1980), 1373–8.
70. T. Freestone, R. J. Turner, A. Coady *et al.*, Inflammation and matrix metalloproteinases in the enlarging abdominal aortic aneurysm. *Arteriosclerosis, Thrombosis and Vascular Biology*, **15**(8) (1995), 1145–51.
71. R. Pyo, J. K. Lee, J. M. Shipley *et al.*, Targeted gene disruption of matrix metalloproteinase-9 (gelatinase B) suppresses development of experimental abdominal aortic aneurysms. *Journal of Clinical Investigation*, **105**(11) (2000), 1641–9.
72. K. M. Newman, A. M. Malon, R. D. Shin *et al.*, Matrix metalloproteinases in abdominal aortic aneurysm: characterization, purification, and their possible sources. *Connective Tissue Research*, **30**(4) (1994), 265–76.
73. E. Irizarry, K. M. Newman, R. H. Gandhi *et al.*, Demonstration of interstitial collagenase in abdominal aortic aneurysm disease. *Journal of Surgical Research*, **54**(6) (1993), 571–4.
74. K. M. Newman, Y. Ogata, A. M. Malon *et al.*, Identification of matrix metalloproteinases 3 (stromelysin-1) and 9 (gelatinase B) in abdominal aortic aneurysm. *Arteriosclerosis and Thrombosis*, **14**(8) (1994), 1315–20.
75. T. W. Carrell, K. G. Burnand, G. M. Wells, J. M. Clements & A. Smith, Stromelysin-1 (matrix metalloproteinase-3) and tissue inhibitor of metalloproteinase-3 are overexpressed in the wall of abdominal aortic aneurysms. *Circulation*, **105**(4) (2002), 477–82.
76. D. Mao, J. K. Lee, S. J. VanVickle & R. W. Thompson, Expression of collagenase-3 (MMP-13) in human abdominal aortic aneurysms and vascular smooth muscle cells in culture. *Biochemical and Biophysical Research Communication*, **261**(3) (1999), 904–10.
77. M. W. Olson, M. M. Bernardo, M. Pietila *et al.*, Characterization of the monomeric and dimeric forms of latent and active matrix metalloproteinase-9. Differential rates for activation by stromelysin 1. *Journal of Biological Chemistry*, **275**(4) (2000), 2661–8.
78. D. Mao, S. J. VanVickle, J. A. Curci & R. W. Thompson, Expression of matrix metalloproteinases and TIMPs in human abdominal aortic aneurysms. *Annals of Vascular Surgery*, **13**(2) (1999), 236–7.
79. J. B. Knox, G. K. Sukhova, A. D. Whittemore & P. Libby, Evidence for altered balance between matrix metalloproteinases and their inhibitors in human aortic diseases. *Circulation* **95**(1) (1997), 205–12.
80. N. A. Tamarina, W. D. McMillan, V. P. Shively & W. H. Pearce, Expression of matrix metalloproteinases and their inhibitors in aneurysms and normal aorta. *Surgery*, **122**(2) (1997), 264–72.
81. S. K. Rao, K. V. Reddy & J. R. Cohen, Role of serine proteases in aneurysm development. *Annals of the New York Academy of Sciences*, **800** (1996), 131–7.
82. G. S. Herron, E. Unemori, M. Wong *et al.*, Connective tissue proteinases and inhibitors in abdominal aortic aneurysms. Involvement of the vasa vasorum in the pathogenesis of aortic aneurysms. *Arteriosclerosis and Thrombosis*, **11**(6) (1991), 1667–77.
83. M. Wassef, B. T. Baxter, R. L. Chisholm *et al*, Pathogenesis of abdominal aortic aneurysms: a multidisciplinary research program supported by the National Heart, Lung, and Blood Institute. *Journal of Vascular Surgery*, **34**(4) (2001), 730–8.
84. S. Anidjar, P. B. Dobrin, M. Eichorst, G. P. Graham & G. Chejfec, Correlation of inflammatory infiltrate with the enlargement of experimental aortic aneurysms. *Journal of Vascular Surgery*, **16**(2) (1992), 139–47.

85. S. Anidjar, P. B. Dobrin, G. Chejfec, J. B. Michel, Experimental study of determinants of aneurysmal expansion of the abdominal aorta. *Annals of Vascular Surgery*, **8**(2) (1994), 127–36.
86. T. Freestone, R. J. Turner, D. J. Higman, M. J. Lever & J. T. Powell, Influence of hypercholesterolemia and adventitial inflammation on the development of aortic aneurysm in rabbits. *Arteriosclerosis, Thrombosis and Vascular Biology*, **17**(1) (1997), 10–7.
87. C. G. Carsten, 3rd, W. C. Calton, J. M. Johanning *et al.*, Elastase is not sufficient to induce experimental abdominal aortic aneurysms. *Journal of Vascular Surgery*, **33**(6) (2001), 1255–62.
88. A. E. Koch, G. K. Haines, R. J. Rizzo *et al.*, Human abdominal aortic aneurysms. Immunophenotypic analysis suggesting an immune-mediated response. *American Journal of Pathology*, **137**(5) (1990), 1199–213.
89. Z. Szekanecz, M. R. Shah, W. H. Pearce & A. E. Koch, Human atherosclerotic abdominal aortic aneurysms produce interleukin (IL)-6 and interferon-gamma but not IL-2 and IL-4: the possible role for IL-6 and interferon-gamma in vascular inflammation. *Agents Actions* **42**(3–4) (1994), 159–62.
90. K. M. Newman, J. Jean-Claude, H. Li, W. G. Ramey & M. D. Tilson, Cytokines that activate proteolysis are increased in abdominal aortic aneurysms. *Circulation* **90**(5 Pt 2) (1994), II224–7.
91. M. A. Ricci, G. Strindberg, J. M. Slaiby *et al.*, Anti-CD 18 monoclonal antibody slows experimental aortic aneurysm expansion. *Journal of Vascular Surgery*, **23**(2) (1996), 301–7.
92. G. Strindberg, M. A. Ricci, R. S. Guibord *et al.*, CD-18 monoclonal antibody blocks the early events of aneurysm expansion. *Annals of the New York Academy of Sciences*, **800** (1996), 266–7.
93. R. R. Keen, K. D. Nolan, M. Cipollone *et al.*, Interleukin-1 beta induces differential gene expression in aortic smooth muscle cells. *Journal of Vascular Surgery*, **20**(5) (1994), 774–86.
94. D. R. Holmes, D. Petrinec, W. Wester, R. W. Thompson & J. M. Reilly, Indomethacin prevents elastase-induced abdominal aortic aneurysms in the rat. *Journal of Surgical Research*, **63**(1) (1996), 305–9.
95. M. Miralles, W. Wester, G. A. Sicard, R. Thompson & J. M. Reilly, Indomethacin inhibits expansion of experimental aortic aneurysms via inhibition of the cox2 isoform of cyclooxygenase. *Journal of Vascular Surgery*, **29**(5) (1999), 884–92.
96. I. J. Franklin, L. J. Walton, R. M. Greenhalgh & J. T. Powell, The influence of indomethacin on the metabolism and cytokine secretion of human aneurysmal aorta. *European Journal of Vascular and Endovascular Surgery*, **18**(1) (1999), 35–42.
97. L. J. Walton, I. J. Franklin, T. Bayston *et al.*, Inhibition of prostaglandin E2 synthesis in abdominal aortic aneurysms: implications for smooth muscle cell viability, inflammatory processes, and the expansion of abdominal aortic aneurysms. *Circulation* **100**(1) (1999), 48–54.
98. I. J. Franklin, L. J. Walton, L. Brown, R. N. Greenhalgh & J. T. Powell, Vascular Surgical Society of Great Britain and Ireland: non-steroidal anti-inflammatory drugs to treat abdominal aortic aneurysm. *British Journal of Surgery*, **86**(5) (1999), 707.
99. A. K. Gregory, N. X. Yin, J. Capella *et al.*, Features of autoimmunity in the abdominal aortic aneurysm. *Archives of Surgery*, **131**(1) (1996), 85–8.
100. M. D. Tilson, K. J. Ozsvath, H. Hirose & S. Xia, A genetic basis for autoimmune manifestations in the abdominal aortic aneurysm resides in the MHC class II locus DR-beta-1. *Annals of the New York Academy of Sciences*, **800** (1996), 208–15.
101. G. Berkenboom, Unstable atherosclerotic plaque. Pathophysiology and therapeutic guidelines. *Acta Cardiologica*, **53**(4) (1998), 235–41.
102. J. W. Heinecke, Mechanisms of oxidative damage by myeloperoxidase in atherosclerosis and other inflammatory disorders. *Journal of Laboratory and Clinical Medicine*, **133**(4) (1999), 321–5.
103. S. Uemura, H. Matsushita, W. Li *et al.*, Diabetes mellitus enhances vascular matrix metalloproteinase activity: role of oxidative stress. *Circulation Research*, **88**(12) (2001), 1291–8.
104. F. J. Miller, Jr., W. J. Sharp, X. Fang *et al.*, Oxidative stress in human abdominal aortic aneurysms: a potential mediator of aneurysmal remodeling. *Arteriosclerosis, Thrombosis and Vascular Biology*, **22**(4) (2002), 560–5.
105. R. J. Chilton, Recent discoveries in assessment of coronary heart disease: impact of vascular mechanisms on development of atherosclerosis. *Journal of the American Osteopathic Association*, **101**(9) (Suppl) (2001), S1–5.
106. I. Escargueil-Blanc, R. Salvayre, N. Vacaresse *et al.*, Mildly oxidized LDL induces activation of platelet-derived growth factor beta-receptor pathway. *Circulation* **104**(15) (2001), 1814–21.

107. Y. Higashi, S. Sasaki, K. Nakagawa *et al.*, Endothelial function and oxidative stress in renovascular hypertension. *New England Journal of Medicine*, **346**(25) (2002), 1954–62.
108. N. Yajima, M. Masuda, M. Miyazaki *et al.*, Oxidative stress is involved in the development of experimental abdominal aortic aneurysm: a study of the transcription profile with complementary DNA microarray. *Journal of Vascular Surgery*, **36**(2) (2002), 379–85.
109. K. Singh, K. H. Bonaa, B. K. Jacobsen, L. Bjork & S. Solberg, Prevalence of and risk factors for abdominal aortic aneurysms in a population-based study: the Tromso study. *American Journal of Epidemiology*, **154**(3) (2001), 236–44.
110. R. H. Gandhi, E. Irizarry, G. B. Nackman *et al.*, Analysis of the connective tissue matrix and proteolytic activity of primary varicose veins. *Journal of Vascular Surgery*, **18**(5) (1993), 814–20.
111. W. D. McMillan, N. A. Tamarina, M. Cipollone, Size matters: the relationship between MMP-9 expression and aortic diameter. *Circulation*, **96**(7) (1997), 2228–32.
112. H. J. Pleumeckers, A. W. Hoes, E. Vander Does *et al.*, Aneursysms of the abdominal aotta in older adults. *American Journal of Epidemiology*, **142** (1995), 1291–9.

15 • Remodelling and AAA

JANET T. POWELL

INTRODUCTION

Smoking is an important risk factor for all forms of cardiovascular disease, but the association between smoking and abdominal aortic aneurysm (AAA) is much stronger than the association between smoking and coronary heart disease. There are other important risk factors for coronary artery disease, e.g. hypercholesterolaemia and elevated plasma fibrinogen concentrations. However, epidemiological studies have provided weak or conflicting evidence for the role of hypercholesterolaemia or elevated plasma fibrinogen in the aetiology of AAA. The cellular and molecular reasons why smoking is such a powerful risk factor for AAA are not clear. Since the smoking of hand-rolled cigarettes is associated with a much higher risk of death from AAA than the smoking of manufactured cigarettes, it is possible that components of the tar fraction of inhaled smoke are implicated in the aortic dilatation [1]. Cadmium and heavy metal deposition, from the inhaled smoke, do not appear to cause aortic dilatation [2]. Atherosclerosis is evident in both coronary heart disease and most cases of AAA, particularly in those over 60 years of age. However, the pathological hallmark of AAA is weakening and thinning of the medial layer of the aorta. The normal aortic media is thick and elastic, providing both the tensile strength and the elastic properties of the vessel that are necessary to conduct the pulse pressure, almost unchanged, from the aortic arch to the iliac bifurcation. With aging, the aorta becomes stiffer, probably associated with extracellular modification of the connective tissue components and diminishing elastin content. The wall of an AAA is even stiffer than the wall of non-dilated aorta in age-matched controls, suggesting more extensive changes to the connective tissue components of the media. These changes include the destruction of elastin and remodelling of the collagen fibres in the aortic wall. The destruction of elastin, with weakening of associated collagen and other fibres, is considered to be a critical process underlying aneurysmal or expansive aortic remodelling. How does this occur? Can constrictive atherosclerotic artery remodelling account for the symptoms of coronary heart disease or aortic occlusive disease, whilst only expansive atherosclerotic artery remodelling is observed in AAA? This chapter will discuss the hypothesis that expansive atherosclerotic remodelling with overcompensation causes AAA (Figure 15.1).

AORTIC ANEURYSMS IN THE ABSENCE OF ATHEROSCLEROSIS

Most aortic aneurysms are found in the infrarenal aorta, proximal to the first major bifurcation (iliac) of the aorta. The infrarenal aorta is an elastic artery, with elastin comprising 30%–35% of the dry weight of the healthy abdominal aorta in young adulthood. The other major protein component of the aorta is collagen, principally types I and III. The thickness of the healthy aortic wall results from the medial structure of vascular smooth muscle cells set in a matrix of elastic connective tissue (Figure 15.2). Apart from elastin and collagen, the connective tissue contains fibrillin, fibrillar glycoproteins and glycosaminoglycans. The media receives its nutrients from luminal perfusion, or vasa vasorum penetrating from the adventitia. However, the density of vasa vasorum and their penetration into the media is much lower in the healthy abdominal aorta than in the thoracic aorta. Therefore, smooth muscle cells in the abdominal aorta may function in a relatively hypoxic environment.

Genetic mutations in several of the protein components of the aorta are associated with AAA, occurring at a relatively young age, in the absence of atherosclerosis. For instance, the Marfan syndrome, where aortic dissection or AAA may be present as early as the third decade, is associated with mutations in the fibrillin-1 gene. Abdominal aortic aneurysm or aortic rupture also

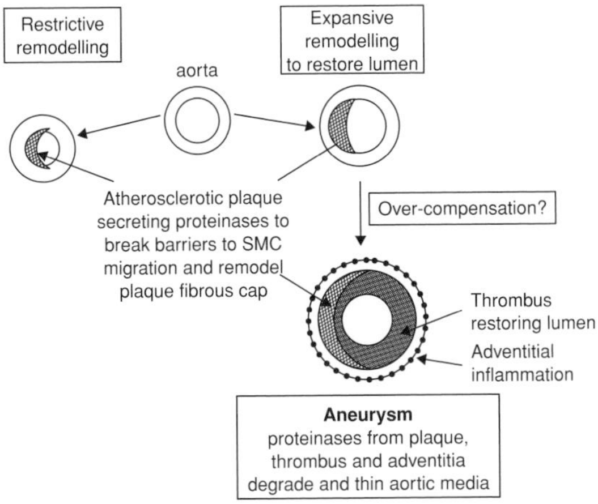

Fig. 15.1. Restrictive and expansive arterial remodelling. Does over-compensation of expansive remodelling lead to aneurysm formation?

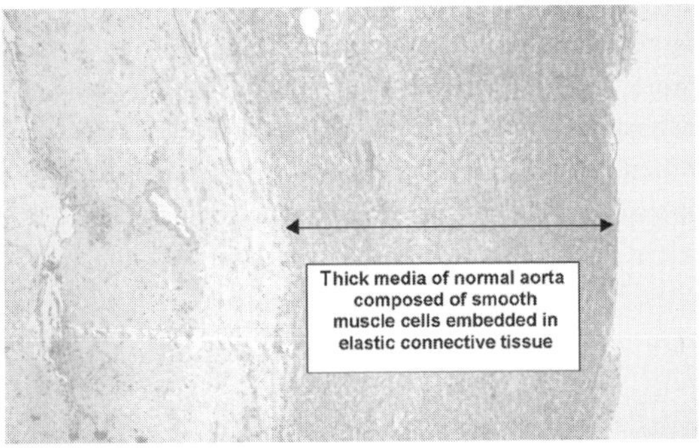

Fig. 15.2. The thick normal aortic media. Haematoxilin and eosin stained section of abdominal aorta showing the thick media (see colour plate section).

may occur in Ehlers–Danlos syndrome type IV, where there are mutations of the type III collagen gene. In both Marfan and Ehlers–Danlos syndromes, weaknesses and loss of aortic connective tissue caused the AAA. There are some other examples of mutations in the type III collagen gene segregating with the AAA phenotype in 30–50 year olds in families without classic Ehlers–Danlos syndrome. These are rare instances and in general there is no evidence that mutations in type III collagen are associated with AAA in the older patients (particularly men over 65 years), where AAA is most prevalent [3]. Mutations in the elastin gene do not appear to be associated with AAA or expansive arterial remodelling. However, mutations in the elastin gene are associated with a form of restrictive arterial remodelling, supravalvular

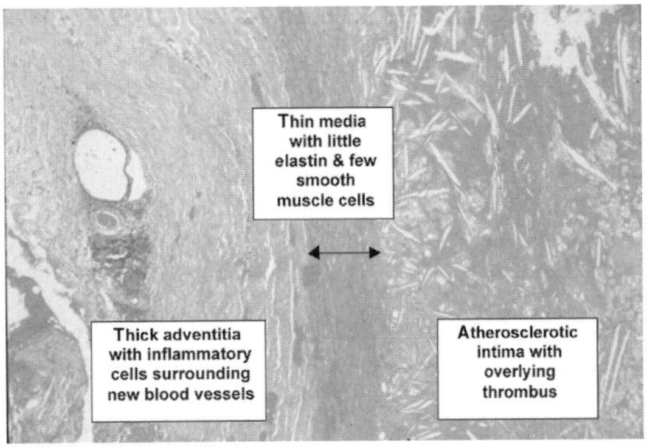

Fig. 15.3. The thin media in an abdominal aortic aneurysm. The section has been stained with haematoxilin and eosin (see colour plate section).

aortic stenosis [4]. Even gene knock-out or gene over-expression studies in mice have provided no evidence to support a role for elastin mutations causing aortic aneurysms.

Infection also may cause aortic aneurysms in the absence of atherosclerosis. The historical example is the syphilitic aneurysm, usually found close to the aortic arch, in the proximal descending aorta. Syphilis is now a very uncommon cause of aneurysms. However, there are interesting examples of mycotic aneurysms in young women in South Africa [5]. The suspected organisms include salmonella and tuberculosis. The pathology shows extensive inflammation in the aneurysm wall.

PATHOLOGICAL PARADIGMS FOR THE FORMATION OF ABDOMINAL AORTIC ANEURYSMS

The examples described above provide the background for contemporary paradigms concerning the pathogenesis of AAA, as elaborated by Shah in 1997 [6]. Weakened connective tissue, resulting from proteolysis, and inflammation, the source of proteinases and other factors stimulating arterial remodelling, lead to AAA (Figure 15.3). Over and above these factors, the apoptosis of the medial smooth muscle cells has been associated with advanced aneurysmal disease [7]. The three biological processes, proteolysis, inflammation and smooth muscle cell apoptosis will be the focus of subsequent sections.

PROTEOLYSIS AND THE FORMATION OF ANEURYSMS

The possible roles of proteolysis in restrictive and expansive arterial remodelling are outlined in Figure 15.1. So is there evidence that the atherosclerotic plaque secretes the enzymes associated with aortic thinning and aneurysmal dilatation? With elastin destruction being a histological hallmark, much of the focus has been on enzymes that can degrade elastin and its associated connective tissue components.

Experimental studies have shown that intra-aortic instillation of pancreatic elastase results in aneurysmal dilatation of the aorta of dogs, rats and mice. Pancreatic elastase has a spectrum of substrates, including elastin. Elastin is usually resistant to proteolytic degradation and is a protein with a half life of 70 years or more in man. In the aorta, particularly the diseased atherosclerotic and aneurysmal aorta, there are several different classes of enzyme with the capacity to degrade elastin and other components of the elastic connective tissue. These include serine, cysteine and metalloproteinases. There is also some information as to whether these different classes of enzyme are localized in the atherosclerotic plaque, in the media, adventitia or whether there is a transmural distribution of the cells synthesizing and secreting these enzymes. Several studies have compared proteolytic activity in the AAA wall and the atherosclerotic wall of age-matched patients with atherosclerotic occlusive disease. Homogenates of both these diseased aortic tissues contain high levels of proteinases and their inhibitors, but most studies have reported much higher proteinase activity levels (particularly against elastin substrates) in the AAA. The possibility that the initiation of expansive remodelling, or aneurysmal dilatation, uses a different spectrum of enzymes than the later stages that provide overcompensation for normal expansive remodelling.

Neutrophils secrete the powerful elastin-degrading enzyme neutrophil elastase. Although there may be transmural infiltration of inflammatory cells in AAA, neutrophils are scant [8]. The principal inflammatory cells are macrophages and lymphocytes. The serine proteinases of the fibrinolytic cascade, urokinase-type plasminogen activator (uPA), tissue-type plasminogen activator (t-PA) and plasmin(ogen) may have a variety of functions in the diseased aorta. Both uPA and t-PA are expressed in macrophages, with particular concentration at the base of the necrotic atheroma [9]. These enzymes were also expressed in other areas of active inflammation and capillary neovascularization, including the adventitia. Urokinase-type plasminogen activator and t-PA are inhibited by plasminogen activator inhibitor-1 (PAI-1), which is also expressed in the aortic wall. However, the expression of PAI-1 was more restricted, and t-PA and uPA were expressed beyond the areas of PAI-1 expression, particularly in the outer aneurysm wall. Where the elastic connective tissue is damaged cryptic domains in a variety of protein components may become exposed. There is recent interesting work to indicate that cryptic domains in the laminin $\alpha 1$ chain can stimulate macrophage expression of both uPA and the matrix metalloproteinase MMP9 [10]. Laminin genes may be differentially expressed in expansive and restrictive aortic remodelling [11]. There is controversy as to whether the laminated thrombus that lines the wall of most aneurysms, is a source of the fibrinolytic enzymes plasmin, uPA and t-PA. The best evidence suggests that the thrombus may be a source of plasmin(ogen), an important enzyme in the activation of matrix metalloproteinase zymogens [12]. There is weak evidence to indicate that the plasma levels of plasmin-antiplasmin complexes predict those small AAAs capable of rapid expansion [13]. Functional polymorphisms in the PAI-1 gene predict the growth rate of small AAAs (*vide infra*) [14].

Cysteine proteinases capable of degrading elastin include the cathepsins S and K. These enzymes are not expressed in normal arteries, but are expressed in atherosclerotic vessels, by both macrophages of atherosclerotic plaques and smooth muscle cells in the sub-adjacent intima [15]. As for most classes of proteinases, cathepsins S and K have specific inhibitors that are synthesized locally, e.g. cystatin C which inhibits both cathepsins S and K. In aortic aneurysms, cystatin C expression was observed in medial smooth muscle and plaque macrophages [16]. However, in the early phases of plaque development, there was noticeably reduced staining for cystatin C. In addition, there appears to be an inverse relationship between plasma cystatin C concentration and aneurysm diameter [16]. Such findings indicate that cysteine proteinases from young atherosclerotic plaques could aggravate elastin destruction in the early phases of AAA development, particularly in AAAs <4 cm in diameter.

The matrix metalloproteinases (MMPs) are the class of proteinases that have received most attention.

Focus has been principally on three soluble members of this family that have broad substrate specificity for matrix proteins and glycoproteins, MMP2, MMP3 and MMP9. Of these, both MMP2 and MMP9 can degrade elastin, whilst MMP3 may have weak activity against elastin. Macrophage elastase, MMP12 also can degrade elastin, whilst MMP1 and MMP8, and other members of this family have fibrillar collagens as their substrate. Other members of this family are membrane bound, e.g. MT1-MMP (MMP14) and have roles in the activation of soluble MMPs. All of the soluble enzymes are synthesized as zymogens and are activated locally, after secretion, by plasmin, MMP3, membrane-bound MMPs or other proteinases in local proteolytic cascades [17]. They are named after the essential zinc atom in their catalytic site and have substantial sequence homologies. The number of metalloproteinases identified has increased rapidly over the last few years and the available evidence could have excluded knowledge of pertinent members of this ever-enlarging family of enzymes. Tissue inhibitors of metalloproteinases (TIMPs), TIMP-1, TIMP-2, TIMP-3 and TIMP-4, are synthesized locally. In the aneurysm wall both MMP3 and MMP9 co-localize to macrophages, that are present transmurally [18; 19]. This contrasts with the localization of MMP2, which is principally found in mesenchymal cells in the media and adventitia. Mesenchymal cells also express MMP1 and MMP9 patchily, but to a lesser extent than MMP2. Macrophage elastase, MMP12, is expressed predominantly by macrophages invading the media of AAAs and on residual elastic tissue: it is not present in the normal aorta [20]. There is no evidence that the expression or concentration of any of these metalloproteinases is higher in the atherosclerotic component of the wall than in the infrarenal media and adventitia. When samples of restrictive and expansive aortic remodelling are compared, there is a selective increase in MMP3 expression in aneurysmal or expansive remodelling [21]. This was accompanied by an increased expression of the inhibitor TIMP-3. Against this background, it becomes increasingly difficult to identify whether over-expression of MMPs by atherosclerotic plaques (that also express TIMPs) contributes to AAA formation. It is also difficult to assess whether the increased expression of specific MMPs is causative or reactive. For these reasons, selective gene targeting in mice has been used to provide complementary evidence. This evidence is summarized in Table 15.1 and discussed later in this chapter. However, there is important evidence from studies of MMP2 and MMP9 in AAAs of different sizes to indicate that MMP2 may play an important role in early aneurysmal remodelling, whilst the activity of MMP9 becomes more important as the aneurysm enlarges beyond 5 cm in diameter [22; 23].

INFLAMMATION

A spectrum of inflammatory changes occurs in AAAs, the most extreme being the inflammatory aortic aneurysm, where the fibrotic adventitia contains dense foci of inflammation with the presence of lymphoid follicles. Lymphoid follicles also are present in 35%–50% of aneurysms with less florid inflammation [24]. Inflammatory cells are present in all layers of the aortic wall, atherosclerotic intima, media and adventitia. These cells include mainly macrophages, T cells and B cells [8; 24]. There is no evidence that the lymphoid follicles contain B cell secreting antibodies to single specific antigens, including oxidized LDL that may arise from the atherosclerotic intima. This has been assessed by examining the clonality of immunoglobulin genes expressed by these B cells. However, all of these inflammatory cells secrete inflammatory mediators and/or proteinases to fuel the proteolytic destruction and progressive weakening of the aortic media of the expanding AAA. Interleukin-Iβ (IL-Iβ) is expressed strongly in atherosclerotic plaques, often co-localizing with cathepsins [15]. Tumour necrosis factor-α (TNFα) is expressed strongly in the endothelial lining of the neovascularized adventitia and in association with inflammatory cells throughout the aneurysm wall. These two cytokines are found at the apex of inflammatory cascades, but only for IL-1β is there any evidence to suggest stronger expression in the atherosclerotic intima than in the remainder of the AAA wall. Other cytokines such as monocyte chemoattractant protein-1 (MCP-1) and interleukin-8 (IL-8) may be secreted by macrophages throughout the AAA wall to recruit additional inflammatory cells and perpetuate the inflammatory process [25]. Whilst the level of inflammation in the aortic wall is variable, observational studies have indicated a strong correlation between adventitial inflammation and AAA diameter, whereas no such relationship was observed for the extent of atherosclerosis and aneurysm diameter (Figure 15.4) [22]. This indicates that adventitial inflammation and TNFα generation may be more important to AAA expansion than the inflammation associated with atherosclerosis, including IL-1β production. The

Table 15.1. *Gene targeting and aortic aneurysm formation in mice*

Gene targeted	Gene product function	Aortic phenotype
Fibrillin mutants and under-expression	Microfibril component	Aortic dissection with inflammation-mediated elastolysis, adult onset
Lysyl oxidase knock-out	Initiates collagen and elastin cross-linking	Aneurysm formation in neonates, with fragmented elastin
Apolipoprotein E knock-out	Clearance of lipoproteins and chylomicrons from circulation	Atherosclerosis with elastin fragmentation and medial destruction. Aneurysm rare
Apolipoprotein E and endothelial nitric oxide synthase double knock-out	Regulates vasomotor tone, anti-adhesive and anti-inflammatory	Aortic dissection in adults, with elastin fragmentation and medial destruction
Apolipoprotein E and uPA double knock-out	uPA is a serine protease, role in fibrinolysis and neovascularization	Atherosclerosis, minimal medial and elastin destruction: no aneurysms
Apolipoprotein E and t-PA double knock-out	t-PA, serine protease with role in fibrinolysis and plasmin activation of MMPs	Atherosclerosis, minimal medial and elastin destruction: no aneurysms
Apolipoprotein E and TIMP-1 double knock-out	TIMP-1 inhibits MMP9 and other MMPs	Atherosclerosis, minimal medial destruction, no aneurysms
MMP2 knock-out	Metalloproteinase degrading elastin and other connective tissue proteins	Normal, but protects from $CaCl_2$ induced aneurysm
MMP9 knock-out	Metalloproteinase degrading elastin and other connective tissue proteins	Normal, but protects from $CaCl_2$ or elastase perfusion induced aneurysm
MMP12 knock-out	Macrophage elastase	Normal, does not prevent aneurysm formation in elastase perfused aorta

importance of inflammation is supported by evidence showing that anti-inflammatory treatments attenuate the development of experimental aneurysms, although such experiments have not dissected out the role of specific inflammatory mediators.

SMOOTH MUSCLE CELL FUNCTION AND APOPTOSIS

Medial smooth muscle cells (SMCs) are the source of elastic connective tissue in the aortic media. The interaction of SMCs with the surrounding connective tissue will control the gene expression and phenotype of these cells. As the elastic connective tissue becomes disordered and degraded, normal signalling processes are disrupted. Experimentally, altered expression of fibrillin leads to increased MMP9 production by SMCs [26]. In addition, the SMCs function in a relatively hypoxic environment. The build up of luminal atheroma is likely to further restrict the supply of oxygen to the medial smooth muscle, and alter the phenotype and synthetic profile of these cells. Decreased SMC density is a key feature of AAA, accompanied by p53 expression [27]. This decreased smooth muscle density is assumed to occur by apoptosis [7; 27]. The macrophages and T lymphocytes of the diseased aortic wall produce perforin, Fas and Fas ligand, all death-promoting molecules. The abdominal aortic aneurysm wall contains CD4+ and

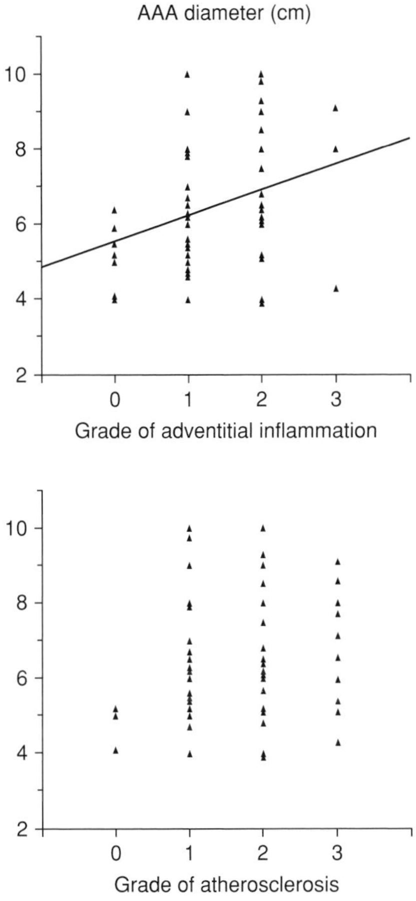

Fig. 15.4. The relationship between adventitial inflammation or atherosclerosis and aneurysm diameter. The data are taken from Freestone (1995) [22].

CD8+ T lymphocytes (not present in normal aorta) that produce perforin, to damage SMC membranes, and Fas. The medial SMCs also express Fas and other signals capable of causing SMC death by apoptosis [28]. Cystic medial degeneration of the aortic wall is also associated with increased expression of p53, Bax and other markers of SMC apoptosis [29], although increases in these specific markers are not confirmed in the medial SMC of AAAs [7; 27]. Atherosclerosis, probably does not have a pivotal role in causing the excessive SMC apoptosis in aorto-aneurysms in comparison to aortic occlusive disease. Therefore signals from CD4+ and CD8+ lymphocytes in the adventitia are more likely to cause thinning of the aortic media and rarefaction of its SMCs in AAA.

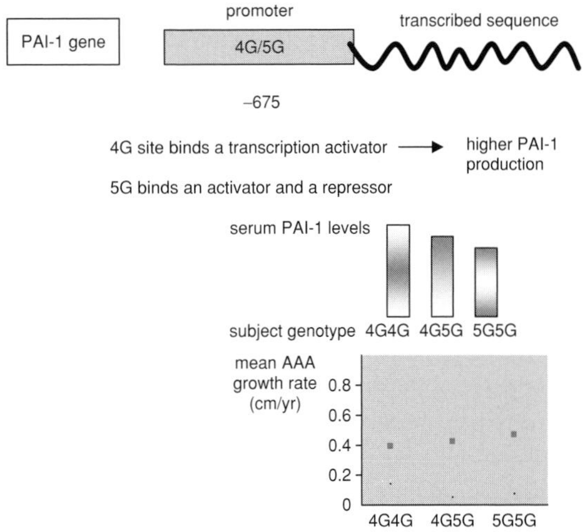

Fig. 15.5. Use of functional polymorphisms to identify the proteolytic cascades involved in the formation of abdominal aortic aneurysm. The example chosen is plasminogen activator inhibitor-1 (PAI-1).

GENETIC VARIATION AND EXPANSIVE ARTERIAL REMODELLING IN MAN

There is a well-documented familial association for AAA. About one-quarter of brothers of patients with AAA have an occult AAA detected by ultrasonographic screening. It is not clear whether this familial association results from environmental or genetic factors, or a combination of these. Population studies have suggested associations between polymorphisms in various genes and AAA. These genes include type III collagen, proteinases and proteins involved in lipid metabolism. The associations have been weak and possibly have arisen as a chance finding from under-powered studies. Scientifically it is more robust to use genetic polymorphisms (common minor variations in genes) for studies in association with AAA growth. To undertake such studies, it is necessary to identify functional polymorphisms associated with altered expression of the gene product. The only such study published to date has focused on PAI-1 [14]. There is a common variation at −675 in the promoter region of this gene, either 4G or 5G, which allows for the differential binding of transcription activators and/or repressors (Figure 15.5). The 5G allele is associated with lower transcription rates of the PAI-1 gene and subjects homozygous for the 5G5G allele have the lowest plasma PAI-1 concentrations. For patients with AAA, those homozygous for the 5G5G allele have significantly faster AAA growth of small aneurysms than patients of the 4G4G or 4G5G genotype. Since this implies that lower concentrations of this protease inhibitor permit slower AAA expansion, it is powerful evidence supporting the role of the serine proteases of the fibrinolytic cascade in AAA pathobiology. There are functional polymorphisms of many of the other candidate proteases involved in expansive aortic remodelling. Whilst there is published evidence associating some of these polymorphisms, including MMP9, with restrictive arterial remodelling in the coronary arteries, there is no available evidence for associations with expansive arterial remodelling.

GENETIC VARIATION AND EXPANSIVE ARTERIAL REMODELLING IN MICE

Many of the gene targeting studies, undertaken in mice, have helped to re-enforce the importance of proteolysis in aneurysm development. The apolipoprotein E double knock-out mouse has been used to generate the appropriate background of aortic atherosclerosis in adults, and the process can be enhanced by feeding the mice an atherogenic diet. Pertinent studies are noted in Table 15.1. The deletion of either uPA or t-PA genes rescues mice from aortic medial degeneration. Similarly TIMP-1 deletion, the relevant physiological inhibitor of MMP9, protects from aortic medial degeneration. Unfortunately, there are no reports of MMP gene deletion in apolipoprotein E deficient mice. The only evidence relates to the role of MMP2, MMP9 or MMP12 in rescuing from the expansive aortic remodelling caused by instillation of a pancreatic elastase or calcium chloride lesion. For expansive remodelling following a calcium chloride lesion of the aorta, there may be evidence that MMP2 and MMP9 work sequentially and/or co-operatively [28]. Other experiments provide support for the key role of connective tissue in expansive remodelling.

CONCLUSIONS

It is possible that atherosclerosis causes early expansive aortic remodelling, with secretion of fibrinolytic proteases, cathepsins and some MMPs by cells of the atherosclerotic plaque. However, there is no strong evidence to indicate that the transition from a minimally dilated aorta (2.5 to 3.9 cm) to a clinically relevant AAA (>4 cm in diameter) is caused by atherosclerosis. In contrast, there is considerable evidence to suggest that pathological inflammation of the adventitia causes the SMC apoptosis and proteolytic destruction of the elastic medial connective tissue that constitute the pathological hallmarks of AAA. Quantification of aneurysm wall thickness shows that wall thickness does not decrease with increasing aneurysm diameter, since there is compensatory adventitial thickening and fibrosis [22]. This is further evidence against the possibility that aneurysms form as a result of overcompensation of expansive remodelling. Frustratingly, there is not yet evidence that there is one pivotal proteolytic enzyme, the inhibition of which would provide a selective, rational target for limiting AAA expansion medically. Given the extent of biological redundancy and the widespread roles of the proteases in homeostasis, a single selective target may not be identified and future strategies may have to focus on local inhibition of classes of enzymes.

REFERENCES

1. D. P. Strachan, Predictors of death from aortic aneurysm among middle-aged men: the Whitehall study. *British Journal of Surgery*, **78** (1991), 401–4.
2. S. Abu-Hayyeh, M. Sian, K. G. Jones, A. Manuel & J. T. Powell, Cadmium accumulation in aortas of smokers. *Arteriosclerosis, Thrombosis and Vascular Biology*, **21** (2001), 863–7.
3. G. Tromp, Y. Wu, D. J. Prockop *et al.*, Sequencing of cDNA from 50 unrelated patients reveals that mutations of triple-helical domain of type III procollagen are an infrequent cause of aortic aneurysms. *Journal of Clinical Investigation*, **91** (1993), 2539–45.
4. A. K. Ewart, W. Jin, D. Atkinson, C. A. Morris & M. T. Keating, Supravalvular aortic stenosis associated with a deletion disrupting the elastin gene. *Journal of Clinical Investigation*, **93** (1994), 1071–7.
5. M. Costa & J. V. Robbs, Abdominal aneurysms in a black population: clinicopathologtical study. *British Journal of Surgery*, **73** (1986), 554–8.

6. P. K. Shah, Inflammation, metalloproteinases, and increased proteolysis: an emerging pathophysiological paradigm in aortic aneurysm. *Circulation*, **96** (1997), 2115–17.
7. A. Lopez-Candales, D. R. Holmes, S. Liao *et al.*, Decreased vascular smooth muscle cell density in medial degeneration of abdominal aortic aneurysms. *American Journal of Pathology*, **150** (1997), 993–1007.
8. A. E. Koch, G. K. Haines, R. J. Rizzo *et al.*, Human abdominal aortic aneurysms. Immunophenotypic analysis suggests immune-mediated response. *American Journal of Pathology*, **137** (1990), 1199–13.
9. J. Schneiderman, G. M. Bordin, I. Engelberg *et al.*, Expression of fibrinolytic genes in atherosclerotic abdominal aneurysm wall. A possible mechanism for aneurysm expansion. *Journal of Clinical Investigation*, **96** (1995), 639–45.
10. K. M. Faisal Khan, G. W. Laurie, T. A. McCaffrey & D. J. Falcone, Exposure of cryptic domains in the alpha 1-chain of laminin elastase stimulates macrophages urokinase and matrix metalloproteinase-9 expression. *Journal of Biological Chemistry*, **277** (2002), 13778–86.
11. W. S. Tung, J. K. Lee & R. W. Thompson, Simultaneous analysis of 1176 gene products in normal human aorta and abdominal aortic aneurysms using a membrane-based complementary DNA expression array. *Journal of Vascular Surgery*, **34** (2001), 143–150.
12. V. Fontaine, M. P. Jacob, X. Houard *et al.*, Involvement of the mural thrombus as a site of protease release and activation in human aortic aneurysms. *American Journal of Pathology*, **161** (2002), 1701–10.
13. J. S. Lindholt, B. Jorgensen, H. Fasting & E. W. Henneberg, Plasma levels of plasmin-antiplasmin-complexes are predictive for small abdominal aortic aneurysms expanding to operation-recommendable size. *Journal of Vascular Surgery*, **34** (2001), 611–15.
14. K. Jones, J. Powell, L. Brown *et al.*, The influence of 4G/5G polymorphism in the plasminogen activator inhibitor-1 gene promoter on the incidence, growth and operative risk of abdominal aneurysm. *European Journal of Vascular and Endovascular Surgery*, **23** (2002), 421–5.
15. G. K. Sukhova, G. P. Shi, D. I. Simon, H. A. Chapman & P. Libby, Expression of the elastolytic cathepsins S and K in human atheroma and regulation of their production in smooth muscle cells. *Journal of Clinical Investigation*, **102** (1998), 576–83.
16. G. P. Shi, G. K. Sukhova, A. Grubb *et al.*, Cystatin C deficiency in human atherosclerosis and aortic aneurysms. *Journal of Clinical Investigation*, **104** (1999), 1191–7.
17. H. Nagase & J. F. Woessner, Jr., Matrix metalloproteinases. *Journal of Biological Chemistry*, **274** (1999), 21491–4.
18. K. M. Newman, J. Jean-Claude, H. Li *et al.*, Cellular localization of matrix metalloproteinases in the abdominal aortic aneurysm wall. *Journal of Vascular Surgery*, **20** (1994), 814–20.
19. R. W. Thompson, D. R. Holmes, R. A. Mertens *et al.*, Production and localization of 92-kilodalton gelatinase in abdominal aortic aneurysms. An elastolytic metalloproteinase expressed by aneurysm-infiltrating macrophages. *Journal of Clinical Investigation*, **96** (1995), 318–26.
20. J. A. Curci, S. Liao, M. D. Huffman, S. D. Shapiro & R. W. Thompson, Expression and localization of macrophage elastase (matrix metalloproteinase-12) in abdominal aortic aneurysms. *Journal of Clinical Investigation*, **102** (1998), 1900–10.
21. T. W. G. Carrell, K. G. Burnand, G. M. A. Wells, J. M. Clements & A. Smith, Stromelysin-1 (matrix metalloproteinase-3) and tissue inhibitor of metalloproteinase-3 are overexpressed in the wall of abdominal aortic aneurysms. *Circulation*, **105** (2002), 477–82.
22. T. Freestone, Inflammation and matrix metalloproteinases in the enlarging abdominal aortic aneurysm. *Arteriosclerosis, Thrombosis and Vascular Biology*, **15** (1995), 1145–51.
23. W. D. McMillan, N. A. Tamarina, M. Cipollone *et al.*, Size matters: the relationship between MMP-9 expression and aortic diameter. *Circulation*, **96** (1997), 2228–32.
24. L. J. Walton, J. T. Powell, D. V. Parums, Unrestricted usage of immunoglobulin heavy heavy chain genes in B cells infiltrating the wall of atherosclerotic abdominal aortic aneurysms. *Atherosclerosis*, **135** (1997), 65–71.
25. A. E. Koch, S. L. Kunkel, W. H. Pearce *et al.*, Enhanced production of the chemotactic cytokines interleukin-8 and monocyte chemoattractant protein-1 in human abdominal aortic aneurysms. *American Journal of Pathology*, **142** (1993), 1423–31.
26. T. E. Bunton, N. J. Biery, L. Myers *et al.*, Phenotypic alteration of vascular smooth muscle cells precedes

elastolysis mouse model of Marfan syndrome. *Circulation Research*, **88** (2001), 37–43.

27. E. L. Henderson, Y. J. Geng, G. K. Sukhova *et al.*, Death of smooth muscle cells and expression of mediators of apoptosis lymphocytes in human abdominal aortic aneurysms. *Circulation*, **99** (1999), 96–104.
28. G. M. Longo, W. Xiong, T. C. Greiner *et al.*, Matrix metalloproteinases 2 and 9 work in concert to produce aortic aneurysms. *Journal of Clinical Investigation*, **110** (2002), 625–32.
29. C. Ihling, T. Szombathy, K. Nampoothiri *et al.*, Cystic medial degeneration of the aorta is associated with p53 accumulation Bax upregulation, apoptotic cell death, and cell proliferation. *Heart*, **82** (1999), 286–93.
30. V. L. Rowe, S. L. Stevens, T. T. Reddick *et al.*, Vascular smooth muscle cell apoptosis in aneurysmal, occlusive and normal human aortas. *Journal of Vascular Surgery*, **31** (2000), 567–76.

16 • Pharmacological treatment of aneurysms

JOHN EVANS, JANET T. POWELL AND MATTHEW M. THOMPSON

BACKGROUND

Abdominal aortic aneurysms (AAAs) are present in 5%–10% of men over the age of 65 [1], and elective surgical intervention has long been the mainstay of treatment. There is a widespread consensus that operative repair is the treatment of choice in larger AAAs, where the risk of rupture increases with the size of the aneurysm [2; 3]. However, even elective operations carry a significant mortality risk, and the UK small aneurysm trial has shown that for smaller aneurysms (between 4 and 5.5 cm) there is no difference in outcome between an operation and no intervention [4]. Currently such patients are treated with the best medical therapy, but there has been considerable research into finding a pharmacological treatment to prevent aneurysm expansion and rupture.

Screening programmes

A major obstacle to the prevention of mortality and morbidity associated with aneurysms has been the fact that the majority are asymptomatic, and therefore often remain undetected. Abdominal aortic aneurysms have tended to present either as emergencies or as a result of their increasing size, and it has been shown that larger aneurysms grow more rapidly than their smaller counterparts and are at greater risk of rupture [3]. These patients would therefore benefit most from operative repair rather than medical intervention. In order for a medical treatment to be of benefit, it needs to be targeted at aneurysms that are small and asymptomatic. The most obvious way of doing this would be the initiation of a mass screening programme, and indeed, the Multicentre Aneurysm Screening Study (MASS) has shown that as many as 88% of screen-detected aneurysms are below the threshold for surgery [66].

The introduction of screening programmes will identify a large population of patients with small aortic aneurysms that are at present untreated. The concept of pharmacotherapy for AAAs has evolved over the past five years, to encompass a medical treatment for aneurysms. Pharmacotherapy aims to reduce the expansion and rupture rate of aortic aneurysms by modifying aortic wall biology. A pharmacotherapeutic approach might be used to reduce the expansion rate of small, screen-detected, abdominal aneurysms and therefore reduce the proportion of patients requiring surgery. Alternatively, effective drug treatment might be able to reduce rupture rates in patients with large aneurysms unsuitable for aneurysm repair. Applications to endovascular aneurysm repair have yet to be explored.

Pathophysiology

Abdominal aortic aneurysms have long been known to be associated with increasing age, male sex, cigarette smoking, chronic lung disease, hypertension and genetic factors [2; 5; 6]. Despite the fact that most of these risk factors are shared with patients with arteriosclerosis, aneurysmal disease appears to be a separate entity. There is good evidence to support this; whilst atherosclerosis is more severe in the Afro-Caribbean population, AAAs occur far more frequently amongst Caucasians [7]. Similarly, diabetes is a strong risk factor for developing atherosclerosis but not for AAAs. The genetic component of aneurysm aetiology is not fully defined at present, but may be due to inborn errors of the connective tissue matrix, such as mutation of the COL3A1 gene coding for the A chain of type III collagen [8].

The detailed pathophysiology of the developing and expanding aneurysm has been covered in Chapter 14. Abdominal aortic aneurysms are characterized by three main inter-related processes; degradation of the extracellular matrix, excessive proteolysis and widespread inflammation. Degradation of the matrix results in early loss of arterial elastin with compensatory collagen remodelling. High levels of matrix metalloproteinases (MMPs) within the arterial wall drive the degradation of the matrix. The MMPs are largely derived from an active inflammatory cell infiltrate which, in addition, secretes high levels of cytokines and inflammatory mediators.

An approach to developing a suitable pharmacotherapy may be considered from one of two perspectives. Firstly, the drug may be targeted to one of the specific processes that have been shown to influence aneurysm development. The second approach hinges on newer theories about the nature of arterial disease. Increasingly it has been recognized that arterial disease is neither a matter of simple deranged lipid metabolism nor of isolated local mechanical effects [9; 10; 11; 12; 13; 14]. The current belief is that arterial disease represents a low-grade systemic inflammation, which can therefore manifest itself at any point – coronary, carotid, aneurysmal or peripheral vascular disease. The Oxford Heart Protection Study [15] has shown that generalized treatment of arteriopathic patients with statin therapy can reduce their chance of undergoing major adverse events, including AAA rupture, regardless of their initial cholesterol level.

The majority of agents proposed to alter aneurysm expansion have been tested in animal models of aneurysm disease. The commonest model was developed in order to investigate the effects of increased proteolysis and the local inflammatory response [16]. The Anidjar rat model utilized an infusion of elastase into the isolated infrarenal rat aorta followed by restoration of flow. Aortas treated this way typically expand to aneurysmal proportions in two to three days.

Therapeutic strategies

Beta-blockade

Hypertension has been known to be associated with AAAs for many years and Gadowski *et al.* have shown that hypertension increases the development of aneurysms in the Anidjar rat model [17]. Comparison of aneurysms induced in normal Wistar-Kyoto rats and those in a strain genetically prone to hypertension proved that those in the hypertensive strain had a growth rate twice that of the control.

Since beta-blockers have been used successfully in the treatment of hypertension, it was not unreasonable to investigate the effect of beta-blockade on aneurysm expansion, as these agents have been shown to slow aneurysm progression in both experimental models and retrospective studies of patients with AAAs [18; 19; 20; 21]. Initially this was thought to be purely due to the drugs' effects on blood pressure, but there is considerable evidence to support the theory that beta-blockers exert their beneficial effects on AAAs by another mechanism.

The broad-breasted white turkey is prone to aortic aneurysms and Boucek *et al.* examined the effect of propanolol administration upon the collagen content of its aorta [19]. After treatment, the tensile strength of the aorta was found to be considerably greater. This was due to stimulation of lysyl oxidase to produce reactive aldehydes for intermolecular cross-links and stabilization of cross-linkages between elastin molecules. In addition, the density of cross-linkages between collagen molecules, which normally increases with age, was reduced. These findings were dose dependent and unrelated to effects on heart rate or blood pressure.

Studies on another animal model of aneurysmal disease, the lysyl oxidase deficient blotchy mouse, have not been quite so conclusive in their support for the collagen/elastin cross-linkage theory. Brophy *et al.* showed that by treating male blotchy mice with propanolol from birth, they could reduce the prevalence of aneurysms at four months from 86% to 32% [20]. A subsequent experiment by the same group looked at the effect treatment with propanolol had on proteins in the skin of the blotchy rat [22]. After 12 weeks treatment with propanolol they found a 147% increase in the content of insoluble elastin and a 54% increase in insoluble collagen. These results suggested that propanolol was exerting its effect via cross-linkage.

By contrast, Moursi *et al.* looked at three groups; normal siblings of blotchy mice, blotchy mice and blotchy mice treated with propanolol [23]. Blotchy mice showed an increase in aortic diameter at harvest, whilst those treated with propanolol showed no significant increase over the controls. Mean heart rate was reduced in the beta-blocked group but blood pressures were similar in all three groups. Significantly, the lysyl oxidase activity of the blotchy mice was reduced to approximately half that of the control and remained low in blotchy mice even when treated with propanolol. Hence the effects seen in this study could not have been attributable to lysyl oxidase activity, nor indeed to a reduction in blood pressure.

The paucity of data on the effect of propanolol on aneurysms in humans prompted Tilson to call for a prospective, randomized clinical trial in 1992 [24]. Such a trial was instigated by the Propanolol Aneurysm Trial Investigators and reported in January 2002 [25]. A total of 548 patients with asymptomatic aneurysms between 3 and 5 cm in diameter were randomized to receive either placebo ($n = 2$) or propanolol ($n = 276$) and were followed for a mean of 2.5 years. The primary criterion was the mean growth rate of the aneurysm, measured by ultrasound scans every six months. Secondary outcomes also measured included death, surgery, withdrawal from study medication and quality of life measured by the standardized short form 36 (SF-36) protocol. There was no significant difference in the growth rates of the two groups, although there was a trend towards more elective operations in the placebo group. There was no difference in death rates, but patients in the treatment arm of the study reported a poorer quality of life, and more of this group stopped taking their medication.

In this robust study it was clear that propanolol has little, if any, effect on the growth rate of AAAs. Crucially, it has also been shown to be poorly tolerated by patients and caused many of them to be non-compliant. Despite promising beginnings and an interesting scientific background, it seems that propanolol has very little potential as a clinical treatment for AAAs.

Modification of the inflammatory response

With considerable evidence to support the theory that aneurysm expansion and rupture are both mediated by the immune system [26; 27], it is unsurprising that there has been interest in modifying this response as a means of attenuating growth. In the rat model of AAA, the effect of treating the animal with cyclosporin and methylprednisolone was investigated [28]. Aneurysm growth was initiated in rats using the elastase infusion technique [16]. Following initiation, the rats were divided into three groups and treated with cyclosporin, methylprednisolone or saline in the case of the control group. Aortas were harvested and examined, macroscopically and histologically, immediately post perfusion, and at five and nine days. Although the diameter of the aorta in all three groups slightly increased immediately following infusion of elastin, there was no significant difference between the groups. Five days post infusion there was still no significant difference in the diameter of the aortas. However, histologically the findings were more varied. The control group showed a marked inflammatory infiltrate throughout all layers of the aortic wall, consisting of monocytes and macrophages with moderate oedema. This was associated with breakage of the elastic lamellae. None of these features were seen in either of the treatment groups.

Furthermore, at nine days post infusion, a significant difference in the diameters of the aortas was seen for the first time. The control group had expanded to approximately three times their pre-infusion size but the treatment groups only grew to around twice their original size. These findings indicate that, at least in this experimental model, preventing the infiltration of inflammatory cells could halt the main spurt of aneurysm growth. Similar results were seen by Ricci *et al.* when using a monoclonal antibody against the macrophage adhesion molecule CD18 [29]. A third experiment using the same model looked at tumour necrosis factor binding protein (TNF-BP) and interleukin-1 receptor antagonist (IL-1RA) [23]. Although IL-1RA failed to slow growth, TNF-BP showed similar results to methylprednisolone and cyclosporin.

The one constant factor in these experiments on immune-modification is that the compounds used have been unacceptable as clinical treatment strategies due to their wide range of action and many side effects. Total immunosuppression is not appropriate, but the use of anti-inflammatories has been examined.

Non steroidal anti-inflammatories

Indomethacin is a powerful anti-inflammatory drug that has been investigated both in the rodent elastase model and in human aortic aneurysmal tissue [30; 31]. Indomethacin reduced both aneurysm growth and MMP9 activity in the rat, and the levels of prostaglandin E2 (PGE-2), interleukin-1 beta (IL-1β) and interleukin-6 (IL-6) in human tissue. However, no effect was seen on MMP9 in human explants. Further evidence that it is the reduction in PGE-2 that is the key step here came from Miralles' group [32]. They who showed that levels of PGE-2 in conditioned media increased with the expansion of the aorta and that indomethacin prevented both of these events. A mixed COX-1 and COX-2 antagonist may therefore be required.

Importantly, in a retrospective analysis of the large group of patients in the UK small aneurysm trial

[4], indomethacin was also shown to inhibit aneurysm growth *in vivo*. The trial was not designed for this purpose and was the result of sub-group analysis, so further trials would be required. Thus we have preliminary evidence that non-selective COX inhibition by indomethacin prevents aneurysm growth, but the side effects of this treatment on the gastrointestinal [33], renal [34] and hepatic [35] systems are well known.

MMP inhibition

Many observers have noted an imbalance between MMPs and their naturally occurring inhibitors, tissue inhibitors of metalloproteinases (TIMPs), in aortic disease [36; 37]. One of the modes of action of indomethacin is to reduce the activity of MMPs. Many other compounds have also been investigated for their anti-MMP properties. For example, BB-94 (or batimastat) has been shown to reduce experimental aneurysm growth in rats [38], and marimastat is a related drug that prevents elastin degradation and MMP2 activity in a porcine model of aneurysms [39]. Vyavahare's group have shown that purified elastin, when injected subdermally into rats, is rapidly calcified and that this calcification is associated with intense MMP2 expression [40]. Administration of the MMP inhibitor BB-1101 prevented elastin calcification, although the effect was more prominent when the drug was injected at the site of calcification rather than given systemically.

Other experimental drugs have been investigated for their anti-MMP activity. Cowan *et al.* demonstrated that the glycoprotein tenascin-C was induced by MMPs and that this caused hypertrophy of the rat pulmonary artery *in vitro* [41]. Addition of the MMP inhibitor GM-6001 caused regression of the hypertrophy and suppression of smooth muscle cell proliferation. Systemic treatment with the hydroxanate-based MMP inhibitor RS132908 reduced aneurysm formation and expansion, and preserved elastin in elastase-perfused rat aortas [42].

Tetracyclines have long been known to prevent connective tissue breakdown by their inhibitory effect on MMPs [43]. Petrinec *et al.* demonstrated that doxycycline reduced the growth of degenerative aneurysms and suppressed MMP9 production in the rat elastase model [44]. Similar results were obtained with four other chemically modified tetracycline derivatives [45; 46]. Using a porcine model of elastase-induced AAA, Boyle *et al.* also showed that doxycycline reduced elastin degradation and MMP9 activity [47]. Tetracycline itself has been proposed as an MMP antagonist and indeed, when given pre-operatively, has been shown to penetrate the aortic wall [48]. However, these experiments used a concentration of 100 μg/ml to produce an effect *in vitro*, but the concentration following a single bolus of 500 mg was 8.3 μg/ml in plasma and 2.8 μg/g of aortic tissue. This suggests that in order to reach therapeutic levels the treatment dose would have to be enormous.

Nevertheless, pre-operative treatment with doxycycline caused a reduction in both the expression of macrophage MMP9 mRNA and the activity of MMP2 in aneurysm tissue [49]. Also, a small double-blinded, randomized and placebo controlled pilot study from Finland has shown that treatment with doxycycline for a three month period significantly reduced the rate of aneurysm growth in a cohort of patients as measured by serial ultrasound scans [50]. At six months, there was also a significant reduction in the serum C-reactive protein levels of the treatment group. Although the sample size was small and pre-operative confounding effects are not taken into consideration, this trial has provided evidence to support further research into this area. In 1999, Thompson and Baxter initiated a randomized, prospective clinical trial of doxycycline in the treatment of small aneurysms in the USA. This is an ongoing, multicentre trial, the results of which have not yet been reported [51].

Anti-chlamydial therapy

The hypothesis that atherosclerosis may have an infective aetiology is not new, and it is clear that AAAs and atherosclerosis share many of the same risk factors. Indeed, Lindholt's group has shown that antibodies against chlamydia are associated with the progression of peripheral vascular disease [52] and that these antibodies may also predict the need for surgery in patients diagnosed with small aneurysms [53]. However, a possible source of error in studies of chlamydial infection has been identified by the same group. Using immunohistostaining to investigate the incidence of chlamydial proteins in the aortas of 20 patients undergoing aneurysm repair, *C. pneumoniae* was not identified in a single one [54]. Nevertheless, what was evident was a high degree of cross-reactivity of non-chlamydial proteins, in particular the human haemoglobin beta chain.

Regardless of this, Mosorin's group has reported a significant decrease in the rate of expansion of AAAs in patients treated with doxycycline in a prospective, double-blinded, randomized and controlled study [50]. As discussed earlier, however, it is unclear whether the effects seen were due to chlamydial eradication or the direct effects of doxycycline as an MMP inhibitor.

Another randomized, controlled trial looked at the effect of roxithromycin on aneurysm growth [55]. Patients with small aneurysms were given either roxithromycin or placebo for four weeks, and subsequently followed up for a mean of 1.5 years. Once adjustments had been made for smoking, blood pressure and IgA, there was a significant difference in aneurysm growth between treatment and placebo groups.

Tambiah *et al.*'s work using rabbit aortas showed that a monocyte chemoattractant protein-1-induced influx of macrophages alone into the aortic wall was insufficient to provoke aortic dilatation [56]. When the macrophages were activated by the presence of chlamydia, however, the aortas did undergo dilatation. Moreover, dilatation that occurred in rabbit aortas due to the interaction of macrophages and chlamydial surface antigens was abolished by the administration of azithromycin [57].

Drugs acting on the renin/angiotensin axis

In 1998 a French group reported the effects of angiotensin converting enzyme (ACE) inhibitors and angiotensin II antagonists in a strain of rat prone to rupture of the internal elastic lamina of the aorta [58]. To ensure any beneficial effects were not due to the anti-hypertensive properties of the drugs, they were compared with hydralazine and two calcium channel antagonists. Both ACE inhibitors and angiotensin II antagonists prevented rupture of the internal elastic lamina, suggesting this was due to the effect on angiotensin II and not on another part of the renin/angiotensin system. However, in all the treatment groups a global reduction of elastin, collagen and cell proteins in the media was noted. This contrasts with the results of Thompson's group, who used both ACE inhibitors and an angiotensin II antagonist in the Anidjar/Dobrin rat model [59]. In these experiments, the ACE inhibitors prevented aneurysm formation and preserved elastin whilst angiotensin II antagonism had no significant effect. There was no effect on the inflammatory infiltrate seen in the aneurysmal wall and the reduction in aneurysm formation was independent of blood pressure effects.

Clearly further work in this field is needed to elucidate the exact mechanism of action.

THE FUTURE

The attempts to inhibit AAA expansion rely on anti-inflammatory action or anti-MMP activity. Work with chemically modified tetracyclines is ongoing. Similarly, work looking at the anti-inflammatory properties of COX inhibitors continues, but perhaps the most exciting prospect is a group of drugs that combine both of these approaches.

The hydroxymethylglutaryl CoA reductase inhibitors (statins) are a group of drugs in which there has been considerable interest recently [60; 61]. The statins have been used successfully for their lipid-lowering properties for some time now, but have also exhibited beneficial effects in cardiovascular disease unrelated to this [62]. In laboratory experiments they have been proven to reduce MMP9 expression by human macrophages [63] and their anti-inflammatory effects are well documented [64; 65].

Preliminary experiments in our laboratories have shown that statins reduce MMP expression in both human aortic explants and a porcine model of aneurysmal disease. Inflammatory cytokines have also been inhibited. The biological effects of statins in patients with AAA is currently being investigated.

REFERENCES

1. R. A. Scott, K. A. Vardulaki, N. M. Walker *et al.*, The long-term benefits of a single scan for abdominal aortic aneurysm (AAA) at age 65. *European Journal of Vascular and Endovascular Surgery*, **21** (2001), 535–40.
2. R. W. Thompson, Basic science of abdominal aortic aneurysms: emerging therapeutic strategies for an unresolved clinical problem. *Current Opinion in Cardiology*, **11** (1996), 504–18.
3. K. A. Vardulaki, T. C. Prevost, N. M. Walker *et al.*, Growth rates and risk of rupture of abdominal aortic aneurysms. *British Journal of Surgery*, **85** (1998), 1674–80.
4. J. T. Powell, R. M. Greenhalgh, C. V. Ruckley & F. G. Fowkes, The UK small aneurysm trial. *Annals of the New York Academy of Sciences*, **800** (1996), 249–51.

5. J. M. Reilly & M. D. Tilson, Incidence and etiology of abdominal aortic aneurysms. *Surgical Clinics of North America*, **69** (1989), 705–11.
6. P. K. Shah, Inflammation, metalloproteinases, and increased proteolysis: an emerging pathophysiological paradigm in aortic aneurysm. *Circulation*, **96** (1997), 2115–7.
7. W. W. LaMorte, T. E. Scott & J. O. Menzoian, Racial differences in the incidence of femoral bypass and abdominal aortic aneurysmectomy in Massachusetts: relationship to cardiovascular risk factors. *Journal of Vascular Surgery*, **21** (1995), 422–31.
8. A. Verloes, N. Sakalihasan, L. Koulischer & R. Limet, Aneurysms of the abdominal aorta: familial and genetic aspects in three hundred thirteen pedigrees. *Journal of Vascular Surgery*, **21** (1995), 646–55.
9. J. Dupuis, Mechanisms of acute coronary syndromes and the potential role of statins. *Atherosclerosis Supplement*, **2** (2001), 9–14.
10. J. W. Heinecke, Mechanisms of oxidative damage by myeloperoxidase in atherosclerosis and other inflammatory disorders. *Journal of Laboratory and Clinical Medicine*, **133** (1999), 321–5.
11. D. M. Yamada & E. J. Topol, Importance of microembolization and inflammation in atherosclerotic heart disease. *American Heart Journal*, **140** (2000), S90–102.
12. J. Ijem & C. Granlie, More than cholesterol: the complexity of coronary artery disease. *South Dakota Journal of Medicine*, **53** (2000), 489–91.
13. P. Weissberg, Mechanisms modifying atherosclerotic disease – from lipids to vascular biology. *Atherosclerosis*, **147** (Suppl 1) (1999), S3–10.
14. G. Berkenboom, Unstable atherosclerotic plaque. Pathophysiology and therapeutic guidelines. *Acta Cardiologica*, **53** (1998), 235–41.
15. MRC/BHF Heart Protection Study of cholesterol lowering with simvastatin in 20 536 high-risk individuals: a randomised placebo-controlled trial. *Lancet*, **360** (2002), 7–22. CORPORATE NAME: Heart Protection Study Collaborative Group.
16. S. Anidjar, P. B. Dobrin, M. Eichorst, G. P. Graham & G. Chejfec, Correlation of inflammatory infiltrate with the enlargement of experimental aortic aneurysms. *Journal of Vascular Surgery*, **16** (1992), 139–47.
17. G. R. Gadowski, M. A. Ricci, E. D. Hendley & D. B. Pilcher, Hypertension accelerates the growth of experimental aortic aneurysms. *Journal of Surgical Research*, **54** (1993), 431–6.
18. S. D. Leach, A. L. Toole, H. Stern, R. W. DeNatale & M. D. Tilson, Effect of beta-adrenergic blockade on the growth rate of abdominal aortic aneurysms. *Archives of Surgery*, **123** (1988), 606–9.
19. R. J. Boucek, Z. Gunja-Smith, N. L. Noble & C. F. Simpson, Modulation by propranolol of the lysyl cross-links in aortic elastin and collagen of the aneurysm-prone turkey. *Biochemical Pharmacology*, **32** (1983), 275–80.
20. C. Brophy, J. E. Tilson & M. D. Tilson, Propranolol delays the formation of aneurysms in the male blotchy mouse. *Journal of Surgical Research*, **44** (1988), 687–9.
21. R. Englund, P. Hudson, K. Hanel & A. Stanton, Expansion rates of small abdominal aortic aneurysms. *Australian and New Zealand Journal of Surgery*, **68** (1998), 21–4.
22. C. M. Brophy, J. E. Tilson & M. D. Tilson, Propranolol stimulates the crosslinking of matrix components in skin from the aneurysm-prone blotchy mouse. *Journal of Surgical Research*, **46** (1989), 330–2.
23. M. M. Moursi, H. G. Beebe, L. M. Messina, T. H. Welling & J. C. Stanley, Inhibition of aortic aneurysm development in blotchy mice by beta adrenergic blockade independent of altered lysyl oxidase activity. *Journal of Vascular Surgery*, **21**(5) (1995), 792–800.
24. M. D. Tilson, Propranolol versus placebo for small abdominal aortic aneurysms. *Journal of Vascular Surgery*, **15** (1992), 872–3.
25. Propanol Aneurysm Trial Investigators, Propranolol for small abdominal aortic aneurysms: results of a randomized trial. *Journal of Vascular Surgery*, **35** (2002), 72–9.
26. A. E. Koch, G. K. Haines, R. J. Rizzo *et al.*, Human abdominal aortic aneurysms. Immunophenotypic analysis suggesting an immune-mediated response. *American Journal of Pathology*, **137** (1990), 1199–213.
27. W. D. McMillan & W. H. Pearce, Inflammation and cytokine signaling in aneurysms. *Annals of Vascular Surgery*, **11** (1997), 540–5.
28. P. B. Dobrin, N. Baumgartner, S. Anidjar, G. Chejfec & R. Mrkvicka, Inflammatory aspects of experimental aneurysms. Effect of methylprednisolone and cyclosporine. *Annals of the New York Academy of Sciences*, **800** (1996), 74–88.
29. M. A. Ricci, G. Strindberg, J. M. Slaiby *et al.*, Anti-CD-18 monoclonal antibody slows experimental aortic

aneurysm expansion. *Journal of Vascular Surgery*, **23**(2) (1996), 301–7.

30. D. R. Holmes, D. Petrinec, W. Wester, R. W. Thompson & J. M. Reilly, Indomethacin prevents elastase-induced abdominal aortic aneurysms in the rat. *Journal of Surgical Research*, **63** (1996), 305–9.
31. I. J. Franklin, L. J. Walton, R. M. Greenhalgh & J. T. Powell, The influence of indomethacin on the metabolism and cytokine secretion of human aneurysmal aorta. *European Journal of Vascular and Endovascular Surgery*, **18** (1999), 35–42.
32. M. Miralles, W. Wester, G. A. Sicard, R. Thompson & J. M. Reilly, Indomethacin inhibits expansion of experimental aortic aneurysms via inhibition of the cox2 isoform of cyclooxygenase. *Journal of Vascular Surgery*, **29** (1999), 884–92.
33. Z. Morise & M. B. Grisham, Molecular mechanisms involved in NSAID-induced gastropathy. *Journal of Clinical Gastroenterology*, **27** (Suppl 1) (1998), S87–90.
34. D. Schlondorff, Renal complications of nonsteroidal anti-inflammatory drugs. *Kidney International*, **44** (1993), 643–53.
35. A. V. Manoukian & J. L. Carson, Nonsteroidal anti-inflammatory drug-induced hepatic disorders. Incidence and prevention. *Drug Safety*, **15** (1996), 64–71.
36. D. Mao, S. J. VanVickle, J. A. Curci & R. W. Thompson, Expression of matrix metalloproteinases and TIMPs in human abdominal aortic aneurysms. *Annals of Vascular Surgery*, **13** (1999), 236–7.
37. J. B. Knox, G. K. Sukhova, A. D. Whittemore & P. Libby, Evidence for altered balance between matrix metalloproteinases and their inhibitors in human aortic diseases. *Circulation*, **95** (1997), 205–12.
38. D. A. Bigatel, J. R. Elmore, D. J. Carey *et al.*, The matrix metalloproteinase inhibitor BB-94 limits expansion of experimental abdominal aortic aneurysms. *Journal of Vascular Surgery*, **29** (1999), 130–9.
39. G. D. Treharne, J. R. Boyle, S. Goodall *et al.*, Marimastat inhibits elastin degradation and matrix metalloproteinase 2 activity in a model of aneurysm disease. *British Journal of Surgery*, **86** (1999), 1053–8.
40. N. Vyavahare, P. L. Jones, S. Tallapragada & R. J. Levy, Inhibition of matrix metalloproteinase activity attenuates tenascin-C production and calcification of implanted purified elastin in rats. *American Journal of Pathology*, **157** (2000), 885–93.
41. K. N. Cowan, P. L. Jones & M. Rabinovitch, Elastase and matrix metalloproteinase inhibitors induce regression, and tenascin-C antisense prevents progression, of vascular disease. *Journal of Clinical Investigation*, **105** (2000), 21–34.
42. G. Moore, S. Liao, J. A. Curci *et al.*, Suppression of experimental abdominal aortic aneurysms by systemic treatment with a hydroxamate-based matrix metalloproteinase inhibitor (RS 132908). *Journal of Vascular Surgery*, **29** (1999), 522–32.
43. L. M. Golub, N. S. Ramamurthy, T. F. McNamara, R. A. Greenwald & B. R. Rifkin, Tetracyclines inhibit connective tissue breakdown: new therapeutic implications for an old family of drugs. *Critical Reviews of Oral Biology and Medicine*, **2** (1991), 297–321.
44. D. Petrinec, S. Liao, D. R. Holmes *et al.*, Doxycycline inhibition of aneurysmal degeneration in an elastase-induced rat model of abdominal aortic aneurysm: preservation of aortic elastin associated with suppressed production of 92 kD gelatinase. *Journal of Vascular Surgery*, **23** (1996), 336–46.
45. J. A. Curci, D. Petrinec, S. Liao, L. M. Golub & R. W. Thompson, Pharmacologic suppression of experimental abdominal aortic aneurysms: a comparison of doxycycline and four chemically modified tetracyclines. *Journal of Vascular Surgery*, **28** (1998), 1082–93.
46. D. Petrinec, D. R. Holmes, S. Liao, L. M. Golub & R. W. Thompson, Suppression of experimental aneurysmal degeneration with chemically modified tetracycline derivatives. *Annals of the New York Academy of Sciences*, **800** (1996), 263–5.
47. J. R. Boyle, E. McDermott, M. Crowther *et al.*, Doxycycline inhibits elastin degradation and reduces metalloproteinase activity in a model of aneurysmal disease. *Journal of Vascular Surgery*, **27** (1998), 354–61.
48. I. J. Franklin, S. L. Harley, R. M. Greenhalgh & J. T. Powell, Uptake of tetracycline by aortic aneurysm wall and its effect on inflammation and proteolysis. *British Journal of Surgery*, **86** (1999), 771–5.
49. J. A. Curci *et al.*, Preoperative treatment with doxycycline reduces aortic wall expression and activation of matrix metalloproteinases in patients with abdominal aortic aneurysms. *Journal of Vascular Surgery*, **31** (2000), 325–42.
50. M. Mosorin, J. Juvonen, F. Blancari *et al.*, Use of doxycycline to decrease the growth rate of abdominal aortic aneurysms: a randomized, double-blind, placebo-controlled pilot study. *Journal of Vascular Surgery*, **34** (2001), 606–10.

51. R. W. Thompson & B. T. Baxter, MMP inhibition in abdominal aortic aneurysms. Rationale for a prospective randomized clinical trial. *Annals of the New York Academy of Sciences*, **878** (1999), 159–78.
52. J. S. Lindholt, S. Vammen, I. Lind, H. Fasting & E. W. Henneberg, The progression of lower limb atherosclerosis is associated with IgA antibodies against *Chlamydia pneumoniae. European Journal of Vascular and Endovascular Surgery*, **18** (1999), 527–9.
53. S. Vammen, J. S. Lindholt, P. L. Andersen, E. W. Henneberg & L. Ostergaard, Antibodies against *Chlamydia pneumoniae* predict the need for elective surgical intervention on small abdominal aortic aneurysms. *European Journal of Vascular and Endovascular Surgery*, **22** (2001), 165–8.
54. S. Vammen, H. Vorum, L. Ostergaard, E. W. Henneberg & J. S. Lindholt, Immunoblotting analysis of abdominal aortic aneurysms using antibodies against *Chlamydia pneumoniae* recombinant MOMP. *European Journal of Vascular and Endovascular Surgery*, **24** (2002), 81–5.
55. S. Vammen, J. S. Lindholt, L. Ostergaard, H. Fasting & E. W. Henneberg, Randomized double-blind controlled trial of roxithromycin for prevention of abdominal aortic aneurysm expansion. *British Journal of Surgery*, **88** (2001), 1066–72.
56. J. Tambiah, I. J. Franklin, N. Trendell-Smith, D. Peston & J. T. Powell, Provocation of experimental aortic inflammation and dilatation by inflammatory mediators and *Chlamydia pneumoniae. British Journal of Surgery*, **88** (2001), 935–40.
57. J. Tambiah & J. T. Powell, *Chlamydia pneumoniae* antigens facilitate experimental aortic dilatation: prevention with azithromycin. *Journal of Vascular Surgery*, **36** (2002), 1011–7.
58. W. Huang, F. Alhenc Gelas & M. J. Osborne-Pellegrin, Protection of the arterial internal elastic lamina by inhibition of the renin-angiotensin system in the rat. *Circulation Research*, **82** (1998), 879–90.
59. G. Moore, S. Liao, J. A. Curci *et al.*, Suppression of experimental abdominal aortic aneurysms in the rat by treatment with angiotensin-converting enzyme inhibitors. *Journal of Vascular Surgery*, **33** (2001), 1057–64.
60. K. K. Koh, Effects of statins on vascular wall: vasomotor function, inflammation, and plaque stability. *Cardiovascular Research*, **47** (2000), 648–57.
61. Z. Kmietowicz, Statins are the new aspirin, Oxford researchers say. *British Medical Journal*, **323** (2001), 1145.
62. W. Palinski, New evidence for beneficial effects of statins unrelated to lipid lowering. *Arteriosclerosis, Thrombosis and Vascular Biology*, **21** (2001), 3–5.
63. S. Bellosta, D. Via, M. Canavesi *et al.*, HMG-CoA reductase inhibitors reduce MMP-9 secretion by macrophages. *Arteriosclerosis, Thrombosis and Vascular Biology*, **18** (1998), 1671–8.
64. W. Ni, K. Egashira, C. Kataoka *et al.*, Antiinflammatory and antiarteriosclerotic actions of HMG-CoA reductase inhibitors in a rat model of chronic inhibition of nitric oxide synthesis. *Circulation Research*, **89** (2001), 415–21.
65. H. Kothe, K. Dalhoff, J. Rupp *et al.*, Hydroxymethylglutaryl coenzyme A reductase inhibitors modify the inflammatory response of human macrophages and endothelial cells infected with *Chlamydia pneumoniae. Circulation*, **101** (2000), 1760–3.
66. H. A. Ashton, M. J. Buxton, N. E. Day *et al.*, The Multicentre Aneurysm Screening Study (MASS) into the effect of abdomiral aortic aneurysm screening on mortality in men: a randomised controlled trial. *Lancet*, **360**(9345) (2002), 1531–9.

17 • SIRS, sepsis and multi-organ failure in vascular surgery

J. IAN SPARK

INTRODUCTION

Sepsis is more common today than ever before. Current estimates indicate that there are over 500 000 cases of sepsis in the USA each year. A substantial number of these patients will develop severe sepsis and septic shock, resulting in approximately 100 000 deaths due to this illness [1]. As the general population ages and technology emerges to further support and prolong life, the incidence will only increase. Systemic inflammatory response syndrome (SIRS)/sepsis is already the commonest cause of death in ICU in Europe and the USA [2]. (Figure 17.1). Many aspects of a patient's risk of serious perioperative complications are perceived as being relatively fixed (genotype, pre-operative health status, surgical difficulty, etc.), but the degree to which these may be improved (e.g. cardiac, respiratory and haemodynamic optimization using pharmacologic support) is still under assessment. The contribution of the inflammatory response to patient outcome is potentially remediable and therefore deserves attention.

DEFINITIONS

In 1992, the American College of Chest Physicians and the Society of Critical Care Medicine (ACCP/SCCM) [3] presented their findings on new definitions of sepsis and organ failure, and the differentiation between sepsis, sepsis syndrome and SIRS. Systemic inflammatory response syndrome was developed to imply a clinical response arising from a non-specific insult and includes two or more defined variables (Table 17.1). Sepsis is defined as the presence of SIRS associated with a confirmed infectious process. The term sepsis syndrome was discarded and severe sepsis was defined as the presence of sepsis with either hypotension or systemic manifestation of hypotension. Septic shock was defined as sepsis with hypotension despite adequate fluid resuscitation and associated hypoperfusion abnormalities that included, but were not limited to, lactic acidosis, oliguria or an acute alteration in mental status. The sequelae of SIRS/sepsis is multiple organ dysfunction syndrome (MODS) which can be defined as failure to maintain homeostasis without intervention. Primary MODS is a direct result of a well defined insult, while secondary MODS develops not in direct response to the insult but as a consequence of a host response.

There is a continuum from the development of SIRS to the onset of sepsis, and progression to septic shock and MODS [4]. In a prospective survey of admissions to a tertiary care facility in the USA, 68% of patients met the criteria for SIRS [5]. Of these, 26% developed sepsis, 18% developed severe sepsis and 4% developed septic shock within 28 days. The interval between the identification of SIRS and the development of sepsis was inversely correlated with the number of SIRS criteria initially identified. Mortality rates in that study were 7%, 16%, 20% and 46% for SIRS, sepsis, severe sepsis and septic shock, respectively. It is important to note that the identification of SIRS alone in a patient in the intensive care unit has a poor specificity for predicting the development of sepsis and septic shock [6].

CAUSES OF SIRS

Eiseman *et al.* coined the term multiple organ failure (MOF) and identified the important risk factors to be, pre-existing disease, shock and sepsis [7]. Soon thereafter, Fry *et al.* and Polk and Shields observed a consistent association between infection and MOF, and concluded that MOF was the 'fatal expression of uncontrolled infection' [8; 9]. As a result, research efforts in the early 1980s were focused on determining how the initial traumatic insult promotes infections and how infections cause MOF. This is particularly relevant to vascular patients for as a group they are elderly and undergo a significant traumatic insult following surgery

Table 17.1. *Criteria for SIRS, sepsis and MODS*

SIRS	Two or more of the following: temperature above 38 °C or below 36 °C (rectal); heart rate above 90 beats per min; respiratory rate above 20 breaths per min or Pa_{CO_2} less than 4.3 kPa; WBC count above 12 000 cells per mm^3, below 4000 cells per mm^3 or 10% immature (bands) forms
Sepsis	SIRS with documented infection
Severe Sepsis	SIRS with documented infection and haemodynamic compromise
MODS	A state of physiological derangement in which organ function is not capable of maintaining homeostasis

Advances in medical practice and technology
- Aggressive use of catheters/lines
- Implantation of prosthetic devices
- Chemotherapy/cancer patients
- Steroids/immunosuppressants to patients with transplants or inflammatory conditions

Elderly population

Fig. 17.1. The increasing incidence of SIRS/sepsis

and reperfusion, and the consequences of an infection are devastating. In the mid-1980s, however, observations by Goris *et al.* made this line of research more relevant to the vascular patient [10]. They observed that a significant portion of blunt trauma patients who developed MOF did not have an identifiable infection. Goris *et al.* also showed, in a retrospective study of 55 trauma patients with MOF, that only 33% had a definite bacterial focus with one or more positive blood cultures [10].

They concluded that MOF can occur as a result of an 'autodestructive inflammatory response' and research efforts refocused on explaining how a variety of non-infectious insults could cause SIRS that would result in MOF, independent of a bacterial infection.

PHYSIOLOGY OF INFLAMMATION

The physiological acute phase response to injury represents a complex interplay among the nervous, endocrine

Vasodilatation Increased microvascular permeability Cellular activation Coagulation	} Calor Rubor Tumor Dolor

Fig. 17.2. The four major local events of inflammation

and immune systems, regulated by an array of peptides and their receptors [11; 12]. This is intended to be an early protective homeostatic immune response to injury produced by mechanical, chemical or microbiological stimuli. It is characterized by a rapid highly amplified controlled humoral and cellular response: the complement, kinin, coagulation and fibrinolytic cascades are triggered in tandem with the activation of phagocytes and endothelial cells [13]. This local response may be considered benign as long as the inflammatory process is regulated appropriately to keep cells and mediators sequestered.

The normal physiological response to stress and injury results in a series of cardiovascular changes (increase in heart rate, contractility and cardiac output) and neuroendocrine changes (increase in release of catecholamines, cortisol, antidiuretic hormone, growth hormone, glucagon and insulin). There are four major local events: vasodilatation, increased microvascular permeability, cellular activation/adhesion and coagulation, leading to the classic clinical condition recognized as calor, rubor, tumor and dolor (Figure 17.2) [14; 15]. The inflammatory cells are the main driving force behind this local process and comprise the circulating leucocytes (neutrophils, monocytes and lymphocytes), in addition to tissue fixed macrophages, dendritic cells, mast cells and eosinophils. Neutrophils and monocytes constitute the bulk of circulating inflammatory cells. They normally exist in a non-activated state and in the absence of stimulation have a life-span limited by apoptosis (or programmed cell death) to a day or so [16]. These cells are rapidly transformed by invading bacteria, specific bacterial products, foreign material, endogenous mediators or, in response to trauma or hypoxia, into highly active phagocytes with a greatly enhanced capacity to release mediators, enzymes and reactive oxygen species [17].

Activation increases the number of neutrophils by speeding the maturation process and increasing the release of precursors from bone marrow. Likewise the number of monocytes entering the circulation from the bone marrow is doubled during inflammation [18]. Chemotactic agents and adhesion molecules focus these cells upon sites of infection where they phagocytose and kill bacteria. Monocytes mature into macrophages, which having engulfed, killed and digested micro-organisms, present their foreign antigen to lymphocytes and engender highly specific adaptive immune responses. These inflammatory cells also release a wide range of mediators which act to regulate the whole inflammatory process. This includes controlling cellular activation and endothelial and leucocyte adhesion molecule expression and function. These mediators also act as chemotaxins, prolonging the life-span of inflammatory cells, stimulating fibroblasts, and promoting wound healing and angiogenesis [19]. Unless a second insult occurs, the peak effect of theses local and systemic physiological changes occurs within 3–5 days after the initial stimulus, and abates by 7–10 days.

PATHOPHYSIOLOGY OF SIRS

In the early 1990s, MOF was interpreted as the most severe derangement of SIRS [1; 8; 9] that develops as a result of a variety of severe clinical insults [3]. It has been hypothesized that it either develops early after a massive insult which consequently results in a severe systemic inflammatory response or develops gradually via a continuum of physiological and metabolic changes caused by an ongoing systemic inflammatory response [20; 21; 22]. Recently, the above theory on the pathogenesis of MOF has been refined. Bone *et al.* have argued that the original insult results initially in the synthesis of pro-inflammatory mediators (tumour necrosis factor (TNF) and interleukin-1 (IL-1)) and, if a critical level of pro-inflammatory mediators is reached locally, that systemic spillover may occur [23]. A systemic compensatory anti-inflammatory response is thereby induced to down-regulate the pro-inflammatory reaction and restore homeostasis. In some patients excessive amounts of pro-inflammatory mediators are released which overwhelm the compensatory anti-inflammatory response, leading to a sustained pro-inflammatory response and organ failure. It has further been hypothesized that in some patients the compensatory anti-inflammatory reaction may be excessive, resulting in immunosuppression. This immunosuppression has been termed 'immunoparalysis' by Volk and coworkers [24] or 'the compensatory anti-inflammatory response syndrome' (CARS) by Bone [25]. Although such a mechanism for the pathogenesis of MOF remains hypothetical, the results of several studies substantiate the theory [26; 27; 28].

THE GENERAL OVERVIEW

A complex array of intersecting pathways in the pathophysiology of sepsis has been described. Vascular endothelial injury, inflammation, activation of coagulation and inhibition of fibrinolysis appear to contribute to the development of organ dysfunction and the risk of death. For example, in a gram-negative infection, lysis of bacteria by white blood cells (WBCs) causes the release of endotoxin, a lipopolysaccharide component of the cell wall. Endotoxin stimulates the release of a variety of inflammatory mediators that serve to activate the host's cellular defences. In vascular surgery, ischaemia-reperfusion injury is known to produce free-radicals, derived from oxygen by a process mediated by xanthine oxidase on the endothelial cell surface (see Chapter 18). Reactive oxygen species can stimulate the neutrophils and endothelial cells to produce further free-radicals, proteolytic enzymes and cytokines. Common cytokines in sepsis include TNFα, a variety of interleukins and inflammatory prostaglandins. The inflammatory response is normally balanced by an anti-inflammatory response, with release of anti-inflammatory mediators. While sepsis and SIRS have been thought to result from an excess of inflammatory mediators, anti-inflammatory mediators may also play a significant role in the outcome of some patients [24]. In CARS, an alteration in the helper T cell ratios may lead to paralysis of the immune system and poor outcomes [25].

Some patients with infection, trauma or burns have only mild sepsis or SIRS, and minor organ dysfunction that resolves rapidly. Others exhibit a massive systemic inflammatory reaction and die early from profound shock. A third group has a less severe initial course but a later deterioration, MODS and often death; this group, that never seems to recover from the initial insult, is thought to have CARS. The spectrum of the responses to sepsis/SIRS is illustrated in Figure 17.3. This diagram shows three of the five stages of sepsis leading to MODS. Stage I represents the initial insult producing local inflammation. Stage II occurs when a severe insult

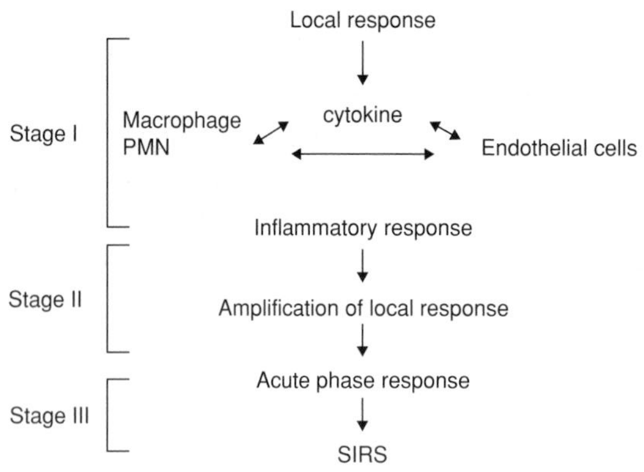

Fig. 17.3. Progression of SIRS

leads to systemic spillover of inflammatory mediators, but there are few clinical signs or symptoms. This amplified response is most likely to be the result of a second insult (second hit) when the macrophages have been primed for an intense cytokine release. In stage III, the systemic reaction becomes apparent, leading to the clinical signs of sepsis or SIRS and early organ dysfunction. It is at this point that most therapies have been tested. Stage IV is characterized by inappropriate immunosuppression or CARS overreaction with increased susceptibility to new infection. Stage V is characterized by an inappropriate, out-of-balance response and either excessive SIRS or CARS along with severe MODS.

Factors influencing incidence, severity and clinical outcome of the inflammatory response, and in particular the reasons why certain patients develop life-threatening perioperative complications, are currently not well understood. To re-cap, three separate perspectives contribute to our understanding of the link between the inflammatory response and adverse clinical sequelae. Firstly, the complex interaction of humoral pro-inflammatory and anti-inflammatory molecules may influence the clinical presentation and course of SIRS, with the balance of pro-inflammatory and anti-inflammatory cytokines determining the clinical course following vascular surgery.

Secondly, a 'multiple-hit' scenario may be seen, whereby serious sequelae develop after vascular surgery as a result of adverse events, such as infection or ongoing organ hypoperfusion [21; 22]. The combination results in the conversion of an inherently self-limiting, tightly controlled homeostatic response to an uncontrolled destructive process resulting in organ dysfunction [13]. Potential mechanistic insights into the pathophysiologic basis for multiple-hits include the ability of ischaemia-reperfusion to 'prime' neutrophils, causing pulmonary leucosequestration [29], and enhanced cytotoxin release following a subsequent insult.

Finally, the pro-inflammatory state, SIRS, may be only one aspect of a multifaceted response. The converse has been termed CARS [30]. Surgery-induced generalized immunosuppression may play an important role in the development of infectious complications [31]. Cumulatively, these responses represent the body's attempt to re-establish homeostasis and may clinically manifest as predominantly pro-inflammatory (SIRS), anti-inflammatory (CARS) or an intermediate mixed response (mixed inflammatory response syndrome (MARS)) [30].

THE ANTI-INFLAMMATORY RESPONSE TO SIRS

The inflammation that is involved in response to surgery is tightly regulated by the expression of anti-inflammatory factors. These include circulating hormones, such as glucocorticoids, and local mediators produced in response to the surgical insult and infiltrating leucocytes.

During the initial stages of the surgical insult the release of chemoattractants by injured tissue triggers the infiltration of leucocytes. Thereafter, the release of pro-inflammatory substances by these cells causes local tissue destruction. These cytokines, TNFα, IL-1β and IL-6 stimulate the release of hypothalamic corticotrophic hormone and pituitary adrenocorticotropic hormone which in turn stimulates the release of cortisol into the circulation. Finally, the generation of anti-inflammatory factors may lead to the attenuation and resolution of disease. These anti-inflammatory factors include cortisol, as well as mediators that are produced at the inflammatory site (see later in the chapter). They block the efficacy of pro-inflammatory substances by inhibiting their production, promoting their degradation or making potential target cells resistant to their actions.

It was recently found that glucocorticoids and anti-inflammatory mediators control inflammatory processes through an efficient cross-talk. Indeed, glucocorticoids provide a very effective means to increase the expression of anti-inflammatory mediators. In turn, anti-inflammatory mediators control glucocorticoid efficacy by modulating glucocorticoid receptor (GR) binding.

These effects of glucocorticoids are generally attributed to the inhibition of synthesis or release of inflammatory mediators, and to the suppression of competence of inflammatory cells. Glucocorticoid responsiveness appears to be mainly due to binding of the hormone to GR in the cytoplasm of target cells. Inside the nucleus, ligand-bound GR regulates gene transcription possibly by interacting directly with other transcription factors, such as activator protein-1, nuclear factor-κ B, or signal transducers and activators of transcription (STAT). This transcriptional interference may either suppress or amplify the efficacy of these factors. The result of this would be a down-regulation of the inflammatory response, with a reduction of TNFα, IL-1β and IL-6, and if excessive possible immune paralysis.

ROLE OF CYTOKINES

Cytokines are soluble proteins and polypeptides that act as paracrine messengers of the immune system, and are produced by a large variety of cell types, including activated monocytes, tissue macrophages, lymphocytes and endothelial cells.

As shown in Table 17.2 many cytokines have more than one action (pleiotropy).

Individual cytokines may exert either pro-inflammatory or anti-inflammatory effects. Cytokines are essential for immunologic and physiologic homeostasis, are normally subject to tight homeostatic control, and are produced in response to a variety of physiologic and pathologic stimuli.

As previously mentioned the cytokines that contribute to pathologic changes in SIRS and sepsis are not unique to infection. Multiple trauma, ischaemia-reperfusion injury, acute transplant rejection, antigen-specific immune responses and various acute inflammatory states (acute hepatitis and pancreatitis), initiate the same cytokine cascade and result in both systemic and local inflammatory processes.

Three cytokines, in particular, play a major role in the pathogenesis of sepsis: TNF, IL-1 and IL-6 [31]. There is also a role for γ-interferon in that this cytokine increases the production of and sensitivity to TNF and IL-1 [31]. All three cytokines activate endothelial cells. In animal models of systemic inflammation (such as in septic shock), specific blockade of either IL-1 or TNF results in a reduction in the severity of the inflammation. Moreover, IL-1 and TNF act synergistically in nearly every *in vitro* and *in vivo* model of local or systemic inflammation. When both cytokines are specifically blocked, the severity of inflammation is reduced further.

Tissue inflammation associated with SIRS is likely to involve another cytokine, IL-8. Interleukin-8 is an example of the family of chemotactic peptides that attracts neutrophils, monocytes and lymphocytes to pass from the circulation into tissues, stimulates the release of enzymes and histamine from phagocytes and mast cells, induces platelet-activating factor (PAF), and contributes to local tissue damage [32; 33].

Nearly each biological property of TNF has also been observed with IL-1. These include fever, haemodynamic shock, the induction of prostaglandin and collagen synthesis, bone and cartilage resorption, inhibition of protein lipase, and increased synthesis of hepatic acute-phase proteins [34; 35; 36; 37; 38]. The shock-like responses to TNF and IL-1 are likely to reflect their effects on the vascular endothelium.

The production of TNF and IL-1 are important in SIRS. Evidence supporting this is derived from studies showing the following:

(1) Injection of IL-1 or TNF into animals or humans causes a fall in systemic blood pressure and coagulopathy often seen in SIRS [35; 39; 40; 41; 42; 43].
(2) Blood levels of these cytokines are often elevated in patients with SIRS/sepsis [35; 40].
(3) Specific blockade of the action of these cytokines in animals with a shock-like syndrome reduces mortality [16; 17; 35; 44; 45; 46].

Interleukin-6 is a family of at least six differentially modified phosphoglycoproteins which are released rapidly within 60 minutes in response to injury [47; 48]. They act as a B cell stimulatory factor, hybridoma/plasmacytoma growth factor, hepatocyte stimulating factor and cytotoxic T cell differentiation factor. Interleukin-6 interacts synergistically with IL-1 to affect thymocyte proliferation. In combination with TNFα-augments T cell proliferation, and promotes polymorphonuclear neutrophils (PMN) activation and accumulation. The temporal relationship of IL-6 appearance within the cytokine cascade suggests

Table 17.2. *Summary of the main features of the best studied cytokines*

Cytokine	Mol wt	Cell source	Main cell target(s)	Main actions
IFN-γ	40–50 000 (dimer)	T cells, NK cells	Lymphocytes, monocytes, tissue cells	Immunoregulation, B cell differentiation, some viral action
IL-1α IL-1β	33 000 17 500	Monocytes, dendritic cells, some B cells, fibroblasts, epithelial cells, endothelial cells, macrophages	Thymocytes, neutrophils, T and B cells, tissue cells	Immunoregulation, inflammation, fever
IL-2	15 000	T cells NK cells	T cells, B cells, monocytes	Proliferation, activation
IL-3	15 000	T cells	Stem cells, progenitors	Pan-specific colony stimulating factor
IL-4	15 000	T cells	B cells, T cells	Division and differentiation
IL-5	15 000	T cells	B cells, eosinophils	Differentiation
IL-6	20 000	Macrophages, T cells, fibroblasts, some B cells	T cells, B cells, thymocytes, hepatocytes	Differentiation, acute phase protein synthesis
IL-8	8000	Macrophages, skin cells	Granulocytes, T cells	Chemotaxis
TNFα TNFβ	50 000 50 000 (trimer)	macrophages, lymphocytes	fibroblasts, endothelium	Inflammation, catabolism, fibrosis, production of other cytokines (IL-1, IL-6, GM-CSF) and adhesion molecules

a strong relationship to antecedent TNFα or IL-1 stimulation [47; 49]. Transcription and production are enhanced in response to TNFα and IL-1. When TNFα or IL-1 activity is attenuated, the subsequent IL-6 response is decreased. Anti-IL-6 monoclonal antibodies protect mice from lethal *Escherichia coli* infection and lethal exposure to TNFα [50].

Interleukin-6 also appears to be associated with the host septic response, probably being released in response to secretion of either TNFα, IL-1 or both cytokines. Infusion of IL-6 itself does not have any effect. Similarly, although direct injection of IL-8 does not produce adverse effects, raised levels of this cytokine have been demonstrated following a challenge of either gram-negative bacteria or endotoxin in experimental models. A great deal of information suggests that this cytokine acts to potentiate the effects of other mediators [51].

ANTI-INFLAMMATORY CYTOKINES

Tumour necrosis factor, IL-1 and the IL-8 family are often grouped together and called 'pro-inflammatory cytokines' to distingiush them from 'anti-inflammatory cytokines'. These latter cytokines include IL-4, IL-10, IL-13, interleukin-1 receptor antagonist (IL-1RA), TNF soluble receptors 1 and 2 (TNFsr 1 and 2) and transforming growth factor-β (TGFβ). They are considered anti-inflammatory because, when administered to animals with infection or inflammation, they reduce the severity of disease, and reduce the production of IL-1 and TNF.

Interleukin-4, IL-10, IL-13 or TGFβ each suppress gene expression and synthesis of IL-1, TNF and other cytokines. *In vitro*, these cytokines can reduce endotoxin-induced gene expression, and synthesis of IL-1 and TNF as much 90%. When given to mice or rats they can reduce lethal endotoxaemia. They are also known to alter monocyte function, impair antigen-presenting activity and reduce the ability of cells to produce pro-inflammatory cytokines. As such, they are potentially useful in some clinical situations. Interleukin-10 appears to be particularly useful because unlike IL-4 or TGFβ, IL-10 has no clinical side effects [52; 53].

Interleukin-1 receptor antagonist is produced primarily from macrophages. Interleukin-1 receptor antagonist binds to IL-1 receptors with nearly the same affinity as IL-1α or IL-1β but does not trigger a response [54]. The cytokine is thus the naturally occurring inhibitor of IL-1.

Unlike IL-1, a naturally occurring receptor antagonist to TNF has not been found. However, soluble receptors to TNF are present in the circulation of healthy humans and may act as naturally occurring inhibitors of TNF activity. The extracellular domains of the TNF receptors are shed from the cell surface by a serine proteinase associated with cell activation and enter the circulation. Increases in the circulating levels of soluble receptors to TNF occur during disease states [55; 56; 57; 58].

Potential mechanisms for the prevention of SIRS and sepsis with regards to cytokines will be covered later in the chapter.

THE ROLE OF THE ENDOTHELIUM

The endothelial cells play an important role in the pathogenesis of sepsis, not only because they may influence the inflammatory cascade but also because upon interaction with excessive amounts of inflammatory mediators, the function of these cells may become impaired. Under physiologic conditions, they exert a number of functions that are important for normal homeostasis. These functions include regulation of intravascular coagulation, orchestration of the migration of blood cells into the tissues by expression of adhesion molecules, production of chemoattractant compounds, regulation of the microcirculation through an extensive array of endogenously produced vasoactive factors and regulation of vasopermeability [59].

Endothelium is considered both a source of and a target for inflammation. Local activation of the endothelium is crucial in walling off infection, whereas systemic activation may result in capillary leakage, hypotension, microvascular thrombosis with resultant tissue hypoxia, and finally organ dysfunction and death.

Adhesion molecules

Exposure of the endothelial cells to endotoxin or pro-inflammatory cytokines (TNF, IL-1, IL-6, IL-8 and γ-interferon) results in endothelial activation and a massive increase in the surface expression of leucocyte adhesion molecules (E-selectin, intercellular adhesion molecule-1 (ICAM-1) and vascular cell adhesion molecule-1 (VCAM-1)) [60]. Two stages of activation occur [61]. The first is endothelial cell stimulation or type I activation, which does not require *de novo* protein synthesis or genotypic up-regulation. Endothelial cells retract from each other, express P-selectin leading to increased neutrophil adhesion and release von Willebrand factor which regulates platelet adherence to the subendothelium. Type II activation requires up-regulation of mRNA expression and *de novo* protein synthesis, particularly of cytokines and adhesion molecules. The endothelium produces VCAM-1 and ICAN-1 and ICAM-2 molecules, and E-selectin, facilitating the firm binding of leucocytes. The selectins are glycoproteins that mediate the initial step of leucocyte adherence and rolling on activated endothelium. Intercellular adhesion moleule-1 is a glycoprotein belonging to the immunoglobulin supergene family [63]. Together with VCAM-1 it mediates firm adhesion between leucocytes and endothelium, and subsequent diapedesis [64; 65]. These adhesion molecules mediate leucocyte activation events that may lead to tissue damage by the release of lysosomal enzymes and the production of reactive oxygen species. Simultaneously, activated neutrophils express a complementary sequence of surface adhesion molecules termed integrins, the most significant of which is the CD11/CD18 complex, which determine the migration of neutrophils into the interstitium.

Nitric oxide

In 1980, an endothelially derived relaxant factor (EDRF) was proposed as the mediator responsible for the vascular smooth muscle relaxation caused by acetylcholine, a process that required an intact endothelium [66; 67]. Endothelially derived relaxant factor was later shown to be pharmacologically identical to

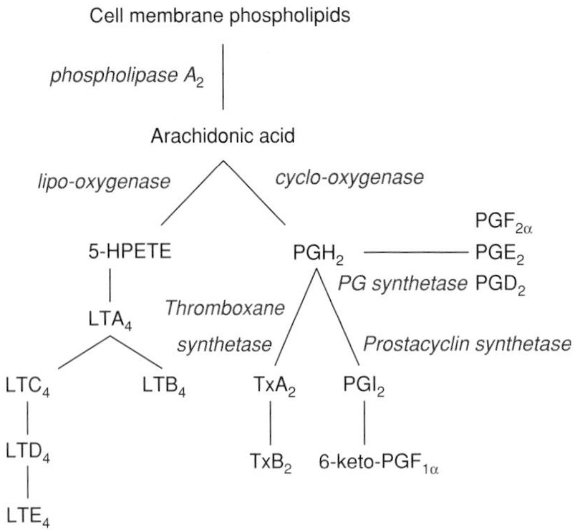

Fig. 17.4. The main pathways of arachidonic acid breakdown. HPETE = hydroperoxyeicosatetraenic acid; LT = leukotriene; Tx = thromboxane and PG = prostaglandin.

nitric oxide (NO). Nitric oxide stimulates guanylate cyclase to form cyclic GMP (cGMP) leading to a reduction in intracellular calcium, thereby modulating dilation in both arterial and venous vascular smooth muscle [68]. Nitric oxide is synthesized from the terminal guanidine nitrogen of the semi-essential amino acid L-arginine by a group of enzymes collectively called NO synthases (NOSs) [66].

In animal models of sepsis up to 1000 times the physiological concentration of NO has been identified [69; 70]. Endotoxin, and the cytokines IL-1, γ-IF and TNF induce NOS in vascular smooth muscle. The sequence of events that actually leads to increased NO production in such circumstances is more difficult to characterize. Nevertheless, the increased production of NO enhances vasodilatation, the formation of oedema and the modulation of sensory nerve endings which are hallmarks of the inflammatory response.

Arachidonic metabolites

Prostaglandins are important regulatory mediators of cardiovascular and pulmonary functions. The known synthetic pathways are summarized in (Figure 17.4).

Of the various derivatives, prostacyclin (PGI_2) and thromboxane (TxA_2) are probably the most important [71; 72; 73]. Prostacyclin is a potent vasodilator, acting on G-protein coupled receptors to increase intracellular cAMP levels. It is also an important inhibitor of platelet aggregation. Thromboxane is a potent constrictor of pulmonary arterioles after endotoxin infusion and is capable of increasing capillary permeability. Conversely, it causes the aggregation of platelets. The most important enzyme appears to be cyclo-oxygenase (COX). Cyclo-oxygenase has two isoforms (COX-1 and COX-2) which are encoded by separate genes. Cyclo-oxygenase-1 is constitutively produced and is thought to contribute to the maintenance of physiological homeostasis, whereas COX-2 is expressed at high levels upon induction [74; 75]. This induction is rapid and the gene encoding COX-2 has been termed an immediate/early or primary response gene. Cyclo-oxygenase-2 leads to the release of a large amount of prostaglandin and TxA_2. Absent from normal tissue, COX-2 is expressed at sites of inflammation, and in monocytes and macrophages stimulated with lipopolysaccharide, TNFα or IL-1. Expression of COX-2 is inhibited by anti-inflammatory glucocorticoids both *in vivo* and *in vitro*, and by anti-inflammatory cytokines such as IL-4 and IL-10 [74].

A variety of other eicosanoids, such as monohydroxy, dihydroxy and epoxy derivatives of arachidonic acid, which are formed by the cyclo-oxygenase-, lipo-oxygenase- and cytochrome P450-dependent mono-oxygenation pathways, also influence vascular tone. Leukotriene B_4 promotes neutrophil chemotaxis and adhesion of neutrophils to endothelium [76].

THE ROLE OF LEUCOCYTES

Polymorphonuclear neutrophil (PMN) cells have been identified as pivotal inflammatory mediators. They are the first immune cells to migrate to sites of inflammation. Their primary functions include phagocytosis of bacteria, elaboration of oxidative and non-oxidative degradative enzymes, and the elaboration of chemotactic factors which recruit other inflammatory cells [77].

Neutrophil priming, adhesion, migration, chemotaxis to inflammatory sites, apoptosis (programmed cell death) or necrosis and cytotoxic activity, continue to be the focus of active research aiming to understand and modulate the inflammatory sequence.

Priming

Polymorphonuclear neutrophil cells may be primed either by pathogenic signals or cytokine mediators. *In vitro* have studies demonstrated that bacterial lipopolysaccharide (LPS), TNFα, ILs, arachidonic acid metabolites, platelet activating factor (PAF), granulocyte-macrophage colony stimulating factor (GM-CSF) and the process of adhesion constitute potent PMN cell primers [78].

Adhesion

As already mentioned the process of adhesion and cell migration involves interaction between primed PMN and endothelial cells. It can be distinguished into three phases: (1) reversible physical rolling of PMN cells along the vessel wall; (2) firm adherence of PMN cells to vascular endothelium; and (3) migration of PMN cells across the endothelium [79].

Apoptosis

Sequestration of PMN cells at the sites of injury has both protective and corrective roles, although the prolonged presence of PMN cells in inflammatory sites may potentially be harmful. Necrosis and disruption of PMN cells releases cytotoxic proteases and reactive oxygen metabolites (ROM), which promote further tissue inflammation and injury. In contrast, apoptosis (regulated cell death) of PMN cells mediates their non-inflammatory disposal. The apoptotic PMN cell retains its cellular membrane intact and does not release its lysosomal enzymes while it is being eliminated by phagocytosis from recruited macrophages. Consequently, apoptosis of PMN cells and their elimination by macrophages contribute to the resolution of the inflammatory process and to the restriction of tissue injury.

Several lines of *in vitro* evidence indicate that apoptosis of neutrophils may limit injury in inflammation. First of all, apoptotic neutrophils have suppressed respiratory burst activity [80]. Apoptotic neutrophils are unable to degranulate and lose important activation associated ligand receptors like ICAM-1 [81]. Phagocytosis of apoptotic neutrophils inhibits the release of pro-inflammatory cytokines from monocytes [82]. Ingestion of necrotic polymorphonuclear cells, however, results in an intense release of these molecules.

It is appealing to project a model in which apoptosis of neutrophils is delayed when inflammatory signals indicate a need for longer activity. One hypothesis linking dysfunction of neutrophil apoptosis with sepsis is that delays in neutrophil apoptosis may allow for the prolonged elaboration of tissue destructive and pro-inflammatory chemotactic factors. A second hypothesis is that delays in neutrophil apoptosis may allow senescent neutrophils to progress to death by necrosis with the detrimental leakage of pro-inflammatory cytosolic proteins, the potentiation of macrophage secretion and the bystander effect of inflammation.

COAGULATION

It has long been suspected that there is a close relationship between coagulant activity and the status of endothelial cells. Whereas unperturbed endothelial cells provide anticoagulant properties, exposure to inflammatory and/or septic stimuli can rapidly lead to procoagulant behaviour.

Endotoxin, a LPS component of the outer membrane of gram-negative bacteria, is involved in the initial activation of the extrinsic pathway of coagulation, which is responsible for the emergence of a procoagulant state [83].

Endothelial cells play an active role in coagulation modulation [84]. Their outer membrane normally expresses various membrane-associated components with anticoagulant properties, including cell surface heparin-like molecules. These molecules accelerate inactivation of coagulation proteases by antithrombin-III and represent a monocyte tissue factor (TF) pathway inhibitor [85]. Tissue factor is a cell surface glycoprotein that mediates initiation of the coagulation serine proteinase cascade.

Thrombomodulin is an endothelial cell surface thrombin-binding protein which is responsible for thrombin activity inhibition. Thrombomodulin, when bound to thrombin, forms a potent protein C activator complex. Loss of thrombomodulin and associated protein C activation represents a key event of decreased endothelial coagulation modulation ability. In addition, release of endothelium-derived factors such as NO and PGI_2 is impaired. Because NO and PGI_2 not only control vascular tone but also have antiadhesive and tissue plasminogen activator-like properties, endothelium dysfunction and/or injury with subendothelium exposure facilitates leucocyte and platelet aggregation, and aggravation of coagulopathy [84].

POTENTIAL STRATEGIES FOR SIRS, SEPSIS AND MODS

Problems with the concept of SIRS

The classification of SIRS leading to sepsis, becoming severe sepsis, and resulting in septic shock and death, as described by Rangel-Frausto *et al.* [4], is really the same as a well person becoming sick, then sicker, finally severely ill and then dead. Such classifications may be acceptable and even worthwhile in describing or categorizing clinical states, but so far they have not been helpful as entry criteria to evaluate therapy.

Even the criteria for entry into SIRS hardly describe what is a very complex pathological process, and gives no indication as to the aetiology and pathophysiology. Hence no information is gained that may be utilized to construct a useful therapeutic strategy.

Multiple organ dysfunction syndrome and the newer more in vogue descriptions MARS and CHAOS are exactly that – mere descriptions or classifications of severity of illness, scoring systems that in themselves are not diseases or even syndromes by definition.

What is of interest is not how we can classify and define the pathological processes of SIRS and sepsis but what is it within that individual that makes them more susceptible to a standard surgical (or not so standard) traumatic insult [86]?

Potential strategies for SIRS/sepsis

- Identification of patients at risk
  - New surgical techniques
    - retroperitoneal approach
    - endovascular
    - vasoactive agents
    - intraluminal agents
  - Modulation of the inflammatory response
    - antioxidant
    - Anticytokine
    - Antiadhesion
    - Antiendotoxin

NEW SURGICAL TECHNIQUES

Retroperitoneal approach for aortic surgery

The progression of SIRS to MODS has been suggested as one of the leading causes (up to 50%) of deaths following elective infrarenal abdominal aortic aneurysm (AAA) repair. Retroperitoneal repair obviates the need to handle or exteriorize the gut. It has been shown to decrease the inflammatory response following AAA repair resulting in decreased neutrophil activation, as measured by elastase alpha-1 anti-trypsin complex formation, attenuated increases in gut mucosal permeability, reduced IL-6 expression and decreased portal endotoxaemia. This has resulted in improved pulmonary function, perioperative oxygenation, and decreased SIRS and MODS scores.

Technical differences in the procedures have been proposed as explanations for differences in the host's response to surgery, including a reduction in the pronounced haemodynamic changes that occur following evisceration of the small intestine and traction on the mesentery. These changes, compounded by cross clamping and mesenteric atherosclerosis, are likely to compromise the splanchnic circulation. This leads to reperfusion injury with loss of mucosal barrier integrity, and translocation of bacteria and endotoxins, as well as the systemic release of cytokines and superoxides leading to SIRS.

Despite this clinical studies have failed to demonstrate a significant difference in mortality [87].

Endovascular repair of aortic aneurysms

Similar reports have demonstrated differences in the inflammatory response following endovascular repair. Decreases in the incidence of intestinal ischaemia, alterations in gut permeability, endotoxaemia, and cytokine and oxygen free radical generation have been reported [88].

One study of patients randomized to open or endovascular AAA repair demonstrated smaller increases in IL-6 and IL-8 with equivalent venous IL-10 levels, revealing a possible pro-/anti-inflammatory imbalance in the open repair group [89].

Other studies have, however, demonstrated conflicting results implying the aetiology of SIRS in these very different procedures in terms of surgical insult is also different [90; 91; 92].

VASOACTIVE AGENTS

Despite early reports of improved splanchnic flow with dopamine and dobutamine, evidence now indicates they may produce or exacerbate bowel ischaemia [93; 94].

Randomized prospective controlled trials (RPCT) of elective AAA patients treated with low dose dopamine demonstrated decreased sigmoid intramucosal pH indicating increased gut ischaemia. A recent review outlined the potential dangers of dopamine use in the treatment of sepsis related acute renal failure. It stated dopamine as being ineffective and potentially dangerous, and recommended it not be used until its efficacy has been established in randomized placebo control trials [95].

Dopexamine and angiotensin converting enzyme inhibitors have, however, shown some promise in the clinical setting. In a multicentre randomized placebo control study of patients undergoing AAA repair, those treated with a perioperative infusion of dopexamine showed significantly less evidence of gastrointestinal ischaemic histological changes compared with the placebo indicating that dopexamine affords protection following AAA surgery.

In a further study of dopexamine vs. prostacyclin, dopexamine produced a significant increase in heart rate, urine output, splanchnic perfusion and oxygen delivery [96].

This is possibly a cause for concern in light of the recent evidence demonstrating the potential benefits of beta-blockade in vascular patients.

INTRALUMINAL THERAPY – INTESTINAL MUCOSAL INTEGRITY

Intraluminal therapy has been studied in an attempt to attenuate the loss of gut mucosal integrity that occurs as a local response to ischaemia and as end organ damage in the case of SIRS. It has the advantage of direct delivery to the site of ischaemia, and may prove important in the prevention of intestinal bacterial and endotoxin translocation [97].

Intraluminal sodium pyruvate has been shown to decrease mucosal injury in animal studies and L-arginine decreases reperfusion injury possibly via a NO mediated mechanism [98].

Selective gut decontamination is widely practised in Europe and the USA, and over 22 PRCT exist that demonstrate a significant reduction in the incidence of pneumonia following trauma. Mortality, however, was not affected [99].

Early total enteral nutrition has also been shown to be beneficial in ischaemic gut injury following burns and severe trauma. In comparison to total parenteral nutrition it showed a reduction in septic mortality. The use of enteral feeding with immune enhancing supplements (glutamine, arginine, omega 3 fatty acids and nucleic acids) has been shown to produce additional clinical benefits by reducing septic morbidity [97].

MODULATION OF THE INFLAMMATORY RESPONSE

Can we block, stimulate or replace the substances and abnormalities of an inflammatory response to avoid sepsis? So far the many clinical trials of agents implicated in the pathophysiology of SIRS to control sepsis or an excessive inflammatory response have been negative. The end point in most, if not all, of these studies was mortality within 28 days. These trials included monoclonal antibodies to endotoxin, anti-TNF antibodies, an IL-1RA, soluble TNF receptors, a TNF receptor-fusion protein, PAF antagonists, a bradykinin antagonist, taurolidine, antithrombin-III concentrate and γ-IF [100; 101; 102; 103; 104].

Four papers recently presented at the Fifth Vienna Shock Forum, suggested that the therapeutic premise of benefit from inhibiting endotoxin or host inflammatory mediators in patients with sepsis or septic shock may be flawed [105]. These studies reported that inhibition of neutrophils by monoclonal antibodies to adhesion molecules may be deleterious. Inhibition of NO may produce more harm than good. Antiendotoxin strategies may work only if used before the insult. A monoclonal antibody to TNF will protect against an injection of endotoxin (an intravascular insult), but anti-TNF monoclonal antibodies increase the mortality of peritonitis in animals. Interleukin-1 receptor antagonist and IL-1 in small doses protected animals from *Klebsiella pneumoniae*, whereas larger doses of IL-1 RA increased lethality. Thus, the complexity and heterogeneity of the underlying disease processes and their life-threatening manifestations, the contradictory underlying pathologic processes, and the complex and redundant mediator-inflammatory system indicate that we have much to learn.

So why have these clinical trials failed to confirm the vast amount of supportive data from animal studies. A number of reasons have been suggested. Flaws in study design such as sampling error, selection bias, heterogeneity of study population, inadequate dose and duration of treatment, and incorrect timing of intervention may be responsible for the lack of improvement seen in some of these trials.

Entering people into trials based on the classification of SIRS or MODS, groups together a heterogeneous population of patients with differing aetiologies, and although helpful in categorizing clinical states is not useful as entry criteria to evaluate therapy. It also begs the question can we control the excess without interfering with what is needed?

Recently the use of multiple agents to modulate rather than block an excessive or continuing response has been recommended, i.e. in view of the complex pathophysiology of sepsis, targeting TNFα alone may be insufficient.

Other recommendations for future trials including the use of:

(1) Specific entry criteria (early recognition of elevated cytokines may help).
(2) Ideal dosing, timing and duration of therapy.
(3) Correct agent (single or multiple) specific to the perceived abnormality.
(4) Standardization of patient management in clinical trials.
(5) The use of different end points, such as decreased MOF or MODS scores, rather than 28-day mortality.

A final reason for failure of human clinical trials is the existence of numerous polymorphisms that exist within human systems altering the initial conditions and making one individual more susceptible to an injury than another. Genotype has been shown to contribute substantially to the outcome in inflammatory and infectious diseases. For example, specific polymorphisms are associated with altered outcome in patients with severe infections, trauma, inflammatory bowel disease and numerous other inflammatory diseases [106; 107].

Polymorphic sites have been demonstrated for some cytokine genes and have been shown to affect cytokine mRNA expression (IL-10, IL-6 and TNFα) [108].

The most studied is a single base substitution in the promoter sequence of TNFα which has been shown in some studies to increase TNFα activity. Tumour necrosis factor-α polymorphisms have been associated with non-survival in septic patients and IL-1RA polymorphisms may impart susceptibility to infection [109].

In conclusion, although sepsis trials have not yet impacted on the care and survival of critically ill patients, there is reason for renewed optimism. Increased understanding of the pathophysiology of sepsis and the emerging identification of the role of genetic susceptibility should translate into effective individualized treatment strategies for sepsis in the future.

REFERENCES

1. D. C. Angus, W. T. Linde-Zwirble, J. Lidicker *et al.*, Epidemiology of severe sepsis in the United States: analysis of incidence, outcome, and associated costs of care. *Critical Care Medicine*, **29** (2001), 1303–10.
2. Centers for Disease Control and Prevention. Increase in national hospital discharge survey rates for septicemia – United States, 1979–87. **39** (1990), 31–4.
3. Consensus Conference Committee. American College of Chest Physicians/Society of Critical Care Medicine consensus conference: definitions for sepsis and organ failure and guidelines for the use of innovative therapies in sepsis. *Critical Care Medicine*, **20** (1992), 864–74.
4. M. S. Rangel-Frausto, D. Pittet, M. Costigan *et al.*, The natural history of the systemic inflammatory response syndrome (SIRS). A prospective study. *Journal of the American Medical Association*, **273** (1995), 117–23.
5. P. R. Miller, D. D. Munn, M. J. Wayne *et al.*, Systemic inflammatory response syndrome in the trauma intensive care unit: who is infected? *Journal of Trauma*, **47** (1999), 1004–8.
6. D. H. Livingston, A. C. Mosenthal & E. A. Deitch, Sepsis and multiple organ dysfunction syndrome: a clinical-mechanistic overview. *New Horizons*, **3** (1995), 257–66.
7. B. Eisman, R. Beart & L. Norton, Multiple organ failure. *Surgery, Gynecology and Obstetrics*, **144** (1977), 323–6.
8. D. E. Fry, L. Pearlstein, R. L. Fulton *et al.*, Multiple system organ failure: the role of uncontrolled infection. *Archives of Surgery*, **115** (1980), 136–40.
9. H. C. Polk & C. L. Shields, Remote organ failure: a valid sign of occult intra-abdominal infection. *Surgery*, **81** (1977), 310–13.
10. R. J. A. Goris, T. P. A. Boekhorst, J. K. S. Nuytinck *et al.*, Multiple organ failure: generalized autodestructive inflammation? *Archives of Surgery*, **120** (1985), 1109–15.
11. C. C. Baker & T. Huynh, Sepsis in the critically ill patient. *Current Problems in Surgery*, **32** (1995), 1015–92.

12. D. R. Dantzker, B. Foresman & G. Gutierrez, Oxygen supply and utilization relationships. A reevaluation. *American Review of Respiratory Diseases*, **143** (1991), 675–9.
13. R. C. Bone, Toward a theory regarding the pathogenesis of the systemic inflammatory response system: what we do and do not know about cytokine regulation. *Critical Care Medicine*, **24** (1996), 163–72.
14. D. Dantzker, Oxygen delivery and utilization in sepsis. *Critical Care Clinics*, **5** (1989), 81–98.
15. D. R. Dantzker, B. Foresman & G. Gutierrez, Oxygen supply and utilization relationships. A reevaluation. *American Review of Respiratory Diseases*, **143** (1991), 675–9.
16. G. J. Slotman, K. W. Burchard, J. J. Williams, A. D'Arezzo & S. A. Yellin, Interaction of prostaglandins, activated complement, and granulocytes in clinical sepsis and hypotension. *Surgery*, **99** (1986), 744–51.
17. S. Fujishima & N. Aikawa, Neutrophil-mediated tissue injury and its modulation. *Intensive Care Medicine*, **21** (1995), 277–85.
18. S. D. Cushing & A. M. Fogelman, Monocytes may amplify their recruitment into inflammatory lesions by inducing monocyte chemotactic protein. *Arteriosclerosis and Thrombosis*, **12** (1992), 78–82.
19. H. A. Pereira, CAP37, a neutrophil-derived multifunctional inflammatory mediator. *Journal of Leukocyte Biology*, **57** (1995), 805–12.
20. C. C. Baker & T. Huynh, Sepsis in the critically ill patient. *Current Problems in Surgery*, **32** (1995), 1015–92.
21. R. Saadia & M. Schein, Multiple organ failure: how valid is the 'two hit' model? *Journal of Accident and Emergency Medicine*, **16** (1999), 163–6.
22. M. G. Davies & P. O. Hagen, Systemic inflammatory response syndrome. *British Journal of Surgery*, **84** (1997), 920–35.
23. R. C. Bone, C. J. Grodzin & R. A. Balk, Sepsis: a new hypothesis for pathogenesis of the disease process. *Chest*, **112** (1997), 235–43.
24. H. D. Volk, M. Thieme, S. Heym *et al.*, Alterations in function and phenotype of monocytes from patients with septic disease: predictive value and new therapeutic strategies. *Behring Institute Mitteilungen*, **88** (1991), 208–15.
25. R. C. Bone, Immunologic dissonance: a continuing evolution in our understanding of the systemic inflammatory response syndrome (SIRS) and the multiple organ dysfunction syndrome (MODS). *Annals of Internal Medicine*, **125** (1996), 680–7.
26. A. S. Goldie, K. C. H. Fearon, J. A. Ross *et al.*, Natural cytokine antagonists and endogenous antiendotoxin core antibodies in sepsis syndrome. The Sepsis Intervention Group. *JAMA*, **274** (1995), 172–7.
27. E. Borelli, P. Roux-Lombard, G. Grau *et al.*, Plasma concentrations of cytokines, their soluble receptors, and antioxidant vitamins can predict the development of multiple organ failure in patients at risk. *Critical Care Medicine*, **24** (1996), 392–7.
28. F. Randow, U. Syrbe, C. Meisel *et al.*, Mechanism of endotoxin desensitization: involvement of interleukin 10 and transforming growth factor beta. *Journal of Experimental Medicine*, **181** (1995), 1887–92.
29. A. L. Picone, C. J. Lutz, C. Finck *et al.*, Multiple sequential insults cause post-pump syndrome. *Annals of Thoracic Surgery*, **67** (1999), 978–85.
30. R. C. Bone, Sir Isaac Newton, sepsis, SIRS and CARS. *Critical Care Medicine*, **24** (1996), 1125–8.
31. A. Billiau & F. Vandekerckhove, Cytokines and their interactions with other inflammatory mediators in the pathogenesis of sepsis and septic shock. *European Journal of Clinical Investigation*, **21** (1991), 559–73.
32. L. Biancone, C. Tetta, E. Turello *et al.*, Platelet-activating factor biosynthesis by cultured mesangial cells is modulated by proteinase inhibitors. *Journal of American Society of Nephrology*, **2** (1992), 1251–61.
33. M. Baggiolini, B. Dewald & A. Waltz, Interleukin-8 and related cytokines. In *Inflammation: Basic Principles and Clinical Correlates*, ed. J. I. Gallin, I. M. Goldstein and R. Synderman (New York, NY: Raven Press, 1992), pp. 247–63.
34. C. A. Dinarello, J. G. Cannon, S. M. Wolff *et al.*, Tumor necrosis factor (cachectin) is an endogenous pyrogen and induces production of interleukin 1. *Journal of Experimental Medicine*, **163** (1986), 1433–50.
35. S. Okusawa, J. A. Gelfand, T. Ikejima, R. J. Connolly & C. A. Dinarello, Interleukin 1 induces a shock-like state in rabbits: synergism with tumor necrosis factor and the effect of cyclooxygenase inhibition. *Journal of Clinical Investigation*, **81** (1988), 1162–72.
36. J. M. Dayer, B. Beutler & A. Cerami, Cachectin/tumor necrosis factor stimulates collagenase and prostaglandin E2 production by human synovial cells and dermal fibroblasts. *Journal of Experimental Medicine*, **162** (1985), 2163–8.

37. B. Beutler & A. Cerami, Cachectin: more than a tumor necrosis factor. *New England Journal of Medicine*, **316** (1987), 379–85.
38. D. H. Perlmutter, C. A. Dinarello, P. I. Punsal, H. R. Colten, Cachectin/tumor necrosis factor regulates hepatic acute-phase gene expression. *Journal of Clinical Investigation*, **78** (1986), 1349–54.
39. P. B. Chapman, T. J. Lester, E. S. Casper *et al.* Clinical pharmacology of recombinant human tumor necrosis factor in patients with advanced cancer. *Journal of Clinical Oncology*, **5** (1987), 1942–51.
40. C. A. Dinarello, Interleukin-1 and its biologically related cytokines. *Advances in Immunology*, **44** (1989), 153–205.
41. J. W. Smith, II, W. Urba, R. Steis *et al.*, Interleukin-1 alpha administered in a phase I trial to patients with advanced malignancies. *Journal of Clinical Oncology*, **10** (1992), 1141–52.
42. T. van der Poll, H. R. Bueller, H. ten Cate *et al.*, Activation of coagulation after administration of tumor necrosis factor to normal subjects. *New England Journal of Medicine*, **322** (1990), 1622–7.
43. E. Fischer, M. A. Marano, A. E. Barber *et al.*, A comparison between the effects of interleukin-1alpha administration and sublethal endotoxemia in primates. *American Journal of Physiology*, **261** (1991), R442–9.
44. W. P. Arend, Interleukin 1 receptor antagonist: a new member of the interleukin family. *Journal of Clinical Investigation*, **88** (1991), 1445–51.
45. J. W. Christman, Potential treatment of sepsis syndrome with cytokine-specific agents. *Chest*, **102** (1992), 613–17.
46. C. A. Dinarello & S. M. Wolff, The role of interleukin-1 in disease. *New England Journal of Medicine*, **328** (1993), 106–13.
47. A. Waage, P. Brandtzaeg, A. Halstensen, P. Kierulf & T. Espevik, The complex pattern of cytokines in serum with meningococcal septic shock. Association between interleukin 6, interleukin 1, and fatal outcome. *Journal of Experimental Medicine*, **169** (1989), 333–8.
48. L. T. May, J. Ghrayeb, U. Santhanam *et al.*, Synthesis and secretion of multiple forms of 'beta2 interferon/B cell differentiation factor BSF-2/hepatocyte stimulating factor' by human fibroblasts and monocytes. *Journal of Biological Chemistry*, **263** (1989), 7760–6.
49. Y. Fong, L. L. Moldawer, M. Marano *et al.*, Endotoxemia elicits increased circulating beta 2-IFN/IL-6 in man. *Journal of Immunology*, **142** (1989), 2321–4.
50. Y. Fong, K. J. Tracey, L. L. Moldawer *et al.*, Antibodies to cachectin/tumor necrosis factor reduce interleukin-1 beta and interleukin-6 appearance during lethal bacteremia. *Journal of Experimental Medicine*, **170** (1989), 1627–33.
51. A. Harada, N. Sekido, T. Akahoshi *et al.*, Essential involvement of interleukin-8 (IL-8) in acute inflammation. *Journal of Leukocyte Biology*, **56** (1994), 559–64.
52. K. W. Moore, A. O'Garra, R. de Waal Malefyt *et al.*, Interleukin-10. *Annual Review of Immunology*, **11** (1993), 165–90.
53. C. Platzer, C. Meisel, K. Vogt, M. Platzer & H. D. Volk, Up-regulation of monocytic IL-10 by tumor necrosis factor-alpha and cAMP elevating drugs. *International Immunology*, **7** (1995), 517–23.
54. C. J. Fisher, Jr, J. F. Dhaihaut, S. M. Opal *et al.*, Recombinant human interleukin 1 receptor antagonist in the treatment of patients with sepsis syndrome. Results from a randomized, double-blind, placebo-controlled trial. Phase III rhIL-1ra Sepsis Syndrome Study Group. *JAMA*, **271** (1994), 1836–44.
55. A. Ayala, P. Wang, Z. F. Ba *et al.*, Differential alterations in plasma IL-6 and TNF levels after trauma and hemorrhage. *American Journal of Physiology*, **260** (Regulatory Integrative Comp. Physiol. 29) (1991), R167–71.
56. A. Ayala, M. M. Perrin, D. R. Meldrum *et al.*, Hemorrhage induced an increase in serum TNF which is not associated with elevated levels of endotoxin. *Cytokine*, **2** (1990), 170–4.
57. A. R. Exley, T. Leese, M. P. Holliday *et al.*, Endotoxaemia and serum tumour necrosis factor as prognostic markers in severe acute pancreatitis. *Gut*, **33** (1992), 1126–8.
58. G. Hamilton, S. Hofbauer & B. Hamilton, Endotoxin, TNF-alpha, interleukin-6 and parameters of the cellular immune system in patients with intraabdominal sepsis. *Scandinavian Journal of Infectious Diseases*, **24** (1992), 361–8.
59. M. G. Davies & P. O. Hagen, The vascular endothelium. A new horizon. *Annals of Surgery*, **218** (1993), 593–609.
60. C. E. Hack & S. Zeerleder, The endothelium in sepsis: source of and a target for inflammation. *Critical Care Medicine*, **29**(Suppl) (2001), S21–7.
61. A. J. Gearing & W. Newman, Circulating adhesion molecules in disease. *Immunology Today*, **14** (1993), 506–12.

62. D. B. Kuhns, G. Alvord & J. Gallin, Increased circulating cytokines, cytokine antagonists, and E-selectin after intravenous administration of endotoxin in humans. *Journal of Infectious Diseases*, **171** (1995), 145–52.
63. N. Hogg, P. A. Bates & J. Harvey, Structure and function of intercellular adhesion molecule-1. *Chemical Immunology*, **50** (1991), 98–115.
64. J. Boldt, M. Muller, D. Kuhn *et al.*, Circulating adhesion molecules in the critically ill: a comparison between trauma and sepsis patients. *Intensive Care Medicine*, **22** (1996), 122–8.
65. M. J. Whalen, L. A. Doughty, T. M. Carlos *et al.*, Intercellular adhesion molecule-1 and vascular cell adhesion molecule-1 are increased in the plasma of children with sepsis-induced multiple organ failure. *Critical Care Medicine*, **28** (2000), 2600–7.
66. A. K. Nussler & T. R. Billiar, Inflammation, immunoregulation, and inducible nitric oxide synthase. *Journal of Leukocyte Biology*, **54** (1993), 171–8.
67. T. A. Wolfe & J. F. Dasta, Use of nitric oxide synthase inhibitors as a novel treatment for septic shock. *Annals of Pharmacotherapy*, **29** (1995), 36–46.
68. S. M. Morris, Jr. & T. R. Billiar, New insights into the regulation of inducible nitric oxide synthesis. *American Journal of Physiology*, **266** (1994), E829–39.
69. H. F. Goode, P. D. Howdle, B. E. Walker & N. R. Webster, Nitric oxide synthase activity is increased in patients with sepsis syndrome. *Clinical Science*, **88** (1995), 131–3.
70. E. Nava, R. M. J. Palmer & S. Moncada, Inhibition of nitric oxide synthesis in septic shock: how much is beneficial? *Lancet*, **338** (1991), 1555–7.
71. J. X. Li, J. R. Oliver, C. Y. Lu & J. B. Philips, 3rd, Delayed thromboxane or tumor necrosis factor-alpha, but not leukotriene inhibition, attenuates prolonged pulmonary hypertension in endotoxemia. *American Journal of Medical Sciences*, **310**(3) (1995), 103–10.
72. H. Zhang, M. Benlabed, H. Spapen, D. N. Nguyen & J. L. Vincent, Prostaglandin E1 increases oxygen extraction capabilities in experimental sepsis. *Journal of Surgical Research*, **57**(4) (1994), 470–9.
73. T. Scheeren, F. Susanto, H. Reinauer, J. Tarnow & P. Radermacher, Prostacyclin improves glucose utilization in patients with sepsis. *Journal of Critical Care*, **9**(3) (1994), 175–84.
74. J. A. Mitchell, S. Larkin & T. J. Williams, Cyclo-oxygenase-2: regulation and relevance in inflammation. *Biochemical Pharmacology*, **50** (1995), 1535–42.
75. S. F. Liu, R. Newton, T. W. Evans & P. J. Barnes, Differential regulation of cyclo-oxygenase-1 and cyclo-oxygenase-2 gene expression by lipopolysaccharide treatment *in vivo* in the rat. *Clinical Science*, **90** (1996), 301–6.
76. A. R. Brash, Arachidonic acid as a bioactive molecule. *Journal of Clinical Investigation*, **107** (2001), 1339–45.
77. S. Fujishima & N. Aikawa, Neutrophil-mediated tissue injury and its modulation. *Intensive Care Medicine*, **21** (1995), 277–85.
78. A. J. Rosenbloom, M. R. Pinsky, J. L. Bryant *et al.*, Leukocyte activation in the peripheral blood of patients with cirrhosis of the liver and SIRS. Correlation with serum interleukin-6 levels and organ dysfunction. *JAMA*, **274** (1995), 58–65.
79. K. Ley, Leukocyte adhesion to vascular endothelium. *Journal of Reconstructive Microsurgery*, **8** (1992), 495–503.
80. M. F. Jimenez, R. W. Watson, J. Parodo *et al.*, Dysregulated expression of neutrophil apoptosis in the systemic inflammatory response syndrome. *Archives of Surgery*, **132** (1997), 1263–70.
81. J. A. Smith, Neutrophils, host defence and inflammation: a double edged sword. *Journal of Leukocyte Biology*, **56** (1994), 672–86.
82. C. Haslett, Resolution of acute inflammation and the role of apoptosis in the tissue fate of granulocytes. *Clinical Science (Colchester)*, **83** (1992), 639–48.
83. S. Gando, S. Nanzaki & O. Kemmotsu, Disseminated intravascular coagulation and sustained systemic inflammatory response syndrome predict organ dysfunctions after trauma: application of clinical decision analysis. *Annals of Surgery*, **229** (1999), 121–7.
84. I. Maruyama, Biology of endothelium. *Lupus*, **7** (1998), S41–3.
85. I. D. McGilvray & O. D. Rotstein, Signaling pathways of tissue factor expression in monocytes and macrophages. *Sepsis*, **3** (1999), 93–101.
86. J. I. Spark & D. J. A. Scott, The role of the neutrophil in sepsis. *British Journal of Surgery*, **88** (2001), 1583–9.
87. M. J. Bown, M. L. Nicholson, P. R. Bell & R. D. Sayers, Cytokines and inflammatory pathways in the pathogenesis of multiple organ failure following abdominal aortic aneurysm repair. *European Journal of Vascular and Endovascular Surgery*, **22**(6) (2001), 485–95.

88. T. E. Rowlands & S. Homer-Vanniasinkam, Pro- and anti-inflammatory cytokine release in open versus endovascular repair of abdominal aortic aneurysm. *British Journal of Surgery*, **88**(10) (2001), 1335–40.
89. A. Odegard, J. Lundbom, H. O. Myhre *et al.*, The inflammatory response following treatment of abdominal aortic aneurysms: a comparison between open surgery and endovascular repair. *European Journal of Vascular and Endovascular Surgery*, **19** (2000), 536–44.
90. J. May, G. H. White, W. Yu *et al.*, Concurrent comparison of endoluminal versus open repair in the treatment of abdominal aortic aneurysms: analysis of 303 patients by life table method. *Journal of Vascular Surgery*, **27** (1998), 213–20.
91. G. H. White, J. May, T. McGahan *et al.*, Historic control comparison of outcome for matched groups of patients undergoing endoluminal versus open repair of abdominal aortic aneurysms. *Journal of Vascular Surgery*, **23** (1996), 201–11.
92. P. Swartbol, L. Norgren, U. Albrechtsson *et al.*, Biological responses differ considerably between endovascular and conventional aortic aneurysm surgery. *European Journal of Vascular Endovascular Surgery*, **12** (1996), 18–25.
93. W. Angehrn, E. Schmid, F. Althaus *et al.*, Effect of dopamine on hepatosplanchnic blood flow. *Journal of Cardiovascular Pharmacology*, **2** (1980), 257–.
94. D. J. Johnson, J. A. Johannigman, R. D. Branson *et al.*, The effect of low dose dopamine on gut hemodynamics during PEEP ventilation for acute lung injury. *Journal of Surgical Research*, **50** (1991), 344–9
95. D. A. Power, J. Duggan & H. R. Brady, Renal-dose (low-dose) dopamine for the treatment of sepsis-related and other forms of acute renal failure: ineffective and probably dangerous. *Clinical and Experimental Pharmacology and Physiology*, **26**(Suppl) (1999), S23–8.
96. A. Thoren, M. Elam & S. E. Ricksten, Differential effects of dopamine, dopexamine, and dobutamine on jejunal mucosal perfusion early after cardiac surgery. *Critical Care Medicine*, **28**(7) (2000), 2338–43.
97. J. MacFie, Enteral versus parenteral nutrition: the significance of bacterial translocation and gut-barrier function. *Nutrition*, **16**(7–8) (2000), 606–11.
98. B. J. Rowlands & K. R. Gardiner, Nutritional modulation of gut inflammation. *Proceedings of the Nutrition Society*, **57**(3) (1998), 395–401.
99. F. A. Moore, The role of the gastrointestinal tract in postinjury multiple organ failure. *American Journal of Surgery*, **178**(6) (1999), 449–53.
100. R. C. Bone, R. A. Balk, A. M. Fein *et al.*, A second large controlled clinical study of E5, a monoclonal antibody to endotoxin: results of a prospective, multicenter, randomized, controlled trial. The E5 Sepsis Study Group. *Critical Care Medicine*, **23**(6) (1995), 989–91.
101. C. C. Baker & T. Huynh, Sepsis in the critically ill patient – in brief. *Current Problems in Surgery*, **32**(12) (1995), 1018–83.
102. J. Cohen & J. Carlet, INTERSEPT: an international, multicenter, placebo-controlled trial of monoclonal antibody to human tumor necrosis factor-alpha in patients with sepsis. International Sepsis Trial Study Group. *Critical Care Medicine*, **24**(9) (1996), 1431–40.
103. O. Laneuville, D. Reynaud, S. Grinstein, S. Nigam & C. R. Pace-Asciak, Hepoxilin A3 inhibits the rise in free intracellular calcium evoked by formyl-methionyl-leucyl-phenylalanine, platelet-activating factor and leukotriene B4. *Biochemical Journal*, **295** (1993), 393–7.
104. A. M. Fein, G. R. Bernard, G. J. Criner *et al.*, Treatment of severe systemic inflammatory response syndrome and sepsis with a novel bradykinin antagonist, deltibant (cp-0127)-results of a randomized, double-blind, placebo-controlled trial. *Journal of the American Medical Association*, **277**(6) (1997), 482–7.
105. Fifth Vienna Shock Forum. Vienna, Austria, May 7–11, 1995. Abstracts. *Shock*, **3** (Suppl) (1995), 1–84.
106. S. Gibot, A. Cariou, L. Drouet *et al.*, Association between a genomic polymorphism within the CD14 locus and septic shock susceptibility and mortality rate. *Critical Care Medicine*, **30** (2002), 969–73.
107. X. M. Fang, S. Schroder, A. Hoeft *et al.*, Comparison of two polymorphisms of the interleukin-1 gene family: interleukin-1 receptor antagonist polymorphism contributes to susceptibility to severe sepsis. *Critical Care Medicine*, **27** (1999), 1330–4.
108. J. P. Mira, A. Cariou, F. Grall *et al.*, Association of TNF2, a TNF-alpha promoter polymorphism, with septic shock susceptibility and mortality: a multicenter study. *Journal of the American Medical Association*, **282** (1999), 561–68.
109. F. Stuber, M. Petersen, F. Bokelmann *et al.*, A genomic polymorphism within the tumor necrosis factor locus influences plasma tumor necrosis factor-alpha concentrations and outcome of patients with severe sepsis. *Critical Care Medicine*, **24** (1996), 381–4.

18 • Pathophysiology of reperfusion injury

PRUE A. COWLED, PETER E. LAWS, DENISE M. ROACH AND ROBERT A. FITRIDGE

INTRODUCTION

Ischaemia-reperfusion injury (IRI) is defined as the paradoxical exacerbation of cellular dysfunction and death following the restoration of blood flow to previously ischaemic tissues. Re-establishment of blood flow is essential to salvage ischaemic tissues, however, reperfusion itself paradoxically causes further damage to the ischaemic tissue, threatening function and viability of the organ. It occurs in a wide range of organs, including the heart, lung, kidney, gut, skeletal muscle and brain, and may involve not only the ischaemic organ but may also have systemic effects on distant organs, leading to multisystem organ failure. Reperfusion injury is a multifactorial process resulting in extensive tissue destruction. The aim of this review is to summarize these molecular and cellular mechanisms, and thus provide an insight into possible windows for therapeutic intervention.

ISCHAEMIA

ATP and mitochondrial function

Ischaemia occurs when the oxygen supply is less than the demand required for normal function. Derangements in metabolic function begin during this ischaemic phase. Initially, mitochondrial anaerobic glycolysis is utilized for the formation of adenosine triphosphate (ATP) resulting in elevation of lactic acid [1; 2] and a decrease in tissue pH, preventing further ATP production (Figure 18.1). Adenosine triphosphate is then sequentially broken down into adenosine diphosphate (ADP), adenosine monophosphate (AMP), and inosine monophosphate (IMP), and then further into adenosine, inosine, hypoxanthine and xanthine (Figure 18.2) [3].

At the cellular level, cessation of ATP synthesis deranges ionic pump function across the cell membranes and the transmembrane ionic gradients are lost. Consequently, cytosolic sodium content rises, drawing with it a volume of water to maintain the osmotic equilibrium. To maintain the ionic balance, potassium ions escape from the cell into the interstitium [4]. Calcium is released from the mitochondria into the cytoplasm and extracellular spaces [5; 6], activating cytosolic proteinases including calpain [7], which convert xanthine dehydrogenase to xanthine oxidase (Figure 18.2) [8]. Phospholipases are also activated during ischaemia, [9; 10], degrading membrane lipids and increasing the levels of polyunsaturated fatty acids [11].

Gene activity

During the ischaemic phase, hypoxia activates a number of genes, particularly transcription factors, including activating protein-1 (AP-1) [12], hypoxia inducible factor-1 (HIF-1) [13] and nuclear factor-κ B (NF-κ B) [14; 15]. Hypoxia inducible factor-1 activates transcription of other genes such as vascular endothelial growth factor (VEGF), erythropoietin and glucose transporter-1 (GLUT-1), which all play an important role in the cells' adaptive response to hypoxia [16]. Both HIF-1 and AP-1 are rapidly activated during liver ischaemia [13]. Expression of both HIF-1 and cyclo-oxygenase-2 (COX-2) are also induced in the lungs of rats subjected to haemorrhagic shock. Cyclo-oxygenase-2 may promote the inflammatory response through the rapid and exaggerated production of nitric oxide (NO) and prostaglandins, contributing to organ damage [17]. Activation of NF-κ B occurs during both the ischaemic and reperfusion phases, and will therefore be discussed below.

REPERFUSION

Reactive oxygen species

Table 18.1 illustrates the major reactive oxygen species (ROS) which play a role in tissue damage during

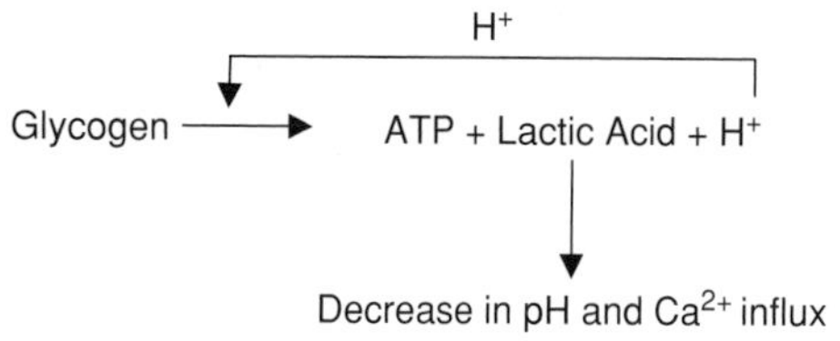

Fig. 18.1. Anaerobic glycolysis during ischaemia results in negative feedback which inhabits ATP production and induces tissue acidosis.

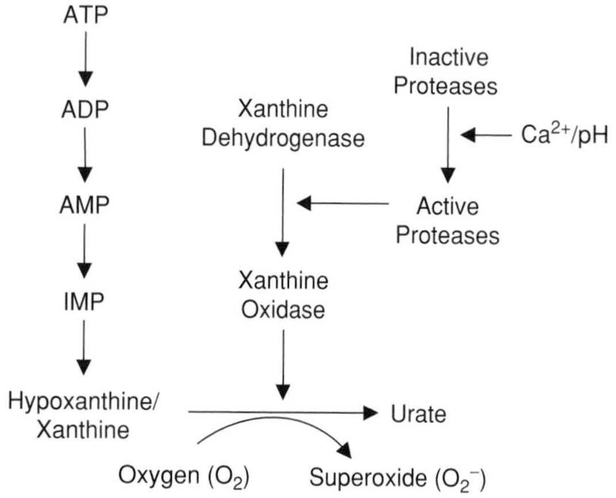

Fig. 18.2. During reperfusion, ATP is degraded and xanthine oxidase catalyses the conversion of hypoxanthine to highly reactive and toxic superoxide anions.

Table 18.1. *Reactive oxygen species involved in IRI*

Major ROS
- Superoxide anion (O_2^-)
- Hydrogen peroxide (H_2O_2)
- Hydroxyl radical (OH)
- Nitric oxide (NO)

Minor ROS
- Lipid hydroperoxide
- Lipid peroxyl radical
- Lipid alkoxyl radical
- Thiol radical

Sources of ROS during IRI
- Xanthine oxidase system
- Activated neutrophils
- Mitochondrial electron transport chain
- Arachidonic acid metabolism
- Auto-oxidation of catecholamines

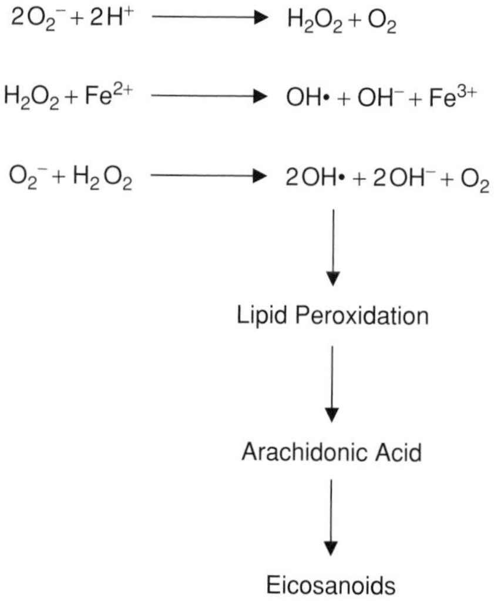

Fig. 18.3. Superoxide reacts with H^+ to initate the production of both hydrogen peroxide and the hydroxyl radical, which ultimately mediates lipid peroxidation.

IRI and the sources of these species. Reactive oxygen species have a potentially destructive role, mediating tissue damage during IRI. Degradation of ATP during ischaemia produces hypoxanthine. During reperfusion, an influx of molecular oxygen catalyses the action of xanthine oxidase, producing uric acid and liberating the highly reactive superoxide anion (O_2^-) (Figure 18.2). Superoxide is subsequently converted to hydrogen peroxide (H_2O_2) and the hydroxyl radical (OH) (Figure 18.3). The major consequence of hydroxyl radical production is peroxidation of the lipid structures of the cell membranes resulting in the production and systemic release of pro-inflammatory eicosanoids, disruption of cell permeability and ultimately cell death. During IRI, ROS activate endothelial cells, elevating the activity of the transcription factor, NF-κ B. Once activated, the endothelial cell produces E-selectin, vascular cell adhesion molecule-1 (VCAM-1), intercellular adhesion molecule-1 (ICAM-1), endothelial leucocyte adhesion molecule-1 (ELAM-1), plasminogen activator inhibitor-1 (PAI-1), tissue factor and interleukin-8 (IL-8). These adhesion molecules contribute to interactions between the neutrophil and the endothelium, and will be discussed in more detail later.

Superoxide anions can be detected within ischaemic muscle and in the venous effluent of reperfused limbs [18], suggesting a role for superoxide damage to distant organs during skeletal muscle reperfusion injury. Xanthine oxidase is located within a spectrum of cell types and tissues to varying degrees [19; 20; 21], indicating widespread distribution and differing susceptibility to oxidant-mediated IRI. Inhibition of xanthine oxidase activity by the administration of allopurinol prior to ischaemia reduces the production of superoxide, and hence reduces the severity of reperfusion injury in animal models using a range of tissues, including skeletal muscle [22], brain [3] and gut [23].

Eicosanoids

As discussed above, ROS initiate the lipid peroxidation of cell membranes, releasing arachidonic acid [24], the main substrate for the production of prostaglandins, thromboxanes and leukotrienes. These derivatives of arachidonic acid are collectively known as the eicosanoids and play a major role in IRI.

Prostaglandins, synthesized from arachidonic acid via the cyclo-oxygenase pathway, have a protective vasodilatory effect in IRI [25]. However, a rapid depletion of prostaglandins leads to uninhibited vasoconstriction, reduced local blood flow and exacerbation of ischaemia [26]. The potential of prostaglandins to ameliorate the degree of metabolic and tissue derangement following IRI has been demonstrated in various tissues. Using experimental models of liver transplantation, administration of prostacyclin (PGI_2) improved post-operative liver graft function [27; 28; 29]. Patients who received prostacyclin demonstrated better post-operative myocardial oxygen consumption after coronary artery bypass surgery [30] and improved muscle blood flow following skeletal muscle IRI [31].

Plasma thromboxane A_2, synthesized from arachidonic acid, promotes vasoconstriction and platelet aggregation, and increases in minutes following skeletal muscle IRI. This coincides with a rapid rise in pulmonary artery pressure and a subsequent increase in pulmonary microvascular permeability [32; 33], which correlates with sequestration of polymorphonuclear cells in the lungs. Thromboxane synthase inhibitors and synthetic thromboxane A_2 receptor antagonists prevent pulmonary leuco-sequestration [34], increase blood flow to reperfused tissues, and preserve organ viability [35] and function [36; 37] in animal models of IRI. These data suggest that administration of thromboxane A_2 antagonists may improve limb salvage rates after surgery for acute ischaemia.

Leukotrienes are synthesized from arachidonic acid through the activation of 5-lipoxygenase and participate in the inflammatory cascade of IRI [24]. Leukotrienes lead to local and systemic injury by their direct action on endothelial and smooth muscle cells, and indirectly by their effects on neutrophils. The leukotrienes C_4, D_4 and E_4 produce changes in the endothelial cytoskeleton leading to increased vascular permeability, and enhance smooth muscle contraction, resulting in vasoconstriction. The lung produces leukotrienes following remote IRI [38]. The direct effects on pulmonary microvessels lead to increased permeability, transient pulmonary hypertension and induction of the endothelium to produce thromboxane. Indirectly this results in additional vasoconstriction. The leukotriene B_4, released by activated neutrophils, leads to further pulmonary neutrophil accumulation.

The administration of a 5-lipoxygenase synthesis inhibitor has been used in animal studies to attenuate IRI. Such agents abolish the elevations in leukotrienes B_4 and C_4, and inhibit neutrophil infiltration normally induced by IRI, reducing mucosal permeability [39].

Nitric oxide

Nitric oxide is a signalling molecule synthesized from L-arginine by nitric oxide synthase (NOS) of which there are three types, neuronal (nNOS), inducible (iNOS) and endothelial (eNOS). The role of NO in reperfusion injury is controversial, dependent on the nature of its generation and appears tissue specific. In some instances it acts as an antioxidant and in others combines with the superoxide anion to form the peroxynitrite radical, a potent promoter of lipid peroxidation and hence cellular membrane disruption. Many studies have examined its role in cerebral, cardiac, intestinal and pulmonary IRI [40; 41; 42; 43; 44; 45]. In skeletal muscle IRI, NO production may be deleterious [46]. However, eNOS-derived NO is necessary for the maintenance of vascular tone. The reduction in NO levels that occurs in IRI may therefore predispose to vasoconstriction [47], a common response seen in IRI [48]. Endothelial dysfunction following

Table 18.2. *Mechanisms of modulation of severity of IRI by nitric oxide*

- Inhibition of platelet aggregation and adhesion
- Inhibition of neutrophil and monocyte adhesion to endothelium
- Reduced microvascular permeability/dysfunction
- Increased resistance of skeletal muscle to fatigue after IRI

cardiac IRI impairs cNOS. This can be ameliorated with L-arginine treatment (a NO donor) [49], which similarly also decreases skeletal muscle necrosis following IRI [50]. Nitric oxide inhibits platelet aggregation and adhesion [51], neutrophil and monocyte endothelial interactions, and reduces microvascular permeability [52]. The NO donor, S-nitroso-N-acetylcysteine administered during IRI also reduces skeletal muscle contractile dysfunction [53]. Taken together, the experimental evidence suggests a protective role for NO during IRI (Table 18.2).

Endothelin

Endothelin-1 is a 21 amino-acid vasoconstrictive peptide produced by endothelial cells. Hypoxia, growth factors, angiotensin II and noradrenalin all stimulate its production resulting in Ca^{2+} mediated vasoconstriction. Endothelin-1 is elevated following skeletal muscle IRI [54], and mediates capillary vasoconstriction, neutrophil aggregation and neutrophil-endothelial interactions [55], indirectly enhancing superoxide production [56]. Endothelin-1 inhibitors increase functional capillary density [57], microvascular perfusion [58], and hence viability and function following IRI [59].

Cytokines

Hypoxia and IRI both induce the expression of numerous cytokines, including tumour necrosis factor-α (TNFα), interleukin-1 (IL-1), interleukin-6 (IL-6), interleukin-8 (IL-8) and platelet activating factor (PAF), in association with elevated NF-κB activity [60]. These cytokines are released systemically and are thus important in the development of multisystem organ failure. The sites of origin and effects of these cytokines are discussed in detail in Chapter 17.

Tumour necrosis factor-α is a 17 kDa pro-inflammatory cytokine produced by activated macrophages, monocytes, T lymphocytes, killer cells and fibroblasts. TNFα is a potent chemoattractant and early response cytokine [61], increasing the levels of expression of IL-1, IL-6 IL-8 and PAF [62]. Elevated serum levels of TNFα have been detected during cerebral [63] and skeletal muscle IRI [64], and are known to increase neutrophil sequestration and permeability following pulmonary IRI [65]. Serum TNFα increases rapidly during lower extremity ischaemia, increasing the production of NO from rat lungs by the up-regulation of iNOS [66]. In the same study, inhibition of TNFα activity prior to limb ischaemia decreased pulmonary NO production and reduced the severity of IRI. Tumour necrosis factor-α induces the generation of ROS [67] and enhances the susceptibility of the vascular endothelium to neutrophil mediated injury, possibly by inducing the expression of ICAM-1 [68].

Numerous studies in animal models attest to the potential of TNFα blockade as a therapeutic modality to reduce the severity of IRI. Anti-TNFα antibody protects against IRI induced pulmonary injury [69], prevents microvascular damage [65] and attenuates no-reflow [70], protecting against both local and systemic IRI [61]. However, clinical trials to test the efficacy of TNFα blockade in human IRI have not yet been reported.

The cytokine, IL-1 is produced by tissue macrophages, neutrophils and the vascular endothelium. Interleukin-1 is a potent chemotactic agent and has been shown to stimulate neutrophil infiltration during hepatic IRI [71]. Both IL-1 and TNFα increase the expression of ICAM-1 on the vascular endothelium [72]. Exposure of endothelial cells in culture to IL-1 and TNFα induces synthesis of E-selectin, which then interacts with L-selectin on the neutrophil surface leading to rolling on the endothelial surface [73; 74]. Further adhesion of the neutrophil to the endothelium requires expression of IL-8 and PAF in the endothelial membranes (Figure 18.4).

Numerous stimuli expressed during IRI, including H_2O_2, thrombin, leukotrienes C_4 and D_4,IL-1, histamine, bradykinin and ATP, induce the synthesis of PAF by monocytes, macrophages, neutrophils, eosinophils, basophils, platelets and endothelial cells.

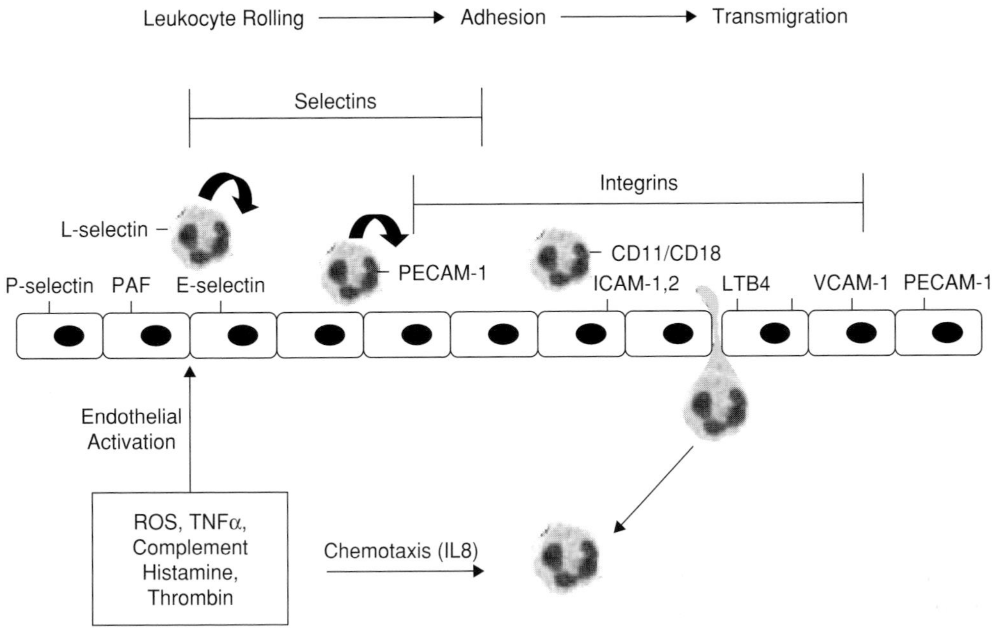

Fig. 18.4. During reperfusion, activated neutrophils adhere to the activated endothelium and subsequently extravaste into surrounding tissue, resulting in proteolytic degradation of basement membranes.

Platelet activating factor (PAF) functions as both inter- and intracellular messenger [75], having three major effects, vasoconstriction, chemoattraction and increased microvascular permeability [76; 77]. Platelet activating factor is produced following skeletal muscle [78] and renal IRI [79], with peak levels after 15 minutes of reperfusion. Platelet activating factor enhances the binding of neutrophils to endothelial cells since a PAF-receptor antagonist (WEB-2086) blocked adhesion to endothelial cells during IRI [78; 80]. Similarly pre-treatment with the PAF inhibitor lexipafant, reduces the severity of intestinal barrier dysfunction, and pulmonary and liver permeability in a rat model of intestinal IRI [81].

Interleukin-6 is a 19–26 kDa protein produced by monocytes, fibroblasts, keratinocytes and endothelial cells in response to IL-1 and TNFα. Interleukin-6 may prime and stimulate the respiratory burst in neutrophils, stimulate endothelial cell expression of ICAM-1 and increase endothelial permeability [82]. Interleukin-6 is produced in hypoperfused skeletal muscle in patients with peripheral arterial disease [83] and is released systemically during reperfusion in aortic aneurysm surgery [84].

Interleukin 8 is a potent neutrophil chemotactic and activating factor. It is produced by monocytes, T cells, NK cells, fibroblasts, endothelial cells, eosinophils and neutrophils in response to IL-1, TNFα, endotoxin, histamine and hypoxia [85]. Elevated levels of serum IL-8 have been detected during early reperfusion following human lung transplantation and predict poor graft function [86]. Anti-IL-8 antibody prevented pulmonary neutrophil infiltration and tissue injury in a rabbit model of lung IRI [87].

Neutrophils and endothelial interactions

Neutrophils play a major role in tissue damage incurred during IRI. Neutrophil infiltration is observed at sites of tissue damage [88; 89; 90] and the depletion of neutrophils reduces the severity of organ damage following IRI. [91; 92] Activated neutrophils generate toxic reactive oxygen species (Figure 18.5) and secrete proteases, including matrix metalloproteinases [93], contributing to the severity of tissue destruction. Depletion of neutrophils during cardiac surgery is recognized as an effective modality to reduce the severity of post-operative cardiac dysfunction [94; 95; 96].

$$2O_2 + NADPH \xrightarrow{\text{NADPH oxidase}} 2O_2^- + NADP^+ + H^+$$

$$2O_2^- + 2H^+ \xrightarrow{\text{Superoxide dismutase}} H_2O_2 + O_2$$

$$H_2O_2 + Cl^- + H^+ \xrightarrow{\text{Myeloperoxidase}} HOCl + H_2O$$

Fig. 18.5. Activated neutrophils generate toxic reactive oxygen species from molecular oxygen, contributing to tissue degradation during reperfusion.

Selectins are a family of transmembrane molecules, expressed on the surface of leucocytes and activated endothelial cells, and in platelets. Selectins mediate the initial phase of neutrophil–endothelial cell interactions, often termed rolling (Figure 18.4), which is essential for their subsequent adhesion and extravasation [97]. L-selectin is expressed constitutively on the surface of neutrophils [98], and initiates the reversible attachment of neutrophils to endothelial cells [99] and platelets [100]. Blocking of L-selectin impairs the ability of neutrophils to roll on endothelial cell monolayers and the endothelial surface of mesenteric venules [101], and reduces neutrophil infiltration following skeletal muscle [102] and pulmonary IRI [103].

P-selectin is stored in the α-granules of platelets and the Wiebel-Palade bodies of endothelial cells, and is rapidly translocated to the cell surface along with PAF in response to thrombin, histamine [104], ROS [105], complement [106; 107] and TNFα [108]. Typically, peak levels of endothelial P-selectin are detected six hours after reperfusion. Mast cells, a major source of PAF, and histamine may therefore also contribute to these interactions [109].

Activation of the endothelium by pro-inflammatory mediators results in de novo transcription and synthesis of E-selectin. Renal and cerebral IRI [110; 111], IL-1 and TNFα [61; 112] all increase the expression of E-selectin. The focal expression of E-selectin at sites of endothelial activation promotes neutrophil adhesion and infiltration into adjacent tissues. Antibodies to E-selectin reduce infarct size following cerebral IRI in mice [113].

The integrin and immunoglobulin supergene families of adhesion molecules mediate the strong adhesion of activated neutrophils, and hence subsequent extravasation during IRI, which may be observed directly with intravital microscopy [114].

The integrins form a large family of cell surface adhesion molecules that mediate intercellular recognition and cellular binding to the extracellular matrix. The neutrophil β_2-integrin adhesion glycoprotein complex consists of a common polypeptide chain, CD18, which is non-covalently linked to three different α-polypeptide chains (CD11a, CD11b, CD11c). CD11a/CD18 is expressed on all leucocytes, and mediates the attachment of stimulated neutrophils to the vascular endothelium through a specific interaction with ICAM-1 and ICAM-2 [115]. Chemotactic agents (including the T lymphocyte surface molecule, CD5a, as well as LTB4 and PAF), cytokines (IL-1, TNFα) and ROS all induce neutrophil adherence to the endothelium by CD11/CD18-dependent mechanisms. The CD11b/18 complex on neutrophils interacts with ICAM-1 on the surface of the endothelial cell to mediate firm adhesion of neutrophils prior to their extravasation. All of these molecules are required for the development of lung injury following skeletal muscle [116] and hepatic IRI [117]. Inhibition of CD18-mediated leucocyte adhesion prevents vasoconstriction [118], increases microvascular permeability and also vascular resistance following IRI [119]. However, the clinical efficacy of blocking CD11/CD18-mediated interactions remains doubtful [120]. Clinical trials in humans have failed to demonstrate that antibodies to CD11/CD18 reduce infarct size following primary coronary angioplasty in the setting of acute myocardial infarction [121].

The immunoglobulin supergene family (ligands for integrins) contains a large number of molecules with multiple immunoglobulin-G-like domains. Several members of this family are involved in leucocyte–endothelial cell interactions including ICAM-1, VCAM-1 and platelet endothelial cell adhesion molecule-1 (PECAM-1). The basal expression of ICAM-1 on endothelial cells is enhanced by exposure to circulating TNFα [122] and following cardiac IRI [123]. Vascular cell adhesion molecule-1 is also elevated in response to renal IRI but occurs independently of TNFα [124]. Platelet endothelial cell adhesion molecule-1 is expressed constitutively on platelets, leucocytes and endothelial cells, and enhances activation of neutrophil–endothelial interactions mediated by β-integrins [125].

The therapeutic potential of blocking the activity of adhesion molecules has been tested in a number of animal models with encouraging results. Immunoneutralization of ICAM-1 and/or PECAM-1 attenuates neutrophil adhesion in the liver [126; 127], pulmonary sequestration and oedema following skeletal muscle IRI [128], and reduces intestinal dysfunction following IRI [129]. Antisense oligonucleotides to ICAM-1 ameliorated renal IRI and prevented delayed graft dysfunction in a rat model of renal transplantation [130]. However, results obtained in clinical trials have not been as positive. A recent clinical trial of anti-ICAM-1 antibody therapy in ischaemic stroke concluded that this was not an effective treatment and may significantly worsen stroke outcome [131], raising significant doubts regarding the efficacy of this therapeutic modality.

Activated neutrophils are a major source of ROS [132], generated through the activity of the membrane-bound nicotinamide adenine dinucleotide phosphate (NADPH) oxidase complex [133] (Figure 18.5). Whilst oxidizing NADPH to $NADP^+$, NADPH oxidase also reduces molecular oxygen to form the superoxide anion. Myeloperoxidase, stored in the azurophilic granules of neutrophils, converts hydrogen peroxide to hypochlorous acid [134], which in addition to its direct effects, is capable of activating proteases [135].

Complement activation

Complement activation and deposition [136] also contribute significantly to the pathogenesis of IRI. Rubin and colleagues have demonstrated that reperfusion of skeletal muscle is associated with systemic depletion of the complement protein, factor B, indicative of activation of the alternative complement pathway [137]. The complex C5b-9 is also deposited into the endothelial cell membrane after IRI, leading to osmotic lysis [136; 138]. Pulmonary damage following bilateral hindlimb ischaemia was significantly reduced when the soluble complement receptor (sCR1) was administered to rats, thus inhibiting complement activity [139]. Complement-dependent mechanisms also stimulated Kupffer cell-mediated hepatic injury following bilateral hindlimb ischaemia [140]. In the clinical setting, a relationship has been demonstrated between the severity of multisystem organ dysfunction and degree of complement activation after aortic cross clamping [141; 142].

Inhibition of the complement cascade has been demonstrated to improve outcomes following IRI in a number of different animal models. Complement depletion of circulating plasma improved the initial blood flow, decreased muscle necrosis and injury after ischaemia, and prolonged reperfusion in dogs [143]. Complement blockade also prevented leucocyte adhesion, leading to better capillary perfusion and muscle cell viability, and attenuated the increase in permeability index in tissues [138; 144]. Unequivocal evidence for the importance of complement activation during skeletal muscle IRI has been provided from experiments where limb ischaemia was induced in C5-deficient mice. These mice had approximately 50% less tissue damage than the wild-type animals [138], demonstrating the multifactorial nature of tissue damage induced during IRI. An additive role of complement and neutrophils in mediating skeletal muscle IRI has also been observed, with a greater reduction in histological damage in neutropenic C5-deficient animals than in neutropenic or C5-deficient mice alone [138].

TISSUE DESTRUCTION

Proteases and metalloproteinases

The matrix metalloproteinases (MMPs) are a family of zinc dependent enzymes that have the ability to degrade components of the extracellular matrix. Together with their inhibitors, the tissue inhibitors of metalloproteinases (TIMPs), they are the major physiological regulators of the extracellular matrix. Matrix metalloproteinases are intimately involved in all processes that necessitate degradation or synthesis of the extracellular matrix. Important roles for these enzymes have been identified in wound healing, periodontal disease, cancer metastasis and, of particular relevance, vascular disease, including the development of aneurysms [145], atherosclerotic plaques [146] and reperfusion injury.

Elevation of MMP2 and MMP9 have been detected following pulmonary [147], hepatic [148] and cardiac IRI [149]. Matrix metalloproteinases are also elevated following cerebral IRI [150], corresponding with degradation of the basal lamina, increased capillary permeability and cerebral oedema [151; 152]. A definitive role for MMP9 has been demonstrated by the use of selective MMP9 inhibitors or MMP9 knock-out mice, which both reduce cerebral infarct size significantly [153; 154]. The role for MMPs in renal IRI is less clear. Matrix metalloproteinase-2 may have a late role in renal IRI with an elevation detected as late as eight weeks after IRI [155]. However, the MMP inhibitor (batimastat) does not alter the severity of IRI induced renal dysfunction [156].

Studies in our laboratory have demonstrated both a local and systemic role for MMP2 and MMP9 in the degradation of type IV collagen in pulmonary tissues and in skeletal muscle following lower limb IRI [90]. Ischaemia alone without reperfusion also results in elevation of MMP2 and MMP9, correlating with destruction of the basement membrane components, type IV collagen and laminin [157].

Other proteases involved in IRI include the Ca^{2+} dependent protease, calpain. Calpain levels are increased in neurons after global and focal brain ischaemia and early reperfusion, and may contribute to postischaemic injury [158; 159]. In support of a role for calpain in mediating tissue damage during IRI, administration of calpain inhibitor-1 to rats subjected to renal IRI reduced the severity of renal dysfunction [7].

Apoptotic cell death during ischaemia-reperfusion injury

Tissue destruction resulting from IRI can be due to either necrotic or apoptotic cell death. Oxidative stress and the production of ROS act as mediators of apoptosis [160], the characteristics of which can be recognized following cerebral IRI [161; 162; 163]. Similarly renal [164], myocytes in culture [165; 166; 167] and *in vivo* cardiac [168; 169; 170] IRI all result in detectable levels of apoptosis. Apoptosis therefore appears to play a fundamental role in cellular damage occurring during IRI in a number of tissues. However, the role of apoptosis in skeletal muscle IRI remains controversial. Studies conducted in our laboratory [89], in agreement with Knight and coworkers [171], have failed to detect any evidence of apoptosis in rat skeletal muscle cells following IRI. This implicates a tissue-specific mechanism of cell death following IRI. Blocking the apoptotic cascade, using specific inhibitors against pro-apoptotic caspase enzymes, has been partially effective in animal models, reducing the severity and infarct size following hepatic [172] and cardiac IRI [173].

No-reflow phenomenon

No-reflow is the failure of microvascular perfusion, following restoration of flow to previously ischaemic tissue. The cause of this phenomenon has not been fully elucidated but is likely to be multifactorial as proposed by Gute and coworkers [174]. Cytokines and activated neutrophils act synergistically to produce microvascular barrier dysfunction. The resultant increase in permeability leads to the exudation of fluids and proteins, increasing the interstitial pressure and decreasing the intravascular pressure. In addition, CD18-dependent leucocyte plugging produces partial occlusion of post-capillary venules, further contributing to no-reflow [119; 174]. Neutrophil depletion virtually abolishes the phenomenon in the myocardium, brain and skeletal muscle [175; 119].

SUMMARY

In summary, IRI is a highly complex series of interwoven pathological events. The production, release and activation of cytokines, ROS, proteinases and complement if left unchecked leads, to both local and systemic injury with potentially fatal consequences. The failure of therapeutic intervention to translate into clinical practice is a reflection of this complexity and redundancy within the system. New therapeutic agents directed towards multiple areas within this cascade may be required to overcome this difficult clinical challenge.

REFERENCES

1. A. Schurr, Lactate, glucose and energy metabolism in the ischemic brain (review). *International Journal of Molecular Medicine*, **10** (2002), 131–6.
2. A. C. Cave, J. S. Ingwall, J. Friedrich *et al.*, ATP synthesis during low-flow ischemia: influence of increased glycolytic substrate. *Circulation*, **101** (2000), 2090–6.
3. H. Akdemir, Z. Asik, H. Pasaoglu *et al.*, The effect of allopurinol on focal cerebral ischaemia: an experimental study in rabbits. *Neurosurgical Review*, **24** (2001), 131–5.
4. D. G. Allen & X. H. Xiao, Activity of the Na+/H+ exchanger contributes to cardiac damage following ischaemia and reperfusion. *Clinical Experimental Pharmacolology and Physiology*, **27** (2000), 727–33.

5. C. A. Schumacher, A. Baartscheer, R. Coronel & J. W. Fiolet, Energy-dependent transport of calcium to the extracellular space during acute ischemia of the rat heart. *Journal of Molecular and Cellular Cardiology*, **30** (1998), 1631–42.
6. T. Ivanics, Z. Miklos, Z. Ruttner *et al.*, Ischemia/reperfusion-induced changes in intracellular free $Ca^{2}+$ levels in rat skeletal muscle fibers – an *in vivo* study. *Pflugers Archives*, **440** (2000), 302–8.
7. P. K. Chatterjee, P. A. Brown, S. Cuzzocrea *et al.*, Calpain inhibitor-1 reduces renal ischemia/reperfusion injury in the rat. *Kidney International*, **59** (2001), 2073–83.
8. M. Saksela, R. Lapatto & K. O. Raivio, Irreversible conversion of xanthine dehydrogenase into xanthine oxidase by a mitochondrial protease. *FEBS Letters*, **443** (1999), 117–120.
9. P. C. Grisotto, A. C. dos Santos, J. Coutinho-Netto, J. Cherri & C. E. Piccinato . Indicators of oxidative injury and alterations of the cell membrane in the skeletal muscle of rats submitted to ischemia and reperfusion. *Journal of Surgical Research*, **92** (2000), 1–6.
10. K. Koike, Y. Yamamoto, Y. Hori & T. Ono, Group IIA phospholipase A2 mediates lung injury in intestinal ischemia-reperfusion. *Annals of Surgery*, **232** (2000), 90–7.
11. D. A. Ford, Alterations in myocardial lipid metabolism during myocardial ischemia and reperfusion. *Progress in Lipid Research*, **41** (2002), 6–26.
12. S. Cho, E. M. Park, Y. Kim *et al.*, Early c-Fos induction after cerebral ischemia: a possible neuroprotective role. *Journal of Cerebral Blood Flow and Metabolism*, **21** (2001), 550–6.
13. L. Tacchini, L. Radice & A. Bernelli-Zazzera, Differential activation of some transcription factors during rat liver ischemia, reperfusion, and heat shock. *Journal of Cell Physiology*, **180** (1999), 255–62.
14. A. Schneider, A. Martin-Villalba, F. Weih *et al.*, NF-kappaB is activated and promotes cell death in focal cerebral ischemia. *Nature Medicine*, **5** (1999), 554–9.
15. N. Blondeau, C. Widmann, M. Lazdunski & C. Heurteaux, Activation of the nuclear factor-kappaB is a key event in brain tolerance. *Journal of Neuroscience*, **21** (2001), 4668–77.
16. C. Michiels, E. Minet, G. Michel, HIF-1 and AP-1 cooperate to increase gene expression in hypoxia: role of MAP kinases. *IUBMB Life*, **52** (2001), 49–53.
17. C. Hierholzer, B. G. Harbrecht, T. R. Billiar & D. J. Tweardy, Hypoxia-inducible factor-1 activation and cyclo-oxygenase-2 induction are early reperfusion-independent inflammatory events in hemorrhagic shock. *Archives of Orthopaedic and Trauma Surgery*, **121** (2001), 219–22.
18. K. Yokoyama, M. Kimura, K. Nakamura & M. Itoman, Time course of post-ischemic superoxide generation in venous effluent from reperfused rabbit hindlimbs. *Journal of Reconstructive Microsurgery*, **15** (1999), 215–21.
19. B. Ibrahim & P. J. Stoward, The histochemical localization of xanthine oxidase. *The Histochemical Journal*, **10** (1978), 615–17.
20. Y. Hellsten-Westing, Immunohistochemical localization of xanthine oxidase in human cardiac and skeletal muscle. *Histochemistry*, **100** (1993), 215–22.
21. N. Linder, J. Rapola & K. O. Raivio, Cellular expression of xanthine oxidoreductase protein in normal human tissues. *Laboratory Investigation*, **79** (1999), 967–74.
22. J. K. Smith, D. L. Carden & R. J. Korthuis, Role of xanthine oxidase in postischemic microvascular injury in skeletal muscle. *American Journal of Physiology*, **257** (1989), H1782–9.
23. R. G. Albuquerque, A. J. Sanson & M. A. Malangoni, Allopurinol protects enterocytes from hypoxia-induced apoptosis *in vivo*. *Journal of Trauma*, **53** (2002), 415–21.
24. A. M. Rao, J. F. Hatcher, M. S. Kindy & R. J. Dempsey, Arachidonic acid and leukotriene C4: role in transient cerebral ischemia of gerbils. *Neurochemical Research*, **24** (1999), 1225–32.
25. T. Ravingerova, J. Styk, V. Tregerova *et al.*, Protective effect of 7-oxo-prostacyclin on myocardial function and metabolism during postischemic reperfusion and calcium paradox. *Basic Research in Cardiology*, **86** (1991), 245–53.
26. J. L. Cracowski, P. Devillier, T. Durand, F. Stanke-Labesque & G. Bessard, Vascular biology of the isoprostanes. *Journal of Vascular Research*, **38** (2001), 93–103.
27. H. M. Chen, M. F. Chen & M. H. Shyr, Prostacyclin analogue (OP-2507) attenuates hepatic microcirculatory derangement, energy depletion, and lipid peroxidation in a rat model of reperfusion injury. *Journal of Surgical Research*, **80** (1998), 333–8.
28. U. P. Neumann, U. Kaisers, J. M. Langrehr *et al.*, Administration of prostacyclin after liver

transplantation: a placebo controlled randomized trial. *Clinical Transplantation*, **14** (2000), 70–4.

29. A. Meyer zu, C. Vilsendorf, Link, A. Jorns, E. Nagel & J. Kohl, Preconditioning with the prostacyclin analog epoprostenol and cobra venom factor prevents reperfusion injury and hyperacute rejection in discordant liver xenotransplantation. *Xenotransplantation*, **8** (2001), 41–7.
30. S. F. Katircioglu, D. S. Kucukaksu, M. Bozdayi, O. Tasdemir & K. Bayazit, Beneficial effects of prostacyclin treatment on reperfusion of the myocardium. *Cardiovascular Surgery*, **3** (1995), 405–8.
31. T. E. Rowlands, M. J. Gough & S. Homer-Vanniasinkam, Do prostaglandins have a salutary role in skeletal muscle ischaemia-reperfusion injury? *European Journal of Vascular and Endovascular Surgery*, **18** (1999), 439–44.
32. H. Anner, R. P. Kaufman, Jr., C. R. Valeri, D. Shepro & H. B. Hechtman, Reperfusion of ischemic lower limbs increases pulmonary microvascular permeability. *Journal of Trauma*, **28** (1988), 607–10.
33. J. M. Klausner, I. S. Paterson, G. Goldman *et al.*, Thromboxane A2 mediates increased pulmonary microvascular permeability following limb ischemia. *Circulation Research*, **64** (1989), 1178–89.
34. H. Anner, R. P. Kaufman, Jr., L. Kobzik *et al.*, Pulmonary leukosequestration induced by hind limb ischemia. *Annals of Surgery*, **206** (1987), 162–7.
35. P. J. Mazolewski, A. C. Roth, H. Suchy, L. L. Stephenson & W. A. Zamboni, Role of the thromboxane A2 receptor in the vasoactive response to ischemia-reperfusion injury. *Plastic and Reconstructive Surgery*, **104** (1999), 1393–6.
36. P. J. Garvin, M. L. Niehoff, S. M. Robinson *et al.*, Evaluation of the thromboxane A2 synthetase inhibitor OKY-046 in a warm ischemia-reperfusion rat model. *Transplantation*, **61** (1996), 1429–34.
37. S. Homer-Vanniasinkam, J. N. Crinnion & M. J. Gough, Role of thromboxane A2 in muscle injury following ischaemia. *British Journal of Surgery*, **81** (1994), 974–6.
38. G. Goldman, R. Welbourn & J. M. Klausner *et al.*, Mast cells and leukotrienes mediate neutrophil sequestration and lung edema after remote ischemia in rodents. *Surgery*, **112** (1992), 578–86.
39. M. J. Mangino, M. K. Murphy & C. B. Anderson, Effects of the arachidonate 5-lipoxygenase synthesis inhibitor A-64077 in intestinal ischemia-reperfusion injury. *Journal of Pharmacology and Experimental Therapeutics*, **269** (1994), 75–81.
40. Y. Gursoy-Y. Ozdemir, H. Bolay, O. Saribas & T. Dalkara, Role of endothelial nitric oxide generation and peroxynitrite formation in reperfusion injury after focal cerebral ischemia. *Stroke*, **31** (2000), 1974–1.
41. P. Liu, B. Xu, L. J. Forman, R. Carsia & C. E. Hock, L-NAME enhances microcirculatory congestion and cardiomyocyte apoptosis during myocardial ischemia-reperfusion in rats. *Shock*, **17** (2002), 185–92.
42. S. Cuzzocrea, P. K. Chatterjee, E. Mazzon *et al.*, Role of induced nitric oxide in the initiation of the inflammatory response after postischemic injury. *Shock*, **18** (2002), 169–76.
43. Y. Naito, T. Yoshikawa, K. Matsuyama *et al.*, Neutrophils, lipid peroxidation, and nitric oxide in gastric reperfusion injury in rats. *Free Radical Biology and Medicine*, **24** (1998), 494–502.
44. H. Abdih, C. J. Kelly, D. Bouchier- Hayes *et al.*, Nitric oxide (endothelium-derived relaxing factor) attenuates revascularization-induced lung injury. *Journal of Surgical Research*, **57** (1994), 39–43.
45. H. Yamagishi, C. Yamashita & M. Okada, Preventive influence of inhaled nitric oxide on lung ischemia-reperfusion injury. *Surgery Today*, **29** (1999), 897–901.
46. L. H. Phan, M. J. Hickey, Z. B. Niazi & A. G. Stewart, Nitric oxide synthase inhibitor, nitro-iminoethyl-L-ornithine, reduces ischemia-reperfusion injury in rabbit skeletal muscle. *Microsurgery*, **15** (1994), 703–7.
47. W. C. Sternbergh, R. G. Makhoul & B. Adelman, Nitric oxide-mediated, endothelium-dependent vasodilation is selectively attenuated in the postischemic extremity. *Surgery*, **114** (1993), 960–7.
48. J. R. Urbaniak, A. V. Seaber & L. E. Chen, Assessment of ischemia and reperfusion injury. *Clinical Orthopaedics*, (1997), 30–6.
49. D. T. Engelman, M. Watanabe, R. M. Engelman *et al.*, Constitutive nitric oxide release is impaired after ischemia and reperfusion. *Journal of Thoracic and Cardiovascular Surgery*, **110** (1995), 1047–53.
50. D. G. Meldrum, L. L. Stephenson & W. A. Zamboni, Effects of L-NAME and L-arginine on ischemia-reperfusion injury in rat skeletal muscle. *Plastic and Reconstructive Surgery*, **103** (1999), 935–40.
51. J. C. de Graaf, J. D. Banga, S. Moncada *et al.*, Nitric oxide functions as an inhibitor of platelet adhesion under flow conditions. *Circulation*, **85** (1992), 2284–90.

52. I. Kurose, R. Wolf, M. B. Grisham & D. N. Granger, Modulation of ischemia/reperfusion-induced microvascular dysfunction by nitric oxide. *Circulation Research*, **74** (1994), 376–82.
53. L. E. Chen, A. V. Seaber, R. M. Nasser, J. S. Stamler & J. R. Urbaniak, Effects of S-nitroso-N-acetylcysteine on contractile function of reperfused skeletal muscle. *American Journal of Physiology*, **274** (1998), R822–9.
54. K. Hvaal, E. Oie, H. Attramadal *et al.*, Endothelin-1 is upregulated during skeletal muscle ischemia and reperfusion. *Journal of Orthopaedic Research*, **16** (1998), 128–35.
55. A. Lopez Farre, A. Riesco, G. Espinosa *et al.*, Effect of endothelin-1 on neutrophil adhesion to endothelial cells and perfused heart. *Circulation*, **88** (1993), 1166–71.
56. M. Huribal, R. Kumar, M. E. Cunningham, B. E. Sumpio & M. A. McMillen, Endothelin-stimulated monocyte supernatants enhance neutrophil superoxide production. *Shock*, **1** (1994), 184–7.
57. K. Hvaal, S. R. Mathisen, A. Svindland, L. Nordsletten & S. Skjeldal, Protective effect of the endothelin antagonist Bosentan against ischemic skeletal muscle necrosis. *Acta Orthopaedica Scandinavica*, **70** (1999), 293–7.
58. K. J. Herbert, M. J. Hickey, D. A. Lepore *et al.*, Effects of the endothelin receptor antagonist Bosentan on ischaemia/reperfusion injury in rat skeletal muscle. *European Journal of Pharmacology*, **424** (2001), 59–67.
59. F. T. Hammad, G. Davis, X. Zhang & A. M. Wheatley, The role of endothelin in early renal cortical reperfusion in renal transplantation. *European Surgical Research*, **32** (2000), 380–8.
60. B. D. Shames, H. H. Barton, L. L. Reznikov *et al.*, Ischemia alone is sufficient to induce TNF-alpha mRNA and peptide in the myocardium. *Shock*, **17** (2002), 114–9.
61. A. Seekamp, J. S. Warren, D. G. Remick, G. O. Till & P. A. Ward, Requirements for tumor necrosis factor-alpha and interleukin-1 in limb ischemia/reperfusion injury and associated lung injury. *American Journal of Pathology*, **143** (1993), 453–63.
62. G. Camussi, F. Bussolino, G. Salvidio & C. Baglioni, Tumor necrosis factor/cachectin stimulates peritoneal macrophages, polymorphonuclear neutrophils, and vascular endothelial cells to synthesize and release platelet-activating factor. *Journal of Experimental Medicine*, **166** (1987), 1390–404.
63. G. Y. Yang, G. P. Schielke, C. Gong *et al.*, Expression of tumor necrosis factor-alpha and intercellular adhesion molecule-1 after focal cerebral ischemia in interleukin-1beta converting enzyme deficient mice. *Journal of Cerebral Blood Flow and Metabolisim*, **19** (1999), 1109–17.
64. G. C. Gaines, M. B. Welborn, L. L. Moldawer, Attenuation of skeletal muscle ischemia/reperfusion injury by inhibition of tumor necrosis factor. *Journal of Vascular Surgery*, **29** (1999), 370–6.
65. P. L. Khimenko, G. J. Bagby, J. Fuseler & A. E. Taylor, Tumor necrosis factor-alpha in ischemia and reperfusion injury in rat lungs. *Journal of Applied Physiology*, **85** (1998), 2005–11.
66. A. K. Tassiopoulos, R. E. Carlin, Y. Gao *et al.*, Role of nitric oxide and tumor necrosis factor on lung injury caused by ischemia/reperfusion of the lower extremities. *Journal of Vascular Surgery*, **26** (1997), 647–56.
67. M. Serteser, T. Koken, A. Kahraman *et al.*, Changes in hepatic TNF-alpha levels, antioxidant status, and oxidation products after renal ischemia/reperfusion injury in mice. *Journal of Surgical Research*, **107** (2002), 234–40.
68. S. J. Klebanoff, M. A. Vadas, J. M. Harlan *et al.*, Stimulation of neutrophils by tumor necrosis factor. *Journal of Immunology*, **136** (1986), 4220–5.
69. C. H. Chiang, C. P. Wu, W. C. Perng, H. C. Yan & C. P. Yu, Use of anti-(tumour necrosis factor-alpha) antibody or 3-deaza-adenosine as additives to promote protection by University of Wisconsin solution in ischaemia/reperfusion injury. *Clinical Science (London)*, **99** (2000), 215–22.
70. W. C. Sternbergh, 3rd, T. M. Tuttle, R. G. Makhoul *et al.*, Postischemic extremities exhibit immediate release of tumor necrosis factor. *Journal of Vascular Surgery*, **20** (1994), 474–81.
71. S. Suzuki & L. H. Toledo-Pereyra, Interleukin 1 and tumor necrosis factor production as the initial stimulants of liver ischemia and reperfusion injury. *Journal of Surgical Research*, **57** (1994), 253–8.
72. J. S. Pober, L. A. Lapierre, A. H. Stolpen *et al.*, Activation of cultured human endothelial cells by recombinant lymphotoxin: comparison with tumor necrosis factor and interleukin 1 species. *Journal of Immunology*, **138** (1987), 3319–24.
73. G. A. Zimmerman, S. M. Prescott & T. M. McIntyre, Endothelial cell interactions with granulocytes:

tethering and signaling molecules. *Immunology Today*, **13** (1992), 93–100.
74. M. Raab, H. Daxecker, S. Markovic *et al.*, Variation of adhesion molecule expression on human umbilical vein endothelial cells upon multiple cytokine application. *Clinica Chimica Acta*, **321** (2002), 11–16.
75. W. Chao & M. S. Olson, Platelet-activating factor: receptors and signal transduction. *Biochemical Journal*, **292** (1993), 617–29.
76. W. N. Duran & P. K. Dillon, Acute microcirculatory effects of platelet-activating factor. *Jouranal of Lipid Mediators*, **2** (1990), S215–27.
77. R. E. Klabunde & D. E. Anderson, Role of nitric oxide and reactive oxygen species in platelet-activating factor-induced microvascular leakage. *Journal of Vascular Research*, **39** (2002), 238–45.
78. D. Silver, A. Dhar, M. Slocum, J. G. Adams, Jr. & S. Shukla, Role of platelet-activating factor in skeletal muscle ischemia-reperfusion injury. *Advances in Experimental Medicine and Biology*, **416** (1996), 217–21.
79. N. Lloberas, J. Torras, I. Herrero-Fresneda *et al.*, Postischemic renal oxidative stress induces inflammatory response through PAF and oxidized phospholipids. Prevention by antioxidant treatment. *FASEB Journal*, **16** (2002), 908–10.
80. W. N. Duran, V. J. Milazzo, F. Sabido & R. W. Hobson, 2nd, Platelet-activating factor modulates leukocyte adhesion to endothelium in ischemia-reperfusion. *Microvascular Resceach*, **51** (1996), 108–15.
81. Z. Sun, X. Wang, X. Deng *et al.*, Beneficial effects of lexipafant, a PAF antagonist on gut barrier dysfunction caused by intestinal ischemia and reperfusion in rats. *Digestive Surgery*, **17** (2000), 57–65.
82. N. Maruo, I. Morita, M. Shirao & S. Murota, IL-6 increases endothelial permeability *in vitro*. *Endocrinology*, **131** (1992), 710–14.
83. M. Testa, E. De Ruvo, A. Russo *et al.*, Induction of interleukin-1beta and interleukin-6 gene expression in hypoperfused skeletal muscle of patients with peripheral arterial disease. *Italian Heart Journal*, **1** (2000), 64–7.
84. A. B. Groeneveld, P. G. Raijmakers, J. A. Rauwerda & C. E. Hack, The inflammatory response to vascular surgery-associated ischaemia and reperfusion in man: effect on postoperative pulmonary function. *European Journal of Vascular and Endovascular Surgery*, **14** (1997), 351–9.
85. N. Hirani, F. Antonicelli, R. M. Strieter *et al.*, The regulation of interleukin-8 by hypoxia in human macrophages – a potential role in the pathogenesis of the acute respiratory distress syndrome (ARDS). *Molecular Medicine*, **7** (2001), 685–97.
86. M. De Perrot, Y. Sekine, S. Fischer *et al.*, Interleukin-8 release during early reperfusion predicts graft function in human lung transplantation. *American Journal of Respiratory Critical Care Medicine*, **165** (2002), 211–15.
87. N. Sekido, N. Mukaida, A. Harada *et al.*, Prevention of lung reperfusion injury in rabbits by a monoclonal antibody against interleukin-8. *Nature*, **365** (1993), 654–7.
88. M. B. Grisham, L. A. Hernandez & D. N. Granger, Xanthine oxidase and neutrophil infiltration in intestinal ischemia. *American Journal of Physiology*, **251** (1986), G567–74.
89. P. A. Cowled, L. Leonardos, S. H. Millard & R. A. Fitridge, Apoptotic cell death makes a minor contribution to reperfusion injury in skeletal muscle in the rat. *European Journal of Vascular and Endovascular Surgery*, **21** (2001), 28–34.
90. D. M. Roach, R. A. Fitridge, P. E. Laws *et al.*, Up-regulation of MMP-2 and MMP-9 leads to degradation of type IV collagen during skeletal muscle reperfusion injury; protection by the MMP inhibitor, doxycycline. *European Jouranal of Vascular and Endovascular Surgery*, **23** (2002), 260–9.
91. Y. Iwahori, N. Ishiguro, T. Shimizu *et al.*, Selective neutrophil depletion with monoclonal antibodies attenuates ischemia/reperfusion injury in skeletal muscle. *Journal of Reconstructive Microsurgery*, **14** (1998), 109–16.
92. G. Martinez-Mier, L. H. Toledo- Pereyra, J. E. McDuffie, R. L. Warner & P. A. Ward, Neutrophil depletion and chemokine response after liver ischemia and reperfusion. *Journal of Investigative Surgery*, **14** (2001), 99–107.
93. M. Lindsey, K. Wedin, M. D. Brown *et al.*, Matrix-dependent mechanism of neutrophil-mediated release and activation of matrix metalloproteinase 9 in myocardial ischemia/reperfusion. *Circulation*, **103** (2001), 2181–7.
94. Y. Sawa & H. Matsuda, Myocardial protection with leukocyte depletion in cardiac surgery. *Seminars in Thoracic and Cardiovascular Surgery*, **13** (2001), 73–81.
95. G. Matheis, M. Scholz, J. Gerber *et al.*, Leukocyte filtration in the early reperfusion phase on cardiopulmonary bypass reduces myocardial injury. *Perfusion*, **16** (2001), 43–9.

96. S. J. Morris, Leukocyte reduction in cardiovascular surgery. *Perfusion*, **16** (2001), 371–80.
97. S. Zahler, B. Heindl & B. F. Becker, Selectin-mediated rolling of neutrophils is essential for their activation and retention in the reperfused coronary system. *Basic Research in Cardiology*, **97** (2002), 359–64.
98. N. Borregaard, L. Kjeldsen, H. Sengelov *et al.*, Changes in subcellular localization and surface expression of L-selectin, alkaline phosphatase, and Mac-1 in human neutrophils during stimulation with inflammatory mediators. *Journal of Leukocyte Biology*, **56** (1994), 80–7.
99. G. S. Kansas, K. Ley, J. M. Munro & T. F. Tedder, Regulation of leukocyte rolling and adhesion to high endothelial venules through the cytoplasmic domain of L-selectin. *Journal of Experimental Medicine*, **177** (1993), 833–8.
100. S. M. Buttrum, R. Hatton & G. B. Nash, Selectin-mediated rolling of neutrophils on immobilized platelets. *Blood*, **82** (1993), 1165–74.
101. K. Ley, P. Gaehtgens, C. Fennie *et al.*, Lectin-like cell adhesion molecule 1 mediates leukocyte rolling in mesenteric venules *in vivo*. *Blood*, **77** (1991), 2553–5.
102. Z. Q. Yan, M. P. Bolognesi, D. A. Steeber *et al.*, Blockade of L-selectin attenuates reperfusion injury in a rat model. *Journal of Reconstructive Microsurgery*, **16** (2000), 227–33.
103. A. J. Levine, K. Parkes, S. J. Rooney & R. S. Bonser, The effect of adhesion molecule blockade on pulmonary reperfusion injury. *Annals of Thoracic Surgery*, **73** (2002), 1101–6.
104. D. E. Lorant, K. D. Patel, T. M. McIntyre *et al.*, Coexpression of GMP-140 and PAF by endothelium stimulated by histamine or thrombin: a juxtacrine system for adhesion and activation of neutrophils. *Journal of Cell Biology*, **115** (1991), 223–34.
105. M. Takano, A. Meneshian, E. Sheikh *et al.*, Rapid upregulation of endothelial P-selectin expression via reactive oxygen species generation. *American Journal of Heart and Circulatory Physiology*, **283** (2002), H2054–61.
106. S. A. Woodcock, C. Kyriakides, Y. Wang *et al.*, Soluble P-selectin moderates complement dependent injury. *Shock*, **14** (2000), 610–15.
107. C. Kyriakides, S. A. Woodcock, Y. Wang *et al.*, Soluble P-selectin moderates complement-dependent reperfusion injury of ischemic skeletal muscle. *American Journal of Physiology – Cell Physiology*, **279** (2000), C520–8.
108. A. Weller, S. Isenmann & D. Vestweber, Cloning of the mouse endothelial selectins. Expression of both E- and P-selectin is inducible by tumor necrosis factor alpha. *Journal of Biological Chemistry*, **267** (1992), 15176–83.
109. C. Mukundan, M. F. Gurish, K. F. Austen, H. B. Hechtman & D. S. Friend, Mast cell mediation of muscle and pulmonary injury following hindlimb ischemia-reperfusion. *Journal of Histochemistry and Cytochemistry*, **49** (2001), 1055–6.
110. K. L. Billups, M. A. Palladino, B. T. Hinton & J. L. Sherley, Expression of E-selectin mRNA during ischemia/reperfusion injury. *Journal of Laboratory and Clinical Medicine*, **125** (1995), 626–33.
111. R. Berti, A. J. Williams, J. R. Moffett *et al.*, Quantitative real-time RT-PCR analysis of inflammatory gene expression associated with ischemia-reperfusion brain injury. *Journal of Cerebral Blood Flow and Metabolisim*, **22** (2002), 1068–79.
112. V. Stangl, C. Gunther, A. Jarrin *et al.*, Homocysteine inhibits TNF-alpha-induced endothelial adhesion molecule expression and monocyte adhesion via nuclear factor-kappaB dependent pathway. *Biochemical and Biophysical Research Communications*, **280** (2001), 1093–100.
113. J. Huang, T. F. Choudhri, C. J. Winfree *et al.*, Postischemic cerebrovascular E-selectin expression mediates tissue injury in murine stroke. *Stroke*, **31** (2000), 3047–53.
114. H. A. Lehr, A. Guhlmann, D. Nolte, D. Keppler & K. Messmer, Leukotrienes as mediators in ischemia-reperfusion injury in a microcirculation model in the hamster. *Journal of Clinical Investigation*, **87** (1991), 2036–41.
115. S. D. Marlin & T. A. Springer, Purified intercellular adhesion molecule-1 (ICAM-1) is a ligand for lymphocyte function-associated antigen 1 (LFA-1). *Cell*, **51**, (1987), 813–19.
116. A. Seekamp, M. S. Mulligan, G. O. Till *et al.*, Role of beta 2 integrins and ICAM-1 in lung injury following ischemia-reperfusion of rat hind limbs. *American Journal of Pathology*, **143** (1993), 464–72.
117. A. Kobayashi, H. Imamura, M. Isobe *et al.*, Mac-1 (CD11b/CD18) and intercellular adhesion molecule-1 in ischemia-reperfusion injury of rat liver. *American*

Journal of Physiology – Gastrointestinal and Liver Physiology, **281** (2001), G577–85.
118. W. A. Zamboni, L. L. Stephenson, A. C. Roth, H. Suchy & R. C. Russell, Ischemia-reperfusion injury in skeletal muscle: CD 18-dependent neutrophil-endothelial adhesion and arteriolar vasoconstriction. *Plastic and Reconstructive Surgery*, **99** (1997), 2002–9.
119. S. N. Jerome, C. W. Smith & R. J. Korthuis, CD18-dependent adherence reactions play an important role in the development of the no-reflow phenomenon. *American Journal of Physiology*, **264** (1993), H479–83.
120. M. E. McKenzie & P. A. Gurbel, The potential of monoclonal antibodies to reduce reperfusion injury in myocardial infarction. *BioDrugs*, **15** (2001), 395–404.
121. D. Faxon, R. Gibbons, N. Chronos, P. Gurbel & F. Sheehan, The effect of blockade of the CD11/CD18 integrin receptor on infarct size in patients with acute myocardial infarction treated with direct angioplasty: the results of the HALT-MI study. *Journal of the American College of Cardiology*, **40** (2002), 1199.
122. L. M. Colletti, A. Cortis, N. Lukacs *et al.*, Tumor necrosis factor up-regulates intercellular adhesion molecule 1, which is important in the neutrophil-dependent lung and liver injury associated with hepatic ischemia and reperfusion in the rat. *Shock*, **10** (1998), 182–91.
123. K. Jaakkola, S. Jalkanen, K. Kaunismaki *et al.*, Vascular adhesion protein-1, intercellular adhesion molecule-1 and P-selectin mediate leukocyte binding to ischemic heart in humans. *Journal of the American College of Cardiology*, **36** (2000), 122–9.
124. M. J. Burne, A. Elghandour, M. Haq *et al.*, IL-1 and TNF independent pathways mediate ICAM-1/VCAM-1 up-regulation in ischemia reperfusion injury. *Journal of Leukocyte Biology*, **70** (2001), 192–8.
125. R. D. Thompson, M. W. Wakelin, K. Y. Larbi *et al.*, Divergent effects of platelet-endothelial cell adhesion molecule-1 and beta 3 integrin blockade on leukocyte transmigration *in vivo*. *Journal of Immunology*, **165** (2000), 426–34.
126. K. Monden, S. Arii, S. Ishiguro *et al.*, Involvement of ICAM-1 expression on sinusoidal endothelial cell and neutrophil adherence in the reperfusion injury of cold-preserved livers. *Transplantation Proceedings*, **27** (1995), 759–61.
127. M. Rentsch, S. Post, P. Palma *et al.*, Anti-ICAM-1 blockade reduces postsinusoidal WBC adherence following cold ischemia and reperfusion, but does not improve early graft function in rat liver transplantation. *Journal of Hepatology*, **32** (2000), 821–8.
128. M. J. Horgan, M. Ge, J. Gu, R. Rothlein & A. B. Malik, Role of ICAM-1 in neutrophil-mediated lung vascular injury after occlusion and reperfusion. *American Journal of Physiology*, **261** (1991), H1578–84.
129. Z. Sun, X. Wang, A. Lasson *et al.*, Effects of inhibition of PAF, ICAM-1 and PECAM-1 on gut barrier failure caused by intestinal ischemia and reperfusion. *Scandinavian Journal of Gastroenterology*, **36** (2001), 55–65.
130. D. Dragun, S. G. Tullius, J. P. Park *et al.*, ICAM-1 antisense oligodesoxynucleotides prevent reperfusion injury and enhance immediate graft function in renal transplantation. *Kidney International*, **54** (1998), 590–602.
131. Enlimomab Acute Stroke Trial Investigators, Use of anti-ICAM-1 therapy in ischemic stroke: results of the Enlimomab Acute Stroke Trial. *Neurology*, **57** (2001), 1428–34.
132. C. Duilio, G. Ambrosio, P. Kuppusamy *et al.*, Neutrophils are primary source of O_2 radicals during reperfusion after prolonged myocardial ischemia. *American Journal of Heart and Circulatory Physiology*, **280** (2001), H2649–57.
133. B. M. Babior, J. D. Lambeth & W. Nauseef, The neutrophil NADPH oxidase. *Archives of Biochemistry and Biophysics*, **397** (2002), 342–4.
134. C. Bergt, G. Marsche, U. Panzenboeck *et al.*, Human neutrophils employ the myeloperoxidase/hydrogen peroxide/chloride system to oxidatively damage apolipoprotein A-I. *European Journal of Biochemistry*, **268** (2001), 3523–31.
135. X. Fu, S. Y. Kassim, W. C. Parks & J. W. Heinecke, Hypochlorous acid oxygenates the cysteine switch domain of pro-matrilysin (MMP-7). A mechanism for matrix metalloproteinase activation and atherosclerotic plaque rupture by myeloperoxidase. *Journal of Biological Chemistry*, **276** (2001), 41279–87.
136. M. S. Wong, T. M. Lara, L. Kobzik *et al.*, Hindlimb ischemia-reperfusion increases complement deposition and glycolysis. *Journal of Surgical Research*, **85** (1999), 130–35.
137. B. B. Rubin, A. Smith, S. Liauw *et al.*, Complement activation and white cell sequestration in postischemic skeletal muscle. *American Journal of Physiology*, **259** (1990), H525–31.

138. C. Kyriakides, W. Austen, Y. Wang *et al.*, Skeletal muscle reperfusion injury is mediated by neutrophils and the complement membrane attack complex. *American Journal of Physiology*, **277** (1999), C1263–8.
139. T. F. Lindsay, J. Hill, F. Ortiz *et al.*, Blockade of complement activation prevents local and pulmonary albumin leak after lower torso ischemia-reperfusion. *Annals of Surgery*, **216** (1992), 677–83.
140. R. W. Brock, R. G. Nie, K. A. Harris & R. F. Potter, Kupffer cell-initiated remote hepatic injury following bilateral hindlimb ischemia is complement dependent. *American Journal of Physiology – Gastrointestinal and Liver Physiology*, **280** (2001), G279–84.
141. A. Bengtson, W. Lannsjo & M. Heideman, Complement and anaphylatoxin responses to cross-clamping of the aorta. Studies during general anaesthesia with or without extradural blockade. *British Journal of Anaesthesia*, **59** (1987), 1093–97.
142. M. Heideman, B. Norder Hansson, A. Bengtson & T. E. Mollnes, Terminal complement complexes and anaphylatoxins in septic and ischemic patients. *Archives of Surgery*, **123** (1988), 188–92.
143. B. Rubin, J. Tittley, G. Chang *et al.*, A clinically applicable method for long-term salvage of postischemic skeletal muscle. *Journal of Vascular Surgery*, **13** (1991), 58–68.
144. C. Kyriakides, Y. Wang, W. G. Austen, Jr. *et al.*, Moderation of skeletal muscle reperfusion injury by a sLe(x)-glycosylated complement inhibitory protein. *American Journal of Physiology – Cell Physiology*, **281** (2001), C224–30.
145. J. R. Elmore, B. F. Keister, D. P. Franklin, J. R. Youkey & D. J. Carey, Expression of matrix metalloproteinases and TIMPs in human abdominal aortic aneurysms. *Annals of Vascular Surgery*, **12** (1998), 221–8.
146. H. R. Lijnen, Plasmin and matrix metalloproteinases in vascular remodeling. *Thrombosis and Haemostasis*, **86** (2001), 324–33.
147. P. M. Soccal, Y. Gasche, J. C. Pache *et al.*, Matrix metalloproteinases correlate with alveolar-capillary permeability alteration in lung ischemia-reperfusion injury. *Transplantation*, **70** (2000), 998–1005.
148. R. Cursio, B. Mari, K. Louis *et al.*, Rat liver injury after normothermic ischemia is prevented by a phosphinic matrix metalloproteinase inhibitor. *FASEB Journal*, **16** (2002), 93–5.
149. V. Falk, P. M. Soccal, J. Grunenfelder *et al.*, Regulation of matrix metalloproteinases and effect of MMP-inhibition in heart transplant related reperfusion injury. *European Journal of Cardiothoracic Surgery*, **22** (2002), 53–8.
150. G. A. Rosenberg, L. A. Cunningham, J. Wallace *et al.*, Immunohistochemistry of matrix metalloproteinases in reperfusion injury to rat brain: activation of MMP-9 linked to stromelysin-1 and microglia in cell cultures. *Brain Research*, **893** (2001), 104–12.
151. G. A. Rosenberg, E. Y. Estrada & J. E. Dencoff, Matrix metalloproteinases and TIMPs are associated with blood-brain barrier opening after reperfusion in rat brain. *Stroke*, **29** (1998), 2189–95.
152. M. Fujimura, Y. Gasche, Y. Morita-Fujimura *et al.*, Early appearance of activated matrix metalloproteinase-9 and blood-brain barrier disruption in mice after focal cerebral ischemia and reperfusion. *Brain Research*, **842** (1999), 92–100.
153. A. M. Romanic, R. F. White, A. J. Arleth, E. H. Ohlstein & F. C. Barone, Matrix metalloproteinase expression increases after cerebral focal ischemia in rats: inhibition of matrix metalloproteinase-9 reduces infarct size. *Stroke*, **29** (1998), 1020–30.
154. M. Asahi, K. Asahi, J. C. Jung *et al.*, Role for matrix metalloproteinase 9 after focal cerebral ischemia: effects of gene knockout and enzyme inhibition with BB-94. *Journal of Cerebral Blood Flow and Metabolism*, **20** (2000), 1681–9.
155. S. Jain, G. R. Bicknell & M. L. Nicholson, Molecular changes in extracellular matrix turnover after renal ischaemia-reperfusion injury. *British Journal of Surgery*, **87** (2000), 1188–92.
156. R. Ziswiler, C. Daniel, E. Franz & H. P. Marti, Renal matrix metalloproteinase activity is unaffected by experimental ischemia-reperfusion injury and matrix metalloproteinase inhibition does not alter outcome of renal function. *Experimental Nephrology*, **9** (2001), 118–24.
157. E. Frisdal, E. Teiger, J. P. Lefaucheur *et al.*, Increased expression of gelatinases and alteration of basement membrane in rat soleus muscle following femoral artery ligation. *Neuropathology and Applied Neurobiology*, **26** (2000), 11–21.
158. R. W. Neumar, F. H. Meng, A. M. Mills *et al.*, Calpain activity in the rat brain after transient forebrain ischemia. *Experimental Neurology*, **170** (2001), 27–35.
159. C. Zhang, R. Siman, Y. Xu *et al.*, Comparison of calpain and caspase activities in the adult rat brain after

transient forebrain ischemia. *Neurobiology of Disease*, **10** (2002), 289.

160. Y. Morita-Fujimura, M. Fujimura, T. Yoshimoto & P. H. Chan, Superoxide during reperfusion contributes to caspase-8 expression and apoptosis after transient focal stroke. *Stroke*, **32** (2001), 2356–61.
161. M. D. Linnik, J. A. Miller, J. Sprinkle- Cavallo *et al.*, Apoptotic DNA fragmentation in the rat cerebral cortex induced by permanent middle cerebral artery occlusion. *Brain Research Molecular Brain Research*, **32** (1995), 116–24.
162. Y. Sei, K. J. Von, Lubitz, A. S. Basile *et al.*, Internucleosomal DNA fragmentation in gerbil hippocampus following forebrain ischemia. *Neuroscience Letters*, **171** (1994), 179–82.
163. Y. Li, M. Chopp, C. Powers & N. Jiang, Apoptosis and protein expression after focal cerebral ischemia in rat. *Brain Research*, **765** (1997), 301–12.
164. M. Schumer, M. C. Colombel, I. S. Sawczuk *et al.*, Morphologic, biochemical, and molecular evidence of apoptosis during the reperfusion phase after brief periods of renal ischemia. *American Journal of Pathology*, **140** (1992), 831–8.
165. M. Tanaka, H. Ito, S. Adachi *et al.*, Hypoxia induces apoptosis with enhanced expression of Fas antigen messenger RNA in cultured neonatal rat cardiomyocytes. *Circulation Research*, **75** (1994), 426–33.
166. R. A. Gottlieb, K. O. Burleson, R. A. Kloner, B. M. Babior & R. L. Engler, Reperfusion injury induces apoptosis in rabbit cardiomyocytes. *Journal of Clinical Investigtion*, **94** (1994), 1621–8.
167. R. A. Gottlieb & R. L. Engler, Apoptosis in myocardial ischemia-reperfusion. *Annals of the New York Academy of Sciences*, **874** (1999), 412–26.
168. N. Maulik, T. Yoshida & D. K. Das, Oxidative stress developed during the reperfusion of ischemic myocardium induces apoptosis. *Free Radical Biology and Medicine*, **24** (1998), 869–75.
169. G. Itoh, J. Tamura, M. Suzuki *et al.*, DNA fragmentation of human infarcted myocardial cells demonstrated by the nick end labeling method and DNA agarose gel electrophoresis. *American Journal of Pathology*, **146** (1995), 1325–31.
170. R. H. Bardales, L. S. Hailey, S. S. Xie, R. F. Schaefer & S. M. Hsu, *In situ* apoptosis assay for the detection of early acute myocardial infarction. *American Journal of Pathology*, **149** (1996), 821–9.
171. K. R. Knight, A. Messina, J. V. Hurley *et al.*, Muscle cells become necrotic rather than apoptotic during reperfusion of ischaemic skeletal muscle. *International Journal of Experimental Pathology*, **80** (1999), 169–75.
172. R. Cursio, J. Gugenheim, J. E. Ricci *et al.*, Caspase inhibition protects from liver injury following ischemia and reperfusion in rats. *Transplantation International*, **13**(Suppl 1) (2000), S568–72.
173. M. M. Mocanu, G. F. Baxter & D. M. Yellon, Caspase inhibition and limitation of myocardial infarct size: protection against lethal reperfusion injury. *British Journal of Pharmacology*, **130** (2000), 197–200.
174. D. C. Gute, T. Ishida, K. Yarimizu & R. J. Korthuis, Inflammatory responses to ischemia and reperfusion in skeletal muscle. *Molecular and Cellular Biochemistry*, **179** (1998), 169–87.
175. D. L. Carden, J. K. Smith & R. J. Korthuis, Neutrophil-mediated microvascular dysfunction in postischemic canine skeletal muscle. Role of granulocyte adherence. *Circulation Research*, **66** (1990), 1436–44.

19 • Compartment syndromes

MATTHEW BOWN AND ROBERT SAYERS

DEFINITION

Compartment syndrome is a clinical and pathological syndrome where the pressure within an anatomical tissue compartment rises above the normal physiological value for that compartment, and detrimentally alters the function of the tissues within that compartment either temporarily or permanently. Acute compartment syndromes affecting the abdominal cavity and the fascial compartments of the limbs are those encountered in vascular surgery.

ACUTE LIMB COMPARTMENT SYNDROME

The importance of acute limb compartment syndrome (LCS) is that, if left untreated, it results in rhabdomyolysis with resultant release of potassium, myoglobin and other toxins into the systemic circulation, which can lead to renal and/or multi-organ failure. The mortality of acute renal failure and multi-organ failure is high. These patients require critical care which may involve dialysis and other organ support. Untreated LCS often necessitates amputation to prevent further acute systemic deterioration. If the immediate insult is survived without the need for amputation a permanently disabling ischaemic contracture may result [1].

Limb compartment syndrome arises due to the anatomical arrangement of muscles surrounded by restrictive, inelastic osteofascial envelopes. Increased pressure within these fascial compartments can occur as a result of extrinsic compression such as that from plaster casts or bandages, or increased volume of the contents of the compartment. The volume within the compartment can be increased as a result of enlargement of those tissues contained within the compartment (e.g. muscle oedema) or due to the presence of a pathological space-occupying mass (such as a haematoma or abscess). In the field of vascular surgery LCS is most commonly encountered following delayed revascularization of an ischaemic limb, fractures with/without vascular injury or following radiological complications such as perforation during angioplasty. It is occasionally seen in conditions such as phlegmasia caerulea dolens where venous hypertension exists.

Incidence

The incidence of LCS after revascularization depends primarily on the type of insult. After elective revascularization of chronically ischaemic limbs the incidence is very low, from 0% to 0.5% [2; 3]. The incidence increases in revascularized acutely ischaemic limbs to approximately 10% to 20% [4; 5; 6]. Revascularization following vascular trauma is the most significant risk factor for LCS, with a reported incidence of up to 62% [7], particularly if this is associated with either a vascular injury at or below the popliteal artery or a fracture (Figure 19.1).

Anatomy/physiology

Limb compartment syndrome develops in the limbs because of their particular anatomical and physiological characteristics. Anatomically this is principally the arrangement of muscles within envelopes of dense, inelastic fibrous fascia. In addition to muscles, each compartment also contains peripheral nerves and blood vessels that traverse these compartments to supply distal parts of the limb and/or supply the structures within that compartment.

The anatomical arrangement of the capillary beds and physiological processes occurring within these also contribute to the development of LCS. Figure 19.2a shows the normal anatomical arrangement and physiological passage of fluid across the capillary wall. Fluid exchange across a capillary wall is affected by the hydrostatic pressure and oncotic pressure. The extracellular

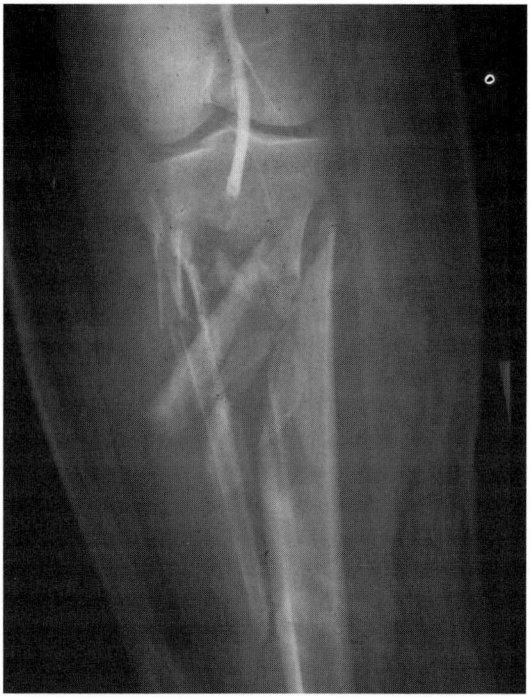

Fig. 19.1. Severe comminuted fracture of the tibia and fibula with distal popliteal artery injury demonstrated angiographically. An injury with a high risk of acute LCS.

compartment has a low hydrostatic and oncotic pressure due to the draining action of the lymphatics. In capillaries hydrostatic and oncotic pressure varies along their length. At the arterial end of the capillary, hydrostatic pressure (35 mm Hg) is greater than tissue hydrostatic pressure (0 mm Hg). Oncotic pressure within the capillary (28 mm Hg) is higher than tissue oncotic pressure (3 mm Hg) (therefore acting to draw fluid back into the capillary) but since the net hydrostatic pressure acting to filter fluid out of the capillary is greater than the net oncotic pressure, fluid is filtered into the extracellular space. As blood passes along the capillary to the venous end fluid is lost. At the venous end of the capillary hydrostatic pressure is much lower (15 mm Hg) and the resultant net force now acts to draw fluid back into the capillary (net oncotic pressure is greater than the net hydrostatic pressure).

Aetiology/pathophysiology

Limb compartment syndrome causes tissue damage due to ischaemia within the affected compartment. This ischaemia is not due to the interruption of the regional blood supply but due to the failure of the microcirculation caused by the elevated compartment pressure (the initial insult may, of course, be due to regional ischaemia). The initial injury causes swelling of the tissues within the compartment that, in turn, results in increased intra-compartmental pressure (ICP).

As ICP increases above physiological levels the first part of the circulation to be affected is the small venules since these vessels have the lowest pressure. These venules collapse and since the arterial side of the capillary beds remains open, the hydrostatic pressure within the capillaries continues to filter plasma out of the blood vessels into the tissues. However, since the venous side of the capillary bed is closed, the normal return of extracellular fluid back into the circulation by combined oncotic and hydrostatic forces cannot occur, and actually reverses due to the venous hypertension in the capillary (Figure 19.2b). Lymphatic drainage is also impaired by the high tissue pressures. The net result is further tissue swelling, with a subsequent increase in ICP and thus the initiation of a vicious cycle. As ICP increases further the arterial side of the capillary bed and eventually the arterioles become affected causing frank ischaemia, and permanent tissue damage shortly follows.

In the initial stages of LCS the principle pathological change in the muscles affected is oedema within and around muscle fascicles. As LCS progresses frank ischaemic changes occur in the muscle fibres [8].

The most common cause of compartment syndrome in vascular surgery is tissue oedema due to the ischaemia-reperfusion injury caused by limb revascularization. The re-establishment of a blood supply to ischaemic tissues has been observed to cause more damage than ischaemia alone. During ischaemia, antioxidant mechanisms are capable of dealing with any oxygen free radicals produced. However, the return of oxygenated blood to ischaemic tissues results in a burst in production of oxygen free radicals due to the action of xanthine oxidase (XO) on tissue hypoxanthine, both of which are produced in ischaemic tissues. The return of oxygen upon reperfusion supplies the final substrate for this reaction to proceed, which results in a burst of superoxide production (Figure 19.3). Free radicals are produced from this superoxide and mediate cell damage largely via lipid peroxidation of cell membranes. Oxygen free radicals also cause activation of microvascular neutrophil

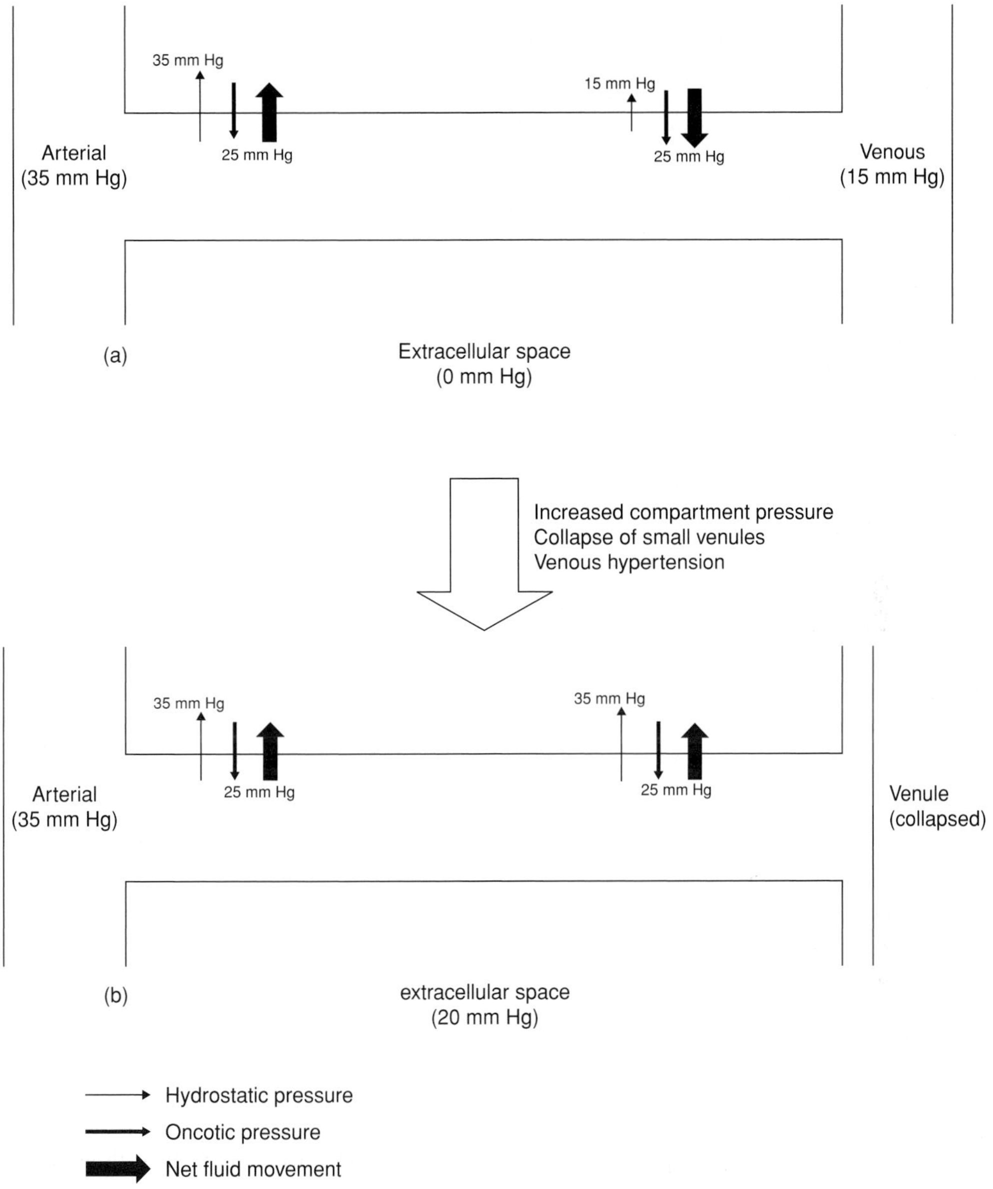

Fig. 19.2. Capillary fluid exchange (a) in normal physiological circumstances and (b) in the case of raised extracellular tissue pressure, as in acute LCS.

polymorphs and endothelial cells. Activated endothelium produces arachidonic acid metabolites, nitric oxide (NO), endothelins, complement and cytokines. These various mediators contribute to the continuation and extension of a local inflammatory response, and the production of a cellular and acellular inflammatory infiltrate with corresponding tissue swelling (Figure 19.4) [9].

Clinical presentation

Different tissues within the osteo-fascial compartments of the limbs are able to tolerate ischaemia to different degrees. The most sensitive to ischaemia are unmyelinated nerve fibres followed by myelinated nerve fibres, skeletal muscle, skin and then bone. Large arteries are

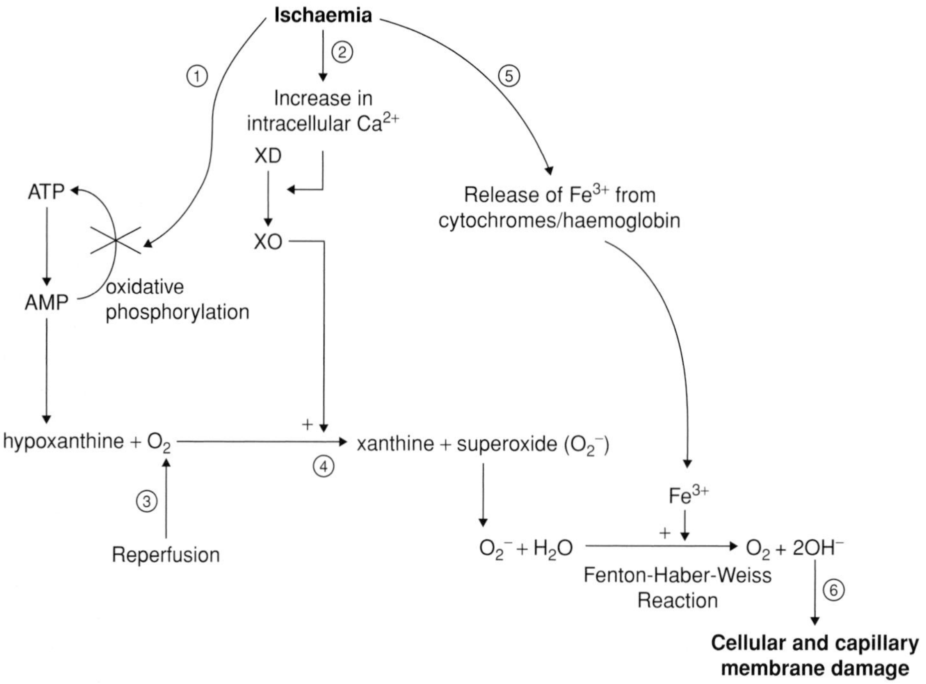

Fig. 19.3. Xanthine oxidase (XO) pathway activation by ischaemia-reperfusion and the production of reactive oxygen species. Ischaemia prevents oxidative phosphorylation (1) and cellular ATP cannot be regenerated. This leads to the accumulation of AMP and, in turn, hypoxanthine. Ischaemia also causes the accumulation of intracellular calcium (2). This catalyses the conversion of xanthine dehydrogenase (XD) to XO. Upon reperfusion oxygen is supplied (3) and this provides the final substrate to allow XO to convert hypoxanthine to xanthine, producing superoxide as a by-product (4). During ischaemia iron is released from cytochrome, haemoglobin and other haem containing molecules (5). This iron catalyses the Fenton-Haber-Weiss reaction producing hydroxyl radicals from superoxide. These hydroxyl radicals damage the cellular and capillary membranes leading to loss of function and cell death (6).

relatively resistant to acute hypoxia and blood flow within them is maintained until late after the onset of LCS since ICP only exceeds systemic blood pressure at the latter stages of the disease process. It is these different hypoxic tolerances of each tissue that lead to the symptoms and clinical signs of LCS.

The most common symptom of LCS is severe pain that is unresolved by analgesics and the degree of which is out of proportion to the injury sustained. Symptoms due to neurological dysfunction include weakness and paraesthesia in the myotomes and dermatomes associated with the peripheral nerves that pass through the affected compartment. These symptoms will progress steadily over a short period of time.

Clinical signs associated with LCS are pain on passive movement of the muscles in the affected compartment, tenderness of the muscle bellies lying within the affected compartment and tenseness of the compartment. There may be muscle weakness and sensory loss (particularly two-point discrimination due to the early loss of the unmyelinated nerve fibres). Commonly foot drop occurs in LCS affecting the lower leg. There may be signs of the injury that has caused LCS to develop such as a fracture, surgical dressings or bruising. Peripheral pulses will be maintained until long after LCS has become established. Signs suggestive of irreversible ischaemic change include fixed, non-blanching skin staining or frank gangrene. In these cases therapy should be directed towards preventing systemic complications and death.

Clinical assessment of suspected LCS is difficult. The majority of these symptoms and signs are only reliably assessed in a fully conscious patient; those at highest risk of LCS often have an altered level of consciousness

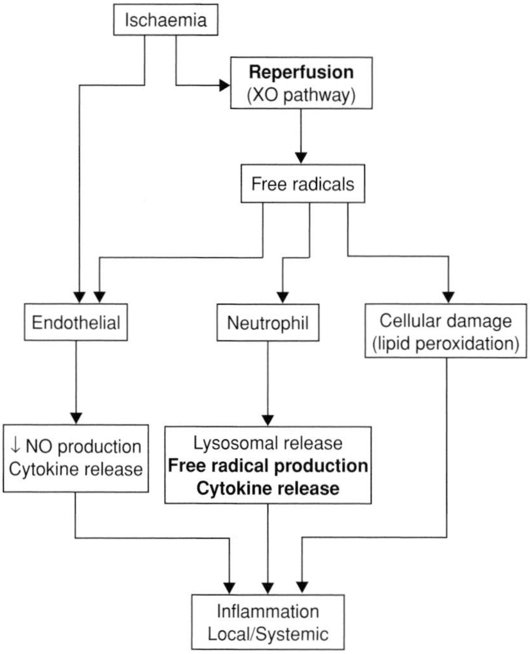

Fig. 19.4. Pathways and effects of ischaemia-reperfusion injury.

due to the injury or operation that has placed them at risk. Also, many patients may have some of these clinical signs present due to the injury that has caused the LCS such as the pulseless, painful, paraesthetic limb of acute ischaemia. The most useful guide to LCS is to maintain a high index of clinical suspicion.

Investigation

Since clinical assessment of a limb at risk of LCS is difficult, a test to give an objective measurement of ICP is desirable. Many methods for measuring ICP exist. Described techniques are wick catheters [10], slit catheters [11], needle manometry [12] and infrared spectroscopy (Figure 19.5) [13]. These various methods all have relative advantages and disadvantages. Catheter techniques allow continuous monitoring of limbs at risk and are more accurate than simple needle manometry [10], but they are more complex and require prior training in their use. Needle manometry can be simply performed using an 18 g needle connected to a mercury manometer, available in any hospital, or small handheld electronic devices are available. Near-infrared spectroscopy is still under evaluation. Whilst it is non-invasive, it requires relatively expensive equipment and the interpretation of the readings from this method are less intuitive than a figure for absolute compartment pressure expressed in mm Hg.

Normal resting ICP is 0–10 mm Hg [2; 14]. Capillary blood pressure varies from 30–40 mm Hg at the arterial side of the capillary bed to 10–15 mm Hg at the venous side [15]. Given the suggested pathophysiological processes underlying the development of LCS discussed above it would be expected that symptoms would first occur at compartment pressures somewhere between these two values. Many authors have suggested absolute cut-off levels of ICP to diagnose LCS. Mubarak *et al.* suggested a value of 30 mm Hg [16], whilst Allen *et al.* suggested a value of 50 mm Hg or a value above 40 mm Hg for longer than six hours [17]. However, in several clinical studies clinical symptoms and signs of LCS have not correlated well with measured compartment pressures. Tissue perfusion is dependent, not only on the interstitial pressure, but also the arterial perfusion pressure. Because of this Whitesides *et al.* suggested that the difference between diastolic blood pressure and ICP should be used to diagnose LCS, with a difference of less than 30 mm Hg being diagnostic [18]. It has been shown than this definition for diagnosing LCS results in less unnecessary fasciotomies than using absolute ICP levels of either 30 mm Hg or 40 mm Hg [19]. An alternative method is to calculate the difference between mean blood pressure and ICP, with a value of less than 40 mm Hg as a diagnostic cut-off [20].

The measurement of ICP may allow a more accurate diagnosis in those patients in whom clinical assessment is difficult due to other injuries or physical attributes. In those who have a clinically evident LCS, time should not be wasted by the measurement of ICP to confirm the diagnosis. In addition, many hospitals will not have the equipment or expertise available to accurately measure ICP. It is also thought that measured ICP may only be the ICP at the tip of the needle/catheter and not the pressure change in the whole compartment. Since any delay in initiating treatment for LCS may result in a worse outcome once diagnosed, LCS should be treated expediently.

Apart from the measurement of ICP there are no specific tests to diagnose LCS. In clinically advanced cases where there is tissue damage, the resulting inflammation may be manifest as a leucocytosis or, if there is significant tissue necrosis, serum creatine phosphokinase will be elevated and a metabolic acidosis occurs.

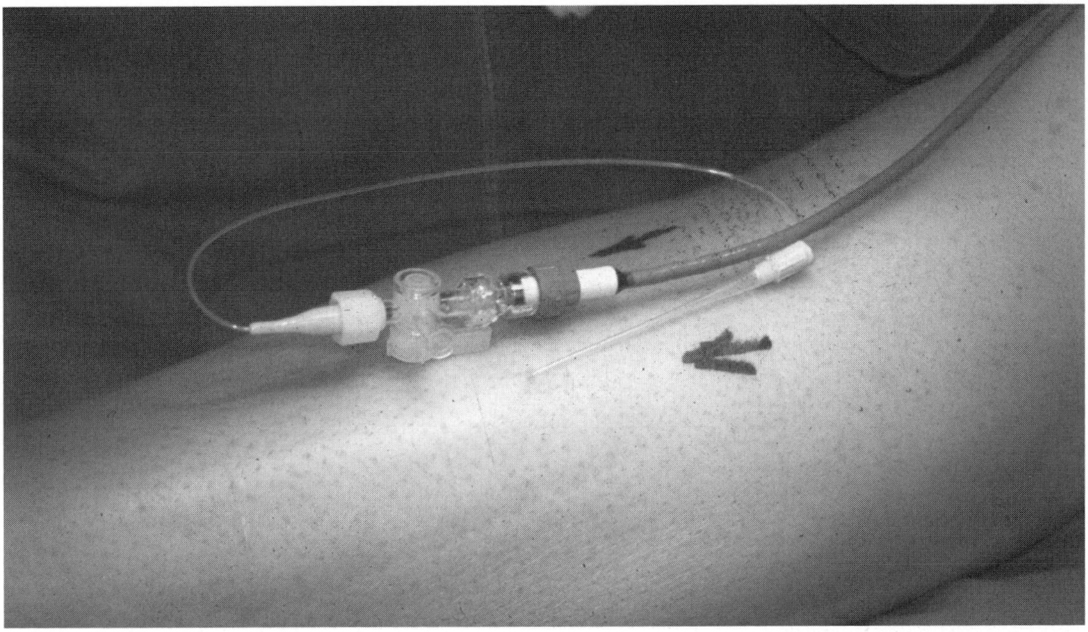

Fig. 19.5. Slit catheter inserted into anterior tibial compartment and connected to a pressure transducer. (Photograph courtesy of Mr M. J. Allen.)

Treatment

The treatment of acute LCS is urgent fasciotomy of all affected compartments (Figure 19.6). In patients who present acutely (within 12 hours of onset of LCS) this should be performed immediately. Delayed fasciotomy (longer than 12 hours after the onset of LCS) results in a significantly poorer outcome in terms of functional loss [21]. In those patients whose presentation is delayed, consideration has to be given as to whether the limb is unsalvageable and the possibility that a fasciotomy in this group of patients may lead to significant morbidity without ultimately improving functional outcome. If fasciotomy is delayed longer than 12 hours but less than 36 hours infection rates increase but limb salvage rates are similar [22]. Beyond 36 hours, rates of amputation, infection, neurological injury and death increase such that early amputation rather than futile attempts at limb salvage should be considered in this group [22; 23].

Fasciotomy should be performed in such a manner so that all constrictive elements surrounding a compartment are released. In the limbs this is the skin and the deep fascia. The area most commonly affected by LCS is the lower leg. This contains four separate compartments, the anterior, lateral (peroneal), superficial posterior and deep posterior. These can be decompressed either via a single lateral incision [24] or via two incisions, one lateral and one medial (Figure 19.7) [25]. The lateral incision is made over the lateral compartment one finger-breadth anterior to the fibula from the fibular head to the ankle. The anterior and lateral compartments are then opened along the length of the incision. The posterior compartments can then be opened either through this incision by dissecting behind the fibula or by removing a piece of the fibula.

Alternatively the deep posterior compartment can be opened by dissecting anteriorly to the fibula through the interosseous membrane. If two incisions are used the second is made on the medial aspect of the lower leg and the two posterior compartments decompressed. The thigh is usually decompressed medially and/or laterally.

In the upper limb the forearm is the most commonly affected by LCS. Both the volar and dorsal compartments can usually be decompressed via a single volar incision over the whole length of the forearm made in a curved fashion to avoid contractures. In other areas of the limbs the incisions should be made based on the

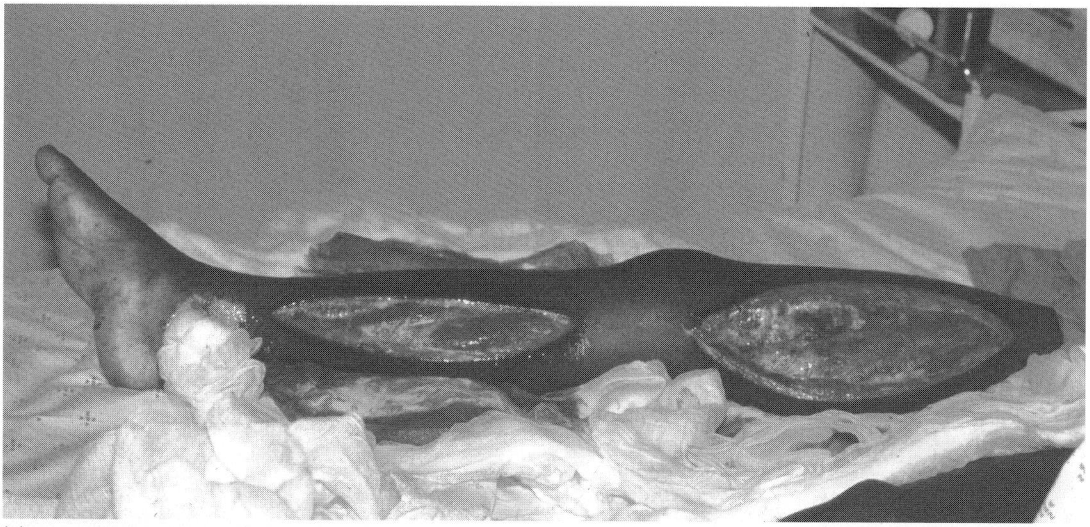

(a)

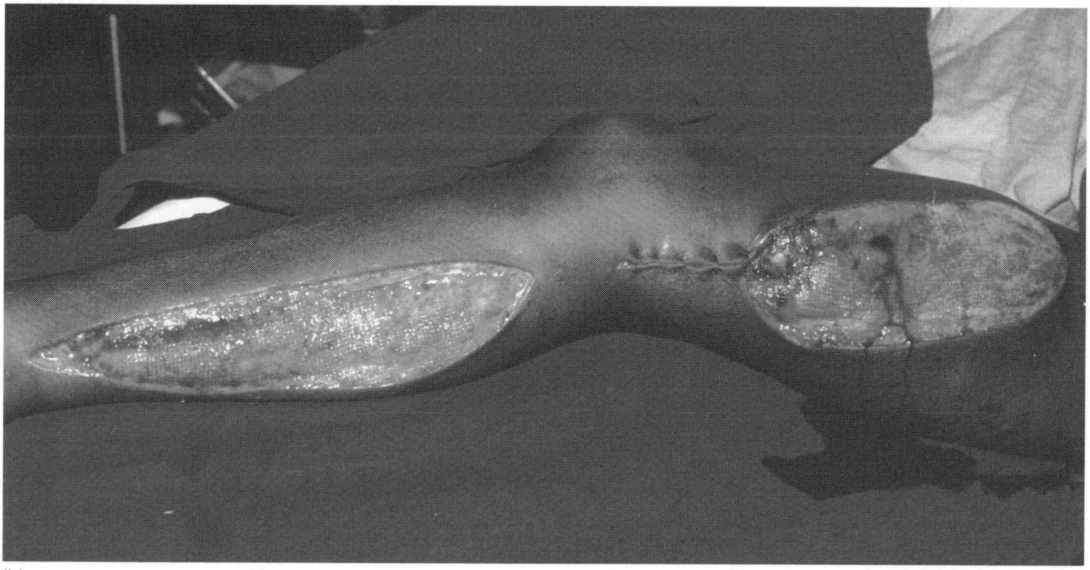

(b)

Fig. 19.6. (a) Medial thigh and calf fasciotomies following lower limb ischaemia after traumatic vascular injury, and (b) the same wounds after five days showing healthy granulation tissue (see colour plate section).

anatomy of that region and positioned so as to open the whole length of the affected compartment. After the fasciotomy has been performed any devitalized or necrotic muscle should be debrided.

Several alternatives exist for the management of fasciotomy wounds after the compartment syndrome has resolved: skin grafting, delayed primary closure, secondary closure, healing by secondary intention and the use of skin flaps. Skin grafting is usually performed between 7 and 21 days, and has been suggested to reduce wound complications when compared to other methods (Figure 19.8) [26].

In addition to fasciotomy, methods directed towards reducing the degree of initial tissue injury causing LCS have been suggested. Free radical scavengers such as mannitol and superoxide dismutase

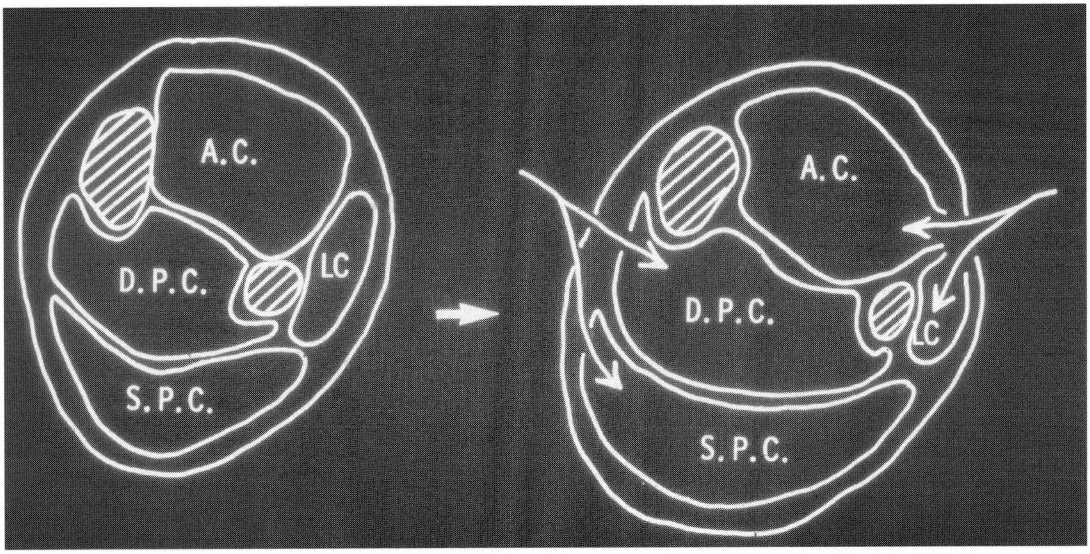

Fig. 19.7. Diagrammatic cross-section through mid-calf showing four osteo-fascial compartments (left). Arrows indicate medial and lateral incisions required for a four-compartment fasciotomy (right). Shaded areas represent the tibia and fibula. AC = anterior compartment; DPC = deep posterior compartment; SPC = superficial posterior compartment; and LC = lateral (peroneal) compartment.

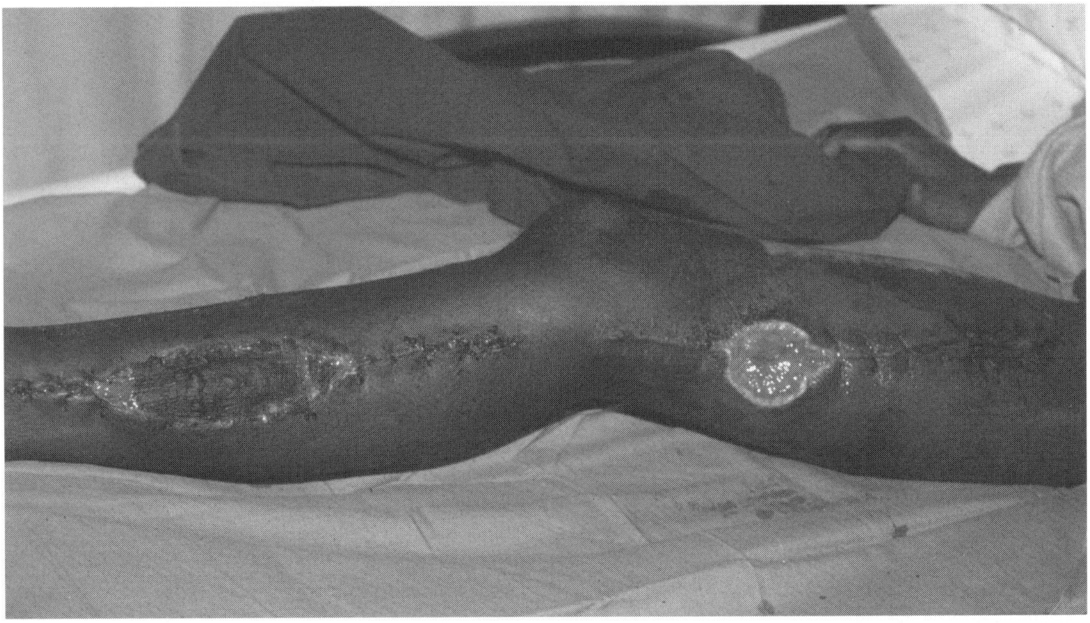

Fig. 19.8. Split skin grafting to calf fasciotomy two weeks post-injury (same patient as figure 19.6). The thigh fasciotomy has been treated by delayed closure leaving a small defect to heal by secondary intention (see colour plate section).

have been shown to be of benefit in LCS caused by ischaemia-reperfusion injury in animals [27; 28]. Some benefit has been shown using these agents in humans [29] although no comparative studies between these treatments and fasciotomy have been performed. Lysine-acetyl-salicylate, a thromboxane A_2 inhibitor has shown some benefit in animals but has not been studied in humans [30]. At present there is not enough evidence to justify the routine use of these compounds in clinical practice. Hyperbaric oxygen therapy has been suggested to be of use in improving the outcome of fasciotomy [31].

Complications of LCS

Locally, LCS, if left untreated, will cause ischaemia and subsequent limb loss. If infection occurs in the devitalized tissues systemic sepsis can occur and may result in multi-organ failure. In addition to infective complications the metabolic consequences of a devitalized limb have to be considered. As skeletal muscle becomes ischaemic and necroses, myoglobin and potassium are released into the circulation. These have nephrotoxic and cardiotoxic effects if released in large enough quantities, and may cause remote organ dysfunction or failure which is discussed in detail in Chapter 17.

Following decompression of LCS, devitalized muscle released myoglobin can cause renal failure due to tubular blockage. Treatment involves optimal fluid therapy and consideration of alkalization of the urine using intravenous sodium bicarbonate, aiming for a urinary pH greater than 6.5 and a plasma pH of greater than 7.4.

In some situations, amputation above the level of ischaemia may be required, a procedure associated with a high risk of mortality and morbidity in an already severely compromised patient.

Outcome

Whilst fasciotomy wounds are associated with a moderate degree of morbidity [26], fasciotomy does not appear to have any effect on long term calf-pump function [32]. If fasciotomy is performed without delay in LCS the outcome in terms of preventing limb loss, systemic complications and long term functional disability is good [33; 34]. Failure to promptly treat LCS risks the development of systemic complications such as multi-organ failure with a corresponding high risk of death.

ACUTE ABDOMINAL COMPARTMENT SYNDROME

The abdominal compartment syndrome (ACS) was first described by Kron *et al.* in 1984 [35]. To date no strict definition on the absolute pressure required to diagnose ACS has been made. Acute elevation of intra-abdominal pressure causes not only dysfunction of those organs within the abdominal cavity (hepatic, gastrointestinal and renal dysfunction) but has effects on more distant organ systems such as the cardiovascular, respiratory and central nervous systems. Whilst it has most commonly been described following abdominal trauma [36], vascular surgical procedures are the next most common cause [37]. Abdominal compartment syndrome is important since it results in dysfunction of multiple organ systems in patients who are already significantly compromised and is a contributory factor in the development of multi-organ failure.

In addition to acute ACS, intra-abdominal pressure may become chronically elevated in patients with obesity or ascites. In this situation, the rise in intra-abdominal pressure occurs over a prolonged period of time and abdominal wall compliance increases concurrently, thus preventing the detrimental physiological effects of acute ACS [38]. This condition is largely irrelevant, except that it may result in falsely high readings when assessing acute changes in intra-abdominal pressure in these patients.

Incidence

The only study to have estimated the incidence of ACS following vascular surgery was that of Fietsam *et al.* [39] where the incidence was 4% following ruptured abdominal aortic aneurysm repair. Abdominal compartment syndrome is rare following elective aortic surgery [40].

Aetiology

In a similar fashion to LCS, raised intra-abdominal pressure can occur as a result of increased intra-abdominal volume (either retroperitoneal or intra-peritoneal) or extrinsic compression, which is usually due to changes in the abdominal wall, either iatrogenic or pathological.

Expansion of retroperitoneal volume can be caused by traumatic bleeding, pancreatitis or sepsis [41; 39]. More commonly intra-abdominal volume expansion is caused by intra-peritoneal expansion by traumatic or iatrogenic bleeding, peritonitis, visceral oedema, or intra-abdominal packing for uncontrollable haemorrhage [42; 43; 44; 45; 46]. Rarely visceral oedema can occur following non-abdominal trauma that is thought to be due to large volume fluid resuscitation [47].

Extrinsic compression of the abdominal cavity can be caused by tight abdominal closure following laparotomy incisions, burns, eschars, pneumatic anti-shock trousers and the repair of large hernias, which result in an effective reduction of abdominal cavity volume [44; 48; 49; 50]. In addition high intra-thoracic pressure may lead to high intra-abdominal pressure [51].

Pathological effects of raised intra-abdominal pressure

Elevated intra-abdominal pressure causes a reduction in mesenteric and hepatic arterial, intestinal and hepatic microcirculatory, and portal venous blood flow [52; 53]. This reduction in the visceral blood flow occurs at pressures as low as 10 mm Hg and further impairment occurs with further increases of intra-abdominal pressure. As visceral blood flow reduces ischaemia occurs, resulting in impaired cellular respiratory function and subsequent cellular damage. The acidosis which follows can be assessed by gastric tonometry. Reduction in gastric pH has been shown to occur early in ACS and this can be reversed by abdominal decompression [54]. Whilst severe tissue damage has been shown to only occur at high intra-abdominal pressures (>40 mm Hg) [55], gastrointestinal bacterial translocation occurs at much lower pressures (25 mm Hg) [56]. Since bacterial translocation has been implicated as a significant contributory factor to the development of multi-organ failure, this is an important effect of relatively low pressure ACS.

Renal impairment was one of the earliest noted effects of ACS [35]. Progressive deterioration in renal function occurs as intra-abdominal pressure increases. Oliguria occurs at pressures above 15 mm Hg whereas pressures of greater than 30 mm Hg cause absolute anuria [40; 57; 58; 40]. Compression of the renal veins and direct renal parenchymal compression causes increased vascular resistance with a secondary reduction in renal perfusion [41; 57]. These changes cause a reduction in glomerular filtration rate, and a subsequent increase in renin, aldosterone and antidiuretic hormone occurs. Further increases in renal vascular resistance occur as a result, and lead to retention of sodium and water. In ACS, ureteral compression does not appear to cause renal dysfunction since the placement of ureteral stents has been shown not to improve renal function [59].

Elevated intra-abdominal pressure affects not only those organs within the abdominal cavity but also has detrimental effects on distant organ systems. Cardiac output decreases as intra-abdominal pressure increases as a result of decreasing preload and increasing afterload [60]. Preload is reduced due to direct compression of the abdominal inferior vena cava and compression of the superior vena cava due to increased intra-thoracic pressure as a result of direct transmission of elevated intra-abdominal pressure across the diaphragm. Elevated intra-thoracic pressure also directly compresses the heart, reducing end diastolic volume. All of the above results in a reduced stroke volume. A compensatory increase in heart rate occurs which only partially restores cardiac output [61]. The reduced cardiac output caused by ACS also causes further impairment of renal function beyond that caused by ACS alone.

Respiratory dysfunction also occurs as intra-abdominal pressure increases [61]. Direct transmission of elevated intra-abdominal pressure across the diaphragm causes elevations in intra-thoracic pressure, which in turn increases pulmonary vascular resistance. The volume of the thoracic cavity is also decreased due to an elevation of the diaphragm, compressing the lungs. This compression results in reduced lung volume and compliance [62]. These changes in the vasculature and physical properties of the lungs reduce respiratory function.

Raised intra-abdominal pressure causes increased intra-cerebral pressure and reduced cerebral perfusion that is thought to be due to reduced cerebral venous drainage [63; 64]. Also, abdominal wall blood flow is reduced in ACS due to direct compression, and leads to ischaemia and muscle swelling [65]. This, in turn, reduces abdominal wall compliance, exacerbating ACS [66].

Clinical presentation

Abdominal compartment syndrome most frequently occurs in patients who are critically ill. In these patients the most important factor to consider is a history of an abdominal injury or intervention that places them at risk of developing ACS. Clinical evaluation of patients with ACS is not reliable [67] and the only physical sign of ACS per se may be a tense, distended abdomen. The majority of clinical signs of ACS are due to the compromise of those organs systems affected by it – respiratory, renal, gastrointestinal and cardiovascular dysfunction.

Investigation

The investigation of choice in a patient with suspected ACS is the measurement of intra-abdominal pressure. The most commonly applied technique is that described by Kron *et al.* [35]. This utilizes an indwelling urinary catheter to obtain a direct measurement of intravesical pressure and has been shown to correlate well with intra-abdominal pressure [68]. A total of 50 ml of saline is introduced into the bladder via the aspiration port of the catheter which is clamped distal to this point. After allowing the pressure within the bladder to equilibrate with that in the abdominal cavity, a pressure transducer (such as that used for measuring central venous pressure) is attached to an 18 g needle inserted into the aspiration port and the pressure measured using the symphysis pubis as a reference point ('zero'). The intra-abdominal pressure can then be measured. Modifications to this technique have been proposed to avoid the repeated disturbance of a closed system with the potential to introduce infection [69]. This method has been shown to be inaccurate at low pressures (<15 mm Hg) [70]. Alternative techniques include intra-gastric pressure measurement [71] and inferior vena caval pressure measurement via femoral vein catheterization [72]. Whilst gastric pressure has shown good correlation with bladder pressure measurements at low intra-abdominal pressure, neither of these methods have been validated against the high bladder pressure measurement in humans with established ACS [73].

Normal intra-abdominal pressure is less than 10.5 mm Hg in men and 8.8 mm Hg in women [74]. An absolute diagnostic pressure at which ACS occurs has not been determined. Pressures above 25 mm Hg have been proposed by some authors, at which ACS should be diagnosed and treatment initiated [35; 45]. However, recent work examining ACS after ruptured abdominal aortic aneurysm repair has suggested that a figure of 15 mm Hg should be used in these patients [75]. An algorithm for the assessment and management of patients after abdominal aortic surgery has been suggested by Loftus & Thompson [76]. They suggest immediate measurement of intra-abdominal pressure in patients at risk after surgery and if the pressure is greater than 20 mm Hg, abdominal closure should be delayed. Following surgery patients should be monitored, if the intra-abdominal pressure rises above 30 mm Hg urgent decompression should be performed. In those with equivocal intra-abdominal pressure (16 to 30 mm Hg) urgent decompression should be considered, especially if there is organ dysfunction. In those patients with an intra-abdominal pressure of less than 15 mm Hg physiological support should be continued.

Treatment

The treatment of ACS is expedient decompressive laparostomy. This has been shown to rapidly reverse the detrimental effects of ACS in the gastrointestinal, renal, cardiovascular, respiratory and central nervous systems [39; 41; 60; 61; 77; 78; 79]. Following formation of the laparostomy consideration has to be given as to the method used to close the resulting defect. Temporary containment of the abdominal contents is achieved using a mesh (silastic, polypropylene or polygalactin), plastic bag (intravenous fluid container or bowel bag) or vacuum systems (Figure 19.9a). Alternatively, the skin can be closed leaving the fascia unapposed. After the patient has recovered from the organ dysfunction associated with ACS delayed primary closure can be considered. Alternatively the abdominal contents can be left to granulate over and then heal by secondary intention or skin grafts applied (Figure 19.9b). If delayed primary closure of the fascia is not achieved the resultant ventral hernia may have to be repaired at a later date.

Outcome

Abdominal compartment syndrome is associated with a high mortality of between 60% and 70%, not solely due to the development of ACS itself but in addition to the insult that caused it [80; 81]. Much of the morbidity of ACS is due to the method used to effect abdominal closure, entero-laparostomy fistulas are not uncommon and once healed the patient is frequently left with a large ventral hernia.

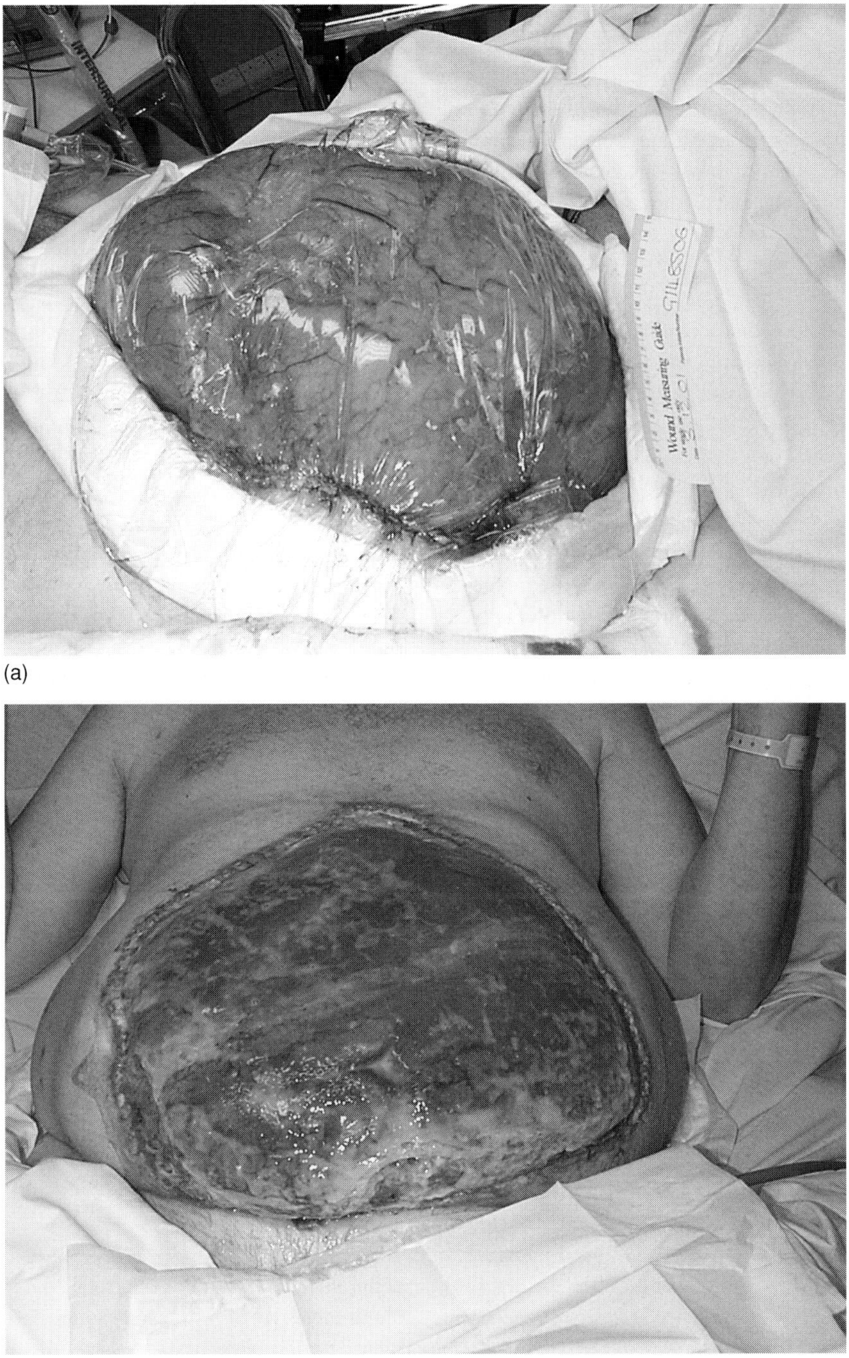

(a)

(b)

Fig. 19.9. (a) Immediate containment of abdominal contents using a plastic bowel bag after decompressive laparostomy following a ruptured abdominal aortic aneurysm repair; and (b) the same wound after four weeks, the viscera having granulated over (see colour plate section).

REFERENCES

1. R. Volkmann, Ischaemic muscle paralyses and contractures. *Clinical Orthopaedics*, **50** (1881), 5–6.
2. D. J. A Scott, M. McShane, M. J. Allen, M. R. Barnes & P. R. F. Bell, Does oedema following lower limb revascularisation cause compartment syndromes? *Annals of the Royal College of Surgeons of England*, **70** (1988), 372–6.
3. R. D. Patman & J. E. Thompson, Fasciotomy in peripheral vascular surgery. *Archives of Surgery*, **101** (1970), 663–72.
4. J. R. Allenberg & H. Meybier, The compartment syndrome from the vascular surgery viewpoint. *Der Chirurg*, **59** (1988), 722–7.
5. S. L. Jensen & J. Sandermann, Compartment syndrome and fasciotomy in vascular surgery. A review of 57 cases. *European Journal of Vascular and Endovascular Surgery*, **13** (1997), 48–53.
6. E. L. Papalambros, Y. P. Panayiotopoulos, E. Bastounis, G. Zavos & P. Balas, Prophylactic fasciotomy of the legs following acute arterial occlusion procedures. *International Angiology*, **8** (1989), 120–4.
7. Z. Abouezzi, Z. Nassoura, R. R. Ivatury, J. M. Porter, W. M. Stahl, A critical reappraisal of indications for fasciotomy after extremity vascular trauma. *Archives of Surgery*, **133** (1998), 547–51.
8. P. Hoffmeyer, J. N. Cox & D. Fritschy, Ultrastructural modifications of muscle in three types of compartment syndrome. *International Orthopaedics*, **11** (1987), 53–9.
9. M. J. Bown, M. L. Nicholson, P. R. F. Bell & R. D. Sayers, Cytokines and inflammatory pathways in the pathogenesis of multi-organ failure after abdominal aortic aneurysm repair. *European Journal of Vascular and Endovascular Surgery*, **22** (2001), 485–95.
10. S. J. Mubarak, A. R. Hargens, C. A. Owen, L. P. Garetto & W. H. Akeson, The wick catheter technique for measurement of intramuscular pressure. A new research and clinical tool. *Journal of Bone and Joint Surgery (American Volume)*, **58** (1976), 1016–20.
11. C. H. Rorabeck, G. S. P. Castle, R. Hardie & J. Logan, Compartmental pressure measurements: an experimental investigation using the slit catheter. *Journal of Trauma*, **21** (1981), 446–9.
12. T. E. Whitesides, T. C. Haney, H. Harada, H. E. Holmes & K. A. Morimoto, Simple method for tissue pressure determination. *Archives of Surgery*, **110** (1975), 1311–13.
13. G. Giannotti, S. M. Cohn, M. Brown *et al.*, Utility of near-infrared spectroscopy in the diagnosis of lower extremity compartment syndrome. *Journal of Trauma*, **48** (2000), 396–9.
14. P. Qvarfordt, J. T. Christenson, B. Eklof & P. Ohlin, Intramuscular pressure after revascularization of the popliteal artery in severe ischaemia. *British Journal of Surgery*, **70** (1983), 39–541.
15. C. E. A. Holden, The pathology and prevention of Volkmann's ischaemic contracture. *Journal of Bone and Joint Surgery*, **61B** (1979), 296–300.
16. S. J. Mubarak, C. A. Owen, A. R. Hargens, L. P. Garetto & W. H. Akeson, Acute compartment syndromes: diagnosis and treatment with the aid of the wick catheter. *Journal of Bone and Joint Surgery (American Volume)*, **60** (1978), 1091–5.
17. M. J. Allen, A. J. Stirling, C. V. Crawshaw & M. R. Barnes, Intracompartmental pressure monitoring of leg injuries. An aid to management. *Journal of Bone and Joint Surgery*, **67B** (1985), 53–7.
18. T. E. Whitesides, T. C. Haney, K. Morimoto & H. Harada, Tissue pressure measurements as a determinant for the need of fasciotomy. *Clinical Orthopaedics*, **113** (1975), 43–51.
19. M. M. McQueen & C. M. Court-Brown, Compartment monitoring in tibial fractures. The pressure threshold for decompressing. *Journal of Bone and Joint Surgery*, **78B** (1996), 99–104.
20. R. A. Moyer, B. P. Boden, P. A. Marchetto, F. Kleinbart & J. D. Kelly, Acute compartment syndrome of the lower extremity secondary to noncontact injury. *Foot and Ankle*, **14** (1993), 534–7.
21. G. W. Sheridan & F. A. Matsen, Fasciotomy in the treatment of the acute compartment syndrome. *Journal of Bone and Joint Surgery (American Volume)*, **58A** (1976), 112–5.
22. A. B. Williams, F. A. Luchette, H. T. Papaconstantinou *et al.*, The effect of early versus late fasciotomy in the management of extremity trauma. *Surgery* **122** (1997), 861–6.
23. J. A. Finkelstein, G. A. Hunter & R. W. Hu, Lower limb compartment syndrome: course after delayed fasciotomy. *Journal of Trauma*, **40** (1996), 342–4.
24. G. G. Cooper, A method of single-incision, four compartment fasciotomy of the leg. *European Journal of Vascular Surgery*, **6** (1992), 659–61.
25. S. J. Mubarak & C. A. Owen, Double-incision fasciotomy of the leg for decompression in compartment syndromes.

Journal of Bone and Joint Surgery (American Volume), **59A** (1977), 184–7.

26. S. B. Johnson, F. A. Weaver, A. E. Yellin, R. Kelly & M. Bauer, Clinical results of decompressive dermotomy-fasciotomy. *American Journal of Surgery*, **164** (1992), 286–90.
27. S. Oredsson, P. Arlock, G. Plate & P. Qvarfordt, Metabolic and electrophysiological changes in rabbit skeletal muscle during ischaemia and reperfusion. *European Journal of Surgery*, **159** (1993), 3–8.
28. B. A. Perler, A. G. Tohmeh & G. B. Bulkley, Inhibition of the compartment syndrome by the ablation of free radical mediated reperfusion injury. *Surgery*, **108** (1990), 40–7.
29. D. M. Shah, D. E. Bock, R. C. Darling *et al.*, Beneficial effects of hypertonic mannitol in acute ischaemia-reperfusion injuries in humans. *Cardiovascular Surgery*, **4** (1996), 97–100.
30. D. Dabby, F. Grief, M. Yaniv *et al.*, Thromboxane A_2 in postischaemic acute compartmental syndrome. *Archives of Surgery*, **133** (1998), 953–6.
31. G. Bouachour, P. Cronier, J. P. Gouello *et al.*, Hyperbaric oxygen therapy in the management of crush injuries: a randomised double-blind placebo-controlled trial. *Journal of Trauma*, **41** (1996), 333–9.
32. H. Ris, M. Furrer, S. Stronsky, B. Walpoth & B. Nachbur, Four-compartment fasciotomy and venous calf-pump function: long term results. *Surgery*, **113** (1993), 55–8.
33. M. M. McQuenn, J. Christie & C. M. Court-Brown, Acute compartment syndrome in tibial diaphysial fractures. *Journal of Bone and Joint Surgery*, **78B** (1996), 95–8.
34. F. A. Matsen, R. A. Winquist & R. B. Krugmire, Diagnosis and management of compartmental syndromes. *Journal of Bone and Joint Surgery (American Volume)*, **62A** (1980), 286–91.
35. I. L. Kron, P. K. Harmon & S. P. Nolan, The measurement of intra-abdominal pressure as a criterion for abdominal re-exploration. *Annals of Surgery*, **199** (1984), 28–30.
36. P. J. Offner, A. L. De Souza, E. E. Moore *et al.*, Avoidance of abdominal compartment syndrome in damage-control laparotomy after trauma. *Archives of Surgery*, **136** (2001), 676–80.
37. M. L. Cheatham, M. W. White, S. G. Sagraves, J. L. Johnson & E. F. J. Block, Abdominal perfusion pressure: a superior parameter in the assessment of intra-abdominal hypertension. *Journal of Trauma*, **49** (2000), 621–7.
38. H. J. Sugerman, A. Windsor, M. Bessos & A. Wolfe, Intra-abdominal pressure, saggital abdominal diameter and obesity comorbidity. *Journal of Internal Medicine*, **241** (1997), 71–9.
39. R. Fietsam, M. Billalba, J. L. Glover & K. Clark, Intra-abdominal compartment syndrome as a complication of ruptured abdominal aortic aneurysm repair. *American Surgery*, **55** (1989), 396–402.
40. C. F. Platell, J. Hall, G. Clark & M. Lawrence-Brown, Intra-abdominal pressure and renal function after surgery to the abdominal aorta. *Australian and New Zealand Journal of Surgery*, **10** (1990), 213–18.
41. T. Jacques & R. Lee, Improvement of renal function after relief of raised intra-abdominal pressure due to traumatic retro-peritoneal haematoma. *Anaesthesia and Intensive Care*, **16** (1988), 478–82.
42. B. H. Saggi, H. J. Sugerman, R. R. Ivatury & G. L. Bloomfield, Abdominal compartment syndrome. *Journal of Trauma*, **45** (1998), 597–609.
43. K. Offenbartl & S. Bengmark, Intra-abdominal infections and gut origin sepsis. *World Journal of Surgery*, **14** (1990), 191–5.
44. P. C. Smith, J. S. Tweddell & P. Q. Bessey, Alternative approaches to abdominal wound closure in severely injured patients with massive visceral edema. *Journal of Trauma*, **32** (1992), 16–20.
45. W. Ertel, A. Oberholzer, A. Platz, R. Stocker & O. Trentz, Incidence and clinical pattern of the abdominal compartment syndrome after 'damage control' laparotomy in 311 patients with severe abdominal and/or pelvic trauma. *Critical Care Medicine*, **28** (2000), 1747–53.
46. K. W. Sharp & R. J. Locieriero, Abdominal packing for surgically uncontrollable haemorrhage. *Annals of Surgery*, **215** (1992), 467–75.
47. R. A. Maxwell, T. C. Fabian, M. A. Croce & K. A. Davis, Secondary abdominal compartment syndrome: an underappreciated manifestation of severe haemorrhagic shock. *Journal of Trauma*, **47** (1999), 995–9.
48. D. G. Greenhalgh & G. D. Warden, The importance of intra-abdominal pressure measurements in burned children. *Journal of Trauma*, **36** (1994), 685–90.
49. N. E. McSwain, Pneumatic anti-shock garment: state of the art. *Annals of Emergency Medicine*, **17** (1981), 506–25.
50. A. Pierri, G. Munegato, L. Carraro *et al.*, Hemodynamic alterations during massive incisional hernioplasty.

Journal of the American College of Surgeons, **181** (1995), 299–302.
51. T. Kopelman, C. Harris, R. Miller & A. Arrillaga, Abdominal compartment syndrome in patients with isolated extra-peritoneal injuries. *Journal of Trauma*, **49** (2000), 744–7.
52. L. N. Diebel, S. A. Dulchavsky & R. F. Wilson, Effect of increased intra-abdominal pressure on mesenteric arterial and intestinal mucosal blood flow. *Journal of Trauma*, **33** (1992), 45–9.
53. L. N. Diebel, R. F. Wilson, S. A. Dulchavsky & S. Saxe, Effect of increased intra-abdominal pressure on hepatic arterial, portal venous, and hepatic microcirculatory blood flow. *Journal of Trauma*, **33** (1992), 279–84.
54. R. R. Ivatury, J. M. Porter, R. J. Simon *et al.*, Intra-abdominal hypertension after life-threatening penetrating abdominal trauma: prophylaxis, incidence and clinical relevance to gastric mucosal pH and abdominal compartment syndrome. *Journal of Trauma*, **44** (1998), 1016–23.
55. F. F. Gudmundsson, H. G. Gislason, A. Dicko *et al.*, Effects of prolonged increased intra-abdominal pressure on gastrointestinal blood flow in pigs. *Surgical Endoscopy*, **15** (2001), 854–60.
56. L. N. Diebel, S. Dulchavsky & W. J. Brown, Splanchnic ischaemia and bacterial translocation in the abdominal compartment syndrome. *Journal of Trauma*, **43** (1997), 852–5.
57. P. K. Harman, I. L. Kron, H. D. McLachlan, A. E. Freedlender & S. P. Nolan, Elevated intra-abdominal pressure and renal function. *Annals of Surgery*, **196** (1982), 594–7.
58. A. J. Kirsch, T. W. Hensle, D. T. Chang *et al.*, Renal effects of CO_2 insufflation: oliguria and acute renal dysfunction in a rat pneumoperitoneum model. *Urology*, **43** (1994), 453–9.
59. R. H. Paramore, The intra-abdominal pressure in pregnancy. *Proceedings of the Royal Society of Medicine*, **6** (1913), 291–334.
60. D. J. Cullen, J. P. Coyle, R. Teplick & M. C. Long, Cardiovascular, pulmonary, and renal effects of massively increased intra-abdominal pressure in critically ill patients. *Critical Care Medicine*, **17** (1989), 118–21.
61. P. C. Ridings, G. L. Bloomfield, C. R. Blocher & H. J. Sugerman, Cardiopulmonary effects of raised intra-abdominal pressure before and after intravascular volume expansion. *Journal of Trauma*, **39** (1995), 1071–5.
62. T. Mutoh, W. J. Lamm & L. J. Embree, Abdominal distension alters regional pleural pressures and chest wall mechanics in pigs *in vivo*. *Journal of Applied Physiology*, **70** (1991), 2611–18.
63. G. L. Bloomfield, P. C. Ridings, C. R. Blocher, A. Marmarou & H. J. Sugerman, Effects of raised intra-abdominal pressure upon intracranial and cerebral perfusion pressure before and after volume expansion. *Journal of Trauma*, **40** (1996), 936–40.
64. G. L. Bloomfield, P. C. Ridings, C. R. Blocher, A. Marmarou & H. J. Sugerman, A proposed relationship between increased intra-abdominal, intra-thoracic and intra-cranial pressure. *Critical Care Medicine*, **25** (1997), 496–501.
65. L. Diebel, J. Saxe & S. Dulchavsky, Effects of intra-abdominal pressure on abdominal wall blood flow. *American Surgeon*, **58** (1992), 573–6.
66. T. Mutoh, W. J. Lamm & L. J. Embree, Volume infusion produces abdominal distension, lung compression, and chest wall stiffening in pigs. *Journal of Applied Physiology*, **72** (1992), 575–82.
67. A. W. Kirkpatrick, F. D. Brenneman, R. F. McLean, T. Rapanos & B. R. Boulanger, Is clinical examination an accurate indicator of raised intra-abdominal pressure in critically injured patients? *Canadian Journal of Surgery*, **43** (2000), 207–11.
68. T. J. Iberti, K. M. Kelly, D. R. Gentili, S. Hirsch & E. Benjamin, A simple technique to accurately determine intra-abdominal pressure. *Critical Care Medicine*, **15** (1987), 1140–2.
69. M. L. Cheatham & K. Safcsak, Intra-abdominal pressure: a revised method for measurement. *Journal of American College of Surgeons*, **186** (1998), 594–5.
70. S. Johna, E. Taylor, C. Brown & G. Zimmerman, Abdominal compartment syndrome: does intra-cystic pressure reflect actual intra-abdominal pressure? A prospective study in surgical patients. *Critical Care*, **3** (1999), 135–8.
71. M. Sugrue, M. D. Buist, A. Lee, D. J. Sanchez & K. M. Hillman, Intra-abdominal pressure measurement using a modified nasogastric tube. Description and validation of a new technique. *Intensive Care Medicine*, **20** (1994), 588–90.
72. S. R. Lacey, J. Bruce & S. P. Brooks, The relative merits of various methods of indirect measurement of intra-abdominal pressure as a guide to closure of abdominal wall defects. *Journal of Paediatric Surgery*, **22** (1987), 1207–11.

73. G. G. Collee, G. G. Lomax, C. Ferguson & G. C. Hanson, Bedside measurement of intra-abdominal pressure (IAP) via an indwelling naso-gastric tube: clinical validation of the technique. *Intensive Care Medicine*, **19** (1993), 478–80.
74. N. C. Sanchez, P. L. Tenofsky, J. M. Dort *et al.*, What is normal intra-abdominal pressure? *American Surgeon*, **67** (2001), 243–8.
75. V. Papavassiliou, M. Anderton, I. M. Loftus *et al.*, The physiological effects of elevated intra-abdominal pressure following aneurysm repair. *European Journal of Vascular and Endovascular Surgery*, **26** (2003), 293–8.
76. I. M. Loftus & M. M. Thompson, The abdominal compartment syndrome following aortic surgery. *European Journal of Vascular and Endovascular Surgery*, **25** (2003), 97–109.
77. M. P. Shelly, A. A. Robinson, J. W. Gesford & G. R. Park, Haemodynamic effects following surgical release of increased intra-abdominal pressure. *British Journal of Anaesthesia*, **59** (1987), 800–5.
78. I. Irgau, Y. Koyfman & J. Tikellis, Elective intraoperative intracranial pressure monitoring during laparoscopic cholecystectomy. *Archives of Surgery*, **130** (1995), 1011–13.
79. G. L. Bloomfield, J. M. Dalton, H. J. Sugerman *et al.*, Treatment of increasing intracranial pressure secondary to the abdominal compartment syndrome in a patient with combined abdominal and head trauma. *Journal of Trauma*, **39** (1995), 1168–70.
80. V. Eddy, C. Nunn & J. A. Morris, Abdominal compartment syndrome. The Nashville experience. *Surgical Clinics of North America*, **77** (1997), 801–12.
81. D. R. Meldrum, F. A. Moore, E. E. Moore *et al.*, Prospective characterization and selective management of abdominal compartment syndrome. *American Journal of Surgery*, **174** (1997), 667–72.

20 • Pathophysiology of pain

STEPHAN A. SCHUG, HELEN C.S. DALY AND KATHRYN J.D. STANNARD

INTRODUCTION

Pain is defined as an unpleasant sensory and emotional experience associated with actual or potential tissue damage [1].

The mechanism by which a damaging stimulus in the body is perceived as painful by the brain is a complex one which is not yet fully understood. The complexity of the process results from the nervous system not being a 'hard wired' system, but exhibiting plasticity which enables it to modify its function under different conditions.

As shown by the definition, pain serves the purpose to prevent tissue damage and protect the body while it is healing. Under certain conditions, pain can become maladaptive and persist as chronic pain. This pain serves no protective function and is described as pathological pain as opposed to physiological pain [2].

In order to adequately treat physiological and pathological pain, an understanding of pain mechanisms is required.

PERIPHERAL MECHANISMS

Nociception

Painful stimuli are detected by nociceptors, which are free nerve endings located in tissues and organs. They have high thresholds and, under normal circumstances, only respond to noxious stimuli [3; 4].

There are two distinct types of nociceptor:

- High threshold mechanoreceptors which stimulate small myelinated Aδ-fibres and transmit a well-localized sharp or pricking sensation that lasts as long as the stimulus.
- Polymodal nociceptors that stimulate small unmyelinated slowly conducting C fibres. As well as responding to mechanical stimuli they are activated by thermal and chemical stimuli, e.g. hydrogen ions, potassium ions, bradykinin, serotonin, adenosine triphosphate (ATP) and prostaglandins.

Conduction

Voltage gated sodium channels mediate conduction along primary sensory afferents. As for all other impulses throughout the body, action potential propagation is dependent on these channels. There are two types of sodium channels, differentiated by their sensitivity to tetrodotoxin. Both types are present in nociceptive neurons, with the tetrodotoxin resistant type only present in nociceptors, which makes it a potential target for novel analgesics [5].

Nociceptors also have voltage gated calcium channels, which are found on the presynaptic membrane and are involved in neurotransmitter release at the dorsal horn.

Pain is transmitted by primary afferents, which have their cell bodies in the dorsal root ganglion (DRG). They terminate in the dorsal horn of the spinal cord. The dorsal horn cells are divided into specific regions or laminae called Rexed's laminae with I being the most superficial [3; 6; 7].

- Aδ-fibres are fast conducting and transmit the first sharp pain on initial stimulation. They terminate mainly in lamina I, but also send some fibres to lamina V of the dorsal horn where they synapse with second order neurones. They contain the neurotransmitter L-glutamate.
- C fibres are unmyelinated slow conducting fibres which transmit a less well-localized persistent aching pain that lasts after the initial stimulus has gone. They terminate in lamina II of the dorsal horn. As well as L-glutamate they contain several other neurotransmitters, including neuropeptides (such as substance P), calcitonin gene-related peptide (CGRP), cholecystokinin (CCK), brain derived neurotrophic factor

and glial derived neurotrophic factor. C fibres express several presynaptic receptors that modulate transmitter release. These include CCK, opioid and gamma-aminobutyric acid subtype B (GABA B) receptors. Apart from the CCK receptor, they inhibit the release of transmitter.

- Aβ-fibres conduct low intensity mechanical stimuli which convey touch and not pain, however, in chronic pain states they are involved in the transmission of pain. They terminate deeper in the dorsal horn in laminae III–VI.

SPINAL CORD MECHANISMS

Primary sensory afferents terminate in the spinal cord where they synapse with cells of the dorsal horn. Nociceptive specific neurons are located mainly in laminae I and II but also lamina V, and respond only to noxious inputs under normal conditions.

There are a number of different cells involved in the relay of painful stimuli including nociceptive specific cells and wide dynamic range neurons. Wide dynamic range neurons are located mainly in lamina V, but also in III and IV to a lesser extent, where they respond to stimuli from Aβ-, Aδ- and C fibres [3].

Cells of the dorsal horn involved in nociception express a number of receptors:

- AMPA (a-amino-3 hydroxy-5-methylisoxazole) which binds glutamate.
- NMDA (N-methyl-D aspartate) which also binds glutamate.
- A neurokinin receptor NK-1 which binds substance P.
- GABA A receptors which are ligand gated calcium channels that hyperpolarize the cell and reduce responsiveness to stimulation.
- Voltage gated calcium channels.
- Glycine receptors that provide an inhibitory function.

The ability to detect a potentially damaging noxious stimulus is mediated by L-glutamate acting on the AMPA receptor following stimulation of Aδ-fibres. The other receptors and neurotransmitters are involved in modulation of the response.

When a high intensity noxious stimulus arrives at the dorsal horn via C fibres, initially L-glutamate is released which acts via the AMPA receptor. As stimulus intensity increases, then other neurotransmitters are released such as substance P. Slow postsynaptic currents are set up which are mediated by a number of receptors including the NMDA receptor. These are also involved in modulation of the pain response [8].

Ascending systems

Noxious information is conveyed from the dorsal horn to the brain via several ascending tracts in the spinal cord. The majority of the wide dynamic range neurons and nociceptive specific neurons are conveyed antero-laterally in three pathways [9]:

- The spinothalamic tract: its fibres cross over to the contralateral side and pass through the brainstem to nuclei in the thalamus, finally terminating in the somatosensory cortex where pain is perceived and localized.
- The spinoreticular tract: it terminates in the reticular formation and has projections, which terminate in the pons, medulla and periaqueductal grey matter. It is involved in descending inhibition of pain.
- The spinomesencephalic tract: it is also involved in the modulation of descending control.

Descending control

The dorsal horn receives inputs from higher centres that modulate the response to nociceptor input [10].

The descending control of output from the dorsal horn comes mainly from areas in the brainstem, namely the periaqueductal grey matter, raphe nuclei and locus coeruleus. Inhibitory tracts descend in the dorsolateral fasciculus and synapse in the dorsal horn. The key neurotransmitters involved are noradrenaline and serotonin. Noradrenaline acts via postsynaptic α-2 receptors, the action of serotonin is less specific. Endogenous opioids are also involved in descending inhibition at a spinal and supraspinal level. These endorphins and encephalins acting via the descending system are thought to be responsible for the analgesia induced by stress.

As well as descending control from the brainstem, nociceptive impulses are attenuated by input via Aβ-fibres (transmitting information on touch), which is the basis for the use of transcutaneous electrical nerve stimulation (TENS) for analgesia and for simply rubbing a hurting body part. This observation formed the basis for the initial gate-control theory of pain [11].

PAIN MODULATION

The above description of pain explains the initial sensation of pain immediately following injury, however, it does not explain the more complex phenomena associated with pathological pain due to neuroplastic changes.

These phenomena have a number of different causal mechanisms, which occur initially in the periphery, but later mainly in the dorsal horn as the main site modulation of painful stimuli.

Peripheral sensitization

Tissue injury results in the release of inflammatory mediators, such as bradykinin, histamine, K^+, H^+, 5-hydroxytryptamine (5-HT), ATP and nitric oxide, from damaged cells [12]. Breakdown of arachidonic acid by cyclo-oxygenase produces leukotrienes and prostaglandins. Immune cell activation results in the release of further mediators, including cytokine and growth factors. These mediators provide an 'inflammatory soup' which produces a painful area of primary hyperalgesia. These inflammatory mediators spread into the tissues surrounding the initial area of injury to produce an area of secondary hyperalgesia [13].

They act either by stimulating the nociceptors themselves or by acting via the inflammatory cells to stimulate the release of additional pain inducing agents. They also modify the response of primary afferents to subsequent stimuli either by changing the sensitivity of the receptors or by modulating the voltage gated ion channels. For example, after tissue and nerve injury, N-type calcium channels become more active resulting in greater release of L-glutamate in the spinal cord [14]. The magnitude of the current generated by sensory-neuron specific sodium channels is also increased.

Chronic inflammation and nerve injury has an effect on the presence and distribution of voltage gated sodium channels, which can become concentrated in areas of injury, and produce ectopic discharges. Sensory-neurone specific sodium channels have a significant role in chronic pain states. Studies have shown them to become concentrated in neurones proximal to a site of nerve injury, and play a role in the hyperalgesia and allodynia of chronic pain states [3].

Not all sensory neurons are active all the time. This peripheral sensitization will recruit 'dormant' nociceptors, thus increasing the receptive fields of dorsal horn neurons, and increasing the intensity and area of pain [6].

Central sensitization in the dorsal horn

Central sensitization is an increase in the excitability of the dorsal horn so that the dorsal horn cells have a lower threshold and respond to low intensity stimuli that are not usually painful. It also results in a greater response to supra-threshold stimuli thus producing the symptoms of allodynia and hyperalgesia.

There are several mechanisms which occur at the dorsal horn and contribute to chronic pathological pain states by central sensitization. These will be discussed in the context of neuropathic pain, as they are most relevant there.

NEUROPATHIC PAIN

Neuropathic pain arises following injury to nerves from a number of aetiologies, e.g. ischaemic, traumatic and infective. Characteristics of neuropathic pain include spontaneous stimulus independent pain, and pain that is stimulus dependent and exhibits the features of allodynia and hyperalgesia. There are a variety of different mechanisms responsible for the generation of symptoms, which may be quite different from patient to patient [5].

Mechanisms of neuropathic pain

The pathophysiology of neuropathic pain involves central and peripheral mechanisms. Usually more than one mechanism may be involved and producing a unifying hypothesis for all neuropathic pain states is inappropriate [15].

Peripheral mechanisms

Electrophysiological evidence over the last 25 years shows that activity in sensory neurones after injury is necessary for the development of neuropathic symptoms. Some proposed mechanisms are:

SPONTANEOUS ECTOPIC DISCHARGE

Normal primary afferent neurones require the input of a stimulus in order to reach firing potential. It has been shown that after a nerve injury spontaneous firing in the afferent neurone occurs [16]. A and C fibres have been shown to demonstrate oscillatory activity resulting in ectopic firing [17]. Cross excitation of other neurones increases this effect. These phenomena may be particularly relevant to the development of hyperalgesia, allodynia and chronic pain after nerve injuries.

Reorganization of expression of ion channels in the peripheral nerves is responsible for the ectopic discharge [18]. Both sodium and calcium channels have been shown to be involved with their altered expression increasing the excitability of neurones. The afferent barrage provided by spontaneous discharge from neurones provides a constant input to the central nervous system that may induce central sensitization [17].

ALTERED GENE EXPRESSION

Damaged peripheral sensory neurones undergo Wallerian degeneration, and lose contact with peripheral targets and the supply of neurotrophic factors. The sensory neurones undergo altered gene expression, the result of which is a change in the type and level of neurotransmitters released in the spinal cord [19]. For example, some Aβ-fibres appear to release transmitters normally associated with nociceptors such as substance P. This seems to contribute to central sensitization [20]. A change in gene expression also results in either up- or down-regulation of ion channels, in particular different types of sodium channel involved in ectopic spontaneous activity.

SPARED SENSORY NEURONES

Changes have also been found in uninjured sensory fibres that are alongside those with a lesion. They frequently show the opposite gene expression changes from their damaged neighbours; possibly due to increased bioavailability of neurotrophic factors. This can result in increased activity in the spared afferents, although the exact mechanism is not understood [19].

INVOLVEMENT OF THE SYMPATHETIC NERVOUS SYSTEM

Some patients exhibit neuropathic pain that is dependent on activity in the sympathetic nervous system. After a peripheral nerve injury, a coupling develops between the sympathetic nervous system and the sensory nervous system. Axons involved develop increased α-adrenoceptors and therefore have an exaggerated response to circulating catecholamines [21]. Morphological changes to the nerve follow with sympathetic axons sprouting into the dorsal root ganglion forming baskets around the cell bodies of sensory neurones [22]. These changes lead to sympathetically maintained pain. Evidence for a sympathetic component to a patient's pain include sympathetically maintained, often unilateral limb pain, oedema, and vasomotor and sudomotor asymmetries.

COLLATERAL SPROUTING

Sprouting of fibres from sensory axons in the skin has been shown to occur in denervated areas, for example, after crush injuries [23]. However, this does not occur in proportion to the degree of neuropathic pain experienced and is likely to be a small if at all significant factor in its pathophysiology.

EFFECTS OF BRADYKININ

This main plasma kinin, a vasodilator peptide, is involved in hyperalgesia associated with inflammatory pain, with a change in expression of its binding sites within the dorsal root ganglion after nerve injury [24].

Central mechanisms

The central mechanisms potentially involved in the generation of neuropathic pain are thought to result in neuroplastic changes in the central nervous system. Central sensitization occurs after peripheral nerve injury. Central sensitization changes the way the neurones respond to subsequent inputs. This may result in spontaneous ongoing pain and abnormally evoked pain (allodynia and hyperalgesia) [6]. The mechanisms that are thought to be responsible occur primarily in the dorsal horn.

WIND-UP

The term wind-up describes the altered response of the dorsal horn neurones to repeated input from C fibres [6; 8; 25]. Following brief, repetitive C fibre stimulation, the dorsal horn cells respond in a linear fashion. However, if the stimulus continues, further C fibre activation produces an amplified response in the dorsal horn to the same intensity of stimulus.

This phenomenon is mediated by the NMDA receptor. Activation by sustained C fibre input leads to opening of the channel, an increased intracellular calcium concentration and an increased response to L-glutamate. L-Glutamate is the main excitatory neurotransmitter released from primary afferent neurones that acts at postsynaptic receptors. The NMDA receptor in its resting state is blocked by magnesium, which is released when the cell is depolarized. Thus the channel in the receptor is opened allowing an influx of sodium and calcium, and further depolarization. When a painful stimulus arrives at the dorsal horn, the cells are initially depolarized by L-glutamate acting at the AMPA receptor thus allowing removal of the magnesium block. Once the stimulus is removed, the dorsal horn cells continue to fire for several seconds.

There is potential for this to be modified pharmacologically, and a number of studies suggest that NMDA antagonists may prevent these phenomena and prevent hyperalgesia [26; 27].

Wind-up is relatively short lived (seconds to minutes), whereas central sensitization persists so the exact relationship remains unclear [28].

CENTRAL SENSITIZATION

Central sensitization is also mediated by the NMDA receptor. Under conditions of prolonged C fibre activation, depolarization of the dorsal horn cells causes the NMDA receptor to lose its magnesium block. Substance P, mediated by the NK-1 receptor, prolongs this depolarization and allows further influx of calcium. The increase of calcium in the dorsal horn activates calcium dependent kinases such as protein kinases A and C, which are then able to phosphorylate amino acids within the NMDA receptor to produce a conformational change in the structure. This permanently removes the magnesium block in the receptor and allows it to be activated by L-glutamate. The process of central sensitization differs from wind-up in that the changes remain long after the C fibre input has ceased. Furthermore, the magnesium is removed by posttranslational changes in the NMDA receptor and is not just depolarization induced [6; 20; 25; 29].

CENTRAL DISINHIBITION

Central disinhibition results from loss of modulatory control mechanisms, which may lead to abnormal excitation of central neurones [30]. The main inhibitory neurotransmitter is gamma-aminobutyric acid (GABA). It has been shown that suppression of this pathway results in allodynia [31]. Within two weeks after a peripheral nerve injury, GABA receptor levels are reduced [32]. Thus it appears that down-regulation of GABA mediated pathways may be in part responsible for central sensitization [33].

EXPANSION IN RECEPTIVE FIELD SIZE (RECRUITMENT)

Receptive fields of dorsal horn neurones contain subliminal areas; these represent a reservoir of activity [34]. With ongoing activation after injury there is an expansion of receptive field size leading to increased perception of pain, resulting in secondary hyperalgesia. This expansion of receptive fields does not reflect peripheral nerve or nerve root distribution, but spinal cord architecture. It might therefore be confusing from a diagnostic point of view, as it transgresses the boundaries imposed by a hard-wired model of the central nervous system [35; 36].

IMMEDIATE EARLY GENE EXPRESSION

Immediate changes in gene expression in dorsal horn cells occur in response to Aδ- and C fibre stimulation. These changes persist for a variable length of time and may contribute to central neuroplasticity.

Noxious stimulation mediated by Aδ- and C fibres produces an immediate change in the expression of certain genes within the dorsal horn cells [37]. These changes are detected within minutes of stimulation and may last for months or even years. The gene c-*fos* encodes a protein, fos, which forms part of a transcription factor. This may control the expression of other genes which produce long term changes in the dorsal horn. *C-fos* activation occurs as a result of increases in intracellular calcium, following release of neurotransmitters like substance P and L-glutamate involved in relay of nociceptive information [38]. This is followed rapidly by the appearance of fos protein which can be detected in laminae I, II and V of the dorsal horn [39]. The presence of fos protein can be used as a marker of noxious stimulation and thus also to determine the effect of agents to reduce noxious stimulation [40; 41; 42].

ANATOMICAL REORGANIZATION OF THE SPINAL CORD

Primary afferent neurones synapse in the laminae of the dorsal horn with second order ascending neurones. Under normal conditions, Aδ- and C fibres terminate in laminae I and II, whereas Aβ-fibres terminate in laminae III and IV.

Following C fibre injury, the large unmyelinated Aβ-fibres sprout terminals into lamina II. Aβ-fibres, which are activated by low intensity non-painful stimuli, can thus stimulate the dorsal horn neurons present in lamina II, usually associated with noxious sensation [43; 44]. This observation could explain allodynia, as Aβ-fibres form synapses with second order neurones and their low-threshold non-noxious inputs will be signalled as nociceptive in origin.

However, doubt surrounds this theory as a main mechanism of allodynia because sprouting is not fully established until two weeks after the injury [15]. Furthermore it has been suggested that this sprouting only occurs in a small sub-group of Aβ neurones [19].

As well as sprouting fibres into lamina II, Aβ-fibres also undergo phenotypic switching, and produce substance P and CGRP. These neurotransmitters are usually produced only by C fibres, but after nerve injury their expression is down-regulated. Aβ-fibres begin to release these at the dorsal horn following low intensity stimulation. This release of substance P can maintain the central sensitization changes in the dorsal horn at the NMDA receptor that is usually only maintained by continued C fibre input [15].

Symptoms of neuropathic pain

Patients with neuropathic pain usually experience persistent and/or paroxysmal pain [5]. The pain often has an abnormal quality, for example, burning, electric shock-like, shooting, lancinating or numbing. Neuropathic pain can occur in an area of neurological deficit, but might also arise from areas still innervated normally. Neuropathic pain exhibits often one or more of the following characteristic features:

- *Dysaesthesia*, an unpleasant abnormal sensation, whether spontaneous or evoked.
- *Hyperalgesia*, an increased response to a painful stimulus.
- *Allodynia*, pain elicited by a normally non-noxious stimulus
- *Hyperpathia*, a painful syndrome characterized by increased reaction to a stimulus, especially a repetitive stimulus, as well as an increased threshold.
- *Hypoalgesia*, diminished pain in response to a normally painful stimulus.

Clinical features of neuropathic pain are often summarized as stimulus dependent, stimulus independent and sympathetically maintained pain.

Stimulus dependent pain

Following nerve injury, increased C fibre activity causes central sensitization within the dorsal horn via activation of the NMDA receptor as described earlier.

Central sensitization produces three main effects:

(1) Enlargement of the sensory field of a dorsal horn neuron (secondary hyperalgesia).
(2) Increase of the response to a suprathreshold stimulus (hyperalgesia).
(3) Generation of a response to a subthreshold stimulus (allodynia).

These phenomena represent stimulus dependent pain, although the relationship between stimulus and response might be widely varying.

Stimulus independent pain

As mentioned earlier, there are two types of sodium channels present on sensory neurons. The tetrodotoxin resistant channels are implicated in the generation of the spontaneous pain of pathological pain states.

Following injury there is reorganization of the expression and location of the various types of sodium channel within the neuron. The tetrodotoxin resistant channels relocate to the neuroma, where it produces areas of hyperexcitability and ectopic discharges. After nerve injury, both injured nerves and uninjured nerves close to the site of injury display spontaneous discharges. The alterations in expression of sodium channels are thought to be due to alterations in the supply of neurotrophins such as nerve growth factor and glial-derived neurotrophic factor [45].

Sympathetically maintained pain (SMP)
In a small but significant proportion of chronic pain sufferers the pain has a definite sympathetic system element to it and is said to be sympathetically maintained.

Following partial nerve injury in these patients, both injured and uninjured primary afferents express α-2 adrenoceptors on their membranes so they become sensitive to circulating catecholamines and noradrenaline release from sympathetic nerve terminals [6; 22].

Direct coupling also occurs between the sympathetic and peripheral nervous systems with sympathetic nerves sprouting axons into the dorsal root ganglion to form baskets around the cell bodies of nociceptor neurons, where they form functional synapses. This sprouting is thought to occur under the influence of nerve growth factor. Other more central mechanisms of somatosensory-sympathetic coupling are also investigated [46].

Neuropathic Pain Syndromes

There are many causes of neuropathic pain including a number of disease states.

Peripheral neuropathies
METABOLIC/ENDOCRINE

Diabetics can develop different types of neuropathies, these include polyneuropathies, autonomic neuropathy, compression neuropathy and focal neuropathies [47]. There are more than 15 million diabetics in the USA and more than half of them over 60 years have neuropathic pain [48].

Many diabetics, especially those with poor blood glucose control develop a distal, symmetrical, proximally spreading and painful neuropathy. Severe pain is often a feature and may be described as burning, aching or have lightning components to it. It seems that the main cause is demyelination and to a lesser extent axonal degeneration. The first stage in prevention and treatment of early neuropathies is good glycaemic control. Additionally, hyperglycaemia may have a direct effect on neuropathic pain by altering pain thresholds, tolerance and affecting opioid receptors.

Mononeuropathies usually involve the motor supply to extraocular muscles and also nerve supply to the limbs. The third cranial nerve is most frequently affected. Pain is often a symptom. Additionally, an asymmetrical proximal predominantly motor neuropathy can occur, especially in older patients with poor glycaemic control [47].

Untreated hypothyroidism may result in neuropathic pain.

TOXIC

Well-known neuropathies here include those caused by alcohol, chemotherapy (where the neuropathy may be the dose limiting factor) and, more recently, anti-AIDS drugs, e.g. isoniazid [49].

POSTINFECTIOUS

The most common problem here is post herpetic neuropathy (PHN), which increases in incidence, intensity and persistence with age. The pain persists in the distribution of a peripheral nerve after herpes zoster infection (shingles). It is thought that chronic inflammatory changes result in damage to sensory nerves resulting in deafferation of nociceptive fibres [50]. The pain is persistent and can become intolerable with associated allodynia. Treatment is very difficult, in particular in later stages [51].

HEREDITARY

Fabry's disease, a rare lipid storage disorder, often presents with a painful neuropathy [52].

MALIGNANT

Neuropathies can occur as a non-metastatic complication of malignant disease, usually a sensory neuropathy that can sometimes be painful. Neuropathic pain can also be caused as the result of direct tumour invasion involving nearby nerves.

IDIOPATHIC

Trigeminal neuralgia (tic douloureux) is defined by the International Association for the Study of Pain (IASP) as a 'sudden, usually unilateral, severe, brief, stabbing, recurrent pains in the distribution of one or more branches of the fifth cranial nerve' [1]. It can occasionally be secondary to an underlying condition, e.g. tumour or multiple sclerosis. The diagnosis is made on clinical grounds as the patients describe a characteristic pain. It occurs most frequently in the maxillary division and least in the ophthalmic division of the trigeminal nerve. The pain is triggered by light touch, eating, talking and the cold. Examination in the absence of other neurological symptoms reveals very little [53]. There is no definitive diagnostic test. Magnetic resonance imaging (MRI) can reveal an underlying cause or nerve compression, but is otherwise not highly sensitive or specific [54]. Magnetic resonance tomographic angiography (MRTA) has been used in delineating the pathophysiological process and may provide a helpful diagnostic image, but there is insufficient evidence at present [55].

The pathophysiology is not completely understood. Most evidence supports vascular compression of the nerve, resulting in hyperexcitability and abnormal neuronal activity, causing pain. This theory is supported by the fact that patients often experience immediate pain relief from microvascular decompression and has been confirmed radiologically in a study utilizing MRTA [56].

Spontaneous remission may occur and thus surgery is reserved for those refractory to medical treatment. Complications of surgical microvascular decompression include facial nerve damage, haematoma, cerebrospinal fluid leak and infection. However, despite its risks microvascular decompression is currently the best option from a variety of surgical procedures [57]. The other surgical techniques include Gasserian ganglion surgery, radiofrequency thermocoagulation [58], percutaneous retro Gasserian glycerol injection or microcompression, posterior fossa surgery, and gamma knife irradiation [59].

Patients should be made aware of the risks associated with the chosen surgical technique and warned that the pain relief may not be permanent. They should balance these against the benefit from potential long term analgesia in cases refractory to medical management [60].

VASCULAR

Vascular pain is a complex issue. Pain can be arterial, microvascular or venous in origin. Neuropathy can in particular follow venous insufficiency [61]. In every vascular disease, sympathetic changes may develop which contribute a neuropathic element to the ischaemic pain. The patient may develop skin hyperalgesia, dystrophic skin with a shiny appearance, muscle atrophy and vasomotor phenomena. Sympathetic blocks may be beneficial [62].

POSTTRAUMATIC

Posttraumatic neuropathies are common and can develop after any nerve injury. Even minor demyelination injuries without neurological sequelae can result in neuropathies [17]. Examples are sciatica, neuroma or nerve entrapment after surgery or trauma, phantom limb pain, complex regional pain syndromes (CRPS) type I (without neurological deficit, previously called reflex sympathetic dystrophy (RSD)) and type II (with neurological deficit, previously called causalgia), and post-thoracotomy pain.

Central neuropathies

Central pain is due to a lesion or dysfunction of the central nervous system. These lesions may have associated symptoms that affect the patient and their pain, e.g. ataxia, motor weakness and hearing/visual loss. Epilepsy and depression are also common with cerebral lesions. These aspects need to be addressed along with treatment of the pain.

Central pain is associated with spinothalamocortical dysfunction, may develop over a length of time and varies widely between individuals regardless of aetiology [63].

VASCULAR LESIONS IN THE BRAIN AND SPINAL CORD

The aetiology here includes infarction, haemorrhage and vascular malformation.

Stroke is the most common cause of central pain due to its high incidence. Some 8% of patients with acute stroke have been shown to suffer from central pain in the following 12 months [64].

MULTIPLE SCLEROSIS

This demyelination process can result in neuropathic pain by a variety of mechanisms. Cranial nerve neuropathies as well as widespread central pain syndromes are common consequences and often difficult to treat [65].

TRAUMA, TUMOURS AND INFECTIONS

Brain injury, but by far more commonly spinal cord injury, can result in a variety of central pain syndromes [66]. Syringomyelia and syringobulbia as a consequence of such injuries can cause further central pain. Tumours of the brain and spine as well as infections and abscesses can cause similar symptoms.

REFERENCES

1. H. Merskey & N. Bogduk (ed.), *Classification of Chronic Pain*, 2nd edn. (Seattle: IASP Press, 1994).
2. C. Woolf, Somatic pain – pathogenesis and prevention. *British Journal of Anaesthesia*, **75**(2) (1995), 169–76.
3. H. Bolay & M. A. Moskowitz, Mechanisms of pain modulation in chronic syndromes. *Neurology*, **59**(5)(Suppl 2) (2002), S2–7.
4. W. Riedel & G. Neeck, Nociception, pain, and antinociception: current concepts. *Zeitschrift für Rheumatologie*, **60**(6) (2001), 404–15.
5. C. J. Woolf & R. J. Mannion, Neuropathic pain: aetiology, symptoms, mechanisms, and management. *Lancet*, **353**(9168) (1999), 1959–64.
6. R. J. Mannion & C. J. Woolf, Pain mechanisms and management: a central perspective. *Clinical Journal of Pain*, **16**(3)(Suppl) (2000), S144–56.
7. F. Riedel & H. B. von Stockhausen, Severe cerebral depression after intoxication with tramadol in a 6-month-old infant. *European Journal of Clinical Pharmacology*, **26**(5) (1984), 631–2.
8. P. K. Eide, Wind-up and the NMDA receptor complex from a clinical perspective. *European Journal of Pain*, **4**(1) (2000), 5–15.
9. M. J. Millan, The induction of pain: an integrative review. *Progress in Neurobiology*, **57**(1) (1999), 1–164.
10. J. A. Stamford, Descending control of pain. *British Journal of Anaesthesia*, **75**(2) (1995), 217–27.
11. R. Melzack & P. D. Wall, Pain mechanisms: a new theory. *Science*, **150** (1965), 971–9.
12. B. L. Kidd & L. A. Urban, Mechanisms of inflammatory pain. *British Journal of Anaesthesia*, **87**(1) (2001), 3–11.
13. W. Kessler, C. Kirchhoff, P. W. Reeh & H. O. Handwerker, Excitation of cutaneous afferent nerve endings *in vitro* by a combination of inflammatory mediators and conditioning effect of substance P. *Experimental Brain Research*, **91**(3) (1992), 467–76.
14. A. H. Dickenson, Gate control theory of pain stands the test of time. *British Journal of Anaesthesia*, **88**(6) (2002), 755–7.
15. D. Bridges, S. W. Thompson & A. S. Rice, Mechanisms of neuropathic pain. *British Journal of Anaesthesia*, **87**(1) (2001), 12–26.
16. P. D. Wall & M. Gutnick, Ongoing activity in peripheral nerves: the physiology and pharmacology of impulses originating from a neuroma. *Experimental Neurology*, **43** (1974), 580–93.
17. M. Devor & Z. Seltzer, Pathophysiology of damaged nerves in relation to chronic pain. In *Textbook of Pain*, 4th edn., ed. P. D. Wall and R. Melzack. (London: Churchill Livingstone, 1999), pp. 129–64.
18. S. G. Waxman, J. D. Kocsis & D. L. Eng, Ligature-induced injury in peripheral nerve: electrophysiological observations on changes in action potential characteristics following blockade of potassium conductance. *Muscle and Nerve*, **8**(2) (1985), 85–92.
19. S. B. McMahon & D. L. H. Bennett, Trophic factors and pain. In *Textbook of Pain*, 4th edn., ed. P. D. Wall, and R. Melzack. (London: Churchill Livingstone, 1999), pp. 105–28.
20. C. J. Woolf & M. W. Salter, Neuronal plasticity: increasing the gain in pain. *Science*, **288**(5472) (2000), 1765–9.
21. W. Jänig, Sympathetic nervous system and pain: ideas, hypotheses, models. *Der Schmerz*, **7** (1993), 226–40.
22. E. M. McLachlan, W. Janig, M. Devor & M. Michaelis, Peripheral nerve injury triggers noradrenergic sprouting within dorsal root ganglia. *Nature*, **363**(6429) (1993), 543–6.
23. M. Devor, D. Schonfeld, Z. Seltzer & P. D. Wall, Two modes of cutaneous reinnervation following peripheral nerve injury. *Journal of Comparative Neurology*, **185**(1) (1979), 211–20.
24. M. Petersen, A. S. Eckert, G. Segond von Banchet *et al.*, Plasticity in the expression of bradykinin binding sites in sensory neurons after mechanical nerve injury. *Neuroscience*, **83**(3) (1998), 949–59.
25. S. Pockett & A. Figurov, Long-term potentiation and depression in the ventral horn of rat spinal cord *in vitro*. *Neuroreport*, **4**(1) (1993), 97–9.
26. T. Kawamata, K. Omote, H. Sonoda, M. Kawamata & A. Namiki, Analgesic mechanisms of ketamine in the presence and absence of peripheral inflammation. *Anesthesiology*, **93**(2) (2000), 520–8.

27. G. Davar, A. Hama, A. Deykin, B. Vos & R. Maciewicz, Mk-801 blocks the development of thermal hyperalgesia in a rat model of experimental painful neuropathy. *Brain Research*, **553**(2) (1991), 327–30.
28. J. Li, D. A. Simone & A. A. Larson, Windup leads to characteristics of central sensitization. *Pain*, **79**(1) (1999), 75–82.
29. C. J. Woolf & M. Costigan, Transcriptional and posttranslational plasticity and the generation of inflammatory pain. *Proceedings of the National Academy of Sciences of the USA*, **96**(14) (1999), 7723–30.
30. N. Attal, Chronic neuropathic pain: mechanisms and treatment. *Clinical Journal of Pain*, **16**(3)(Suppl) (2000), S118–30.
31. T. Yaksh, J. Howe & G. Harty, Pharmacology of spinal pain modulatory systems. *Advances in Pain Research and Therapy*, **7** (1984), 57–70.
32. J. M. Castro-Lopes, I. Tavares & A. Coimbra, GABA decreases in the spinal cord dorsal horn after peripheral neurectomy. *Brain Research*, **620**(2) (1993), 287–91.
33. L. Sivilotti & C. J. Woolf, The contribution of GABA A and glycine receptors to central sensitization: disinhibition and touch-evoked allodynia in the spinal cord. *Journal of Neurophysiology*, **72**(1) (1994), 169–79.
34. P. D. Wall, Recruitment of ineffective synapses after injury. *Advances in Neurology*, **47** (1988), 387–400.
35. R. C. Coghill, D. J. Mayer & D. D. Price, The roles of spatial recruitment and discharge frequency in spinal cord coding of pain: a combined electrophysiological and imaging investigation. *Pain*, **53** (1993), 295–309.
36. A. J. Cook, C. J. Woolf, P. D. Wall & S. B. McMahon, Dynamic receptive field plasticity in rat spinal cord dorsal horn following C-primary afferent input. *Nature*, **325** (1987), 151–3.
37. R. Munglani & S. Hunt, Molecular biology of pain. *British Journal of Anaesthesia*, **75**(2) (1995), 186–92.
38. R. Munglani, B. G. Fleming & S. P. Hunt, Rememberance of times past: the significance of c-*fos* in pain (editorial). *British Journal of Anaesthesia*, **76** (1996), 1–3.
39. R. J. Traub, P. Pechman, M. J. Iadarola & G. F. Gebhart, *Fos*-like proteins in the lumbosacral spinal cord following noxious and non-noxious colorectal distention in the rat. *Pain*, **49** (1992), 393–403.
40. P. Honore, J. Buritova & J. M. Besson, Aspirin and acetaminophen reduced both *fos* expression in rat lumbar spinal cord and inflammatory signs produced by carrageenin inflammation. *Pain*, **63**(3) (1995), 365–75.
41. C. J. Kovelowski, R. B. Raffa & F. Porreca, Tramadol and its enantiomers differentially suppress c-*fos*-like immunoreactivity in rat brain and spinal cord following acute noxious stimulus. *European Journal of Pain*, **2**(3) (1998), 211–19.
42. T. R. Tölle, J. M. Castro-Lopez, A. Coimbra & W. Zieglgansberger, Opiates modify induction of c-*fos* proto-oncogene in the spinal cord of the rat following noxious stimulation. *Neuroscience Letters*, **111** (1990), 46–51.
43. C. J. Woolf, P. Shortland, M. Reynolds *et al.*, Reorganization of central terminals of myelinated primary afferents in the rat dorsal horn following peripheral axotomy. *Journal of Comparative Neurology*, **360**(1) (1995), 121–34.
44. H. R. Koerber, K. Mirnics, P. B. Brown & L. M. Mendell, Central sprouting and functional plasticity of regenerated primary afferents. *Journal of Neuroscience*, **14**(6) (1994), 3655–71.
45. S. G. Waxman, T. R. Cummins, S. D. Dib-Hajj & J. A. Black, Voltage-gated sodium channels and the molecular pathogenesis of pain: a review. *Journal of Rehabilitation Research and Development*, **37**(5) (2000), 517–28.
46. W. Janig & H. J. Habler, Sympathetic nervous system: contribution to chronic pain. *Progress in Brain Research*, **129** (2000), 451–68.
47. T. H. Wein & J. W. Albers, Diabetic neuropathies. *Physical Medicine and Rehabilitation Clinics of North America*, **12**(2) (2001), 307–20, ix.
48. P. G. Jensen, J. R. Larson, Management of painful diabetic neuropathy. *Drugs and Aging*, **18**(10) (2001), 737–49.
49. M. Koltzenburg, Painful neuropathies. *Current Opinion in Neurology*, **11**(5) (1998), 515–21.
50. F. T. Scott, M. E. Leedham-Green, W. Y. Barrett-Muir *et al.*, A study of shingles and the development of postherpetic neuralgia in East London. *Journal of Medical Neurology*, **70**(Suppl 1) (2003), S24–30.
51. L. M. Panlilio, P. J. Christo & S. N. Raja, Current management of postherpetic neuralgia. *Neurology*, **8**(6) (2002), 339–50.
52. L. A. Lockman, D. B. Hunninghake, W. Krivit & R. J. Desnick, Relief of pain of Fabry's disease by diphenylhydantoin. *Neurology*, **23**(8) (1973), 871–5.

53. J. D. Loeser, Tic douloureux. *Pain Research and Management*, **6**(3) (2001), 156–65.
54. J. Yang, T. M. Simonson, A. Ruprecht *et al.*, Magnetic resonance imaging used to assess patients with trigeminal neuralgia. *Oral Surgery, Oral Medicine, Oral Pathology, Oral Radiology and Endodontics*, **81**(3) (1996), 343–50.
55. F. Umehara, K. Kamishima, N. Kashio *et al.*, Magnetic resonance tomographic angiography: diagnostic value in trigeminal neuralgia. *Neuroradiology*, **37**(5) (1995), 353–5.
56. J. F. Meaney, P. R. Eldridge, L. T. Dunn *et al.*, Demonstration of neurovascular compression in trigeminal neuralgia with magnetic resonance imaging. Comparison with surgical findings in 52 consecutive operative cases. *Journal of Neurosurgery*, **83**(5) (1995), 799–805.
57. A. Kondo, Microvascular decompression surgery for trigeminal neuralgia. *Stereotactic and Functional Neurosurgery*, **77**(1–4) (2001), 187–9.
58. J. H. Petit, J. M. Herman, S. Nagda, S. J. DiBiase & L. S. Chin, Radiosurgical treatment of trigeminal neuralgia: evaluating quality of life and treatment outcomes. *International Journal of Radiation Oncology, Biology, Physics*, **56**(4) (2003), 1147–53.
59. A. G. Shetter, C. L. Rogers, F. Ponce *et al.*, Gamma knife radiosurgery for recurrent trigeminal neuralgia. *Journal of Neurosurgery*, **97**(5)(Suppl) (2002), 536–8.
60. H. L. Fields, Treatment of trigeminal neuralgia. *New England Journal of Medicine*, **334**(17) (1996), 1125–6.
61. F. Reinhardt, T. Wetzel, S. Vetten *et al.*, Peripheral neuropathy in chronic venous insufficiency. *Muscle and Nerve*, **23**(6) (2000), 883–7.
62. A. Mailis & A. Furlan, Sympathectomy for neuropathic pain (Cochrane Review). *Cochrane Database Systematic Reviews*, (2) (2003), CD002918.
63. T. J. Nurmikko, Mechanisms of central pain. *Clinical Journal of Pain*, **16**(2 Suppl) (2000), S21–5.
64. G. Andersen, K. Vestergaard, M. Ingeman-Nielsen & T. S. Jensen, Incidence of central post-stroke pain. *Pain*, **61**(2) (1995), 187–93.
65. R. D. Kerns, M. Kassirer & J. Otis, Pain in multiple sclerosis: a biopsychosocial perspective. *Journal of Rehabilitation Research and Development*, **39**(2) (2002), 225–32.
66. P. J. Siddall, J. M. McClelland, S. B. Rutkowski & M. J. Cousins, A longitudinal study of the prevalence and characteristics of pain in the first 5 years following spinal cord injury. *Pain*, **103**(3) (2003), 249–57.

21 • Post-amputation pain syndromes

STEPHAN A. SCHUG AND GAIL GILLESPIE

INTRODUCTION

The phenomenon of pain in a missing limb has puzzled patients, doctors and the lay public for centuries. In the sixteenth century the French military surgeon Ambroise Paré published a medical description of the enigmatic affliction, while in the seventeenth century the great philosopher Rene Descartes looked at its potential pathophysiology. The most famous 'first' description of the condition is attributed to the great neurologist Charles Bell [1], but it was only in the later part of the nineteenth century that the US military surgeon Silas Weir Mitchell introduced the term 'phantom limb':

> There is something almost tragical, something ghastly, in the notion of these thousands of spirit limbs, haunting as many good soldiers, and every now and then tormenting them . . .

We now know that post-amputation syndromes can occur with any amputated body part apart from limbs, e.g. breast, tongue, teeth, genitalia and even inner organs such as the rectum [2; 3; 4].

CLASSIFICATION AND INCIDENCE

Following amputation (or deafferentiation injury such as brachial plexus avulsion) a number of phenomena can develop, which require differentiation.

Stump pain

This is pain localized to the site of amputation. It can be acute (usually nociceptive) or chronic (usually neuropathic). Stump pain is most common in the immediate post-operative period [5; 6]. The overall incidence of stump pain is uncertain due to the previous lack of universal definitions for post-amputation pain syndromes causing considerable confusion. The incidence of early stump pain is increased by the presence of severe pre-amputation pain [7]. The cause is unclear but probably multifactorial. Stump pain is problematic and can interfere with prosthesis use.

Phantom sensation

This is defined as any sensory perception of the missing body part with the exclusion of pain. Almost all patients who have undergone amputation experience such phantom sensations [8]. These sensations range from a vague awareness of the presence of the organ via associated paraesthesia to complete sensation, including size, shape, position, temperature and movement. Phantom sensations usually diminish in intensity or size over time, but may persist for a long time. 'Telescoping' of the phantom part can occur with time in up to 30% of patients [9] such that the phantom limb gradually shrinks proximally to approach the stump. Eventually the phantom limb is felt to be within the stump itself.

Phantom limb pain (PLP)

This is defined as any noxious sensory phenomenon of the missing limb or organ. The incidence of PLP is estimated to be 60%–80% after limb amputation [5; 6]. The pain is independent of gender, level or side of amputation [6]. There is, however, a lower incidence among children and congenital amputees [10]. Pain can be immediate or delayed in onset. It is typically intermittent and changes with time. Typical characteristics of PLP are burning, shooting, crushing, throbbing, cramping, aching, tingling or boring. Often the limb is described as being in a hyperextended or otherwise unnatural position. The pain usually occurs in the distal portion of the missing limb [5; 6]. The incidence of pain may be increased if pre-amputation pain was present and may then resemble the pre-amputation pain in character and localization [11]. However, the exact relationship between pre-amputation pain and PLP is not a simple one, especially as patient pain perceptions alter and may be exaggerated with time [5; 6]. The incidence of phantom pain diminishes with time after amputation, as does the frequency and intensity, being highest immediately following surgery [5; 6].

It is important to realize, that the terms for noxious syndromes, 'stump pain', 'phantom sensation' and PLP, are subjective descriptive terms that do not make assumptions on differences in pathophysiology. There is, in fact, a strong correlation between phantom pain and stump pain, and they may be inter-related phenomena [8; 12]. All three phenomena can co-exist [7].

PATHOPHYSIOLOGY

The pathophysiology of post-amputation pain syndromes is in the process of being uncovered. It is most likely to be a combination of peripheral and central factors which interplay subsequent to the significant trauma of an amputation.

Peripheral factors

The following changes occur after peripheral nerve injury such as cutting of a nerve [13]:

(1) Sensitization of peripheral nociceptors with a decreased threshold to noxious stimulation.
(2) Increased response to supra-threshold stimulation.
(3) Spontaneous activity of peripheral receptors due to sensitization, including ectopic pacemaker sites, possibly as a result of the increase in sodium channels, α-adrenergic channels, calcium channels and stretch-activated channels that follows nerve injury.
(4) Sensitization of non-nociceptive receptors to nociceptive impulses.

These changes contribute to hyperalgesia and allodynia in the stump; therefore stump manipulation and revision can worsen pain due to repeated deafferentation injuries. The dorsal root ganglion may also be the site of ectopic neuronal activity subsequent to deafferentation, thereby contributing to pain syndromes.

Furthermore, regrowth of severed nerves often produces nodules called 'neuromas'. Neuronal activity originating from peripheral neuromas either spontaneously or in response to mechanical, chemical or electrical stimulation, may cause increased sensitivity of the stump to different stimuli [13].

Other peripheral factors include increased muscle tension in the stump correlated with cramping and spasmodic pain, and decreased blood flow to the stump correlates with descriptions of phantom pain such as burning or tingling. Low stump temperature correlates with a burning pain.

Overall, while physical stimulation of the stump may accentuate PLP, current evidence suggests that peripheral mechanisms do not cause, but at most modulate or perpetuate PLP.

Spinal factors

The combination of increased afferent input from sensitized nerve endings and the dorsal root ganglion may contribute to central sensitization.

The following changes occur in the dorsal horn of the spinal cord after nerve injury [13]:

(1) Increased spontaneous activity of dorsal horn neurones.
(2) Increased response to afferent input.
(3) After-discharges following repetitive stimulation.
(4) Expansion of peripheral receptive fields.
(5) Wind-up (increased neuronal activity in dorsal horn neurons following repetitive C fibre stimulation), mainly mediated by N-methyl-D aspartate (NMDA) receptors.

These factors play an important role in many chronic pain syndromes, but to which extent these factors are involved in the perpetuation of phantom syndromes is currently unclear, although involvement is likely.

Supraspinal factors

The presence of pain prior to amputation is thought to increase the likelihood of phantom pain [11]. In 1971, Melzack proposed that the painful extremity had created a painful central 'engram' [50]. An engram is the schematic representation of body parts in the central nervous system (CNS) caused by consistent sensory input. This engram was thought to persist after amputation causing phantom pain.

On the basis of these observations, the **neuromatrix theory** was proposed by Melzack in 1990 [14]. In this theory, the body's physical self is represented by a matrix, a complex network of neurones connecting the somatosensory cortex, thalamus and limbic system.

This *neuromatrix* is genetically determined and subsequently modulated by sensory input, thereby creating a *neurosignature* for each body part. This neurosignature determines how a body part is consciously perceived; phantom sensations are the result of persistence of the neurosignature after the loss of the limb. The genetic determination of the neurosignature is confirmed by the observation, that children who are born with a missing limb may feel phantom sensations of the missing part.

In this theory, PLP is the result of abnormal reorganization in the matrix, either due to a pre-existing pain state or the amputation process itself [15].

By analysing neuromagnetic fields, Flor *et al.* have been able to show a close correlation between the degree of neuromatrix reorganization and the development of PLP [16]. Reorganization of the somatosensory cortex occurs with neighbouring representation zones moving into the deafferented zone [17]. Here it is also of note that many of the sites of amputation that commonly lead to phantom sensation and pain are sites with a relatively large cortical somatosensory representation.

An alternative theory discussed in the literature is the **dynamic reverberation theory**. This originated from the observation that selective stereotactic cortectomies of the corona radiata or focal brain lesions in the parietal cortex, thalamus or cortico-thalamic fibres on the contralateral side have resulted in permanent relief of phantom pain. This led Canavero, in 1994, to the theory that phantom pain and sensation were a result of a localized dynamic reverberation loop between cortex and thalamus. He postulated that this loop could operate with or without sensory activation [18].

Current pathophysiological model

A comprehensive model incorporating the current state of knowledge has been proposed by Flor *et al.* It includes peripheral as well as central factors as relevant contributors to development and perpetuation of PLP [19]. In principle, it suggests that somatosensory pain memories and a subsequently altered homuncular representation in the somatosensory cortex are the underlying factors of phantom limb pain, which can be sustained by peripheral factors. This model assumes that memories of pain established before an amputation are powerful causative contributors to PLP generation. In analogy to findings in other chronic pain patients, such pain memories increase the representation zone in the primary somatosensory cortex. The changes are then perpetuated after the amputation by selective C fibre deafferentation, random input from stump neuromas, abnormal changes in the dorsal root ganglia and dorsal horn of the spinal cord, and sympathetic activation [19].

PREVENTION

In view of the immense difficulties of treating PLP once it is established, considerable efforts have been made to identify techniques to prevent the syndrome. Regrettably, none of the evidence on the methods tried is conclusive, although overall the results on epidural anaesthesia and possibly ketamine administration are promising.

Perioperative lumbar epidural blockade

In 1988, Bach *et al.* demonstrated that lumbar epidural blockade (LEB) with bupivacaine plus morphine, started 72 hours *prior to surgery*, reduced the incidence of PLP in the first year after surgery [20].

This promising result initiated a number of similar studies. Schug *et al.* investigated the use of pre-emptive lumbar epidural anaesthesia/analgesia pre-operatively for 24 hours and post-operatively for 72 hours in a small sample of patients. At an interview one year after amputation, those patients with epidural analgesia had significantly less severe PLP than those receiving general anaesthesia [21].

Another study comparing pre-operative and intra-operative analgesia using LEB showed no difference between groups. The duration of pre-operative LEB, however, was variable between patients with a median pre-operative infusion of 18 hours [22]. However, this study has been criticized for its quality of analgesia and the inclusion of pain of any intensity in the results.

More recently, Lambert and colleagues compared pre-operative epidural with perineural analgesia. The LEB was started 24 hours before surgery and continued for three days post-operatively. No difference was found in stump or phantom pain or in phantom sensation at six and 12 months [23]. Although this was a randomized trial, the numbers were small and it is questionable whether the study had sufficient power for phantom pain outcome measurements.

In conclusion, there have been several studies looking at pre-emptive analgesia using LEB. The results are conflicting and further trials are required to clarify the benefits or otherwise of this technique. However, overall the results are promising and a protective effect has again been confirmed in a recent audit at our institution.

Peripheral nerve blockade

Infusions of local anaesthetics via peripheral nerve sheath catheters, usually inserted by the surgeon during the amputation, are a safe method providing excellent analgesia for the immediate post-operative wound pain. They are, however, of no proven benefit in the prevention of phantom pain or stump pain [23; 24].

NMDA antagonists

The use of pre-incision ketamine as pre-emptive analgesia has been described previously in other settings. A small observational study suggests that the incidence of severe PLP may be reduced with the use of ketamine as a bolus, followed by an infusion started prior to skin incision and continued for 72 hours post-operatively [25]. This promising study was small and used historical controls; larger randomized controlled trials are required to evaluate the use of ketamine for prophylaxis here.

EVALUATION OF THE PATIENT WITH POST-AMPUTATION PAIN SYNDROMES

Phantom sensation requires pre- and post-operative counselling and education but it should not generally pose a diagnostic problem clinically.

Examination

Examine the stump to exclude common causes:

(1) **Prosthogenic pain**
- (a) Due to an improperly fitting prosthesis:
  - (i) Poor socket fit, cushioning or alignment.
- (b) Inappropriate suspension resulting in pistoning.
- (c) Painful adductor roll in the above-knee amputee.
- (d) Distal residual limb weight bearing.
- (e) Poor trim line.

2. **Neurogenic pain**
- (a) Caused by neuroma formation
- (b) Test for presence of wind-up by examining for Tinel's sign – shooting pains elicited by repeated tapping over the area

(3) **Arthrogenic pain**
- (a) Pain originating in neighbouring joint or surrounding soft tissue, ligaments or tendons.

(4) **Referred pain**

Excessive biomechanical stress in amputees may cause painful musculoskeletal conditions such as sacroiliac dysfunction, piriformis syndrome, facet syndrome or radiculopathy [26]. Therefore it is important to examine posture and gait.

Furthermore, it is of value to examine: the skin for areas of ulceration and infection; palpate for areas of tenderness, bony exostosis, heterotropic ossification and adherent scar tissue; and evaluate muscle strength and range of movement of neighbouring joints to exclude contracture formation.

THERAPY

A survey by Sherman *et al.* in 1980 identified over 50 different therapies currently in use for the treatment of PLP [27]. This clearly suggests that a successful treatment regime for PLP has not been established and that 'the results are poor and usually below the expected rate of cure of pain with placebo treatment alone'.

Few treatment strategies have been subjected to randomized controlled trials to assess their effectiveness. However, as early treatment is more effective and often multidisciplinary approaches are needed, patients with severe post-amputation pain should be promptly referred to a multidisciplinary pain clinic to ensure optimal and timely pain management.

Calcitonin

Calcitonin parenterally is a proven treatment for PLP and, in our experience, the most effective in the early stages [28]. After initial anecdotal reports [29], a randomized double-blind cross-over study by Jaeger and Maier showed excellent effectiveness [30]. Some 200 IU of salmon calcitonin was given as an intravenous infusion over 20 minutes and provided complete pain relief for 76% of patients; 71% did not experience a recurrence of their phantom pain.

Calcitonin may also be given subcutaneously or intra-nasally [28]. The mechanism of action of calcitonin in inhibition or modulation of pain perception is unknown. However, anecdotal descriptions of its effectiveness in a number of states of central sensitization are published [29; 51].

Side effects including dysaesthesia, nausea and vomiting have been described, but most are transient and can be prevented by prophylactic use of anti-emetics [30]. The risk of an anaphylactic reaction is very low, but needs to be considered.

Ketamine

Ketamine, an antagonist of the NMDA receptor, is another proven treatment of stump pain and PLP. In a randomized trial of patients with existing pain, ketamine has been shown to significantly reduce phantom pain and stump pain. It was also shown to decrease wind-up like pain (pain evoked by repetitive mechanical stimuli), and to increase the pain-pressure threshold in patients with phantom pain and stump pain. It was given as a bolus of 0.1 mg/kg per 5 minutes followed by an infusion of 7 mcg/kg per minute. Pain recurred 30 minutes after discontinuation of the infusion in most patients [13]. Over-activity of NMDA receptors may be a factor in the maintenance of stump pain and phantom pain.

Analgesic and co-analgesic compounds

Analgesic and co-analgesic agents can play an important role in pain due to nerve injury, but have only variable effects in PLP.

Opioids

Generally, neuropathic pain is less responsive to opioids than nociceptive pain [31]. However, a randomized double-blind study of oral retarded morphine sulphate (MST) showed a significant reduction in phantom pain in opioid-sensitive patients, with pain reduction of over 50% occurring in 42% of patients. Neuromagnetic source imaging of three patients suggested reduced cortical reorganization may be occurring with the use of MST [32].

A study comparing the effects of intravenous lidocaine with intravenous morphine showed that morphine given as 0.05 mg/kg bolus followed by 0.2 mg/kg infusion over 40 minutes, given on three consecutive days, significantly reduced both stump and phantom pain [33].

Further larger studies are needed to confirm these results.

Gabapentin

In a randomized double-blind placebo-controlled crossover study, six weeks of gabapentin monotherapy was better than placebo in relieving post-amputation PLP. Pain intensity reduction was significantly greater for gabapentin than for placebo [34].

Clonazepam

Anecdotal evidence suggests that clonazepam may be useful in the treatment of phantom pain [35]. There are, however, no studies to confirm this.

Lidocaine

A randomized double-blind study comparing the effects of intravenous lidocaine with intravenous morphine showed that lidocaine given as 1 mg/kg bolus followed by 4 mg/kg infusion, given on three consecutive days, significantly reduced stump pain but had no effect on phantom pain [33].

Carbamazepine

There is only anecdotal evidence for the use of carbamazepine in the treatment of post-amputation syndromes [36]. It has been extensively used in the treatment of other neuropathic pain states. Side effects can be problematic. Randomized trials are required.

Tricyclic antidepressants (TCAs)

In a randomized trial, chlorimipramine, a serotonin reuptake inhibitor, was found to be significantly better than nortriptyline, a noradrenaline reuptake inhibitor, in the treatment of central pain syndromes [37]. However, no TCA has been studied in a randomized controlled trial of post-amputation syndromes.

Selective serotonin reuptake inhibitors

Venlafaxine is a serotonin and noradrenaline reuptake inhibitor with a side effect profile significantly better than TCAs [38]. There are no randomized controlled trials of its effect on post-amputation pain syndromes.

Baclofen
This gamma-aminobutyric acid (GABA) agonist, when given intrathecally, has been shown to reduce chronic musculoskeletal pain [39]. It may therefore be of some benefit if muscle spasm is the source of the pain. It has not been proven to be of use in PLP.

Capsaicin
Capsaicin depletes the neurotransmitter substance P from sensory nerves and may give relief to some patients with stump pain when used topically [40].

Symptomatic treatment of pain components

The burning component of PLP alone can be decreased by pharmacological and behavioural therapies that increase the temperature of the stump, such as sympathectomy, α- or β-blockade, or biofeedback.

Cramping can be relieved by treatments that reduce muscle tension, for example, with the use of baclofen or again biofeedback.

Non-pharmacological therapies

The following therapies are thought to relieve phantom pain by causing increased sensory inflow into the stump area:

- Transcutaneous electrical nerve stimulation (TENS)
- Acupuncture
- Physical therapy

With the development of theories on cortical reorganization as a cause for PLP, there are now experimental therapies tried, which are based on the concept of reversing such reorganization. Sensory discrimination training programmes show promise here. This is a process during which patients have to discriminate the frequency or location of high intensity, non-painful electrical stimuli applied through electrodes on their stump in an attempt to separate merged regions on their cortical somatosensory map.

A recent study using this technique showed that PLP was significantly decreased in the group who underwent the training process compared with controls. Cortical reorganization, assessed by neuroelectric source imaging and structural magnetic resonance imaging, was also reduced in this group [41].

Similarly, early data suggest that use of a myoelectric prosthesis may prevent cortical reorganization and PLP [42].

These approaches are among the most promising therapeutic concepts in this difficult area and the findings may have implications for chronic pain treatment in general [43].

Invasive therapies

Elecroconvulsive therapy (ECT)
This psychiatric treatment is thought to interrupt the dynamic reverberations that maintain central and phantom pain in the thalamocortical pathway [18] and has been used in the treatment of refractory phantom pain [44]. There have been no trials in this area.

Nerve blockade
There is only anecdotal evidence for the use of peripheral nerve blockade in the treatment of phantom pain syndromes [45]. There have been no trials in this area.

Spinal cord stimulation
This treatment, thought to facilitate inhibitory descending pathways, has been described in the treatment of phantom pain. The overall success rate of this expensive and invasive approach is less than 50% [46; 47].

Implantable intrathecal delivery systems
Infusing clonidine, local anaesthetic, baclofen or opioids, usually in a combination, may be beneficial in selected patients with PLP, although there are no definitive studies.

Dorsal root entry zone lesions
Dorsal root entry zone lesioning has a limited effect for a limited time only in PLP [48]; this is in line with clinical experience of this neurodestructive approach. Other types of surgery and neuroablation often make pain worse because of repeated stimulation and/or deafferentation of the affected nerves.

Psychological therapy

Pre-amputation counselling is mandatory as amputees go through normal grieving processes. It is important to identify anxiety and depression early, as these can magnify pain perception.

Behavioural, cognitive and group therapy, and pain management programmes are all useful methods of helping patients cope with their pain. Hypnosis, biofeedback and muscular relaxation training to disrupt the pain-anxiety-tension cycle are important components of chronic pain therapy [49].

FUTURE AIMS

Future aims in the management of post-amputation syndromes focus on:

(1) Further prospective randomized trials to evaluate the benefits of current pharmacological therapies.
(2) Clarification of the role of pre-emptive analgesia in the prevention of phantom pain.
(3) Evaluation of the promising methods that attempt to revert the cortical reorganization that occurs following amputation towards normal.
(4) A multi-modal and multidisciplinary approach to pain management.

REFERENCES

1. T. Furukawa, Charles Bell's description of the phantom phenomenon in 1830. *Neurology*, **40** (1990), 1830.
2. K. Kroner, U. B. Knudsen, L. Lundby & H. M. Hvid, [Phantom breast syndrome]. *Ugeskrift for Laeger*, **156**(7) (1994), 977–80.
3. R. E. Bates, Jr. & C. M. Stewart, Atypical odontalgia: phantom tooth pain. *Oral Surgery, Oral Medicine, Oral Pathology*, **72**(4) (1991), 479–83.
4. R. A. Boas, S. A. Schug & R. H. Acland, Perineal pain after rectal amputation: a 5-year follow-up. *Pain*, **52**(1) (1993), 67–70.
5. T. S. Jensen, B. Krebs, J. Nielsen & P. Rasmussen, Immediate and long-term phantom limb pain in amputees: incidence, clinical characteristics and relationship to pre-amputation limb pain. *Pain*, **21**(3) (1985), 267–78.
6. L. Nikolajsen & T. S. Jensen, Phantom limb pain. *British Journal of Anaesthesia*, **87**(1) (2001), 107–16.
7. L. Nikolajsen, S. Ilkjaer, K. Kroner, J. H. Christensen & T. S. Jensen, The influence of preamputation pain on postamputation stump and phantom pain. *Pain*, **72**(3) (1997), 393–405.
8. T. S. Jensen, B. Krebs, J. Nielsen & P. Rasmussen, Phantom limb, phantom pain and stump pain in amputees during the first 6 months following limb amputation. *Pain*, **17**(3) (1983), 243–56.
9. T. S. Jensen, B. Krebs, J. Nielsen & P. Rasmussen, Non-painful phantom limb phenomena in amputees: incidence, clinical characteristics and temporal course. *Acta Neurologica Scandinavica*, **70**(6) (1984), 407–14.
10. K. L. Wilkins, P. J. McGrath, G. A. Finley & J. Katz, Phantom limb sensations and phantom limb pain in child and adolescent amputees. *Pain*, **78**(1) (1998), 7–12.
11. J. Katz & R. Melzack, Pain 'memories' in phantom limbs: review and clinical observations. *Pain*, **43**(3) (1990), 319–36.
12. C. M. Kooijman, P. U. Dijkstra, J. H. Geertzen, A. Elzinga & C. P. van der Schans, Phantom pain and phantom sensations in upper limb amputees: an epidemiological study. *Pain*, **87**(1) (2000), 33–41.
13. L. Nikolajsen, C. L. Hansen, J. Nielsen *et al.*, The effect of ketamine on phantom pain: a central neuropathic disorder maintained by peripheral input. *Pain*, **67**(1) (1996), 69–77.
14. R. Melzack, Pain – an overview. *Acta Anaesthesiologica Scandinavica*, **43**(9) (1999), 880–4.
15. R. Melzack, From the gate to the neuromatrix. *Pain*, (Suppl 6) (1999), S121–6.
16. H. Flor, T. Elbert, S. Knecht *et al.*, Phantom-limb pain as a perceptual correlate of cortical reorganization following arm amputation. *Nature*, **375**(6531) (1995), 482–4.
17. E. Huse, W. Larbig, N. Birbaumer *et al.*, Kortikale reorganisation und schmerz: empirische befunde und therapeutische implikationen am beispiel des phantomschmerzes. *Schmerz*, **15**(2) (2001), 131–7.
18. S. Canavero, Dynamic reverberation. A unified mechanism for central and phantom pain. *Medical Hypotheses*, **42**(3) (1994), 203–7.
19. H. Flor, N. Birbaumer, R. A. Sherman, Phantom limb pain. *Pain Clinical Updates*, **8**(3) (2000), 1–7.
20. S. Bach, M. F. Noreng & N. U. Tjellden, Phantom limb pain in amputees during the first 12 months following limb amputation, after preoperative lumbar epidural blockade. *Pain*, **33**(3) (1988), 297–301.
21. S. A. Schug, R. Burrell, J. Payne & P. Tester, Pre-emptive epidural analgesia may prevent phantom limb pain. *Regional Anesthesia*, **20**(3) (1995), 256.

22. L. Nikolajsen, S. Ilkjaer, J. H. Christensen, K. Kroner & T. S. Jensen, Pain after amputation. *British Journal of Anaesthesia*, **81**(3) (1998), 486.
23. A. Lambert, A. Dashfield, C. Cosgrove *et al.*, Randomized prospective study comparing preoperative epidural and intraoperative perineural analgesia for the prevention of postoperative stump and phantom limb pain following major amputation. *Regional Anesthesia and Pain Medicine*, **26**(4) (2001), 316–21.
24. M. S. Pinzur, P. G. Garla, T. Pluth, L. Vrbos, Continuous postoperative infusion of a regional anesthetic after an amputation of the lower extremity. A randomized clinical trial. *Journal of Bone and Joint Surgery (American Volume)*, **78**(10) (1996), 1501–5.
25. R. Dertwinkel, C. Heinrichs, I. Senne *et al.*, Prevention of severe phantom limb pain by perioperative administration of ketamine – an observational study. *Acute Pain*, **4**(1) (2002), 9–13.
26. R. W. Davis, Phantom sensation, phantom pain, and stump pain. *Archives of Physical Medicine and Rehabilitation*, **74**(1) (1993), 79–91.
27. R. A. Sherman, C. J. Sherman & N. G. Gall, A survey of current phantom limb pain treatment in the United States. *Pain*, 8 (1980), 85–99.
28. G. C. Wall & C. A. Heyneman, Calcitonin in phantom limb pain. *Annals of Pharmacotherapy*, **33**(4) (1999), 499–501.
29. H. Jaeger, C. Maier & J. Wawersik, [Postoperative treatment of phantom pain and causalgias with calcitonin]. *Anaesthetist*, **37**(2) (1988), 71–6.
30. H. Jaeger & C. Maier, Calcitonin in phantom limb pain: a double-blind study. *Pain*, **48**(1) (1992), 21–7.
31. S. Arner & B. A. Meyerson, Lack of analgesic effect of opioids on neuropathic and idiopathic forms of pain. *Pain*, **33**(1) (1988), 11–23.
32. E. Huse, W. Larbig, H. Flor & N. Birbaumer, The effect of opioids on phantom limb pain and cortical reorganization. *Pain*, **90**(1–2) (2001), 47–55.
33. C. L. Wu, P. Tella, P. S. Staats *et al.*, Analgesic effects of intravenous lidocaine and morphine on postamputation pain: a randomized double-blind, active placebo-controlled, crossover trial. *Anesthesiology*, **96**(4) (2002), 841–8.
34. M. Bone, P. Critchley & D. J. Buggy, Gabapentin in postamputation phantom limb pain: a randomized, double-blind, placebo-controlled, cross-over study. *Regional Anesthesia and Pain Medicine*, **27**(5) (2002), 481–6.
35. S. L. Bartusch, B. J. Sanders, J. G. D'Alessio & J. R. Jernigan, Clonazepam for the treatment of lancinating phantom limb pain. *Clinical Journal of Pain*, **12**(1) (1996), 59–62.
36. J. F. Patterson, Carbamazepine in the treatment of phantom limb pain. *Southern Medical Journal*, **81**(9) (1988), 1100–2.
37. A. E. Panerai, G. Monza, P. Movilia *et al.*, A randomized, within-patient, cross-over, placebo-controlled trial on the efficacy and tolerability of the tricyclic antidepressants chlorimipramine and nortriptyline in central pain. *Acta Neurologica Scandinavica*, **82**(1) (1990), 34–8.
38. C. Mattia, F. Paoletti, F. Coluzzi & A. Boanelli, New antidepressants in the treatment of neuropathic pain. A review. *Minerva Anestesiologica*, **68**(3) (2002), 105–14.
39. P. G. Loubser & N. M. Akman, Effects of intrathecal baclofen on chronic spinal cord injury pain. *Journal of Pain and Symptom Management*, **12**(4) (1996), 241–7.
40. D. T. Cannon & Y. Wu, Topical capsaicin as an adjuvant analgesic for the treatment of traumatic amputee neurogenic residual limb pain. *Archives of Physical Medicine and Rehabilitation*, **79**(5) (1998), 591–3.
41. H. Flor, C. Denke, M. Schaefer & S. Grusser, Effect of sensory discrimination training on cortical reorganisation and phantom limb pain. *Lancet*, **357**(9270) (2001), 1763–4.
42. M. Lotze, W. Grodd, N. Birbaumer *et al.*, Does use of a myoelectric prosthesis prevent cortical reorganization and phantom limb pain? *Nature Neuroscience*, **2**(6) (1999), 501–2.
43. H. Flor, Cortical reorganisation and chronic pain: implications for rehabilitation. *Journal of Rehabilitation Medicine*, **41**(Suppl) (2003), 66–72.
44. K. G. Rasmussen & T. A. Rummans, Electroconvulsive therapy for phantom limb pain. *Pain*, **85**(1–2) (2000), 297–9.
45. P. Lierz, K. Schroegendorfer, S. Choi, P. Felleiter & H. G. Kress, Continuous blockade of both brachial plexus with ropivacaine in phantom pain: a case report. *Pain*, **78**(2) (1998), 135–7.
46. Y. Katayama, T. Yamamoto, K. Kobayashi *et al.*, Motor cortex stimulation for phantom limb pain: comprehensive therapy with spinal cord and thalamic stimulation. *Stereotactic and Functional Neurosurgery*, **77**(1–4) (2001), 159–62.

47. K. Kumar, C. Toth & R. K. Nath, P. Laing, Epidural spinal cord stimulation for treatment of chronic pain – some predictors of success. A 15-year experience. *Surgical Neurology*, **50**(2) (1998), 110–20.
48. G. Garcia-March, M. J. Sanchez-Ledesma, P. Diaz *et al.*, Dorsal root entry zone lesion versus spinal cord stimulation in the management of pain from brachial plexus avulsion. *Acta Neurochirurgica Supplement (Wien)*, **39** (1987), 155–8.
49. R. A. Sherman, N. Gall & J. Gormly, Treatment of phantom limb pain with muscular relaxation training to disrupt the pain-anxiety-tension cycle. *Pain*, **6**(1) (1979), 47–55.
50. R. Melzack, Phantom limb pain: implications for treatment of pathologic pain. *Anesthesiology*, **35** (1971), 409–19.
51. E. J. Visser, A review of calcitonin and its use in the treatment of acute pain. *Acute Pain*, **7**(4) (2005), 185–9.

22 • Treatment of neuropathic pain

STEPHAN A. SCHUG AND KATHRYN J.D. STANNARD

INTRODUCTION

Neuropathic pain is defined by The International Association for the Study of Pain (IASP) as pain following a primary lesion or dysfunction of the nervous system [1]. It is caused either by peripheral damage with lesions involving the peripheral nerves, dorsal root ganglia and dorsal roots, or by central damage which may involve injury caused by infarction or trauma of the spinal cord or brain.

Neuropathic pain results in persistent pain syndromes that have no biological function, but are difficult to treat and cause great distress to the individual. Neuropathic pain is also referred to as neurogenic pain, deafferentation pain, neuralgia, neuralgic pain or nerve pain.

Neuropathic pain may develop immediately after a nerve injury or after a variable interval. It may be maintained by factors different from the initial cause. It can persist for a long time and is frequently not explained by underlying pathology. Patients are frequently seen by many different specialists and their treatment often fails to resolve the pain. As the pain persists other factors such as environmental, psychological and social stressors become relevant contributors to the overall presentation.

PRINCIPLES OF TREATMENT

Treatment of neuropathic pain is not straightforward. The pain is often refractory to conventional analgesic regimens such as non-steroidal anti-inflammatory drugs (NSAIDs). Opioids have only limited efficacy in neuropathic pain as outlined later in this chapter; therefore so called co-analgesics, medications which are not typically used as analgesics, are often the first-line treatment of neuropathic pain.

Except in a few specific conditions, the treatment is usually empirical. However, increasing data from randomized controlled trials (RCTs) and meta-analysis are leading to improvements in management, and a more evidence-based approach.

It is important that patients have realistic expectations regarding treatment efficacy and potential side effects in order to improve compliance with medication [2]. A balance between these should be achieved on an individual basis. A single drug therapy should be tried before combinations of drugs are started. Non-pharmacological treatments are available that may be appropriate for certain cases. For optimal results a multidisciplinary approach to treatment should be adopted that addresses affective and behavioural changes, and disability.

PHARMACOLOGICAL TREATMENT

Opioids

The use of opioids to treat neuropathic pain is controversial. In 1988 a study implied that patients with neuropathic pain did not experience pain relief from opioids [3]. However, this study has been criticized for possible selection bias as most non-responders had previously used morphine without effective results and there was no individual titration of morphine.

Since then several RCTs in neuropathic pain have been conducted with morphine, fentanyl and oxycodone [4; 5; 6]. The general consensus is that pain intensity may be relieved by opioids titrated for that individual. In 1990 a review was conducted of opioid responsiveness in neuropathic pain. It was suggested that there was a continuum of opioid responsiveness in which patients with neuropathic pain may simply require higher drug doses to achieve analgesia [7]. This concept was confirmed in a study in which dose responses of opioids in nociceptive and neuropathic pain were compared, and higher doses were indeed required in neuropathic pain [8].

A number of reasons have been suggested for this relative opioid resistance. These include amongst others, down-regulation of peripheral and spinal opioid receptors [5; 9], and physiological antagonism with up-regulation of cholecystokinin [10].

There is also evidence in animal experiments that long term use of opioids induces a state of central nervous system (CNS) hyperexcitability implying that tolerance to opioids may have a pharmacology similar to hyperalgesia [11]. Studies in humans have so far not confirmed these experimental data. In an unblinded study of patients with post-herpetic neuralgia analgesic efficacy was reported at two and six month intervals with oral opioids [12]. In a similar study with oxycodone administered for two months in patients with post-herpetic neuralgia, the treatment group received significantly more analgesia than the placebo group [6]. Prolonged pain relief has also been reported in cases of neuropathic pain with intrathecal morphine administration [13].

The issue of tolerance relates to a drug having decreasing effect and/or increasing dosage to maintain the same effect [14]. Some research suggests that ongoing nociceptive input may result in tolerance [15]. However, many cancer patients are maintained on stable doses of opioids [16]. Studies of patients with non-cancer pain without ongoing nociceptive input have not inevitably resulted in rapidly increasing doses of opioids, although some dose increase is observed [17].

Recommendations for clinical use of opioids in neuropathic pain

There is now a general consensus that a subset of patients with neuropathic pain does benefit from treatment with opioids [18]. Guidelines exist to identify these patients and make a treatment plan for management and eventual withdrawal of opioids. Such guidelines include a past/present history of drug addiction as a relative contraindication, the need for regular follow-up visits, and opioids to be prescribed and supervised by the same doctor. Legal issues with opioid prescriptions are associated with their controlled status, the risk of addiction and abuse, and the potential for diversion into illegal channels by selling or passing on to others [19; 20].

Methadone, due to its additional monoaminergic and N-methyl-D aspartate (NMDA) receptor effects, might be a particularly useful opioid in the setting of neuropathic pain [21; 22]. Detailed guidelines for the use of opioids in chronic pain of non-malignant origin are now published in most countries. Summarizing these is beyond the scope of this chapter [20; 23; 24; 25; 26; 27].

TRAMADOL

Mechanism of action

Tramadol is a centrally acting synthetic analogue of codeine. However, it is not a conventional opioid as it has a relatively low affinity for μ-opioid receptors and is classified by the Food and Drug Administration (FDA) as an atypical centrally acting analgesic.

Tramadol together with its primary active metabolite has three synergistic mechanisms of action to provide analgesia. It combines weak effects on opioid receptors with monoaminergic mechanisms. Reuptake inhibition of 5-hydroxytryptamine (5-HT) and noradrenaline contribute to the anti-nociceptive action of tramadol [28; 29]. Tramadol is a racemate. Opioid receptor activity and 5-HT reuptake inhibition are mainly associated with the (+)-tramadol enantiomer, whereas (−)-tramadol is a reuptake inhibitor of noradrenaline [30; 31]. The monaminergic effects suggest a higher analgesic potency of tramadol in neuropathic than in nociceptive pain states; this has been recently confirmed by our group.

Efficacy

Tramadol has had some evaluation for the treatment of chronic pain in the past. More recently, two randomized placebo controlled trials of tramadol in patients with neuropathic pain have been completed. The first involved 131 patients with diabetic neuropathic pain. Some 37% of patients withdrew, mainly due to the adverse effects in the tramadol group and the lack of efficacy in the placebo group. The tramadol group had significantly more pain relief than placebo [32]. In a subsequent randomized placebo controlled cross-over trial 45 patients with neuropathic pain were studied. Significant reductions in spontaneous and touch evoked pain were achieved with tramadol [33]. Further trials are needed to assess the full potential of this agent in neuropathic pain.

Adverse effects

Tramadol causes less respiratory depression and constipation than conventional opioids. Physical dependence to tramadol use is extremely rare and occurs in the range of 1 in 100 000 users [34]. Similarly, tramadol has a low abuse potential [35] and its risk of addiction has been rated in the range of 1 in 100 000 [34]. For these reasons, tramadol is not under special regulatory control in most countries.

Phase IV clinical trials have reported the overall incidence of side effects from tramadol to be 15.3% [36]. The majority of side effects were found to be dose dependent.

Recommendations for clinical use of tramadol in neuropathic pain

Although sufficient data are still lacking, experimental evidence and limited trial data suggest tramadol to be a particularly useful analgesic in neuropathic pain with a low incidence of adverse effects, mainly of a benign nature.

In our experience (and that of many other pain clinics) it is gaining increasing usage in this indication, in particular as a background analgesic in a slow-release preparation.

ANTIDEPRESSANTS

Tricyclic antidepressants (TCAs)

In 1960, Paoli *et al.* made the incidental discovery that the TCA imipramine had an analgesic effect [37]. Since then other TCAs and newer agents have been evaluated, and used for the treatment of neuropathic pain.

The role of TCAs in the treatment of neuropathic pain is now well established and has the best documented evidence. Tricyclic antidepressants are the first class of medication proven to be effective for neuropathic pain in a double-blind placebo controlled trial [38]. No other group of drugs has to date been proven to be more effective.

Amitriptyline is established as the 'gold standard' as it has the most evidence available, especially for the treatment of painful diabetic neuropathy and post-herpetic neuralgia [39].

Other TCAs have been evaluated for the relief of pain in diabetic neuropathy, post-herpetic neuralgia, peripheral neuropathies and central post-stroke pain [40; 41; 42].

In comparative trials no single TCA has been found to be superior for neuropathic pain, except in post-herpetic neuralgia where amitriptyline was found to be superior to maprotiline [38].

Mechanism of action

Initially it was thought that the analgesic action of TCAs was related to their antidepressant activity. However, it is now clear that there is an independent specific analgesic effect. The doses used to relieve neuropathic pain are smaller and the onset of analgesic efficacy is faster than an antidepressant effect, and analgesia does not appear to depend upon mood improvement in depressed patients [40; 42]. In addition, pain relief was found to be independent of any sedative effect.

Tricyclic antidepressants inhibit the reuptake of monoaminergic transmitters and this mechanism mediates their analgesic effect by the following presumed mechanisms [39]:

(1) Central blockade of monoamine reuptake, particularly serotonin and noradrenaline, leads to enhancement of the descending inhibitory monoaminergic pathways in the dorsal horn of the spinal cord.
(2) Anticholinergic activity reduces firing of central neurones involved in pain, especially after deafferentation.

Additionally there may be a number of other contributing mechanisms: moderation of NMDA and opioid receptor activity; increase in dopamine or endorphin levels; blockade of central or peripheral histamine receptors; sodium channel blockade; and blockade of adrenergic receptors on regenerating sprouts [39; 43].

Adverse effects

The TCAs have at best moderate efficacy but their optimum analgesic dose can often not be reached due to unpleasant side effects.

A systematic review of randomized controlled trials of TCAs used to treat neuropathic pain found that out of 100 patients, 30 had significant pain relief, 30 had minor side effects and 4 had to discontinue their therapy due to side effects [44]. These include:

(1) Anticholinergic: dry mouth, constipation, urinary retention and blurred vision.
(2) Antihistaminergic: confusion and sedation (the latter may be of benefit).
(3) Anti α-adrenergic: postural hypotension and sexual dysfunction.

Cardiac conduction abnormalities may also arise due to the muscarinic anticholinergic actions. Patients at risk should have a pre-treatment ECG and cardiac conduction defects are a contraindication to treatment with TCAs. Another potential problem is overdose in suicidal ideation, where TCAs are more dangerous than other groups of antidepressants, and may be fatal due to severe cardiac arrhythmias and convulsions.

Desipramine, imipramine and nortriptyline are more specific to noradrenergic blockade, and are associated with less anticholinergic and antihistamine side effects. They may be useful in patients who are not able to tolerate amitriptyline, before progressing to another class of drug. In post-herpetic neuralgia and painful diabetic neuropathy, they were found to be as effective as amitriptyline [38; 42; 45], but associated with less side effects.

Physical withdrawal reactions have been described for most antidepressants, but psychological addiction is not an issue [39].

Other antidepressants

The selective serotonin reuptake inhibitors (SSRIs) such as fluoxetine and paroxetine, have not been found to be as useful as TCAs in neuropathic pain. They alter serotonergic (5-HT) far more than noradrenergic (NA) neurotransmission. Due to their selectivity they do not interfere as much with adrenergic, histaminergic or muscarinic receptors and therefore have fewer side effects. Although evidence is increasing for some analgesic efficacy in neuropathic pain, there is currently insufficient evidence to make generalizations regarding their use for this indication [46].

Studies to date in diabetic neuropathy have shown paroxetine to be more effective than placebo, but not more effective than imipramine [47], and fluoxetine was found to be ineffective [45].

There is no evidence that they are more efficacious than the older antidepressants [48], which have a more consistent anti-nociceptive effect [49]. Venlafaxine is a novel antidepressant that is not a TCA or SSRI. It is classified as a serotonin and noradrenergic reuptake inhibitor (SNARI), but has no anticholinergic effects. It has been found to have a potential analgesic effect [50]. It seems better than placebo and possibly as effective as the TCAs with fewer side effects, which may result in improved compliance [51]. However, further evidence is required before its usefulness as an adjunct in pain can be confirmed [52].

Recommendations for clinical use of antidepressants as analgesics

Evidence-based decisions to use antidepressants in neuropathic pain states are usually based on a number-needed-to-treat (NNT) approach [44; 53; 54]

- TCAs for post-herpetic neuralgia: NNT 2.3.
- TCAs for atypical face pain: NNT 2.8.
- Amitriptyline, imipramine and desipramine for diabetic neuropathy: NNT 3.
- TCAs and SSRIs for chronic headaches: NNT 3.2.
- TCAs and SSRIs for fibromyalgia: NNT 4.

It is difficult to generalize a dosage regimen for antidepressants in neuropathic pain, due to significant inter-individual variability [47]. McQuay *et al.* have demonstrated a dose response relation for amitriptyline with a greater analgesic response at 75 mg/day than either 25 or 50 mg/day [55].

Current recommendations for prescribing TCAs are [2]:

(1) Start with a low dose (5–10 mg/day), especially in the elderly, and increase this weekly to analgesic efficacy or unacceptable side effects.
(2) Once the optimal dose is achieved analgesic efficacy usually takes up to a week to achieve.
(3) There have not been any trials conducted for longer than six weeks, so there is no evidence base for optimum duration of treatment. The current practice is to continue the same effective dose for several months and then to try to reduce it.
(4) If a therapeutic dose of a TCA fails to provide pain relief, other antidepressants are also likely to fail.
(5) If a TCA provides pain relief at the expense of unacceptable side effects then other antidepressants with a lower side effect profile should be tried.

(6) If due to contraindications or unacceptable side effects a patient is unable to be treated with TCAs, other antidepressants should be tried before excluding this drug category.

ANTICONVULSANTS

In the 1960s phenytoin was found to have an analgesic effect in the treatment of painful diabetic neuropathy [56]. Since then anticonvulsants have been evaluated and used in neuropathic pain states including old agents (carbamazepine, sodium valproate and phenytoin), and newer agents (gabapentin, lamotrigine, felbamate and pregabalin).

Anticonvulsants have a specific indication in the treatment of trigeminal neuralgia with carbamazepine the first line therapy. They may prove effective in conditions that have proved intractable to other treatments.

Mechanism of action

The neuronal hyperexcitability and corresponding molecular changes in neuropathic pain have many features in common with the cellular changes in certain forms of epilepsy [57]. The pain relieving effect of anticonvulsants is thought to be due to dampening of abnormal central nervous system activity that follows nerve damage [58]. This may occur by [59; 60]:

(1) Sodium channel blockade resulting in a reduction of ectopic firing in both peripheral nerves and the dorsal root ganglion.
(2) Indirect or direct enhancement of inhibitory GABAergic neurotransmission.
(3) Inhibition of excitatory glutaminergic neurotransmission.

Overall effects may be due to a combination of these mechanisms and longer term neuroplastic effects [60].

The process of ectopic impulse generation is so sensitive to sodium channel blockade that these agents have an action at much lower concentrations than that required to block normal neuronal transmission [61].

Individual medications

Clonazepam

Clonazepam is a benzodiazepine anticonvulsant, acting as a GABA agonist. Several studies suggest a role for clonazepam in lancinating neuropathic pain in oncology patients, trigeminal neuralgia, headaches and post-traumatic neuralgia. Bartusch and colleagues, in an uncontrolled study, reported two patients treated with clonazepam achieving effective relief from lancinating phantom limb pain for more than six months [62]. The cross-over trial by Swerdlow and Cundill shows clonazepam to be superior to carbamazepine, phenytoin and sodium valproate with regard to efficacy in neuropathic pain and adverse effects [63].

This reflects our clinical experience, where clonazepam has been shown to be an easy to use agent with excellent efficacy and minimal side effects, in particular sedation.

Lorazepam, nitrazepam and diazepam have also been used in chronic pain. They have anxiolytic and anticonvulsant properties. However, with the exception of clonazepam, benzodiazepines are not generally felt to have specific analgesic activity, and their use is not encouraged for this purpose due to their addictive nature, tolerance and cognitive impairment [64].

Gabapentin

Gabapentin is a relatively new anticonvulsant, available in the USA since 1995. It is a lipophilic GABA analogue but does not interact with $GABA_A$ or $GABA_B$ receptors or directly affect GABA uptake. The mechanisms of action are unknown, although there are numerous proposed ones [65; 66; 67; 68]:

(1) It indirectly increases the levels of GABA and decreases the level of glutamate in the CNS.
(2) That there is involvement of a specific gabapentin-binding protein, a subunit of a calcium channel protein found in the CNS. Gamma-aminobutyric acid itself does not appear to bind at this site, but gabapentin analogues bind to the $\alpha_2\delta$ subunit and appear to have analgesic actions at the postsynaptic dorsal horns.

There is increasing evidence for analgesic efficacy in a variety of neuropathic states. Large scale RCTs have demonstrated efficacy in post-herpetic neuralgia and diabetic neuropathy at target doses of 3600 mg/day [66; 69; 70]. The Cochrane review reported NNTs of 3.2 in post-herpetic neuralgia and 3.8 for painful diabetic neuropathy [71]. Results indicate a similar efficacy of gabapentin and TCAs [72]. Rice and Maton recently found gabapentin to be efficacious at lower doses in post-herpetic neuralgia [73].

A case report cited a significant improvement with gabapentin treatment in a patient with central post-stroke pain that had failed to respond to a variety of analgesics [74].

Gabapentin is a popular choice amongst the anticonvulsants used for neuropathic pain as it has less serious side effects (including in the elderly), is easier to monitor and drug–drug interactions are far less of a problem. It is the first medication with a specific indication for use in neuropathic pain states. It is considered to be the first choice in this group for the treatment of painful diabetic neuropathy and post-herpetic neuralgia [75]. It may prove to be useful in a wide range of other neuropathic pain states [2].

The most commonly reported side effects are somnolence, fatigue, ataxia and dizziness. A dose adjustment is required in renal failure but not in hepatic disorders as gabapentin is excreted unchanged by the kidneys. The effective analgesic dose of gabapentin is variable, with some patients responding at low doses and others requiring high doses (more than 3600 mg/day) for the same benefit. It has been suggested that treatment failure may be due to inadequate dosage, although rapid dose escalation can be responsible for the high incidence of CNS side effects [76].

Pregabalin, an analogue to gabapentin, is currently under development for neuropathic pain and has been shown to have antihyperalgesic and anti-nociceptive properties, but results from clinical trials are awaited [67; 75].

Carbamazepine

Carbamazepine has been the first line treatment for trigeminal neuralgia for many years [77]. A recent Cochrane review found that three placebo controlled trials of carbamazepine in trigeminal neuralgia demonstrated a combined NNT of 2.5 [71]. It has not, however, been shown to be efficacious in post-herpetic neuralgia or central pain and its use in other neuropathic states has been reported only in small uncontrolled studies.

Evidence shows carbamazepine inhibits spontaneous and evoked responses of spinal neurones, and increases brain serotonin. Doses of up to 1200 mg/day can be used.

Side effects are the main limitation to its use, including sedation, ataxia, drug interactions and liver dysfunction [78]. Serious but rare side effects are irreversible aplastic anaemia and Steven-Johnson-Syndrome. With carbamazepine therapy regular haematological and liver function monitoring is required. Occasional monitoring of serum sodium is also recommended because hyponatraemia can occur. The sustained release preparations of carbamazepine may limit the side effects.

Sodium valproate

This is structurally unrelated to other anticonvulsants and does not block sodium channels. The exact mechanism of action is unknown but may be related to increased GABA synthesis and release, and hence potentiated GABAergic inhibition. In addition valproate attenuates the neuronal excitation caused by glutamate activation of NMDA receptors [79].

There is evidence for its use in migraine prophylaxis [80] and as a second line therapy in trigeminal neuralgia [81]. It can be used in doses up to 800 mg/day.

Again side effects and the risk of serious toxicity limit its use. These include sedation, gastrointestinal disturbance, altered liver function with potentially fatal hepatotoxicity, decreased platelet aggregation and other haematological effects, and drug interactions. Close follow-up is mandatory.

Phenytoin

Phenytoin can be of help in patients with neuropathic pain but less so than carbamazepine. It has fallen from favour mainly due to its extensive side effect profile, complex kinetics and drug interactions.

Side effects include sedation, gingival hypertrophy, hirsutism and coarsening of facial features. At high blood levels neurotoxicity occurs and cardiac conduction is affected, therefore close blood drug level monitoring is required. Results from RCTs have shown an analgesic effect in diabetic neuropathy and Fabry's disease [82; 83]. The Cochrane review found that NNT for diabetic neuropathy with phenytoin was 2.1 [71].

Lamotrigine

This new anticonvulsant appears to act on voltage gated cation channels (calcium and potassium) as well as inhibiting glutamate release [84]. Studies (open and double-blind) have indicated that lamotrigine can be effective in diabetic neuropathy, central post-stroke pain, human immunodeficiency virus (HIV) associated polyneuropathy and trigeminal neuralgia [57; 64; 85]. It may be useful in cases of trigeminal neuralgia that have proved refractory to carbamazepine and phenytoin, in doses of 50–400 mg/day [64]. However, other evidence suggests that it may not be more effective than placebo in many other cases of neuropathic pain [84].

Side effects have restricted the use of lamotrigine: dizziness, constipation, nausea, somnolence and diplopia [64]. It is associated with Steven-Johnson-Syndrome, with 1 in 1000 patients requiring hospitalization and can rarely be fatal. These side effects can be lessened and the incidence of a rash significantly decreased by slow titration of lamotrigine, starting at a dose of 12.5 to 25 mg per day and slowly increasing to 100 to 200 mg per day over one to two months.

Recommendations for clinical use of anticonvulsants as analgesics

Anticonvulsants are typically used for neuropathic pain that has a shooting, burning or lancinating character. Empirically they are used in combination with a TCA, although the evidence for using both classes of drug in combination is not strong.

Systematic reviews suggest efficacy of anticonvulsants generally for trigeminal neuralgia, diabetic neuropathy, central post-stroke pain and migraine. Number-needed-to-treat for the therapeutic efficacy of anticonvulsants in these conditions are as follows [86]:

- Trigeminal neuralgia: NNT 2.6.
- Diabetic neuropathy: NNT 2.5.
- Migraine prophylaxis: NNT 1.6.

Although few trials exist for the treatment of central pain, e.g. after stroke, current opinion is that lamotrigine and gabapentin may be helpful [87]. As with antidepressants, titration should start with low doses gradually increasing to a dose that either produces analgesic efficacy or unacceptable side effects.

The Cochrane review of anticonvulsants for acute and chronic pain concludes that in chronic pain syndromes other than trigeminal neuralgia, anticonvulsants should be withheld until other interventions have been tried [71]. While gabapentin is increasingly being used for neuropathic pain, the evidence would suggest that it is not superior to carbamazepine with regard to efficacy, although it does have a much more favourable side effect profile. In our experience, the first-line anticonvulsant for trigeminal neuralgia only is carbamazepine. Clonazepam and gabapentin are preferred for all other neuropathic pain states, due to their benign side effect profile. Gabapentin might become the first-line agent here due to its efficacy and low adverse effect rate, but has the disadvantage of high costs and is not reimbursed in a number of countries.

LOCAL ANAESTHETICS AND ANTIARRHYTHMICS

In 1948 systemic procaine was identified as beneficial in the treatment of neuropathic pain. This led to the evaluation of other local anaesthetics for the treatment of neuropathic pain.

Mechanism of action

The mechanism of analgesic action is thought to be due to membrane stabilizing effects, through the blockade of voltage-dependent sodium channels and hence reduced ectopic activity in damaged afferent nerves [59]. In addition there may be a central action on sodium channels and at the spinal level a blocking of the actions of glutamate [88; 89].

Lignocaine

Over the last 35 years there have been reports of the analgesic efficacy of intravenous lignocaine in a wide range of neuropathic pain states, including diabetic neuropathy, peripheral nerve lesions, post-herpetic neuralgia and central pain [4; 90; 91; 92; 93; 94]. Sakurai and Kanazawa have reported its effectiveness in multiple sclerosis associated pain [95]. There is a large variation in reported duration of analgesic effect, varying from no residual effect to 20 weeks benefit in patients with central pain. A beneficial response to a lignocaine infusion may suggest a similar benefit from oral mexiletine, but does not predict this reliably [96].

Mexiletine

This antiarrhythmic is an oral analogue of lignocaine that has been used in neuropathic pain with mixed results. Effectiveness has been demonstrated in treating pain after peripheral nerve injuries and painful diabetic neuropathy. However, these findings are not consistent and the effects are less than that provided by TCAs and anticonvulsants [97; 98; 99]. Optimal dosing may be a problem with a poor therapeutic ratio and potential cardiotoxicity [2].

Recommendations for clinical use of lignocaine and mexiletine in neuropathic pain

Side effects of both substances are CNS (dizziness, nausea, perioral numbness, convulsions and coma) and cardiovascular system effects (arrhythmias). Contraindications include therefore cardiac conduction abnormalities, left ventricular failure and ischaemic heart disease. An ECG should be obtained before and during treatment to monitor any cardiac effects. If there is a question regarding safety in a patient, a cardiologist's opinion should be sought, prior to starting treatment.

For lignocaine the recommended starting dose is 1–1.5 mg/kg as a slow IV bolus; this is an ideal agent for the neuropathic pain emergency. Maintenance is by IV infusion of 1–3 mg/minute with measurement of blood concentrations. The recommended starting dose for mexiletine is 150 mg three times a day, with a slow increase to 600–1200 mg per day to optimal results.

NMDA RECEPTOR ANTAGONISTS

N-methyl-D aspartate receptors are activated by the excitatory neurotransmitter glutamate. They are thought to play an important role in the development of central sensitization following a peripheral nerve lesion. The NMDA antagonists may block this hyperactivity responsible for the maintenance of pain. Drugs with NMDA receptor antagonist activity include ketamine, dextromethorphan, memantine and amantadine.

Ketamine

Ketamine is the most commonly used NMDA antagonist. Its original use was as an anaesthetic agent, particularly 'in the field' and other difficult locations and situations. It has also been used for the treatment of severe asthma and for sedation. However, ketamine is known to have analgesic properties at subanaesthetic doses.

Analgesic efficacy has been demonstrated in RCTs for post-herpetic neuralgia, peripheral nerve injuries, phantom limb pain and post-stroke central pain [100; 101; 102; 103; 104]. There are individual case reports, including successful management of central post-stroke pain and post-herpetic neuralgia with oral ketamine [105; 106]. However, oral ketamine has not been used widely in clinical practice and results of RCTs have not been promising [107].

Ketamine may in part provide analgesia by reversing opioid tolerance [21]. A case has been reported where ketamine provided pain relief and a reduction in oral morphine requirements in a patient with neuropathic cancer pain that had failed to respond to increasing doses of both oral and spinal morphine [108]. Unpleasant side effects limit its use. These are mostly psychometric: sedation-reduced reactions, hallucinations, dysphoria, unpleasant sensations (dissociation) and paranoid feelings. It is important to warn patients in advance of these potential effects; they can be reduced by co-prescribing benzodiazepines such as midazolam if needed.

Other NMDA antagonists

Dextromethorphan, amantadine and memantine have been shown to have weaker actions than ketamine. In a blinded trial, Nelson *et al.* demonstrated an analgesic effect with a high dose of dextromethorphan in painful diabetic neuropathy [109], but this has not been reproduced in other neuropathic pain states [110]. Parenteral amantadine has been shown to relieve pain and allodynia in cancer patients with surgical neuropathic pain [111]. Memantine was recently shown to be ineffective in phantom limb pain treatment [112].

MISCELLANEOUS COMPOUNDS FOR SYSTEMIC USE

Clonidine

Clonidine is an α_2-agonist with analgesic activity. Its analgesic action is thought to occur centrally and at a spinal level, mediated by activation of α_2-adrenoceptors in the dorsal horn of the spinal cord. This results in direct inhibition of postsynaptic spinal dorsal horn neurones or by decreasing the release of noradrenaline from sympathetic nerve terminals. Only a small number of studies have been conducted to look at a potential role in the treatment of neuropathic pain. Significant improvement was reported in patients with post-herpetic neuralgia treated with clonidine [113].

Transdermal clonidine (0.1 to 0.3 mg per day) has been used with success in patients with diabetic neuropathies [114; 115]. A double-blind cross-over study in 20 chronic pain patients, comparing epidural clonidine, and an epidural combination of clonidine and lignocaine, found epidural clonidine to be as effective as epidural morphine in all 20 patients [116].

It is registered in the USA as an adjuvant in combination with epidural local anaesthetics and opioids for resistant neuropathic pain. Side effects include drowsiness, dizziness and dry mouth.

Baclofen

Baclofen is a GABA receptor agonist, capable of crossing the blood brain barrier. It is an agonist at $GABA_B$ receptors and has presynaptic action in the spinal cord preventing the release of excitatory neurotransmitters [117].

Baclofen causes muscle relaxation and is used to treat muscle spasticity. It has been shown to have antinociceptive action and used to treat neuropathic pain [118]. It was first used for this purpose to treat trigeminal neuralgia [119]. Its efficacy has not, however, been confirmed in other neuropathic pain conditions [120]. Baclofen has been administered intrathecally and may be useful for pain related to spinal cord injuries [121].

Side effects include sedation, nausea, confusion, convulsions, hypotension, gastrointestinal upset, visual disturbances and occasionally hepatic impairment. After prolonged use, baclofen requires a gradual dose reduction in order to minimize the risk of a withdrawal syndrome [117].

Levodopa

Ertas *et al.* found levodopa to be better than placebo in treating painful diabetic neuropathy [122]. A review of placebo controlled trials by Sindrup and Jensen in patients with diabetic neuropathy showed that the NNT was 3.4 for levodopa, compared with 6.7 for SSRIs [123]. A placebo controlled trial has demonstrated efficacy in acute herpes zoster pain [124].

Cannabinoids

There has been recent interest in the use of cannabis and cannabinoids as analgesics in chronic pain. Cannabinoid receptors are located in the central and peripheral nervous system, although their role is as yet unclear. Animal models have shown that cannabinoid receptors do not undergo down-regulation after nerve lesions (unlike opioid receptors) and that cannabinoids may attenuate the associated sensory changes [10].

Cannabis has been used for thousands of years for medicinal and recreational purposes. There is much interest surrounding its legalization and its potential role as an analgesic.

However, the evidence for analgesic efficacy in humans is very thin, based mostly on retrospective reports. In a qualitative systematic review of RCTs, there were no large trials in neuropathic pain but there was some suggestion of efficacy (from very small numbers) [125]. A more recent open trial did not, however, reveal any significant efficacy of D9-tetrahydrocannabinol in a small cohort of patients with chronic refractory neuropathic pain. It showed an unfavourable and poorly tolerated side effect profile [126].

Adverse effects associated with cannabinoids are common, the main being sedation, disorientation, ataxia, memory impairment, dry mouth and blurred vision.

Larger blinded, RCTs are required before it can be ascertained whether cannabinoids are efficacious in neuropathic pain. The development of new safe and effective agonists that separates the psychotropic effects from the therapeutic ones would improve trial designs.

TOPICAL TREATMENTS

Allodynia is frequently a feature of neuropathic pain especially in post-herpetic neuralgia, traumatic neuropathies and causalgia. It may therefore be helpful to consider the use of topical medications for the treatment of cutaneous hyperalgesia in these cases.

There are a few options in the form of capsaicin, local anaesthetics (and NSAIDs as there are some reports of good pain relief from post-herpetic neuralgia with topical aspirin preparations) [127; 128; 129].

Topical application of local anaesthetics

In patients with post-herpetic neuralgia success has been reported using lignocaine patches or topically applied gel to painful areas [61; 130; 131]. The mechanism is thought to involve suppression of ectopic discharges from sensory afferents and from providing mechanical protection to underlying allodynic skin [132]. In 1999 the FDA approved the use of 5% topical lignocaine patches for first-line treatment of post-herpetic neuralgia.

The advantages of this route of administration are its effectiveness, duration of analgesia, ease of application without dose titration and lack of systemic side effects. The safety profile is particularly advantageous in the elderly population whom are most affected by post-herpetic neuralgia. The area of pain has, however, to be of limited size for practical application.

There have been conflicting reports regarding the efficacy of the topical eutectic mixture of local anaesthetics (EMLA), an emulsification of lignocaine and prilocaine, in patients with paroxysmal pain and mechanical allodynia [2].

Capsaicin

Capsaicin is the pungent component to chilli peppers. The chilli pepper has been recognized by various cultures for many years for its medicinal qualities [133]. It is neurotoxic and has analgesic properties. When capsaicin is applied topically it initially causes a burning sensation and heat hyperalgesia that decreases with subsequent applications.

Mechanism of action

Capsaicin acts on receptors on the terminals of primary nociceptive afferents. In 1997 a specific receptor occurring on C fibres was cloned, a vanilloid receptor, the VR-1 receptor. When capsaicin binds to this receptor, it induces initial activation of the nociceptors, hence the burning sensation. It depletes substance P from the sensory nerve terminals of peripheral nociceptors. With repeated or prolonged application, this is followed by desensitization and inactivation of the receptive terminals of the nociceptors [134]. There is also evidence that it causes depletion of substance P in epidermal nerve fibres [135].

Efficacy

Several RCTs have demonstrated analgesic efficacy of capsaicin cream in painful diabetic neuropathy [136; 137] and post-herpetic neuralgia [138], although this has not been a consistent result [139; 140]. These contradictory results in double-blind trials of capsaicin might have been caused by the high placebo effect, as the burning effect results in the patient effectively being unblinded. This criticism is confirmed by one double-blind trial using a placebo with a similar burning sensation and finding no difference in analgesic efficacy between placebo and capsaicin [141].

Biesbroeck *et al.* in a double-blind comparison of topical capsaicin and oral amitriptyline in painful diabetic neuropathy found them to be of equal efficacy [142]. It has even been applied to the nasal mucosa to prevent cluster headaches [143].

The use of capsaicin has been limited by this unpleasant burning sensation occurring in 60%–70% of patients, the need for frequent applications and uncertain efficacy [2]. There is some suggestion that a higher concentration (5% or more) can produce longer pain relief in patients with neuropathic pain, although a spinal anaesthetic was required to make its application tolerable [144]. Co-administration of lignocaine gel has been used in order to improve compliance [2].

Capsaicin is seen as an adjuvant treatment and second-line therapy. It seems that its main role is in pain and hyperalgesia caused by C fibre sensitization.

NON-PHARMACOLOGICAL THERAPY

Transcutaneous electrical nerve stimulation (TENS)

This technique applies cutaneous electrodes to stimulate peripheral nerves to relieve pain [145]. This is based on the gate control theory of pain transmission, so that by stimulating Aβ- and Aδ- fibres, pain transmission by C fibres is inhibited. It utilizes a pulse generator that provides a range of currents, frequencies and pulse widths. The surface electrodes are placed either side of the painful area or the nerves supplying that area. The current is then increased until a tingling sensation is felt in the painful area. The timing and duration of pulses is a matter of titration to maximal response. Transcutaneous electrical nerve stimulation may reduce analgesic requirements [146]. It has few side effects and complications, allergic dermatitis may occur at the contact sites and its use is contraindicated in patients with pacemakers. Its efficacy can be assessed quickly (there is a significant placebo effect) and can therefore be easily trialled for any potential benefit to an individual [147]. Unfortunately tolerance may develop resulting in loss of previously effective analgesia; changing the stimulation variables can sometimes attenuate this.

Spinal cord stimulation (SCS)

This techniques requires an implantable device with electrodes positioned under direct vision at open laminectomy or via a needle in the epidural space percutaneously. The electrodes are placed above the level of the pain and connected to an inductance coil placed on the abdominal wall; an implantable power source can also be used. The mechanism of action is not yet clear, but it seems not to be effective in nociceptive pain, but only in neuropathic pain [148]. It seems that this device can be useful for a variety of neuropathic and chronic pain states [149]. Complications include infection, bleeding, dural puncture and hardware failure. Decisions on the use of this invasive and expensive approach should be made ideally by a multidisciplinary team experienced in the use of such techniques.

Deep brain stimulation has also been used to treat neuropathic pain [150].

Sympathetic nerve blocks

The diagnosis of sympathetically maintained pain can be confirmed by the response to a sympatholytic procedure. This may be helpful, if there is a significant sympathetic component to the patient's pain. A patient should receive sustained pain relief after administration of a sympathetic chain or sympathetic plexus local anaesthetic block, or accumulative relief from a number of procedures. If the patient fails to respond, a systematic pharmacological approach is tried. However, a block may be incorrectly thought to be successful. This can happen for one of two reasons: either, the local anaesthetic is absorbed and provides a systemic analgesic effect, or it diffuses locally and acts on nearby somatic nerves [151].

In case of effectiveness, progression to a sympatholytic procedure can be chosen. Techniques then involve the use of neurolytic substances or radiofrequency ablation; regrettably the current scientific basis for this approach is poor [152].

Neurosurgical destructive techniques

There has been increasing awareness that destructive techniques may in fact increase pain in the long term due to the plasticity of the nervous system, sometimes resulting in incapacitating side effects. Therefore these techniques, which include neurectomy and dorsal root entry zone lesions, are now rarely used [153]. The exception being in the treatment of trigeminal neuralgia, which has proved refractory to pharmacological treatments. In this situation a variety of surgical procedures can provide rapid pain relief, the most effective option being microvascular decompression. Recurrence is still a risk but appears to be more frequent after percutaneous radiofrequency rhizotomy or compression with a percutaneously positioned balloon, than the more invasive microvascular decompression technique [154].

Cognitive-behavioural therapy

Chronic neuropathic pain is best managed in a multidisciplinary pain clinic [155]. This is because the patient often has cognitive, affective and behavioural factors influencing their pain. However, new understandings of the physiology of cortical reorganization in chronic pain might also lead to new psychological approaches [156]. A multidisciplinary approach will address both the somatic and psychological aspects of the patient's condition. The main methods are cognitive-behavioural therapy and operant conditioning.

The cognitive-behavioural approach aims to identify and modify the patient's thoughts, feelings, beliefs and behaviour. Common problems are anxiety, depression and the development of fear-avoidance. Behavioural therapy procedures are utilized to bring about change. The aims are to enable patients to take a positive and active role in coping with their pain, and to change maladaptive behaviour that may be aggravating the problem.

Operant conditioning uses continuous reinforcement to encourage positive behaviour from the patient that is then stepped down later on. This is based on the belief that the consequence of certain behaviour determines whether it is likely to recur.

Psychotherapy may increase levels of activity and decrease medication requirements, but an actual reporting in pain reduction may be more modest. In addition the therapy may need to be extended to the carers of the patient in order to change their response to the patients beliefs and behaviour.

REFERENCES

1. H. Merskey & N. Bogduk (eds.), *Classification of Chronic Pain*, 2nd edn (Seattle: IASP Press, 1994).
2. N. Attal, Chronic neuropathic pain: mechanisms and treatment. *Clinical Journal of Pain*, **16**(3)(Suppl) (2000), S118–30.
3. S. Arner & B. A. Meyerson, Lack of analgesic effect of opioids on neuropathic and idiopathic forms of pain. *Pain*, **33** (1988), 11–23.
4. M. C. Rowbotham, L. A. Reisner-Keller & H. L. Fields, Both intravenous lidocaine and morphine reduce the pain of postherpetic neuralgia. *Neurology*, **41** (1991), 1024–8.
5. P. L. Dellemijn & J. A. Vanneste, Randomised double-blind active-placebo-controlled crossover trial of intravenous fentanyl in neuropathic pain. *Lancet*, **349**(9054) (1997), 753–8.
6. C. P. Watson & N. Babul, Efficacy of oxycodone in neuropathic pain: a randomized trial in postherpetic neuralgia. *Neurology*, **50**(6) (1998), 1837–41.
7. R. K. Portenoy, K. M. Foley & C. E. Inturrisi, The nature of opioid responsiveness and its implications for neuropathic pain: new hypotheses derived from studies of opioid infusions. *Pain*, **43**(3) (1990), 273–86.
8. F. Benedetti, S. Vighetti, M. Amanzio *et al.*, Dose-response relationship of opioids in nociceptive and neuropathic postoperative pain. *Pain*, **74**(2–3) (1998), 205–11.
9. D. Besse, M. C. Lombard & J. M. Besson, Autoradiographic distribution of mu, delta and kappa opioid binding sites in the superficial dorsal horn, over the rostrocaudal axis of the rat spinal cord. *Brain Research*, **548**(1–2) (1991), 287–91.
10. D. Bridges, S. W. Thompson & A. S. Rice, Mechanisms of neuropathic pain. *British Journal of Anaesthesia*, **87**(1) (2001), 12–26.
11. D. S. Rohde, D. J. Detweiler & A. I. Basbaum, Spinal cord mechanisms of opioid tolerance and dependence: fos-like immunoreactivity increases in subpopulations of spinal cord neurons during withdrawal [corrected]. *Neuroscience*, **72**(1) (1996), 233–42.
12. M. Pappagallo & J. N. Campbell, Chronic opioid therapy as alternative treatment for post-herpetic neuralgia. *Annals of Neurology*, **35**(Suppl) (1994), S54–6.
13. I. F. Angel, H. J. Gould, Jr. & M. E. Carey, Intrathecal morphine pump as a treatment option in chronic pain of nonmalignant origin. *Surgical Neurology*, **49**(1) (1998), 92–9.
14. H. B. Gutstein & H. Akil, Opioid analgesics. In *The Pharmaceutical Basis of Therapeutics*, 10th edn, ed. J. C. Hardman, L. E. Limbird and A. G. Gilman. (New York: McGraw Hill, 2001), pp. 569–621.
15. B. J. Collett, Opioid tolerance: the clinical perspective. *British Journal of Anaesthesia*, **81**(1) (1998), 58–68.
16. S. A. Schug, D. Zech, S. Grond *et al.*, A long-term survey of morphine in cancer pain patients. *Journal of Pain and Symptom Management*, **7** (1992), 259–66.
17. M. Zenz, M. Strumpf & M. Tryba, Long-term oral opioid therapy in patients with chronic nonmalignant pain. *Journal of Pain and Symptom Management*, **7**(2) (1992), 69–77.
18. R. K. Portenoy, Opioid therapy for chronic nonmalignant pain: a review of the critical issues. *Journal of Pain and Symptom Management*, **11**(4) (1996), 203–17.
19. B. J. Collett, Chronic opioid therapy for non-cancer pain. *British Journal of Anaesthesia*, **87**(1) (2001), 133–43.
20. S. A. Schug, A. F. Merry & R. H. Acland, Treatment principles for the use of opioids in pain of nonmalignant origin. *Drugs*, **42**(2) (1991), 228–39.
21. D. J. Hewitt, The use of NMDA-receptor antagonists in the treatment of chronic pain. *Clinical Journal of Pain*, **16**(2)(Suppl) (2000), S73–79.
22. A. Bulka, A. Plesan, X. J. Xu & Z. Wiesenfeld-Hallin, Reduced tolerance to the anti-hyperalgesic effect of methadone in comparison to morphine in a rat model of mononeuropathy. *Pain*, **95**(1–2) (2002), 103–9.
23. P. J. Graziotti & C. R. Goucke, The use of oral opioids in patients with chronic non-cancer pain. Management strategies. *Medical Journal of Australia*, **167**(1) (1997), 30–4.
24. D. Jones & S. Schug, Opioids in chronic pain of non-malignant origin: an interim consensus (letter). *New Zealand Medical Journal*, **108** (1995), 492.
25. Kentucky Board of Medical Licensure. Model guidelines for the use of controlled substances in pain treatment. *Journal of the Kentucky Medical Association*, **99**(7) (2001), 291–4.
26. M. Skinner, Aspects of the problems in treating chronic pain: Florida pain management guidelines. *Journal of the Florida Medical Association*, **84**(2) (1997), 85–6.

27. N. Hagen, P. Flynne, H. Hays & N. MacDonald, Guidelines for managing chronic non-malignant pain. Opioids and other agents. College of Physicians and Surgeons of Alberta. *Canadian Family Physician*, **41** (1995), 49–53.
28. R. B. Raffa, E. Friderichs, W. Reimann *et al.*, Opioid and nonopioid components independently contribute to the mechanism of action of tramadol, an 'atypical' opioid analgesic. *Journal of Pharmacology and Experimental Therapeutics*, **260**(1) (1992), 275–85.
29. R. B. Raffa & E. Friderichs, The basic science aspect of tramadol hydrochloride. *Pain Reviews*, **3** (1996), 249–71.
30. B. Driessen & W. Reimann, Interaction of the central analgesic, tramadol, with the uptake and release of 5-hydroxytryptamine in the rat brain *in vitro*. *British Journal of Pharmacology*, **105**(1) (1992), 147–51.
31. B. Driessen, W. Reimann & H. Giertz, Effects of the central analgesic tramadol on the uptake and release of noradrenaline and dopamine *in vitro*. *British Journal of Pharmacology*, **108**(3) (1993), 806–11.
32. Y. Harati, C. Gooch, M. Swenson *et al.*, Double-blind randomized trial of tramadol for the treatment of the pain of diabetic neuropathy. *Neurology*, **50**(6) (1998), 1842–6.
33. S. H. Sindrup, G. Andersen, C. Madsen *et al.*, Tramadol relieves pain and allodynia in polyneuropathy: a randomised, double-blind, controlled trial. *Pain*, **83**(1) (1999), 85–90.
34. T. J. Cicero, E. H. Adams, A. Geller *et al.*, A postmarketing surveillance program to monitor ultram (tramadol hydrochloride) abuse in the United States. *Drug and Alcohol Dependence*, **57**(1) (1999), 7–22.
35. K. L. Preston, D. R. Jasinski & M. Testa, Abuse potential and pharmacological comparison of tramadol and morphine. *Drug and Alcohol Dependence*, **27**(1) (1991), 7–17.
36. M. Cossmann & C. Kohnen, General tolerability and adverse event profile of tramadol. *Revisions of Contemporary Pharmacotherapy*, **6** (1995), 513–31.
37. P. Onghena & B. Van Houdenhove, Antidepressant-induced analgesia in chronic non-malignant pain: A meta-analysis of 39 placebo-controlled studies. *Pain*, **49**(2) (1992), 205–19.
38. C. P. Watson, M. Chipman, K. Reed, R. J. Evans & N. Birkett, Amitriptyline versus maprotiline in postherpetic neuralgia: a randomized, double-blind, crossover trial. *Pain*, **48**(1) (1992), 29–36.
39. M. B. Max, Antidepressants as analgesics. In *Progress in Pain Research and Therapy*, ed. H. L. Fields and J. C. Liebesking. (Seattle: IASP Press, 1994) pp. 229–46.
40. M. B. Max, M. Culnane, S. C. Schafer *et al.*, Amitriptyline relieves diabetic neuropathy pain in patients with normal or depressed mood. *Neurology*, **37**(4) (1987), 589–96.
41. M. B. Max, R. Kishore-Kumar, S. C. Schafer *et al.*, Efficacy of desipramine in painful diabetic neuropathy: a placebo-controlled trial. *Pain*, **45**(1) (1991), 1–9.
42. R. Kishore-Kumar, M. B. Max, S. C. Schafer *et al.*, Desipramine relieves postherpetic neuralgia. *Clinical Pharmacology and Therapeutics*, **47**(3) (1990), 305–12.
43. A. M. Gray, P. S. Spencer & R. D. Sewell, The involvement of the opioidergic system in the antinociceptive mechanism of action of antidepressant compounds. *British Journal of Pharmacology*, **124**(4) (1998), 669–674.
44. H. J. McQuay, M. Tramer, B. A. Nye *et al.*, A systematic review of antidepressants in neuropathic pain. *Pain*, **68**(2–3) (1996), 217–27.
45. M. B. Max, S. A. Lynch, J. Muir *et al.*, Effects of desipramine, amitriptyline, and fluoxetine on pain in diabetic neuropathy. *New England Journal of Medicine*, **326**(19) (1992), 1250–6.
46. A. Ansari, The efficacy of newer antidepressants in the treatment of chronic pain: A review of current literature. *Harvard Review of Psychiatry*, **7**(5) (2000), 257–77.
47. S. H. Sindrup, E. Grodum, L. F. Gram & H. Beck-Nielsen, Concentration-response relationship in paroxetine treatment of diabetic neuropathy symptoms: a patient-blinded dose-escalation study. *Therapeutic Drug Monitoring*, **13**(5) (1991), 408–14.
48. S. L. Collins, R. A. Moore, H. J. McQuay & P. Wiffen, Antidepressants and anticonvulsants for diabetic neuropathy and postherpetic neuralgia: a quantitative systematic review. *Journal of Pain and Symptom Management*, **20**(6) (2000), 449–58.
49. D. Fishbain, Evidence-based data on pain relief with antidepressants. *Annals of Medicine*, **32**(5) (2000), 305–16.
50. T. P. Enggaard, N. A. Klitgaard, L. F. Gram, L. Arendt-Nielsen & S. H. Sindrup, Specific effect of venlafaxine on single and repetitive experimental painful stimuli in humans. *Clinical Pharmacology and Therapeutics*, **69**(4) (2001), 245–51.

51. T. Tasmuth, B. Hartel & E. Kalso, Venlafaxine in neuropathic pain following treatment of breast cancer. *European Journal of Pain*, **6**(1) (2002), 17–24.
52. R. L. Barkin & J. Fawcett, The management challenges of chronic pain: the role of antidepressants. *American Journal of Therapy*, **7**(1) (2000), 31–47.
53. G. E. Tomkins, J. L. Jackson, P. G. O'Malley, E. Balden & J. E. Santoro, Treatment of chronic headache with antidepressants: a meta-analysis. *American Journal of Medicine*, **111**(1) (2001), 54–63.
54. P. G. O'Malley, E. Balden, G. Tomkins *et al.*, Treatment of fibromyalgia with antidepressants: a meta-analysis. *Journal of General Internal Medicine*, **15**(9) (2000), 659–66.
55. H. J. McQuay, D. Carroll & C. J. Glynn, Dose-response for analgesic effect of amitriptyline in chronic pain. *Anaesthesia*, **48**(4) (1993), 281–5.
56. M. Ellenberg, Treatment of diabetic neuropathy with diphenylhydantoin. *New York State Journal of Medicine*, **68**(20) (1968), 2653–5.
57. T. S. Jensen, Anticonvulsants in neuropathic pain: rationale and clinical evidence. *European Journal of Pain*, **6**(Suppl A) (2002), 61–8.
58. R. R. Tasker, T. Tsuda & P. Hawrylyshyn, Clinical neurophysiological investigation of deafferation pain. In *Advances in Pain Research and Therapy*, ed. J. J. Bonica (New York: Raven Press, 1983), pp. 713–38.
59. D. L. Tanelian & W. G. Brose, Neuropathic pain can be relieved by drugs that are use-dependent sodium channel blockers: lidocaine, carbamazepine, and mexiletine. *Anesthesiology*, **74**(5) (1991), 949–51.
60. B. Soderpalm, Anticonvulsants: aspects of their mechanisms of action. *European Journal of Pain*, **6**(Suppl A) (2002), 3–9.
61. M. C. Rowbotham, P. S. Davies & H. L. Fields, Topical lidocaine gel relieves postherpetic neuralgia. *Annals of Neurology*, **37**(2) (1995), 246–53.
62. S. L. Bartusch, B. J. Sanders, J. G. D'Alessio & J. R. Jernigan, Clonazepam for the treatment of lancinating phantom limb pain. *Clinical Journal of Pain*, **12**(1) (1996), 59–62.
63. M. Swerdlow & J. G. Cundill, Anticonvulsant drugs used in the treatment of lancinating pain. A comparison. *Anaesthesia*, **36**(12) (1981), 1129–32.
64. M. M. Backonja, Use of anticonvulsants for treatment of neuropathic pain. *Neurology*, **59**(5)(Suppl 2) (2002), S14–17.
65. C. P. Taylor, Emerging perspectives on the mechanism of action of gabapentin. *Neurology*, **44**(6)(Suppl 5) (1994), S10–16.
66. M. Rowbotham, N. Harden, B. Stacey, P. Bernstein & L. Magnus-Miller, Gabapentin for the treatment of postherpetic neuralgia: a randomized controlled trial [see comments]. *JAMA*, **280**(21) (1998), 1837–42.
67. J. S. Bryans & D. J. Wustrow, 3-substituted GABA analogs with central nervous system activity: a review. *Medical Research Reviews*, **19**(2) (1999), 149–77.
68. M. A. Rose & P. C. Kam, Gabapentin: pharmacology and its use in pain management. *Anaesthesia*, **57**(5) (2002), 451–62.
69. M. Backonja, A. Beydoun, K. R. Edwards *et al.*, Gabapentin for the symptomatic treatment of painful neuropathy in patients with diabetes mellitus: A randomized controlled trial [see comments]. *JAMA*, **280**(21) (1998), 1831–6.
70. M. M. Backonja, Gabapentin monotherapy for the symptomatic treatment of painful neuropathy: a multicenter, double-blind, placebo-controlled trial in patients with diabetes mellitus. *Epilepsia*, **40**(Suppl 6) (1999), S57–9.
71. P. Wiffen, S. Collins, H. McQuay *et al.*, Anticonvulsant drugs for acute and chronic pain. *Cochrane Database Systematic Reviews*, (3) (2000), CD001133.
72. C. M. Morello, S. G. Leckband, C. P. Stoner, D. F. Moorhouse & G. A. Sahagian, Randomized double-blind study comparing the efficacy of gabapentin with amitriptyline on diabetic peripheral neuropathy pain. *Archives of Internal Medicine*, **159**(16) (1999), 1931–7.
73. A. S. Rice & S. Maton, Gabapentin in postherpetic neuralgia: a randomised, double blind, placebo controlled study. *Pain*, **94**(2) (2001), 215–24.
74. B. Chen, T. P. Stitik, P. M. Foye, S. F. Nadler & J. A. DeLisa, Central post-stroke pain syndrome: yet another use for gabapentin? *American Journal of Physical Medicine and Rehabilitation*, **81**(9) (2002), 718–20.
75. I. W. Tremont-Lukats, C. Megeff & M. M. Backonja, Anticonvulsants for neuropathic pain syndromes: mechanisms of action and place in therapy. *Drugs*, **60**(5) (2000), 1029–52.
76. M. A. Mellegers, A. D. Furlan & A. Mailis, Gabapentin for neuropathic pain: systematic review of controlled and uncontrolled literature. *Clinical Journal of Pain*, **17**(4) (2001), 284–95.

77. F. G. Campbell, J. G. Graham & K. J. Zilkha, Clinical trial of carbamazepine (tegretol) in trigeminal neuralgia. *Journal of Neurology, Neurosurgery and Psychiatry*, **29**(3) (1966), 265–7.
78. J. M. Killian & G. H. Fromm, Carbamazepine in the treatment of neuralgia. Use and side effects. *Archives of Neurology*, **19**(2) (1968), 129–36.
79. W. Loscher, Valproate: a reappraisal of its pharmacodynamic properties and mechanisms of action. *Progress in Neurobiology*, **58**(1) (1999), 31–59.
80. S. D. Silberstein, Divalproex sodium in headache: literature review and clinical guidelines. *Headache*, **36**(9) (1996), 547–55.
81. J. B. Peiris, G. L. Perera, S. V. Devendra & N. D. Lionel, Sodium valproate in trigeminal neuralgia. *Medical Journal of Australia*, **2**(5) (1980), 278.
82. V. S. Chadda & M. S. Mathur, Double blind study of the effects of diphenylhydantoin sodium on diabetic neuropathy. *Journal of the Association of Physicians of India*, **26**(5) (1978), 403–6.
83. L. A. Lockman, D. B. Hunninghake, W. Krivit & R. J. Desnick, Relief of pain of Fabry's disease by diphenylhydantoin. *Neurology*, **23**(8) (1973), 871–5.
84. G. McCleane, 200 mg daily of lamotrigine has no analgesic effect in neuropathic pain: a randomised, double-blind, placebo controlled trial. *Pain*, **83**(1) (1999), 105–7.
85. E. Eisenberg, N. Alon, A. Ishay, D. Daoud & D. Yarnitsky, Lamotrigine in the treatment of painful diabetic neuropathy. *European Journal of Neurology*, **5**(2) (1998), 167–73.
86. H. McQuay, D. Carroll, A. R. Jadad, P. Wiffen & A. Moore, Anticonvulsant drugs for management of pain: a systematic review. *British Medical Journal*, **311**(7012) (1995), 1047–52.
87. N. B. Finnerup, H. Gottrup & T. S. Jensen, Anticonvulsants in central pain. *Expert Opinion on Pharmacotherapy*, 3(10) (2002), 1411–20.
88. G. Biella & M. L. Sotgiu, Central effects of systemic lidocaine mediated by glycine spinal receptors: an iontophoretic study in the rat spinal cord. *Brain Research*, **603**(2) (1993), 201–6.
89. C. J. Woolf & Z. Wiesenfeld-Hallin, The systemic administration of local anaesthetics produces a selective depression of C-afferent fibre evoked activity in the spinal cord. *Pain*, **23**(4) (1985), 361–74.
90. R. A. Boas, B. G. Covino & A. Shahnarian, Analgesic responses to i.v. lignocaine. *British Journal of Anaesthesia*, **54**(5) (1982), 501–5.
91. P. Marchettini, M. Lacerenza, C. Marangoni *et al.*, Lidocaine test in neuralgia. *Pain*, **48**(3) (1992), 377–82.
92. M. S. Wallace, J. B. Dyck, S. S. Rossi & T. L. Yaksh, Computer-controlled lidocaine infusion for the evaluation of neuropathic pain after peripheral nerve injury. *Pain*, **66**(1) (1996), 69–77.
93. A. P. Baranowski, J. De Courcey & E. Bonello, A trial of intravenous lidocaine on the pain and allodynia of postherpetic neuralgia. *Journal of Pain and Symptom Management*, **17**(6) (1999), 429–33.
94. N. Attal, V. Gaude, L. Brasseur *et al.*, Intravenous lidocaine in central pain: a double-blind, placebo-controlled, psychophysical study. *Neurology*, **54**(3) (2000), 564–74.
95. M. Sakurai & I. Kanazawa, Positive symptoms in multiple sclerosis: their treatment with sodium channel blockers, lidocaine and mexiletine. *Journal of the Neurological Sciences*, **162**(2) (1999), 162–8.
96. B. S. Galer & J. Harle & M. C. Rowbotham, Response to intravenous lidocaine infusion predicts subsequent response to oral mexiletine: a prospective study. *Journal of Pain and Symptom Management*, **12**(3) (1996), 161–7.
97. C. Chabal, L. Russell & K. Burchiel, The effect of intravenous lidocaine, tocainide and mexiletine on spontaneously active fibres originating in rat sciatic neuromas. *Pain*, **38** (1989), 333–8.
98. A. Dejgard, P. Petersen & J. Kastrup, Mexiletine for treatment of chronic painful diabetic neuropathy. *Lancet*, **1**(8575–6) (1988), 9–11.
99. P. Oskarsson, J. G. Ljunggren & P. E. Lins, Efficacy and safety of mexiletine in the treatment of painful diabetic neuropathy. The mexiletine study group. *Diabetes Care*, **20**(10) (1997), 1594–7.
100. S. Felsby, J. Nielsen, L. Arendt-Nielsen & T. S. Jensen, NMDA receptor blockade in chronic neuropathic pain: a comparison of ketamine and magnesium chloride. *Pain*, **64**(2) (1996), 283–91.
101. P. K. Eide, E. Jorum, A. Stubhaug, J. Bremnes & H. Breivik, Relief of post-herpetic neuralgia with the N-methyl-D-aspartate receptor antagonist ketamine: a double blind, cross-over comparison with morphine and placebo. *Pain*, **58** (1994), 347–54.
102. P. K. Eide, A. Stubhaug, I. Oye & H. Breivik, Continuous subcutaneous administration of the N-methyl-D-aspartic acid (NMDA) receptor

antagonist ketamine in the treatment of post-herpetic neuralgia. *Pain*, **61**(2) (1995), 221–8.
103. M. Backonja, G. Arndt, K. A. Gombar, B. Check, M. Zimmermann, Response of chronic neuropathic pain syndromes to ketamine: A preliminary study. *Pain*, **56** (1994), 51–7.
104. L. Nikolajsen, C. L. Hansen, J. Nielsen *et al.*, The effect of ketamine on phantom pain: a central neuropathic disorder maintained by peripheral input. *Pain*, **67**(1) (1996), 69–77.
105. P. G. Vick & T. J. Lamer, Treatment of central post-stroke pain with oral ketamine. *Pain*, **92**(1–2) (2001), 311–13.
106. V. Hoffmann, H. Coppejans, M. Vercauteren & H. Adriaensen, Successful treatment of postherpetic neuralgia with oral ketamine. *Clinical Journal of Pain*, **10**(3) (1994), 240–2.
107. D. R. Hainesz & S. P. Gaines, N of 1 randomised controlled trials of oral ketamine in patients with chronic pain. *Pain*, **83**(2) (1999), 283–7.
108. S. Mercadante, F. Lodi, M. Sapio, M. Calligara & R. Serretta, Long-term ketamine subcutaneous continuous infusion in neuropathic cancer pain. *Journal of Pain and Symptom Management*, **10**(7) (1995), 564–8.
109. K. A. Nelson, K. M. Park, E. Robinovitz, C. Tsigos & M. B. Max, High-dose oral dextromethorphan versus placebo in painful diabetic neuropathy and postherpetic neuralgia. *Neurology*, **48**(5) (1997), 1212–18.
110. H. J. McQuay, D. Carroll, A. R. Jadad *et al.*, Dextromethorphan for the treatment of neuropathic pain: a double-blind randomised controlled crossover trial with integral n-of-1 design. *Pain*, **59**(1) (1994), 127–33.
111. D. Pud, E. Eisenberg, A. Spitzer *et al.*, The NMDA receptor antagonist amantadine reduces surgical neuropathic pain in cancer patients: a double blind, randomized, placebo controlled trial. *Pain*, **75**(2–3) (1998), 349–54.
112. C. Maier, R. Dertwinkel, N. Mansourian *et al.*, Efficacy of the NMDA-receptor antagonist memantine in patients with chronic phantom limb pain – results of a randomized double-blinded, placebo-controlled trial. *Pain*, **103**(3) (2003), 277–83.
113. M. B. Max, S. C. Schafer, M. Culnane, R. Dubner & R. H. Gracely, Association of pain relief with drug side effects in postherpetic neuralgia: a single-dose study of clonidine, codeine, ibuprofen, and placebo. *Clinical Pharmacology and Therapeutics*, **43**(4) (1988), 363–71.
114. D. Zeigler, S. A. Lynch, J. Muir, J. Benjamin & M. B. Max, Transdermal clonidine versus placebo in painful diabetic neuropathy. *Pain*, **48**(3) (1992), 403–8.
115. M. G. Byas-Smith, M. B. Max, J. Muir & A. Kingman, Transdermal clonidine compared to placebo in painful diabetic neuropathy using a two-stage 'enriched enrollment' design. *Pain*, **60**(3) (1995), 267–74.
116. C. Glynn, D. Dawson & R. Sanders, A double-blind comparison between epidural morphine and epidural clonidine in patients with chronic non-cancer pain. *Pain*, **34** (1988), 123–8.
117. G. H. Fromm, Baclofen as an adjuvant analgesic. *Journal of Pain and Symptom Management*, **9**(8) (1994), 500–9.
118. R. Hering-Hanit, Baclofen for prevention of migraine. *Cephalalgia*, **19**(6) (1999), 589–91.
119. G. H. Fromm, C. F. Terrence, A. S. Chattha, Baclofen in the treatment of trigeminal neuralgia: double-blind study and long-term follow-up. *Annals of Neurology*, **15**(3) (1984), 240–4.
120. C. F. Terrence, G. H. Fromm & R. Tenicela, Baclofen as an analgesic in chronic peripheral nerve disease. *European Neurology*, **24**(6) (1985), 380–5.
121. R. M. Herman, S. C. D'Luzansky & R. Ippolito, Intrathecal baclofen suppresses central pain in patients with spinal lesions. A pilot study. *Clinical Journal of Pain*, 8(4) (1992), 338–45.
122. M. Ertas, A. Sagduyu, N. Arac, B. Uludag & C. Ertekin, Use of levodopa to relieve pain from painful symmetrical diabetic polyneuropathy. *Pain*, **75**(2–3) (1998), 257–9.
123. S. H. Sindrup & T. S. Jensen, Efficacy of pharmacological treatments of neuropathic pain: an update and effect related to mechanism of drug action. *Pain*, **83**(3) (1999), 389–400.
124. S. Kernbaum & J. Hauchecorne, Administration of levodopa for relief of herpes zoster pain. *JAMA*, **246**(2) (1981), 132–4.
125. F. A. Campbell, M. R. Tramer, D. Carroll *et al.*, Are cannabinoids an effective and safe treatment option in the management of pain? A qualitative systematic review. *British Medical Journal*, **323**(7303) (2001), 13–16.
126. S. Clermont-Gnamien, S. Atlani, N. Attal *et al.*, The therapeutic use of D9-tetrahydrocannabinol

(dronabinol) in refractory neuropathic pain.] *Presse Medicale*, **31**(39 Pt 1) (2002), 1840–5.
127. R. B. King, Concerning the management of pain associated with herpes zoster and of postherpetic neuralgia. *Pain*, **33** (1988), 73–8.
128. G. De Benedittis, F. Besana & A. Lorenzetti, A new topical treatment for acute herpetic neuralgia and post-herpetic neuralgia: the aspirin/diethyl ether mixture. An open-label study plus a double-blind controlled clinical trial. *Pain*, **48**(3) (1992), 383–90.
129. G. De Benedittis & A. Lorenzetti, Topical aspirin/diethyl ether mixture versus indomethacin and diclofenac/diethyl ether mixtures for acute herpetic neuralgia and postherpetic neuralgia: a double-blind crossover placebo-controlled study. *Pain*, **65**(1) (1996), 45–51.
130. M. C. Rowbotham, P. S. Davies, C. Verkempinck & B. S. Galer, Lidocaine patch: double-blind controlled study of a new treatment method for post-herpetic neuralgia. *Pain*, **65**(1) (1996), 39–44.
131. B. S. Galer, Advances in the treatment of postherpetic neuralgia: the topical lidocaine patch. *Today's Therapeutic Trends*, **18**(1) (2000), 1–20.
132. C. E. Argoff, Lidocaine patch 5% and the management of chronic pain. *Southern Medical Journal*, **95**(7) (2002), 781.
133. W. Robbins, Clinical applications of capsaicinoids. *Clinical Journal of Pain*, **16**(2)(Suppl) (2000), S86–9.
134. P. Bjerring, L. Arendt-Nielsen & U. Soderberg, Argon laser induced cutaneous sensory and pain thresholds in post-herpetic neuralgia. Quantitative modulation by topical capsaicin. *Acta Dermato-Venereologica*, **70**(2) (1990), 121–5.
135. B. Lynn, Capsaicin: actions on nociceptive C-fibres and therapeutic potential. *Pain*, **41**(1) (1990), 61–9.
136. R. Tandan, G. A. Lewis, P. B. Krusinski, G. B. Badger & T. J. Fries, Topical capsaicin in painful diabetic neuropathy. Controlled study with long-term follow-up. *Diabetes Care*, **15**(1) (1992), 8–14.
137. N. M. Scheffler, P. L. Sheitel & M. N. Lipton, Treatment of painful diabetic neuropathy with capsaicin 0.075%. *Journal of the American Podiatric Medical Association*, **81**(6) (1991), 288–93.
138. J. E. Bernstein, N. J. Korman, D. R. Bickers, M. V. Dahl & L. E. Millikan, Topical capsaicin treatment of chronic postherpetic neuralgia. *Journal of the American Academy of Dermatology*, **21**(2) (Pt 1) (1989), 265–70.
139. D. A. Chad, N. Aronin, R. Lundstrom *et al.*, Does capsaicin relieve the pain of diabetic neuropathy? *Pain*, **42**(3) (1990), 387–8.
140. C. P. Watson, K. L. Tyler, D. R. Bickers *et al.*, A randomized vehicle-controlled trial of topical capsaicin in the treatment of postherpetic neuralgia. *Clinical Therapeutics*, **15**(3) (1993), 510–26.
141. P. A. Low, T. L. Opfer-Gehrking, P. J. Dyck, W. J. Litchy & P. C. O'Brien, Double-blind, placebo-controlled study of the application of capsaicin cream in chronic distal painful polyneuropathy. *Pain*, **62**(2) (1995), 163–8.
142. R. Biesbroeck, V. Bril, P. Hollander *et al.*, A double-blind comparison of topical capsaicin and oral amitriptyline in painful diabetic neuropathy. *Advances in Therapy*, **12**(2) (1995), 111–120.
143. D. R. Marks, A. Rapoport, D. Padla *et al.*, A double-blind placebo-controlled trial of intranasal capsaicin for cluster headache. *Cephalalgia*, **13**(2) (1993), 114–16.
144. W. R. Robbins, P. S. Staats, J. Levine *et al.*, Treatment of intractable pain with topical large-dose capsaicin: preliminary report. *Anesthesia and Analgesia*, **86**(3) (1998), 579–83.
145. M. Tulgar, Advances in electrical nerve stimulation techniques to manage chronic pain: an overview. *Advances in Therapy*, **9**(6) (1992), 366–72.
146. M. A. Hamza, P. F. White, W. F. Craig *et al.*, Percutaneous electrical nerve stimulation: A novel analgesic therapy for diabetic neuropathic pain. *Diabetes Care*, **23**(3) (2000), 365–70.
147. K. Kumar, C. Toth, R. K. Nath & P. Laing, Epidural spinal cord stimulation for treatment of chronic pain – some predictors of success. A 15-year experience. *Surgical Neurology*, **50**(2) (1998), 110–120.
148. B. A. Meyerson & B. Linderoth, Mechanisms of spinal cord stimulation in neuropathic pain. *Neurological Research*, **22**(3) (2000), 285–92.
149. S. H. Kim, R. R. Tasker & M. Y. Oh, Spinal cord stimulation for nonspecific limb pain versus neuropathic pain and spontaneous versus evoked pain. *Neurosurgery*, **48**(5) (2001), 1056–64.
150. R. R. Tasker & O. Vilela Filho, Deep brain stimulation for neuropathic pain. *Stereotactic and Functional Neurosurgery*, **65**(1–4) (1995), 122–4.
151. P. L. Dellemijn, H. L. Fields, R. R. Allen, W. R. McKay & M. C. Rowbotham, The interpretation of pain relief

and sensory changes following sympathetic blockade. *Brain*, **117**(6) (1994), 1475–87.

152. A. Mailis & A. Furlan, Sympathectomy for neuropathic pain (Cochrane review). *Cochrane Database Systematic Reviews*, (2) (2003), CD002918.

153. M. Sindou & P. Mertens, Neurosurgical management of neuropathic pain. *Stereotactic and Functional Neurosurgery*, **75**(2–3) (2000), 76–80.

154. H. L. Fields, Treatment of trigeminal neuralgia. *New England Journal of Medicine*, **334**(17) (1996), 1125–6.

155. C. R. Goucke, The management of persistent pain. *Medical Journal of Australia*, **178**(9) (2003), 444–7.

156. H. Flor, Cortical reorganisation and chronic pain: implications for rehabilitation. *Journal of Rehabilitation Medicine*, **41**(Suppl) (2003), 66–72.

23 • Principles of wound healing

GREGORY S. SCHULTZ, GLORIA A. CHIN, LYLE MOLDAWER AND ROBERT F. DIEGELMANN

INTRODUCTION

Acute wounds normally heal in an orderly and efficient manner. They progress smoothly through the four distinct, but overlapping phases of wound healing: haemostasis, inflammation, proliferation and remodelling (Figure 23.1) [1; 2; 3]. In contrast, chronic wounds will similarly begin the healing process, but will have prolonged inflammatory, proliferative or remodeling phases, resulting in tissue fibrosis and non-healing ulcers [4]. The process of wound healing is complex and involves a variety of specialized cells, such as platelets, macrophages, fibroblasts, and epithelial and endothelial cells. These cells interact with each other and the extracellular matrix. In addition to the various cellular interactions, healing is also influenced by the action of proteins and glycoproteins, such as cytokines, chemokines, growth factors, inhibitors and their receptors. Each stage of wound healing has certain milestones that must occur in order for normal healing to progress. In order to identify the differences inherent in chronic wounds that prevent healing, it is important to review the process of healing in normal wounds.

PHASES OF ACUTE WOUND HEALING

Haemostasis

Haemostasis occurs immediately following an injury [5]. To prevent exsanguination, vasoconstriction occurs and platelets undergo activation, adhesion and aggregation at the site of injury. Platelets become activated when exposed to extravascular collagen (such as type I collagen). They detect this via specific integrin receptors which are cell surface receptors that mediate a cell's interactions with the extracellular matrix. Once in contact with collagen, platelets release the soluble mediators (growth factors and cyclic AMP) and adhesive glycoproteins, which signal them to become sticky and aggregate. The key glycoproteins released from the platelet alpha granules include fibrinogen, fibronectin, thrombospondin and von Willebrand factor. As platelet aggregation proceeds, clotting factors are released resulting in the deposition of a fibrin clot at the site of injury. The fibrin clot serves as a provisional matrix [6]. The aggregated platelets become trapped in the fibrin web and provide the bulk of the clot (Figure 23.2). Their membranes provide a surface on which inactive clotting enzyme proteases are bound, become activated and accelerate the clotting cascade.

Growth factors are also released from the platelet alpha granules, including platelet-derived growth factor (PDGF), transforming growth factor-β (TGFβ), transforming growth factor-α (TGFα), basic fibroblast growth factor (bFGF), insulin-like growth factor-I (IGF-I) and vascular endothelial growth factor (VEGF). Major growth factor families are presented in Table 23.1. Neutrophils and monocytes are then recruited by PDGF and TGFβ from the vasculature to initiate the inflammatory response. A breakdown fragment generated from complement, C5a and a bacterial waste product, f-Met-Leu-Phe, also provide additional chemotactic signals for the recruitment of neutrophils to the site of injury. Meanwhile, endothelial cells are activated by VEGF, TGFα and bFGF to initiate angiogenesis. Fibroblasts are then activated and recruited by PDGF to migrate to the wound site. They also begin production of collagen and glycosaminoglycans, as well as proteins in the extracellular matrix which facilitate cellular migration, and interactions with the matrix supporting framework. Thus, the healing process begins with haemostasis, platelet deposition at the site of injury, and interactions of soluble mediators and growth factors with the extracellular matrix, to set the stage for subsequent healing events [1; 2; 7].

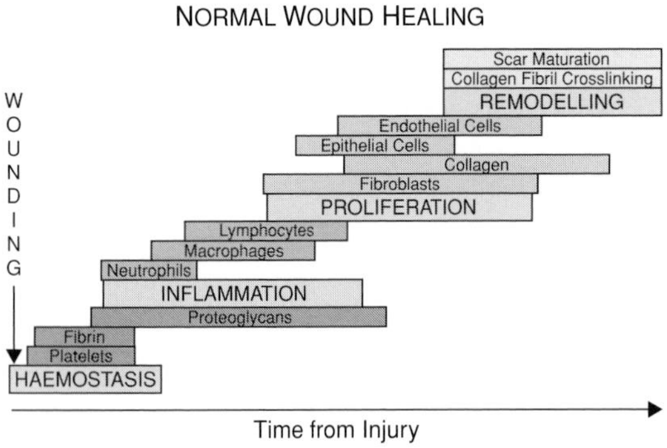

Fig. 23.1. Phase of normal wound healing. Cellular and molecular events during normal wound healing progress through four major, integrated, phases: haemostasis, inflammation, proliferation and remodelling.

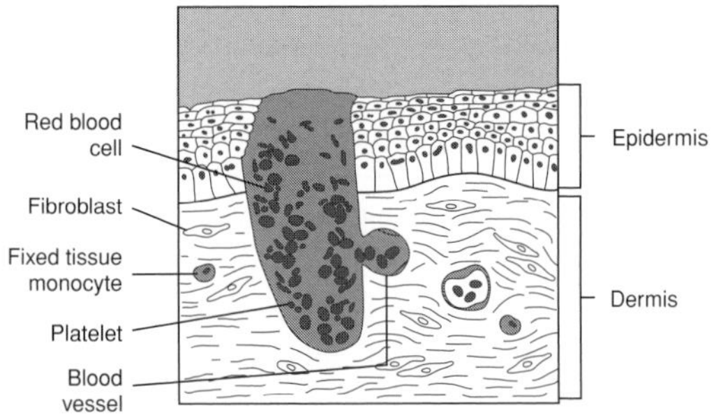

Fig. 23.2. Haemostasis phase. At the time of injury, the fibrin clot forms the provisional wound matrix and platelets release multiple growth factors which initiate the repair process.

Inflammation

Inflammation, the next stage of wound healing occurs within the first 24 hours after injury. It can last for up to two weeks in normal wounds and significantly longer in chronic non-healing wounds (Figure 23.3). Mast cells release granules filled with enzymes, histamine and other active amines. These are responsible for the characteristic signs of inflammation: *rubor* (redness), *calor* (heat), *tumor* (swelling) and *dolor* (pain) around the wound site. Neutrophils, monocytes and macrophages are the key cells during the inflammatory phase. They cleanse the wound of infection and debris, and release soluble mediators such as pro-inflammatory cytokines (including interleukin-1 (IL-1), IL-6, IL-8 and tumour necrosis factor-α (TNFα) and growth factors (such as PDGF, TGFβ, TGFα, IGF-1 and FGF). These are involved in the recruitment and activation of fibroblasts and epithelial cells in preparation for the next phase in healing. Cytokines that play important roles in regulating inflammation in wound healing are described in Table 23.2.

In addition to the growth factors and cytokines, a third important group of small regulatory proteins, listed in Table 23.3, has been identified. They are collectively named chemokines, from a contraction of chemoattractive cytokine(s) [8; 9; 10]. The structural and functional similarities among chemokines were not initially appreciated. This has led to an idiosyncratic nomenclature consisting of many acronyms that were based on their biological functions (e.g. monocyte chemoattractant protein-1 (MCP-1), macrophage inflammatory protein-1 (MIP-1)), their source for isolation (platelet factor-4 (PF-4)) or their biochemical properties (interferon-inducible protein of 10 kDa (IP-10), regulated upon activation normal T cell expressed and secreted (RANTES)). As their biochemical properties were established, it was recognized that the approximately 40 chemokines could be grouped into four major classes based on the pattern of cysteine residues located near the N-terminus. In fact, there has been a recent trend to re-establish a more organized nomenclature system based on these four major classes. In general, chemokines have two primary functions: (1) they regulate the trafficking of leucocyte populations during normal health and development; and (2) they direct the recruitment and activation of neutrophils, lymphocytes, macrophages, eosinophils and basophils during inflammation.

Neutrophils

Neutrophils are the first inflammatory cells to respond to the soluble mediators released by platelets and the coagulation cascade. They serve as the first line of defence against infection by phagocytosing and killing bacteria, and by removing foreign materials and devitalized tissue. During the process of extravasation of inflammatory cells into a wound, important interactions occur between adhesion molecules (selectins, cell adhesion molecules (CAMs) and cadherins) and receptors (integrins) that are associated with the plasma membranes of circulating leucocytes and vascular endothelial cells [11; 12]. Initially, leucocytes weakly adhere

Table 23.1. *Major growth factor families*

Growth factor family	Cell source	Actions
Transforming growth factor: TGFβ-1, TGFβ-2	Platelets, fibroblasts, macrophages	Fibroblast chemotaxis and activation ECM deposition collagen synthesis TIMP synthesis MMP synthesis
TGFβ-2		Reduces scarring collagen fibronectin
Platelet-derived growth factor: PDGF-AA, PDGF-BB, VEGF	Platelets, macrophages, keratinocytes, fibroblasts	Activation of immune cells and fibroblasts, ECM deposition collagen synthesis TIMP synthesis MMP synthesis Angiogenesis
Fibroblast growth factor: acidic FGF, basic KGF	Macrophages, endothelial cells, fibroblasts	Angiogenesis, endothelial cell activation keratinocyte proliferation and migration, ECM deposition
Insulin-like growth factor: IGF-I, IGF-II, insulin	Liver skeletal muscle, fibroblasts, macrophages, neutrophils	Keratinocyte proliferation, fibroblast proliferation, endothelial cell activation, angiogenesis, collagen synthesis, ECM deposition, cell metabolism
Epidermal growth factor: EGF, HB-EGF, TGF-α, amphiregulin, betacellulin	Keratinocytes, macrophages	Keratinocyte proliferation and migration, ECM deposition
Connective tissue growth factor: CTGF	Fibroblasts, endothelial cells, epithelial cells	Mediates action of TGFβs on collagen synthesis

KGF = keratinocyte growth factor; ECM = extracellular matrix; TIMP = tissue inhibitor of matrix metalloproteinases; MMP = matrix metalloproteinases

to endothelial cells via their selectin molecules which causes them to decelerate and begin to roll on the surface of endothelial cells. While rolling, leucocytes can become activated by chemoattractants (cytokines, growth factors or bacterial products). After activation, leucocytes firmly adhere to endothelial cells as a result of the binding between their integrin receptors and ligands, such as vascular cell adhesion molecule (VCAM) and intercellular adhesion molecule (ICAM), that are expressed on activated endothelial cells. Chemotactic signals present outside the venule and then induce leucocytes to squeeze between endothelial cells of the venule. They then migrate into the wounded tissue using their integrin receptors to recognize and bind to extracellular matrix components. The inflammatory cells release elastase and collagenase to help them migrate through the endothelial cell basement membrane, and to migrate into the extracellular matrix at the site of the wound. Neutrophils also produce and release inflammatory mediators, such as TNFα and IL-1, that further recruit and activate fibroblasts and epithelial cells. After the neutrophils migrate into the wound site, they generate oxygen free radicals which kill phagocytized bacteria. They release high levels of proteases (neutrophil

Table 23.2. *Cytokines involved in wound healing*

Cytokine	Cell source	Biological activity
Pro-inflammatory cytokines		
TNF-α	Macrophages	PMN margination and cytotoxicity, ± collagen synthesis; provides metabolic substrate
IL-1	Macrophages, keratinocytes	Fibroblast and keratinocyte chemotaxis, collagen synthesis
IL-2	T lymphocytes	Increases fibroblast infiltration and metabolism
IL-6	Macrophages, PMNs fibroblasts	Fibroblast proliferation, hepatic acute-phase protein synthesis
IL-8	Macrophages, fibroblasts	Macrophage and PMN chemotaxis, keratinocyte maturation
IFN-γ	T lymphocytes, macrophages	Macrophage and PMN activation; retards collagen synthesis and cross-linking; stimulates collagenase activity
Anti-inflammatory cytokines		
IL-4	T lymphocytes, basophils, mast cells	Inhibition of TNF, IL-1, IL-6 production; fibroblast proliferation, collagen synthesis
IL-10	T lymphocytes, macrophages, keratinocytes	Inhibition of TNF, IL-1, IL-6 production; inhibits macrophage and PMN activation

PMN = polymorphonuclear leucocytes

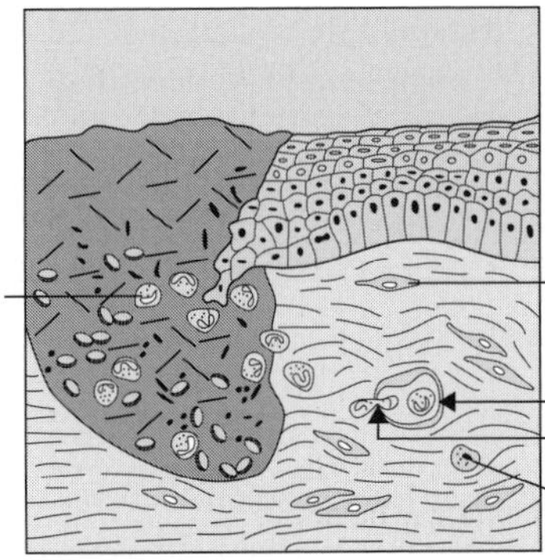

Fig. 23.3. Inflammation phase. Within a day following injury, the inflammatory phase is initiated by neutrophils that attach to endothelial cells in the vessel walls surrounding the wound (margination), change shape and move through the cell junctions (diapedesis) and migrate to the wound site (chemotaxis).

elastase and neutrophil collagenase) which remove components of the extracellular matrix that were damaged by the injury. The persistent presence of bacteria in a wound may contribute to chronicity through continued recruitment of neutrophils and their release of proteases, cytokines and reactive oxygen species. Usually neutrophils are depleted in the wound after two to three days by the process of apoptosis and they are replaced by tissue monocytes.

Macrophages

Activated macrophages play pivotal roles in the regulation of healing and the healing process does not proceed normally without macrophages. Macrophages begin as circulating monocytes that are attracted to the wound site beginning about 24 hours after injury (Figure 23.4). They extravasate by the mechanism described for neutrophils, and are stimulated to differentiate into activated tissue macrophages in response to chemokines, cytokines, growth factors and soluble fragments of extracellular matrix components produced by proteolytic degradation of collagen and fibronectin [13]. Similar to neutrophils, tissue macrophages have a dual role in the healing process. They patrol the wound area ingesting and killing bacteria, and removing devitalized tissue through the actions of secreted matrix metalloproteinases (MMPs) and elastase. Macrophages differ

Table 23.3. *Chemokine families involved in wound healing.*

Chemokines	Cells affected
α-Chemokines (α-CXC)	Neutrophils
with glutamic acid-leucine-arginine near the N-terminal	
Interleukin-8 (IL-8)	
α-Chemokines (α-CXC)	
without glutamic acid-leucine-arginine near the N-terminal	Activated T lymphocytes
Interferon-inducible protein of 10 kDa (IP-10)	
Monokine induced by interferon-gamma (MIG)	
Stromal-cell-derived factor-1 (SDF-1)	
β-Chemokines (β-CC)	
Monocyte chemoattractant proteins (MCPs): MCP-1, 2, 3, 4, 5	Eosinophils, basophils, monocytes, activated T lymphocytes
Regulated upon activation normal T cell expressed and secreted (RANTES)	
Macrophage inflammatory protein (MIP-1)	
Eotaxin	
γ-Chemokines (γ-C)	Resting T lymphocytes
Lymphotactin	
δ-Chemokines (δ-CXXXC)	
Fractalkine	Natural killer cells

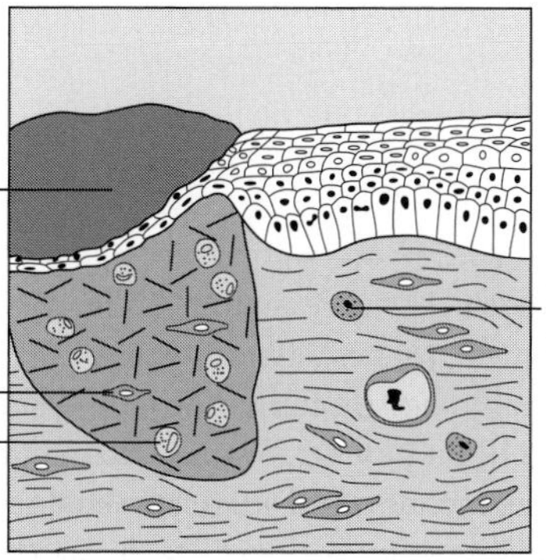

Fig. 23.4. Proliferation phase. Fixed tissue monocytes activate and move into the site of injury. They transform into activated wound macrophages that kill bacteria and release proteases that remove denatured extracellular matrix. They also secrete growth factors that stimulate fibroblasts, epidermal cells and endothelial cells to proliferate, and produce scar tissue.

from neutrophils in their ability to more closely regulate the proteolytic destruction of wound tissue by secreting inhibitors for the proteases. As important as their phagocytic role, macrophages also mediate the transition from the inflammatory phase to the proliferative phase of healing. They release a wide variety of growth factors and cytokines including PDGF, TGFβ, TGFα, FGF, IGF-1, TNFα, IL-1 and IL-6. Some of these soluble mediators recruit and activate fibroblasts, which will then synthesize, deposit and organize the new tissue matrix, while others promote angiogenesis. The absence of neutrophils and a decrease in the number of macrophages in the wound is an indication that the inflammatory phase is nearing an end and that the proliferative phase is beginning.

Proliferative phase

The milestones during the proliferative phase include replacement of the provisional fibrin matrix with a new matrix of collagen fibres, proteoglycans and fibronectin to restore the structure and function to the tissue. Another important event in healing is angiogenesis, the in-growth of new capillaries to replace the previously damaged vessels and restore circulation. Other significant events in this phase of healing are the formation of granulation tissue and epithelialization. Fibroblasts are the key cells in the proliferative phase of healing.

Fibroblast migration

Fibroblasts migrate into the wound in response to multiple soluble mediators released initially by platelets and later by macrophages (Figure 23.4). Fibroblast migration in the extracellular matrix depends on precise recognition and interaction with specific components of the matrix. Fibroblasts in normal dermis are typically quiescent and sparsely distributed, whereas in the provisional matrix of the wound site and in the granulation tissue, they are quite active and numerous. Their migration and accumulation in the wound site requires them to change their morphology, as well as to produce and secrete proteases to clear a path for their movement from the extracellular matrix into the wound site.

Fibroblasts begin moving by first binding to matrix components such as fibronectin, vitronectin and fibrin via their integrin receptors. Integrin receptors attach to specific amino acid sequences (such as R-G-D or arginine-glycine-aspartic acid) or binding sites in these matrix components. While one end of the fibroblast remains bound to the matrix component, the cell extends a cytoplasmic projection to find another binding site. When the next site is found, the original site is released (apparently by local protease activity) and the cell uses its cytoskeleton network of actin fibers to pull itself forward.

The direction of fibroblast movement is determined by the concentration gradient of chemotactic growth factors, cytokines and chemokines, and by the alignment of the fibrils in the extracellular matrix and provisional matrix. Fibroblasts tend to migrate along these fibrils as opposed to across them. Fibroblasts secrete proteolytic enzymes locally to facilitate their forward motion through the matrix. The enzymes secreted by the fibroblasts include three types of MMPs, collagenase (MMP1), gelatinases (MMP2 and MMP9) which degrade gelatin substrates, and stromelysin (MMP3) which has multiple protein substrates in the extracellular matrix.

Collagen and extracellular matrix production

The collagen, proteoglycans and other components that comprise granulation tissue are synthesized and deposited primarily by fibroblasts. Platelet-derived growth factor and TGFβ are two of the most important growth factors that regulate fibroblast activity. Platelet-derived growth factor, which predominantly originates from platelets and macrophages, stimulates a number of fibroblast functions, including proliferation, chemotaxis and collagenase expression. Transforming growth factor-β, also secreted by platelets and macrophages, is considered to be the master control signal that regulates extracellular matrix deposition. Through the stimulation of gene transcription for collagen, proteoglycans and fibronectin, TGFβ increases the overall production of matrix proteins. At the same time, TGFβ down-regulates the secretion of proteases responsible for matrix degradation, and stimulates the synthesis of tissue inhibitors of metalloproteinases (TIMPs), to further inhibit breakdown of the matrix. Recent data indicate that a new growth factor, named connective tissue growth factor (CTGF), mediates many of the effects of TGFβ on the synthesis of extracellular matrix [14].

Once the fibroblasts have migrated into the matrix they again change their morphology, settle down and begin to proliferate, as well as to synthesize granulation tissue components including collagen, elastin and proteoglycans. Fibroblasts attach to the cables of the provisional fibrin matrix and begin to produce collagen. At least 20 individual types of collagen have been identified to date. Type III collagen is initially synthesized at high levels, along with other extracellular matrix proteins and proteoglycans. After transcription and processing of the collagen mRNA, it is attached to polyribosomes on the endoplasmic reticulum where the new collagen chains are produced. During this process, there is an important step involving hydroxylation of proline and lysine residues. Three protein chains associate and begin to form the characteristic triple helical structure of the fibrillar collagen molecule. The nascent chains undergo further modification by the process of glycosylation. Hydroxyproline in collagen is important because it plays a major role in stabilizing the triple helical conformation of collagen molecules. Fully hydroxylated collagen has a higher melting temperature. When levels of hydroxyproline are low, for example, in vitamin C-deficient conditions (scurvy), the collagen triple helix has an altered structure and denatures (unwinds) much more rapidly at lower temperatures. To ensure optimal wound healing, wound care specialists should be sure patients are receiving good nutritional support in the form of a diet with ample protein and vitamin C.

Finally, procollagen molecules are secreted into the extracellular space where they undergo further processing by proteolytic cleavage of the short, non-helical segments at the N- and C-termini. The collagen molecules then spontaneously associate in a head-to-tail and side-by-side arrangement forming collagen fibrils, which associate into larger bundles that form collagen fibres. In the extracellular spaces an important enzyme, lysyl oxidase, acts on the collagen molecules to form stable, covalent cross-links. As the collagen matures and becomes older, more and more of these intramolecular and intermolecular cross-links are placed in the molecules. This important cross-linking step gives collagen its strength and stability, and the older the collagen the more cross-link formation has occurred.

Dermal collagen on a per weight basis approaches the tensile strength of steel. In normal tissue, it is a strong molecule and highly organized. In contrast, collagen fibres formed in scar tissue are much smaller and have a random appearance. Scar tissue is always weaker and will break apart before the surrounding normal tissue.

Angiogenesis

Damaged vasculature must be replaced to maintain tissue viability. The process of angiogenesis is stimulated by local factors in the microenvironment, including low oxygen tension, low pH and high lactate levels [15]. Also, certain soluble mediators are potent angiogenic signals for endothelial cells. Many of these are produced by epidermal cells, fibroblasts, vascular endothelial cells and macrophages, and include bFGF, TGFβ and VEGF. It is now recognized that oxygen levels in tissues directly regulate angiogenesis by interacting with oxygen sensing proteins that regulate transcription of angiogenic and anti-angiogenic genes. For example, synthesis of VEGF by capillary endothelial cells is directly increased by hypoxia through activation of the recently identified transcription factor, hypoxia-inducible factor (HIF), which binds oxygen [16]. When oxygen levels surrounding capillary endothelial cells drop, levels of HIF increase inside the cells. Hypoxia-inducible factor-1 binds to specific DNA sequences and stimulates transcription of specific genes such as VEGF that promote angiogenesis. When oxygen levels in wound tissue increase, oxygen binds to HIF, leading to the destruction of HIF molecules in cells and decreased synthesis of angiogenic factors. Regulation of angiogenesis involves both stimulatory factors like VEGF and anti-angiogenic factors like angiostatin, endostatin, thrombospondin and pigment epithelium-derived factor (PEDF).

Binding of angiogenic factors causes endothelial cells of the capillaries adjacent to the devascularized site to begin to migrate into the matrix and then proliferate to form buds or sprouts. Once again the migration of these cells into the matrix requires the local secretion of proteolytic enzymes, especially MMPs. As the tip of the sprouts extend from endothelial cells and encounter another sprout, they develop a cleft that subsequently becomes the lumen of the evolving vessel and complete a new vascular loop. This process continues until the capillary system is sufficiently repaired, and the tissue oxygenation and metabolic needs are met. It is these new capillary tufts that give granulation tissue its characteristic bumpy or granular appearance.

Granulation

Granulation tissue is a transitional replacement for normal dermis, which eventually matures into a scar during the remodelling phase of healing. It is characterized from unwounded dermis by an extremely dense network of blood vessels and capillaries, an elevated cellular density of fibroblasts and macrophages, and randomly organized collagen fibres. It also has an elevated metabolic rate compared to normal dermis, which reflects the activity required for cellular migration and division, and protein synthesis.

Epithelialization

All dermal wounds heal by three basic mechanisms: contraction, connective tissue matrix deposition and epithelialization. Wounds that remain open heal by contraction; the interaction between cells and matrix results in the movement of tissue toward the centre of the wound. As previously described, matrix deposition is the process by which collagen, proteoglycans and attachment proteins are deposited to form a new extracellular matrix. Epithelialization is the process where epithelial cells around the margin of the wound or in residual skin appendages such as hair follicles and sebaceous glands lose contact inhibition. Then by the process of epiboly begin to migrate into the wound area. As migration proceeds, cells in the basal layers begin to proliferate to provide additional epithelial cells.

Epithelialization is a multi-step process that involves epithelial cell detachment, and change in their internal structure, migration, proliferation and differentiation [17]. The intact mature epidermis consists of five layers of differentiated epithelial cells, ranging from the cuboidal basal keratinocytes nearest the dermis, up to the flattened, hexagonal, tough keratinocytes in the uppermost layer. Only the basal epithelial cells are capable of proliferation. These basal cells are normally attached to their neighbouring cells by intercellular connectors called desmosomes and to the basement membrane by hemi-desmosomes. When growth factors, such as EGF, keratinocyte growth factor (KGF) and TGFα, are released during the healing process, they bind to receptors on these epithelial cells, and stimulate migration and proliferation. The binding of the growth factors triggers the desmosomes and hemi-desmosomes to dissolve so the cells can detach in preparation for migration. Integrin receptors are then expressed and the normally cuboidal basal epithelial cells flatten in shape and begin to migrate as a monolayer over the newly deposited granulation tissue, following along collagen fibres. Proliferation of the basal epithelial cells near the wound margin supply new cells to the advancing monolayer apron of cells (cells that are actively migrating are incapable of proliferation). Epithelial cells in the leading edge of the monolayer produce and secrete proteolytic enzymes (MMPs), which enable the cells to penetrate scab, surface necrosis or eschar. Migration continues until the epithelial cells contact other advancing cells to form a confluent sheet. Once this contact has been made, the entire epithelial monolayer enters a proliferative mode, and the stratified layers of the epidermis are re-established and begin to mature to restore barrier function. Transforming growth factor-β is one growth factor that can speed up the maturation (differentiation and keratinization) of the epidermal layers. The intercellular desmosomes and hemi-desmosome attachments to the newly formed basement membrane are also re-established. Epithelialization is the clinical hallmark of healing but it is not the final event – remodelling of the granulation tissue is yet to occur.

Remodelling

Remodelling is the final phase of the healing process in which the granulation tissue matures into scar, and tissue tensile strength is increased (Figure 23.5). The maturation of granulation tissue also involves a reduction in the number of capillaries via aggregation into larger vessels. In addition it involves a decrease in the amount of glycosaminoglycans, and the water associated with the glycosaminoglycans and proteoglycans. Cell density and metabolic activity in the granulation tissue decrease during maturation. Changes also occur in the type, amount and organization of collagen, which enhance tensile strength. Initially, type III collagen is synthesized at high levels, but it becomes replaced by type I collagen, the dominant fibrillar collagen in skin. The tensile strength of a newly epithelialized wound is only about 25% of normal tissue. Healed or repaired tissue is never as strong as normal tissues that have never been wounded. Tissue tensile strength is enhanced primarily by the reorganization of collagen fibres that were deposited randomly during granulation and increased covalent cross-linking of collagen molecules by the enzyme, lysyl oxidase, which is secreted into the extracellular matrix by fibroblasts. Over several months or more, changes in collagen organization in the repaired tissue slowly increases the tensile strength to a maximum of about 80% of normal tissue.

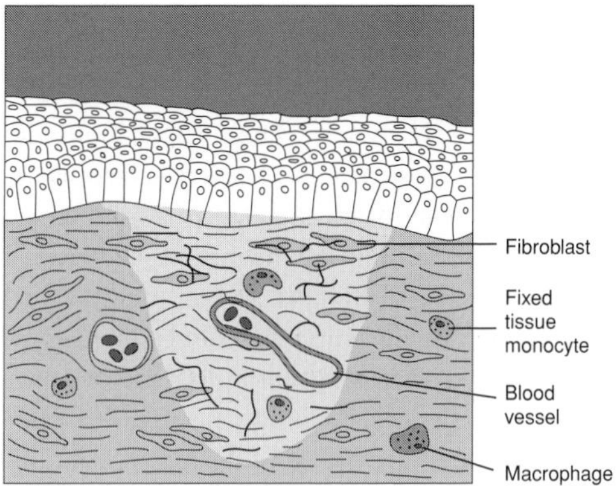

Fig. 23.5. Remodelling phase. This initial, disorganized scar tissue is slowly replaced by a matrix that more closely resembles the organized extracellular matrix of normal skin.

Remodelling of the extracellular matrix proteins occurs through the actions of several different classes of proteolytic enzymes produced by cells in the wound bed at different times during the healing process. Two of the most important families are MMPs and serine proteases. Specific MMP proteases that are necessary for wound healing are the collagenases (which degrade intact fibrillar collagen molecules), gelatinases (which degrade damaged fibrillar collagen molecules) and stromelysins (which very effectively degrade proteoglycans). An important serine protease is neutrophil elastase which can degrade almost all types of protein molecules. Under normal conditions, the destructive actions of the proteolytic enzymes are tightly regulated by specific enzyme inhibitors, which are also produced by cells in the wound bed. The specific inhibitors of MMPs are TIMPs and specific inhibitors of serine protease are α 1-protease inhibitor (α 1PI) and α 2 macroglobulin.

Summary of acute wound healing

Four phases of wound healing:

- Haemostasis – establishes the fibrin provisional wound matrix, and platelets provide the initial release of cytokines and growth factors in the wound.
- Inflammation – mediated by neutrophils and macrophages that remove bacteria and denatured matrix components that retard healing, and are the second source of growth factors and cytokines. Prolonged, elevated inflammation retards healing due to excessive levels of proteases and reactive oxygen that destroy essential factors.
- Proliferation – fibroblasts, supported by new capillaries, proliferate and synthesize disorganized extracellular matrix. Basal epithelial cells proliferate and migrate over the granulation tissue to close the wound surface.
- Remodelling – fibroblast and capillary density decreases, and initial scar tissue is removed and replaced by extracellular matrix that is more similar to normal skin. Extracellular matrix remodelling is the result of the balanced, regulated activity of proteases.

Cellular functions during the different phases of wound healing are regulated by key cytokines, chemokines and growth factors. Cell actions are also influenced by interaction with components of the extracellular matrix through their integrin receptors and adhesion molecules. Matrix metalloproteinases produced by epidermal cells, fibroblasts and vascular endothelial cells assist in migration of the cells. Also proteolytic enzymes produced by neutrophils and macrophages remove denatured extracellular matrix components and assist in remodelling of initial scar tissue.

COMPARISON OF ACUTE AND CHRONIC WOUNDS

Normal and pathological responses to injury

Pathological responses to injury can result in non-healing wounds (ulcers), inadequately healing wounds (dehiscence) or excessively healing wounds (hypertrophic scars and keloids). Normal repair is the response that re-establishes a functional equilibrium between scar formation and scar remodelling, and is the typical response that most humans experience following injury. The pathological responses to tissue injury stand in sharp contrast to the normal repair response. In excessive healing there is too much deposition of connective tissue that results in altered structure, and thus, loss of function. Fibrosis, strictures, adhesions, keloids, hypertrophic scars and contractures are examples of excessive healing. Contraction is part of the normal process of healing, but if excessive it becomes pathologic and is known as a contracture. Deficient healing is the opposite of fibrosis. It occurs when there is insufficient deposition of connective tissue matrix and the tissue is weakened to the point where scars fall apart under minimal tension. Chronic non-healing ulcers are examples of severely deficient healing.

Biochemical differences in the molecular environments of healing and chronic wounds

The healing process in chronic wounds is generally prolonged, incomplete and unco-ordinated, resulting in a poor anatomic and functional outcome. Chronic, non-healing ulcers are a prime clinical example of the importance of the wound cytokine profile and the critical balance necessary for normal healing to proceed. Since cytokines, growth factors, proteases and endocrine hormones play key roles in regulating acute wound healing, it is reasonable to hypothesize that alterations in the actions of these molecules could contribute to the failure of wounds to heal normally. Several methods are used to assess differences in molecular environments of healing and chronic wounds. Messenger ribonucleic acid (mRNA) and protein levels can be measured in homogenates of wound biopsies. The proteins in wounds can be immunolocalized in histological sections of biopsies. Wound fluids collected from acute surgical wounds and chronic skin ulcers are used to analyse the molecular environment of healing and chronic wounds. From these studies, several important concepts have emerged from the molecular analyses of acute and chronic wound environments.

The first major concept to emerge from analysis of wound fluids is that the molecular environments of chronic wounds have reduced mitogenic activity compared with the environments of acute wounds [4]. Fluids collected from acute mastectomy wounds when added to cultures of normal human skin fibroblasts, keratinocytes or vascular endothelial cells, consistently stimulated DNA synthesis of the cultured cells. In contrast, addition of fluids collected from chronic leg ulcers typically did not stimulate DNA synthesis of the cells in culture. Also, when acute and chronic wound fluids were combined the mitotic activity of acute wound fluids was inhibited. Similar results were reported by several groups of investigators who also found that acute wound fluids promoted DNA synthesis while chronic wound fluids did not stimulate cell proliferation [18; 19; 20].

The second major concept to emerge from wound fluid analysis is the elevated levels of pro-inflammatory cytokines observed in chronic wounds as compared with the molecular environment of acute wounds. The ratios of two key inflammatory cytokines, TNFα and IL-1β, and their natural inhibitors, P55 and IL-1 receptor antagonist, in mastectomy fluids were significantly higher in mastectomy wound fluids than in chronic wound fluids. Trengove and colleagues also reported high levels of the inflammatory cytokines IL-1, IL-6 and TNFα in fluids collected from venous ulcers of patients admitted to the hospital [21]. More importantly, levels of the cytokines significantly decreased in fluids collected two weeks after the chronic ulcers had begun to heal. Harris and colleagues also found cytokine levels were generally higher in wound fluids from non-healing ulcers than healing ulcers [20]. These data suggest that chronic wounds typically have elevated levels of pro-inflammatory cytokines and that the molecular environment changes to a less pro-inflammatory cytokine environment as chronic wounds begin to heal.

The third important concept that emerged from wound fluid analysis was the elevated levels of protease activity in chronic wounds compared to acute wounds [4; 22; 23]. For example, the average level of protease activity in mastectomy fluids determined using the general MMP substrate, azocoll, was low (0.75 μg collagenase equivalents/ml, $n = 20$) with a range of 0.1 to 1.3 μg collagenase equivalents/ml [24]. This suggests that protease activity is tightly controlled during the early phase of wound healing. In contrast, the average level of protease activity in chronic wound fluids (87 μg collagenase equivalents/ml, $n = 32$) was approximately 116-fold higher ($p < 0.05$) than in mastectomy fluids. Also, the range of protease activity in chronic wound fluids is rather large (from 1 to 584 μg collagenase equivalents/ml). More importantly, the levels of protease activity decrease in chronic venous ulcers two weeks after the ulcers begin to heal [24]. Yager and colleagues also found 10-fold higher levels of MMP2 protein, 25-fold higher levels of MMP9 protein and 10-fold higher collagenase activity in fluids from pressure ulcers compared with surgical wound fluids, using gelatin zymography and cleavage of a radioactive collagen substrate [25]. Other studies using immunohistochemical localization observed elevated levels of MMPs in granulation tissue of pressure ulcers, along with elevated levels of neutrophil elastase and cathepsin-G [26]. Tissue inhibitor of matrix metalloproteinases-1 levels were found to be decreased while MMP2 and MMP9 levels were increased in fluids from chronic venous ulcers compared with mastectomy wound fluids [27]. Recently, Ladwig and colleagues reported that the ratio of active MMP9/TIMP-1 was closely correlated with

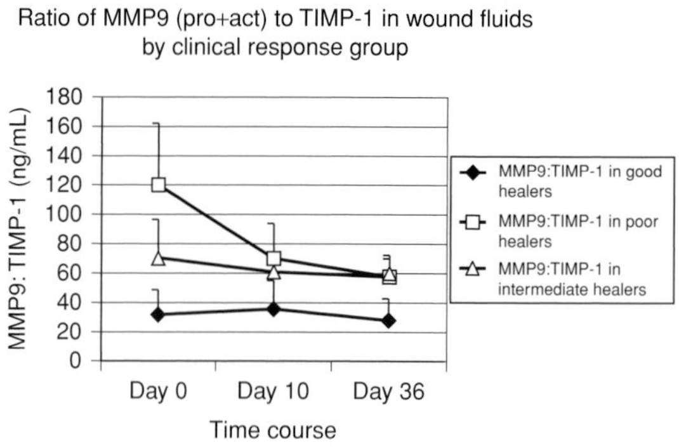

Fig. 23.6. Low protease/inhibitor ratios correlate with healing. Low values of the MMP9/TIMP-1 ratio in wound fluids from patients with chronic pressure ulcers correlate with healing of chronic pressure ulcers over 36 days of treatment. This supports the concept that high protease/inhibitor ratios prevent healing of chronic wounds.

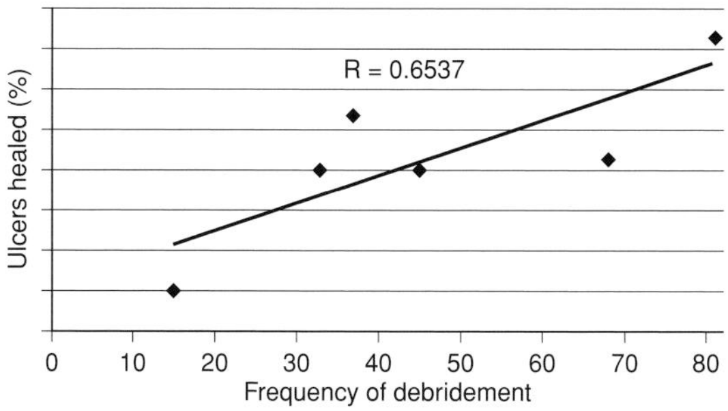

Fig. 23.7. Frequency of wound debridement correlates with improved healing. There was a strong correlation between the frequency of debridement and healing of chronic diabetic foot ulcers. This supports the concept that the abnormal cellular and molecular environment of chronic wounds impairs healing.

healing outcome of pressure ulcers, treated by a variety of protocols (Figure 23.6) [28].

It is interesting to note that the major collagenase found in non-healing chronic pressure ulcers was MMP8, the neutrophil-derived collagenase. Thus, the persistent influx of neutrophils releasing MMP8 and elastase appears to be a major underlying mechanism resulting in tissue and growth factor destruction, and thus impaired healing. This suggests that chronic inflammation must decrease if pressure ulcers are to heal.

Other classes of proteases also appear to be elevated in chronic wound fluids. It has been reported that fluids from skin graft donor sites or breast surgery patients contained: intact α1-antitrypsin, a potent inhibitor of serine proteases; very low levels of neutrophil elastase activity; and intact fibronectin [29]. In contrast, fluids from the chronic venous ulcers contained degraded α1-antitrypsin, as well as 10–40-fold higher levels of neutrophil elastase activity, and degraded fibronectin. Chronic leg ulcers were found to contain elevated MMP2 and MMP9. Also fibronectin degradation in chronic wounds was dependent on the relative levels of elastase, α 1PI and α 2 macroglobulin [30; 31].

Besides being implicated in degrading essential extracellular matrix components like fibronectin, proteases in chronic wound fluids also have been reported to degrade exogenous growth factors *in vitro* such as EGF, TGFα or PDGF [1; 24; 32; 33]. In contrast, exogenous growth factors were stable in acute surgical wound fluids *in vitro*. Supporting this general concept of increased degradation of endogenous growth factors by proteases in chronic wounds, the average immunoreactive levels of some growth factors such as EGF, TGFβ and PDGF were found to be lower in chronic wound fluids than in acute wound fluids. However, PDGF-AB, TGFα and IGF-1 were not lower [32; 34].

In general, these results suggest that many chronic wounds contain elevated MMP and neutrophil elastase activities. The physiological implications of these data are that elevated protease activities in some chronic wounds may directly contribute to the failure of wounds to heal. This occurs by degrading proteins which are necessary for wound healing, such as extracellular matrix proteins, growth factors, their receptors and protease inhibitors. Interestingly, Steed and colleagues [35] reported that extensive debridement of diabetic foot ulcers improved healing in patients treated with placebo or with recombinant human PDGF (Figure 23.7). It is likely that frequent sharp debridement of diabetic ulcers helps to convert the detrimental molecular environment of a chronic wound into a pseudo-acute wound molecular environment.

Biological differences in the response of chronic wound cells to growth factors

The biochemical analyses of healing and chronic wound fluids, and biopsies have suggested that there are important molecular differences in the wound environments. However, these data only indicate half of the picture. The other essential component is the capacity of the wound cells to respond to cytokines and growth factors. Interesting new data are emerging suggesting that fibroblasts in skin ulcers which have failed to heal for many years, may not be capable of responding to growth factors and divide as fibroblasts in healing wounds. Ågren and colleagues [36] reported that fibroblasts from chronic venous leg ulcers grew to a lower density than fibroblasts from acute wounds from uninjured dermis. Also, fibroblasts from venous leg ulcers that had been present more than three years, grew slowly and responded poorly to PDGF compared with fibroblasts from venous ulcers that had been present for less than three years. These results suggest that fibroblasts in ulcers of long duration may approach senescence and have a decreased response to exogenous growth factors.

FROM BENCH TO BEDSIDE

Role of endocrine hormones in the regulation of wound healing

Classical endocrine hormones are molecules that are synthesized by a specialized tissue and secreted into the bloodstream. They are then carried to distant target tissue where they interact with specific cellular receptor proteins and influence the expression of genes that ultimately regulate the physiological actions of the target cell. It has been known for decades that alterations in endocrine hormones can alter wound healing. Diabetic patients frequently develop chronic wounds due to multiple direct and indirect effects of the inadequate insulin action on wound healing. Patients receiving anti-inflammatory glucocorticoids for extended periods are also at risk of developing impaired wound healing due to the direct suppression of collagen synthesis in fibroblasts and the extended suppression of inflammatory cell function. The association of oestrogen with healing was recently reported by Ashcroft and colleagues [37] when they observed that healing of skin biopsy sites in healthy, postmenopausal women was significantly slower than in healthy premenopausal women. Molecular analyses of the wound sites indicated that TGFβ protein and mRNA levels were dramatically reduced in postmenopausal women in comparison to sites from premenopausal women. However, the rate of healing of wounds in postmenopausal women taking oestrogen replacement therapy occurred as rapidly as in premenopausal women. Furthermore, molecular analyses of wounds in postmenopausal women treated with oestrogen replacement therapy demonstrated elevated levels of TGFβ protein and mRNA that were similar to levels in wounds from premenopausal women. Aging was also associated with elevated levels of MMPs and decreased levels of TIMPs in skin wounds, which were reversed by oestrogen treatment [38; 39]. The beneficial effects of oestrogen on wound healing could be achieved with topical oestrogen and were also observed in healthy older men [40]. These data indicate the significant interactions that can occur between endocrine hormones and growth factors in the regulation of wound healing.

Molecular basis of chronic non-healing wounds

Conditions that promote chronic wounds are repeated trauma, foreign bodies, pressure necrosis, infection, ischaemia and tissue hypoxia. These wounds share a chronic inflammatory state characterized by an increased number of neutrophils, macrophages and lymphocytes, which produce inflammatory cytokines, such as TNFα, IL-1 and IL-6. *In vitro* studies have shown that TNFα and IL-1 increase the expression of MMPs and down-regulate the expression of tissue inhibitors of matrix metalloproteinases (TIMPs) in a variety of cells, including macrophages, fibroblasts, keratinocytes and endothelial cells. All MMPs are synthesized as inactive proenzymes and they are activated by proteolytic cleavage of the pro-MMP. Serine proteases, such as plasmin, as well as the membrane type MMPs can activate MMPs. Another serine protease, neutrophil elastase, is also present in increased concentrations in chronic wounds. It is very important in directly destroying extracellular matrix components and in destroying the TIMPs, which indirectly increases the destructive activity of MMPs [4; 22; 25; 33]. Thus, the general molecular profile that appears in various types of chronic ulcers is: (1) increased levels of inflammatory cytokines which leads to; (2) increased levels of proteases and decreased levels of protease inhibitors which; (3) degrade molecules that are essential for healing, including growth factors, their receptors and extracellular matrix proteins which; (4) prevents wounds from healing normally. Nwomeh and colleagues [23] further describe this common pathway of chronic wounds as a self-perpetuating environment in which chronic inflammation produces elevated levels of reactive oxygen species and degradative enzymes. These eventually exceed their beneficial actions of destroying bacteria and debriding the wound bed, and produce destructive effects that help to establishs a chronic wound.

Based on these biochemical analyses of the molecular environment of acute and chronic human wounds, it is possible to propose a general model of differences between healing and chronic wounds. As shown in Figure 23.8, the molecular environment of healing wounds promotes mitosis of cells, has low levels of inflammatory cytokines and proteases, and high levels of growth factors and cells capable of rapid division. In contrast, the molecular environment of chronic wounds does not promote mitosis of cells, has elevated levels of inflammatory cytokines and proteases, and low levels of growth factors and cells that are approaching senescence [21; 24; 41]. If these general concepts are correct, then it may be possible to develop new treatment

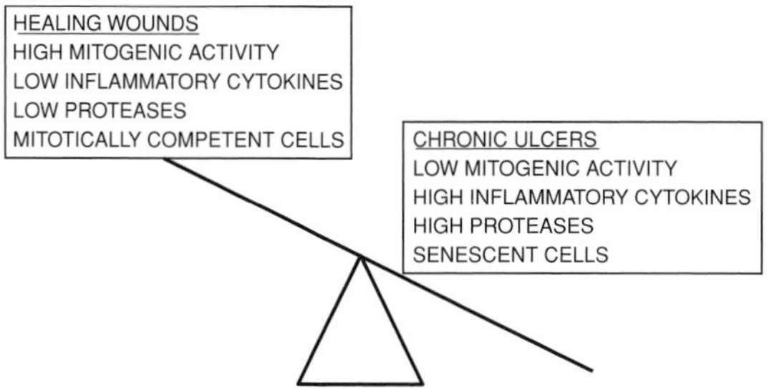

Fig. 23.8. Comparison of the molecular and cellular environments of healing and chronic wounds. Elevated levels of cytokines and the proteases in chronic wounds reduce mitogenic activities and the response of wound cells, impairing healing.

strategies which would re-establish in chronic wounds the balance of cytokines, growth factors, proteases, their natural inhibitors and competent cells found in healing wounds.

Chronic venous stasis ulcers

Mechanisms involved in the creation and perpetuation of chronic wounds are varied, and depend on the individual wounds. In general, the inability of chronic venous stasis ulcers to heal appears to be related to impairment in wound epithelialization. The wound edges show a hyperproliferative epidermis under microscopy, even though further immunohistochemical studies reveal optimal conditions for keratinocyte recruitment, proliferation and differentiation. The extracellular matrix and expression of integrin receptors by keratinocytes that allow it to translocate, play an important regulatory role in epithelialization. After receiving the signal to migrate, epidermal cells begin by disassembling their attachments from basement membrane and neighbouring cells. They then travel over a provisional matrix containing fibrinogen, fibronectin, vitronectin and tenascin, and stop when they encounter laminin. During this process, keratinocytes produce fibronectin and continue to do so until the epithelial cells contact, at which time they again begin manufacturing laminin to regenerate the basement membrane.

There is evidence that the interaction between integrin receptors on keratinocytes with the extracellular matrix transforms resting cells to a migratory phenotype. Integral in this transformation is the alteration in the pattern of integrin receptors expressed. After epithelialization is completed, integrin expression reverts back to the resting pattern. To further complicate this process, growth factors are involved in mediating keratinocyte activation, integrin expression and alterations in the matrix. Growth factors are able to differentially affect these processes, for example, TGFβ is able to promote epithelial migration while inhibiting proliferation. Although TGFβ induces the necessary integrin expression for migration, the cells behind those at the leading edge have little proliferative ability and so epithelial coverage of the wound is inhibited. Some chronic wounds may be deficient in TGFβ and its receptor [42].

Pressure ulcers

Chronic wounds have also been demonstrated to have elevated matrix degrading enzymes and decreased levels of inhibitors for these enzymes. Pressure ulcers unlike chronic venous stasis ulcers appear to have difficulty in healing related to the impairment of extracellular matrix production. Studies have indicated that neutrophil elastase present in chronic wounds can degrade peptide growth factors and is responsible for degrading fibronectin [31; 33]. Pressure ulcers have also shown an increase in MMPs and plasminogen activators in tissue [26]. Chronic wound fluids demonstrate increased levels of gelatinases MMP2 and MMP9 [30]. Levels of MMP1 and MMP8 were also found to be higher in pressure ulcers and venous stasis ulcers than acute healing wounds [25]. In addition, several of the endogenous proteinase inhibitors were shown to be decreased in chronic wounds [27]. Proteinase inhibitors serve a regulatory role in matrix degradation by containing the matrix degrading enzymes. Factors that promote MMP production or activation could counteract the effectiveness of proteinase inhibitors, for example, the destruction of TIMPs by neutrophil elastase. The tissue inhibitor level to MMP ratio may indicate an imbalance which contributes to the wound chronicity.

Future concepts for the treatment of chronic wounds

Although the aetiologies and physical characteristics of the various types of chronic wounds are different, there is a common trend in their biochemical profiles. The precise pattern of growth factor expression in the different types of chronic wounds is not yet known; but it

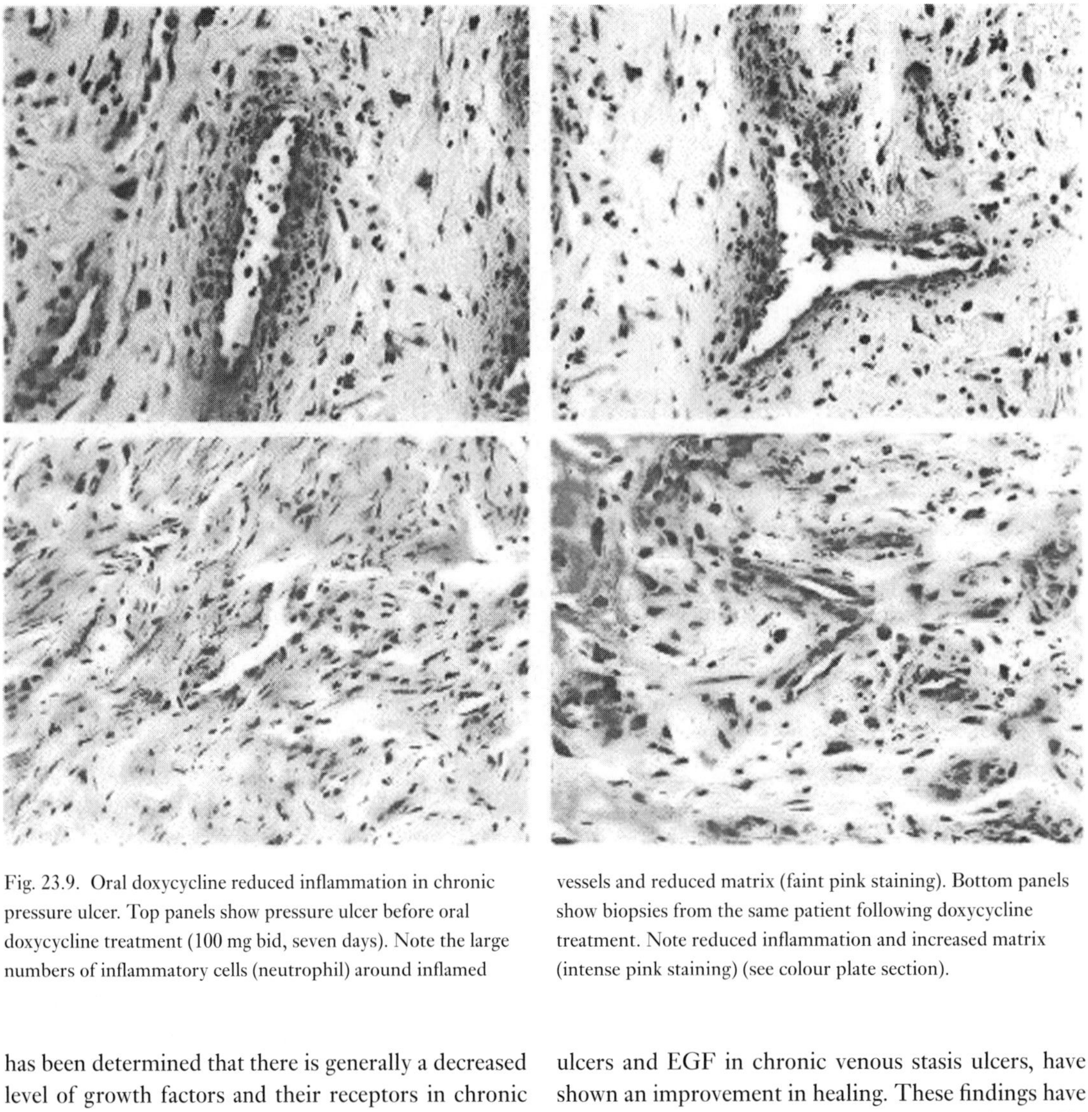

Fig. 23.9. Oral doxycycline reduced inflammation in chronic pressure ulcer. Top panels show pressure ulcer before oral doxycycline treatment (100 mg bid, seven days). Note the large numbers of inflammatory cells (neutrophil) around inflamed vessels and reduced matrix (faint pink staining). Bottom panels show biopsies from the same patient following doxycycline treatment. Note reduced inflammation and increased matrix (intense pink staining) (see colour plate section).

has been determined that there is generally a decreased level of growth factors and their receptors in chronic wound fluids. The absolute levels of growth factors may not be as important as the relative concentrations necessary to replace the specific deficiencies in the tissue repair processes. For the treatment of chronic wounds, Robson [43] proposed that growth factor therapy be tailored to the deficiency in the repair process. Therefore, the effectiveness of the therapy is predicted on adequate growth factor levels and the expression of their receptors, balanced against receptor degradation by proteases and the binding of growth factors by macromolecules such as macroglobulin and albumin.

Studies that evaluated topical growth factor treatment of chronic wounds, such as PDGF in diabetic foot ulcers and EGF in chronic venous stasis ulcers, have shown an improvement in healing. These findings have led us to hypothesize that altering the cytokine profile of chronic wounds through the use of MMP inhibitors, the addition of growth factors, and the elimination of inflammatory tissue and proteases by debridement, would shift the wound microenvironment towards that of an acute wound and thereby improve healing.

Current treatment strategies are being developed to address the deficiencies (growth factor and protease inhibitor levels) and excesses (MMPs, neutrophil elastase and serine protease levels) in the chronic wound microenvironment. The more specific and sophisticated treatments remain in the laboratory at this time, such as the new potent, synthetic inhibitors of MMPs and the naturally occurring protease inhibitors, TIMP-1 and α1-antitrypsin, available by recombinant DNA technology. However, use of gene therapy in the treatment of chronic diabetic foot ulcers is currently being evaluated in a clinical trial. A phase III clinical trial is underway to determine the efficacy of KGF-2 in the treatment of chronic venous stasis ulcers. The treatment strategy which is to add growth factor to a chronic wound has been in place for the past several years. Regranex®, human recombinant PDGF-BB, has been available for the treatment of diabetic foot ulcers and demonstrated approximately 20% improvement in healing compared to controls [44]. In keeping with the strategy to restore a deficient wound environment, Dermagraph® and Apligrapf®, engineered tissue replacements, have been applied to chronic diabetic ulcers [45; 46]. Although Apligrapf® is no longer available, both tissue replacements have proven to be effective in selected types of ulcers. Other approaches to the treatment of chronic wounds have been to remove the increased protease levels. This is in part the strategy of a vacuum-assisted negative pressure wound dressing [47], and the recent development of dressings that bind and remove MMPs from the wound fluid, such as Promogran® [48; 49].

Another strategy is to use synthetic protease inhibitors to decrease the activities of MMPs in the wound environment. Doxycycline, a member of the tetracycline family of antibiotics, is a moderately effective inhibitor of MMPs, including the TNFα converting enzyme (TACE). As shown in Figure 23.9, treatment of a patient with chronic pressure ulcers with oral doxycycline (100 mg, bid, for 7 days), improved the histological appearance of biopsies. Specifically, the top panels of Figure 23.9 show the pressure ulcers before oral doxycycline treatment. Note the large numbers of inflammatory cells (neutrophils) around the inflamed vessels and the reduced amount of extracellular matrix, which is indicated by faint pink staining. The bottom panels show biopsies from the same patient following doxycycline treatment. Note the reduced level of inflammation (fewer numbers of leucocytes) and increased amount of extracellular matrix (intense pink staining). Low dose doxycycline (20 mg, bid) has been proven to be beneficial in other pathologic states such as periodontitis that are characterized by chronic, neutrophil-driven inflammation and matrix destruction [50]. In the future, treatment of chronic wounds may require the use of specific growth factors or inhibitors unique to the type of ulcer, or the use of combinations of selective inhibitors of proteases, growth factors and tissue replacements to act synergistically to promote healing.

As previously described, endocrine hormones, such as insulin, glucocorticoids and oestrogen, play important roles in regulating wound healing. Although there is no current therapy that specifically addresses the molecular deficits created by type I or type II diabetes (inadequate insulin levels or insulin resistance), system insulin injections may improve the local wound microenvironment. For patients receiving long term corticosteroids, the use of vitamin A seems to facilitate wound healing. Studies are underway to determine the efficacy of topical oestrogen applications on skin aging.

CONCLUSION

The molecular environment of chronic wounds contains elevated levels of inflammatory cytokines and proteases, low levels of mitogenic activity and cells that often respond poorly to growth factors compared with acute healing wounds. As chronic wounds begin to heal, this molecular pattern shifts to one that resembles a healing wound. As more information is learned about the molecular and cellular profiles of healing and chronic wounds, new therapies will be developed that selectively correct the abnormal aspects of chronic wounds and promote healing of these costly clinical problems.

REFERENCES

1. N. T. Bennett & G. S. Schultz, Growth factors and wound healing: part II. Role in normal and chronic wound healing. *The American Journal of Surgery*, **166** (1993), 74–81. (1995), 3–16.
2. N. T. Bennett & G. S. Schultz, Growth factors and wound healing: biochemical properties of growth factors and their receptors. *The American Journal of Surgery*, **165** (1993), 728–37.
3. W. T. Lawrence, Physiology of the acute wound. *Clinical Plastic Surgery*, **25** (1998), 321–40.
4. B. A. Mast & G. S. Schultz, Interactions of cytokines, growth factors, and proteases in acute and chronic wounds. Wound *Repair and Regeneration*, **4** (1996), 411–20.
5. G. S. Schultz, Molecular regulation of wound healing. In *Acute and Chronic Wounds: Nursing Management*,

2nd edn, ed. R. A. Bryant. (Philadelphia: Mosby, 2000), pp. 413–29.
6. J. Gailit & R. A. F. Clark, Wound repair in context of extracellular matrix. *Current Opinion in Cell Biology*, **6** (1994), 717–25.
7. V. K. Rumalla & G. L. Borah, Cytokines, growth factors, and plastic surgery. *Plastic and Reconstructive Surgery*, **108** (2001), 719–33.
8. A. D. Luster, Chemokines – chemotactic cytokines that mediate inflammation. *New England Journal of Medicine*, **338** (1998), 436–45.
9. R. Gillitzer & M. Goebeler, Chemokines in cutaneous wound healing. *Journal of Leukocyte Biology*, **69** (2001), 513–21.
10. C. A. Dinarello & L. L. Moldawer, *Chemokines and Their Receptors. Proinflammatory and Anti-inflammatory cytokines in Rheumatoid Arthritis*. (Thousand Oaks, CA: Amgen Inc., 2000), pp. 99–110.
11. P. S. Frenette & D. D. Wagner, Adhesion molecules, blood vessels and blood cells. *New England Journal of Medicine*, **335** (1996), 43–5.
12. P. S. Frenette & D. D. Wagner, Molecular medicine, adhesion molecules. *New England Journal of Medicine*, **334** (1996), 1526–9.
13. R. F. Diegelmann, I. K. Cohen & A. M. Kaplan, The role of macrophages in wound repair: a review. *Plastic and Reconstructive Surgery*, **68** (1981), 107–13.
14. M. R. Duncan, K. S. Frazier, S. Abramson *et al.*, Connective tissue growth factor mediates transforming growth factor beta-induced collagen synthesis: down-regulation by cAMP. *FASEB Journal*, **13** (1999), 1774–86.
15. M. Bhushan, H. S. Young, P. E. Brenchley & C. E. Griffiths, Recent advances in cutaneous angiogenesis. *British Journal of Dermatology*, **147** (2002), 418–25.
16. G. L. Semenza, HIF-1 and tumor progression: pathophysiology and therapeutics. *Trends in Molecular Medicine*, **8** (2002), S62-7.
17. E. A. O'Toole, Extracellular matrix and keratinocyte migration. *Clinical and Experimental Dermatology*, **26** (2001), 525–30.
18. B. Bucalo, W. H. Eaglstein & V. Falanga, Inhibition of cell proliferation by chronic wound fluid. *Wound Repair and Regeneration*, **1** (1993), 181–6.
19. M. H. Katz, A. F. Alvarez, R. S. Kirsner, W. H. Eaglstein & V. Falanga, Human wound fluid from acute wounds stimulates fibroblast and endothelial cell growth. *Journal of the American Academy of Dermatology*, **25** (1991), 1054–8.
20. I. R. Harris, K. C. Yee, C. E. Walters *et al.*, Cytokine and protease levels in healing and non-healing chronic venous leg ulcers. *Experimental Dermatology*, **4** (1995), 342–9.
21. N. J. Trengove, H. Bielefeldt-Ohmann & M. C. Stacey, Mitogenic activity and cytokine levels in non-healing and healing chronic leg ulcers. *Wound Repair and Regeneration*, **8** (2000), 13–25.
22. D. R. Yager & B. C. Nwomeh, The proteolytic environment of chronic wounds. *Wound Repair and Regeneration*, **7** (1999), 433–41.
23. B. C. Nwomeh, D. R. Yager & I. K. Cohen, Physiology of the chronic wound. *Clinical Plastic Surgery*, **25** (1998), 341–56.
24. N. J. Trengove, M. C. Stacey, S. Macauley *et al.*, Analysis of the acute and chronic wound environments: the role of proteases and their inhibitors. *Wound Repair and Regeneration*, **7** (1999), 442–52.
25. D. R. Yager, L. Y. Zhang, H. X. Liang, R. F. Diegelmann & I. K. Cohen, Wound fluids from human pressure ulcers contain elevated matrix metalloproteinase levels and activity compared to surgical wound fluids. *The Journal of Investigative Dermatology*, **107** (1996), 743–8.
26. A. A. Rogers, S. Burnett, J. C. Moore, P. G. Shakespeare & W. Y. J. Chen, Involvement of proeolytic enzymes – plasminogen activators and matrix metalloproteinases – in the pathophysiology of pressure ulcers. *Wound Repair and Regeneration*, **3** (1995), 273–83.
27. E. C. Bullen, M. T. Longaker, D. L. Updike *et al.*, Tissue inhibitor of metalloproteinases-1 is decreased and activated gelatinases are increased in chronic wounds. *The Journal of Investigative Dermatology*, **104** (1995), 236–40.
28. G. P. Ladwig, M. C. Robson, R. Liu *et al.*, Ratios of activated matrix metalloproteinase-9 to tissue inhibitor of matrix metalloproteinase-1 in wound fluids are inversely correlated with healing of pressure ulcers. *Wound Repair and Regeneration*, **10** (2002), 26–37.
29. C. N. Rao, D. A. Ladin, Y. Y. Liu *et al.*, Alpha 1-antitrypsin is degraded and non-functional in chronic wounds but intact and functional in acute wounds: the inhibitor protects fibronectin from degradation by chronic wound fluid enzymes. *The Journal of Investigative Dermatology*, **105** (1995), 572–8.
30. A. B. Wysocki, L. Staiano-Coico & F. Grinnell, Wound fluid from chronic leg ulcers contains elevated levels of

metalloproteinases MMP-2 and MMP-9. *The Journal of Investigative Dermatology*, **101** (1993), 64–8.

31. F. Grinnel & M. Zhu, Fibronectin degradation in chronic wounds depends on the relative levels of elastase, α 1-proteinase inhibitor, and α 2-macroglobulin. *The Journal of Investigative Dermatology*, **106** (1996), 335–41.
32. R. W. Tarnuzzer & G. S. Schultz, Biochemical analysis of acute and chronic wound environments. *Wound Repair and Regeneration*, **4** (1996), 321–5.
33. D. R. Yager, S. M. Chen, S. I. Ward *et al.*, Ability of chronic wound fluids to degrade peptide growth factors is associated with increased levels of elastase activity and diminished levels of proteinase inhibitors. *Wound Repair and Regeneration*, **5** (1997), 23–32.
34. E. A. Baker & D. J. Leaper, Proteinases, their inhibitors, and cytokine profiles in acute wound fluid. *Wound Repair and Regeneration*, 8 (2000), 392–8.
35. D. L. Steed, D. Donohoe, M. W. Webster & L. Lindsley, Effect of extensive debridement and treatment on the healing of diabetic foot ulcers. *Journal of the American College of Surgeons*, **183** (1996), 61–4.
36. M. S. Agren, W. H. Eaglstein, M. W. Ferguson *et al.*, Causes and effects of the chronic inflammation in venous leg ulcers. *Acta Dermato-Venerologica*, **210** (Suppl) (2000), 3–17.
37. G. S. Ashcroft, J. Dodsworth, E. van Boxtel *et al.*, Estrogen accelerates cutaneous wound healing associated with an increase in TGF-beta1 levels. *Nature Medicine*, **3** (1997), 1209–15.
38. G. S. Ashcroft, M. A. Horan, S. E. Herrick *et al.*, Age-related differences in the temporal and spatial regulation of matrix metalloproteinases (MMPs) in normal skin and acute cutaneous wounds of healthy humans. *Cell and Tissue Research*, **290** (1997), 581–91.
39. G. S. Ashcroft, S. E. Herrick, R. W. Tarnuzzer *et al.*, Human ageing impairs injury-induced *in vivo* expression of tissue inhibitor of matrix metalloproteinases (TIMP)-1 and -2 proteins and mRNA. *Journal of Pathology*, **183** (1997), 169–76.
40. G. S. Ashcroft, T. Greenwell-Wild, M. A. Horan, S. Wahl & M. W. Ferguson, Topical estrogen accelerates cutaneous wound healing in aged humans associated with an altered inflammatory response. *American Journal of Pathology*, **155** (1999), 1137–46.
41. N. J. Trengove, S. R. Langton & M. C. Stacey, Biochemical analysis of wound fluid from nonhealing and healing chronic leg ulcers. *Wound Repair and Regeneration*, **4** (1996), 234–9.
42. A. J. Cowin, N. Hatzirodos, C. A. Holding *et al.*, Effect of healing on the expression of transforming growth factor beta(s) and their receptors in chronic venous leg ulcers. *The Journal of Investigative Dermatology*, **117** (2001), 1282–9.
43. M. C. Robson, The role of growth factors in the healing of chronic wounds. *Wound Repair and Regeneration*, **5** (1997), 12–17.
44. J. M. Smiell, T. J. Wieman, D. L. Steed *et al.*, Efficacy and safety of becaplermin (recombinant human platelet-derived growth factor-BB) in patients with nonhealing, lower extremity diabetic ulcers: a combined analysis of four randomized studies. *Wound Repair and Regeneration*, **7** (1999), 335–46.
45. V. Falanga, D. Margolis, O. Alvarez *et al.*, Rapid healing of venous ulcers and lack of clinical rejection with an allogeneic cultured human skin equivalent. Human Skin Equivalent Investigators Group [see comments]. *Archives of Dermatology*, **134** (1998), 293–300.
46. R. S. Kirsner, V. Falanga & W. H. Eaglstein, The development of bioengineered skin. Trends *in Biotechnology*, **16** (1998), 246–9.
47. L. C. Argenta & M. J. Morykwas, Vacuum-assisted closure: a new method for wound control and treatment: clinical experience. *Annals of Plastic Surgery*, **38** (1997), 563–76.
48. B. Cullen, R. Smith, E. McCulloch, D. Silcock & L. Morrison, Mechanism of action of PROMOGRAN, a protease modulating matrix, for the treatment of diabetic foot ulcers. *Wound Repair and Regeneration*, **10** (2002), 16–25.
49. A. Veves, P. Sheehan & H. T. Pham, A randomized, controlled trial of promogran (a collagen/oxidized regenerated cellulose dressing) vs standard treatment in the management of diabetic foot ulcers. *Archives of Surgery*, **137** (2002), 822–7.
50. L. M. Golub, T. F. McNamara, M. E. Ryan, *et al.*, Adjunctive treatment with subantimicrobial doses of doxycycline: effects on gingival fluid collagenase activity and attachment loss in adult periodontitis. *Journal of Clinical Periodontology*, **28** (2001), 146–56.

24 • Varicose veins: principles and vascular biology

RACHEL C. SAM, STANLEY H. SILVERMAN AND
ANDREW W. BRADBURY

INTRODUCTION

Chronic venous insufficiency (CVI) is the commonest condition affecting the lower limb, with varicose veins (VVs) representing the bulk of the operative workload. Vascular vein surgery is the single largest cause of medico-legal action against general and vascular surgeons in the UK [1; 2]. As such, it would be fair to say that the treatment of VVs remains unsatisfactory, at least in part because many clinicians lack a clear understanding of the underlying anatomy and pathophysiology.

ANATOMY

Venous blood from the lower limbs returns to the right heart against gravity through the superficial and deep venous systems. The superficial venous system of the lower limb is made up of the long (LSV) and short saphenous (SSV) veins, and their tributaries. The LSV originates from the dorsal venous arch, passing anterior to the medial malleolus to cross the tibia. From there it continues along the medial aspect of the tibia and up the medial aspect of the thigh to enter the common femoral vein in the groin at the saphenofemoral junction (SFJ). The SSV commences on the lateral border of the foot, passes posterior to the lateral malleolus and then up the back of the calf between the heads of the gastrocnemius muscle into the popliteal fossa. It is joined variably by the gastrocnemius veins and then enters the popliteal vein at the saphenopopliteal junction (SPJ). The SPJ may be absent in which case the SSV continues up the postero-medial aspect of the thigh (Giacomini vein) to enter the LSV. These two systems also interconnect at many other (highly variable) points through an extensive network of tributaries. The deep system veins, often paired, accompany each named artery. The superficial and deep systems connect at numerous points at various non-junctional perforators in addition to the SFJ and SPJ. These systems and interconnections are interdependent, both anatomically and functionally in health and disease.

In health, the deep venous system transmits 90% of the venous return from the leg. The superficial system drains only the skin and subcutaneous tissues, with most of that blood draining immediately into the deep system via perforators in the foot, calf and thigh. It also plays a role in thermoregulation.

HISTOLOGY

Veins consist of three tunica layers, as in arteries, but these are less well defined. The intima is thin and surrounded by a fine elastic lamina. The media is made up of three layers of muscular bundles that are arranged in different orientations, with the amount of smooth muscle varying with the calibre and working pressure of the vein. Beyond this, the adventitia merges with the perivenous connective tissue, which contains nerve fibres and vasa vasorum. With age the arrangement of the layers becomes progressively disorganized. There is thickening of the intima and disorientation of the elastic fibres. The outer muscle layer of the media becomes hypertrophied with dystrophic elastic fibres and the adventitia is increasingly fibrous [3].

PHYSIOLOGY

Venous return against gravity is primarily dependent on muscle pumps located in the foot and calf. Pressure on the sole of the foot and muscular contraction (systole) in the fascial compartments of the calf, compress the sinusoidal intramuscular veins directing blood into the deep system and thence up the leg. Superficial veins collect blood from the superficial tissues and during muscle relaxation (diastole) this blood enters the deep system through the perforating veins down a pressure gradient, filling the sinuses. Reverse flow (reflux) during muscle relaxation is prevented by the closure of valves. These are delicate but strong bicuspid leaflets at the base of a localized dilated sinus in the vein. In both superficial and deep systems the density of valves is greatest in the calf and reduces gradually up the lower limb, with the iliac and inferior vena cava frequently lacking valves altogether. Valves are present in venules down to ~0.15 mm diameter.

During systole, blood is prevented from re-entering the superficial system through the closure of non-junctional perforators. This was originally thought to occur through the closure of valves but several studies have failed to demonstrate such valves. Instead, external pressure from the fascia and muscle through which the perforators pass is thought to be responsible for limiting outward blood flow. This is somewhat akin to the 'pinch-cock' mechanism that prevents reflux at the gastro-oesophageal junction. Importantly, this also protects the superficial veins, subcutaneous tissues and skin from the extremely high deep venous pressures (up to 250 mm Hg) generated by the calf muscle pump in systole.

When standing motionless, with venous valves in the neutral position, the pressure in the foot veins gradually increases as blood continues to enter the veins from the arterial side (*vis a tergo*). As soon as the pressure in one segment exceeds that in the segment just above, the valve opens. Eventually the hydrostatic pressure in the veins of the foot is that developed by an unbroken column from the foot to the right atrium – perhaps 90 mm Hg in a person of average height. With active movement, deep veins and sinuses are compressed raising venous pressure and moving blood cranially and, initially, caudally (Figure 24.1). However, valve closure prevents retrograde flow within 0.5–1.0 seconds. At this point, these closed valves divide the high-pressure, single column of venous blood described above into a large number of low-pressure, shorter columns. As a result the pressure in the foot veins falls in health to less than 25 mm Hg on walking – ambulatory venous pressure (AVP) (Figure 24.2). This reduces venous pooling and lowers capillary hydrostatic pressure, reducing the tendency for the accumulation of interstitial fluid (oedema) in the feet. Patients with muscle pump and/or venous valve failure and/or venous outflow obstruction, demonstrate raised AVP. It is this raised AVP that underlies all the symptoms and signs of CVI.

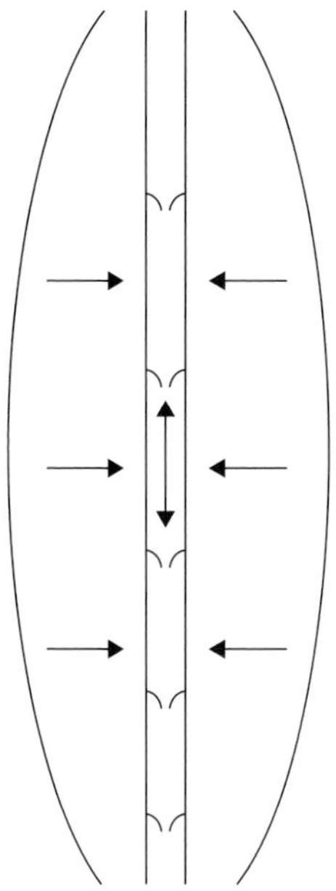

Fig. 24.1. The calf muscle pump. Calf muscle contraction in systole compresses the deep veins and causes cranial venous flow. Caudal flow (known as venous reflux or incompetence) during systole and calf muscle relaxation is prevented by valve closure. These mechanisms deliver the venous return from the legs to the heart. Also the valves divide the column of venous blood into small segments, resulting in lower resting and ambulatory venous pressures.

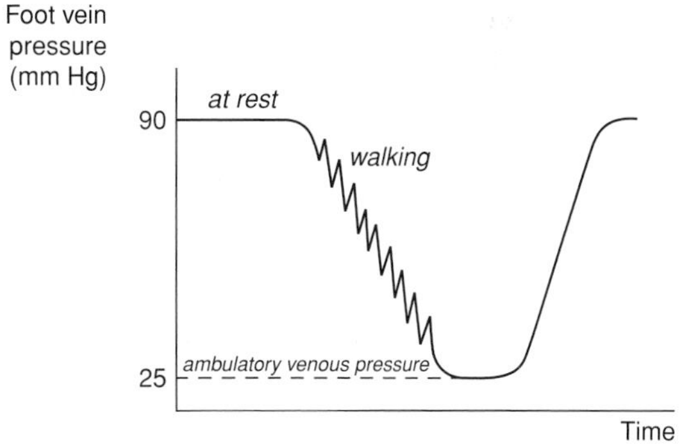

Fig. 24.2. Resting and ambulatory venous pressure at the ankle in health. With the legs completely motionless, and thus the valves open, the venous pressure at the ankle equates to the weight of the column of blood between the foot and the right atrium. Upon movement, the venous pressure falls dramatically as a result of the muscle pumps and valve closure.

VARICOSE VEINS

Varicose veins are dilated, tortuous subcutaneous veins that permit reverse flow. They are most commonly found in the lower limb, and may be primary or secondary to deep venous pathology. The LSV system is most frequently affected with the SSV being involved in <20% of cases. The aetiology of VVs at a microscopic level is still disputed but the essential defect macroscopically is generally agreed to be the failure of venous valve closure, resulting in the superficial veins becoming elongated and tortuous. The main factor contributing to the development and progression of VVs is sustained venous hypertension that increases the diameter of superficial veins resulting in further valve incompetence.

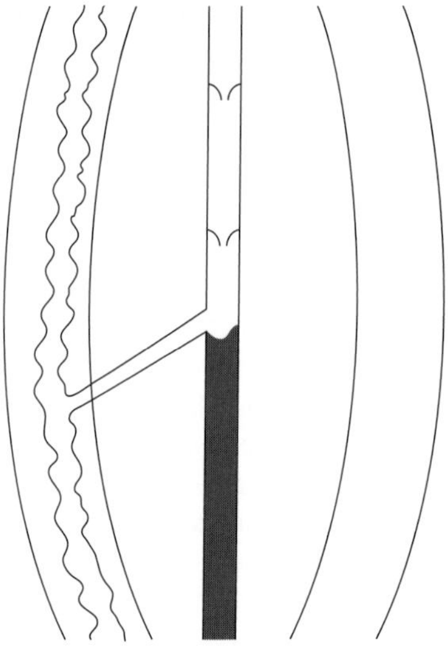

Fig. 24.3. Secondary varicose veins caused by deep venous obstruction. Venous return from the leg is transmitted via 'incompetent' perforators to the superficial vein, which may become dilated and appear varicose. However such varicosities must not be removed or ligated as such action will increase ambulatory venous pressure.

VALVULAR ABNORMALITIES

Failure of valve closure leading to valve incompetence and reflux may affect the deep and/or superficial venous systems, and may be primary or secondary. Primary valvular incompetence (PVI) is believed to be due to loss of mural elastin and collagen, which leads to dilatation and separation of the valve leaflets. The commonest clinical consequence of this process is the development of VVs. As investing fascia supports the main LSV trunk, it is usually the tributaries that become varicose. Primary valvular incompetence may also affect the deep venous system, although because other tissues support the deep veins, the clinical consequences of PVI are less obvious and certain.

Secondary valvular incompetence may be due to a developmental weakness in the vein wall, leading to secondary widening of the valve commissures, incompetence and clinically, primary VVs. It also follows thrombosis, most commonly in the deep venous system; deep venous thrombosis (DVT). Blood flowing within the lumen of the vein provides the vascular endothelium with its oxygen and nutrition. Deep venous thrombosis prevents this, therefore leading to endothelial destruction and inflammation within and around the affected veins. Although most (90%) of the venous segments occluded by DVT recanalize over the subsequent months, the vein is usually scarred, narrowed and, because the valves have been destroyed, incompetent. In about 10% of cases, recanalization does not occur, in which case blood is forced to find an alternative drainage route. For example, blood may be forced out of the deep venous system via non-junctional calf perforators leading to dilatation of the superficial veins (secondary VVs) (Figure 24.3). Obstruction of the iliac veins may lead to the development of groin and pelvic collaterals. Venous reflux and obstruction secondary to DVT leads to the so-called post-thrombotic syndrome (PTS), which represents the most severe form of CVI. The superficial venous system may also be affected by thrombosis, either in isolation or in combination with DVT, leading to superficial thrombophlebitis (SVT).

Rarely, VVs and CVI may be due to congenital valve hypoplasia or agenesis, or due to arterio-venous malformations. In Klippel-Trenaunay syndrome, for example, there is sometimes deep venous hypoplasia and a laterally placed venous complex that acts as the main venous outflow of the limb. All the symptoms and signs of CVI are due to ambulatory venous hypertension, resulting from these various pathological processes acting upon the microvasculature of the skin and subcutaneous tissues.

MUSCLE PUMP FAILURE

Any cause of chronic debility or immobility is associated with calf muscle pump dysfunction; for example, old age, stroke, neuromuscular conditions, arthritis and trauma. Injuries that limit or prevent ankle movement have a particularly adverse effect upon the calf muscle pump.

VENOUS RECIRCULATION

In patients with VVs there is often a recirculation of venous blood within the leg. During calf relaxation abnormally large volumes of blood enter the muscle pump from the superficial varices (increased preload). During exercise the muscle pump expels blood from the leg only for it to re-enter the lower limb by refluxing down the LSV and/or SSV VVs (akin to an increase in afterload due to aortic regurgitation). This blood then re-enters the muscle pump through the perforating veins in the lower calf and so on. The effect is that the same blood can re-circulate up and down the leg several times before eventually finding its way up the iliac veins to the heart.

Patients with mild superficial reflux and/or an efficient calf pump are able to compensate for this by increasing their calf muscle pump 'stroke volume' and output. This allows them to still reduce their AVP to (near) normal levels on walking. However, severe reflux and/or a weak muscle pump may overwhelm the deep system and lead to the development of the sustained venous hypertension and skin changes of CVI. This accounts for two important clinical observations:

- CVI and ulceration can develop without primary deep venous pathology.
- In a proportion of patients with VVs and deep venous reflux the latter disappears following eradication of superficial disease [4].

RECURRENT VARICOSE VEINS

Recurrent varicose veins after surgery are common (20%–80%) leading to a re-operation rate of around 20% at between a five and 20 year follow-up [5]. The origin of these recurrent VVs may be classified into three groups:

(1) *New varicose veins.* This is the development of new VVs, often in a second system, since the original operation. This may be due to the fact that their presence was not recognized as assessment was inadequate, or that they were 'subclinical' at that time. For example, duplex assessment (had it been undertaken) at the time of an original LSV system operation may have detected reflux in, for example, the SSV in addition. In the course of time the untreated SSV reflux can lead to recurrent VVs. Alternatively a previously competent site of potential deep to superficial reflux may become incompetent.
(2) *Persistent VVs.* This is due to inadequate treatment of VVs at the original operation. In prolonged procedures requiring multiple avulsions of extensive VVs, prominent varicosities may be missed. These may be tackled at a later date by injection sclerotherapy or phlebectomy under local anaesthetic.
(3) *True recurrent VVs.* Unsuccessful previous VV surgery results in the development of further VVs in the same system [6]. These VVs may be connected to the deep system via a leash of small vessels through the site of previous junctional surgery, or via thigh perforators. This allows a further classification:
    (a) *Type I* saphenofemoral venous complex intact.
    (b) *Type II* saphenofemoral complex obliterated.

The majority of recurrent VVs are due to the failure to perform flush SFJ ligation and failure to remove the LSV in the thigh through which perforator incompetence subsequently becomes apparent [7]. Type I recurrence with an intact SFJ is always due to a failure to properly expose the SFJ and adjacent femoral vein at the original operation. The concept of neovascularization, 'development of new vessels connecting previously ligated superficial veins to the deep venous system' is thought by some to be responsible for groin recurrence, where the SFJ has previously been ligated. Support for this idea originates from the appearance of numerous venous channels seen on duplex connecting the stump of the LSV in the groin, through scar tissue of previous surgery, to the recurrent VVs in the thigh [8; 9]. There can be no doubt that this happens in some patients. However, its significance in the development of clinically apparent recurrent VVs remains unproven. These tiny new vessels have high resistance to blood flow making it unlikely for them to cause significant recurrence on their own. In practice, neovascularization at the groin rarely leads to significant lower limb VVs unless the LSV or a major (often the anterolateral thigh) tributary has been left behind after the first operation. These observations underscore the absolute requirement to strip the LSV in the thigh and the lateral thigh branch if it is a significant vessel at the first operation in order to prevent clinically significant recurrence.

CONCLUSION

Despite the very large numbers of patients affected by CVI and VVs, research into venous disease is generally given low priority and so there are still significant gaps in our knowledge. Further work is needed if we are to improve our understanding of the aetiology of the disease and improve the results of treatment.

REFERENCES

1. W. B. Campbell, F. France & H. M. Goodwin, Medicolegal claims in vascular surgery. *Annals of the Royal College of Surgeons of England*, **84** (2002), 181–4.
2. W. G. Tennant, Medicolegal action following treatment for varicose veins. *British Journal of Surgery*, **8** (1996), 291–2.
3. M. P. Goldman & A. Fronek, Anatomy and pathophysiology of varicose veins. *Journal of Dermatologic Surgery and Oncology*, **15**(2) (1989), 138–45.
4. J. C. Walsh, J. J. Bergan, S. Beeman & T. P. Comer, Femoral vein reflux abolished by greater saphenous vein stripping. *Annals of Vascular Surgery*, **10**(2) (1996), 186–9.
5. M. R. Perrin, J. Terome Guex, C. V. Ruckley *et al.*, Recurrent varices after surgery (REVAS), a consensus document. *Cardiovascular Surgery*, **8**(4) (2000), 233–45.
6. P. A. Stonebridge, N. Chalmers, I. Beggs, A. W. Bradbury & C. V. Ruckley, Recurrent varicose veins: a varicographic analysis leading to a new practical classification. *British Journal of Surgery*, **82** (1995), 60–2.
7. S. Dwerryhouse, B. Davies, K. Harradine & J. J. Earnshaw, Stripping the long saphenous vein reduces the rate of reoperation for recurrent varicose veins: five year results of a randomized trial. *Journal of Vascular Surgery*, **29** (1999), 589–92.
8. L. Jones, B. D. Braithwaite, D. Selwyn, S. Cooke & J. J. Earnshaw, Neovascularisation and recurrent varicose veins. *European Journal of Vascular and Endovascular Surgery*, **12** (1996), 422–5.
9. I. Nyamekye, N. A. Shephard, B. Davies, B. P. Heather & J. J. Earnshaw, Clinicopathological evidence that neovascularisation is a cause of recurrent varicose veins. *European Journal of Vascular and Endovascular Surgery*, **15** (1998), 412–15.

25 • Chronic venous insufficiency and leg ulceration: principles and vascular biology

MICHAEL STACEY

DEFINITIONS

Chronic venous insufficiency

Chronic venous insufficiency is a term that is used to describe changes in the leg that include a variety of different clinical problems, caused by several types of abnormalities in the veins, that may occur at a number of different locations [1]. For these reasons it has been difficult to make accurate comparisons of reports of chronic venous insufficiency from different institutions. As a result attempts have been made to formulate systems of classification that enable accurate comparisons to be made.

The most recent classification, referred to as the CEAP classification, was devised by an international panel and encompasses features of some of the earlier classifications [2]. This classification has four categories which include – Clinical (C), Etiology (E), Anatomy (A) and Pathophysiology (P). Within each category the different levels are each given a number or a letter or both. The Clinical classification has seven levels from no visible or palpable signs of venous disease through to skin changes with active ulceration (Table 25.1). In addition the clinical categories are further characterized according to the presence or absence of symptoms. The Etiological classification recognizes the roles of congenital (E_c), primary (E_p) and secondary (E_s) causes in venous dysfunction. The Anatomical classification can be represented as a simple or more detailed form. The simple form refers to the site at which the veins are involved as superficial (A_s), deep (A_d) or perforating (A_p). The more detailed form identifies the specific veins that are involved and has 18 segments that can be identified. The Pathophysiologic classification identifies the cause of venous dysfunction being either reflux (P_R) or obstruction (P_O), or both (P_{RO}). This classification can be used in part or in whole when describing the patients in a published report.

Leg ulceration

Leg ulceration may occur as a result of many different aetiological factors (Table 25.2). For patients presenting with an ulcer on the leg it is imperative to determine the aetiology since the treatment may differ according to the cause. For ulcers on the leg, not including the foot, the commonest aetiology is chronic venous disease either alone or in common with another cause of impaired healing such as arterial disease, diabetes or rheumatoid arthritis. The venous abnormality that leads to venous leg ulceration may involve abnormalities at different locations in the venous system, of different extent and different aetiologies.

EPIDEMIOLOGY

A number of epidemiological studies of leg ulceration have been conducted in different Western countries and have found a similar prevalence of leg ulceration ranging from 0.11% to 0.18% of the population [3; 4; 5; 6]. These studies have confirmed that chronic venous disease is the commonest cause, representing approximately 65% of ulcers on the leg. These occur most commonly in elderly people with a mean age in excess of 65 years. There are nearly twice as many women as men with leg ulcers, however, when these are related to age, the prevalence for males and females is similar because there are more women than men in the older age groups [3].

An Australian epidemiological study found that venous ulcers are associated with delayed healing (with a median duration of 26 weeks) and tend to recur in over 70% of patients [3].

PATHOPHYSIOLOGY

Venous abnormality

The basic underlying physiological abnormality in chronic venous disease is altered return of blood in the

Table 25.1. *Clinical classification of chronic venous disease of the lower extremity*

Class	Definition
0	No visible or palpable signs of venous disease
1	Telangiectases or reticular veins
2	Varicose veins
3	Oedema
4	Skin changes ascribed to venous disease (e.g. pigmentation, eczema, lipodermatosclerosis)
5	Skin changes as above in conjunction with healed ulceration
6	Skin changes as above in conjunction with active ulceration

The presence or absence of symptoms is denoted by the addition of 's' for symptomatic, or 'a' for asymptomatic

Table 25.2. *Commonest causes of leg ulceration*

Venous disease
Arterial disease
Rheumatoid arthritis
Diabetes
Vasculitis
Scleroderma
Pyoderma gangrenosum
Trauma
Infective
Ulcerating skin cancer

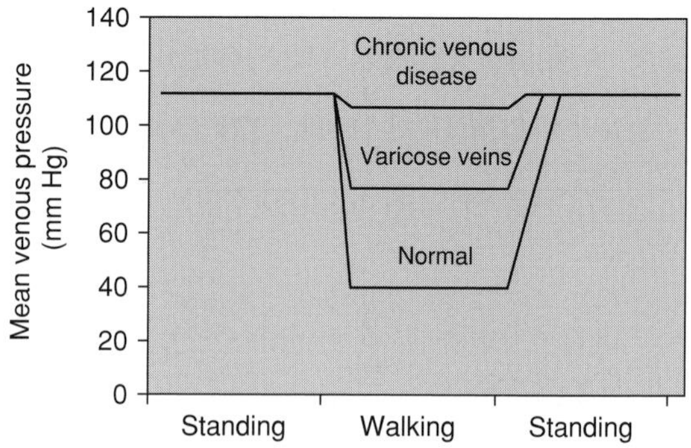

Fig. 25.1. Superficial venous pressures in normal legs and legs with chronic venous disease.

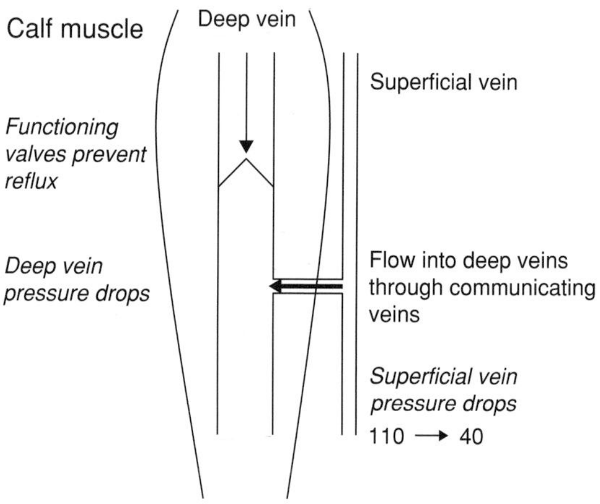

Fig. 25.2. Pressure in the deep and superficial veins in a normal leg after calf muscle contraction.

veins of the leg, which results in ambulatory venous hypertension in the superficial veins [7]. When venous pressures are measured in the surface veins of the foot or ankle, the pressure is normally highest (approximately 100 mm Hg) when standing immobile, and drops to 25 to 40 mm Hg when walking (Figure 25.1). This occurs because the 'calf muscle pump' assists the return of blood from the leg by compression of the deeper veins during muscle contraction. When the muscles relax, the emptied deeper veins have a lower pressure which allows more blood to flow into them from the surface veins, thereby reducing the pressure in those veins (Figure 25.2).

In patients with chronic venous insufficiency the pressure in the surface veins drops only a small amount, hence the term 'ambulatory' venous hypertension (Figure 25.1). An increase in the pressure in the surface veins above that present on standing is very uncommon and only occurs when there is extensive proximal venous occlusion. The failure to reduce superficial venous pressure on exercise occurs when there is reflux in either the deep or surface veins. Reflux in the deep veins results in rapid refilling of the deep veins when the calf muscles relax (Figure 25.3). This results in only a small increase in the amount of blood that flows from the surface veins into the deep veins. If the reflux is primarily in the superficial veins, the superficial veins refill quickly as the blood flows into the deep veins and the ambulatory

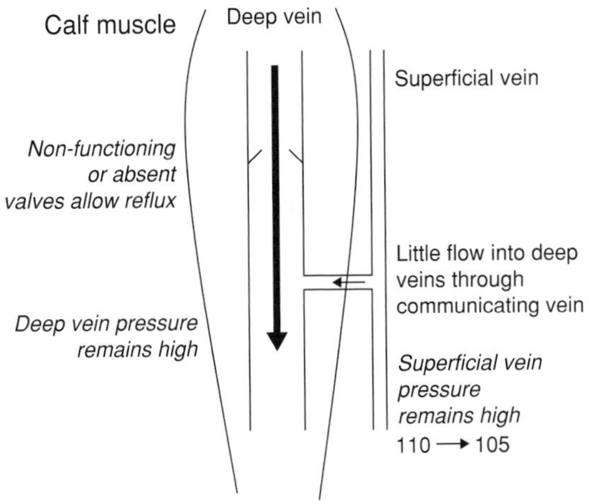

Fig. 25.3. Pressure in the deep and superficial veins in a leg with chronic venous disease after contraction of the calf muscle.

venous pressure remains elevated even though more blood may be flowing into the deep veins [8].

Reflux in veins is caused either by destruction of the valves when a venous thrombosis recanalizes or by primary incompetence of the valves. The relative proportions of the two causes in the deep veins remain a point of debate. Definite evidence of previous deep vein thrombosis has been reported in 40%–50% of patients with venous ulceration [9; 10]. In chronic venous insufficiency the venous reflux may involve the deep veins or may involve only the surface and perforating veins. Involvement of the deep veins has also been variously reported at between 40% and 90% [9; 10]. The major reason for this variation in reporting is the use of different techniques for assessing the deep veins. The rate of deep vein involvement was reported to be higher when the standard method of assessing veins was venography [9]. Duplex scanning has now become the major method for assessing veins and the quoted rates of deep vein involvement have dropped [10]. This possibly relates to the difficulty in visualizing the calf veins with duplex scanning.

Effect of ambulatory venous hypertension on the tissues in the leg

The obvious clinical finding in chronic venous insufficiency is the pigmentation and fibrosis that occurs in the skin at the gaiter region of the leg, referred to as lipodermatosclerosis (Figure 25.4). Histologically there is also an increase in the extent of the capillary bed in the skin, although there is some debate as to whether the capillaries are all perfused. This is particularly the case in areas of atrophie blanche (white atrophy) in which there are tufts of capillaries interspersed within relatively avascular skin (Figure 25.5). This condition is common in venous ulceration, but may also be present in other conditions such as vasculitis [11].

A number of hypotheses have been proposed over the years to try to explain how ambulatory venous hypertension affects the tissues and thereby leads to impaired healing. It has generally been acknowledged that there must be some impairment to the nutrition of the skin cells either due to reduced nutrients or reduced oxygenation. To date such reduced skin nutrition has not been conclusively demonstrated. Many studies have shown reduced transcutaneous oxygen measurements, however, because of the change to the structure of the skin this may not be an accurate reflection of tissue oxygenation.

Theories that have been proposed to support the concept of reduced nutrition to the skin are arterio-venous shunting [12], the presence of a diffusion barrier to oxygen by fibrin and other proteins that deposit around skin capillaries [13], and the occlusion of capillaries by activated white cells becoming ‘trapped’ in the capillary bed [14]. Other theories have hypothesized that growth factors are trapped in the pericapillary protein deposits, therefore impeding the healing process (Figure 25.6) [15]. Other hypotheses have focused on the presence of factors that directly damage the tissue by activation of white cells, these subsequently release factors and substances that can impede healing [14; 16]. To date there is no conclusive support for any given hypothesis, although the presence of an excessive inflammatory response has been repeatedly demonstrated in venous ulcers.

Influence of venous disease on the wound healing process

The cause of impaired healing in venous ulceration remains uncertain. This is in spite of the clinical observation that non-healing venous ulcers begin to heal once patients are admitted to hospital for bed rest. Efforts are continuing to try to determine what is occurring at a cellular and molecular level to impede the healing process. These have demonstrated a highly

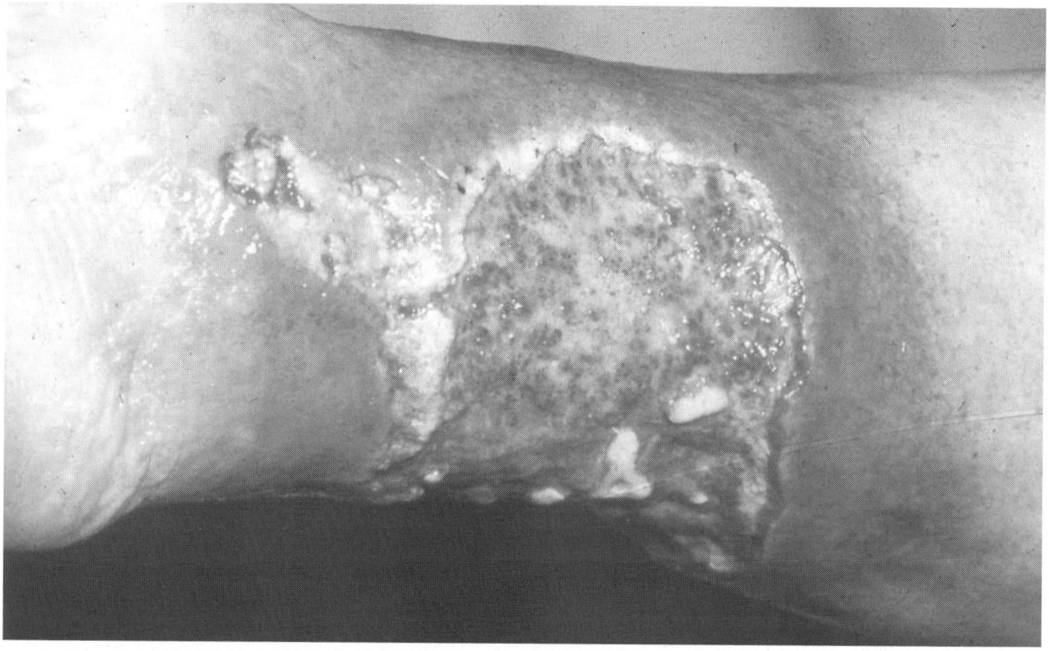

Fig. 25.4. Lipodermatosclerosis and ulceration in a leg with chronic venous disease.

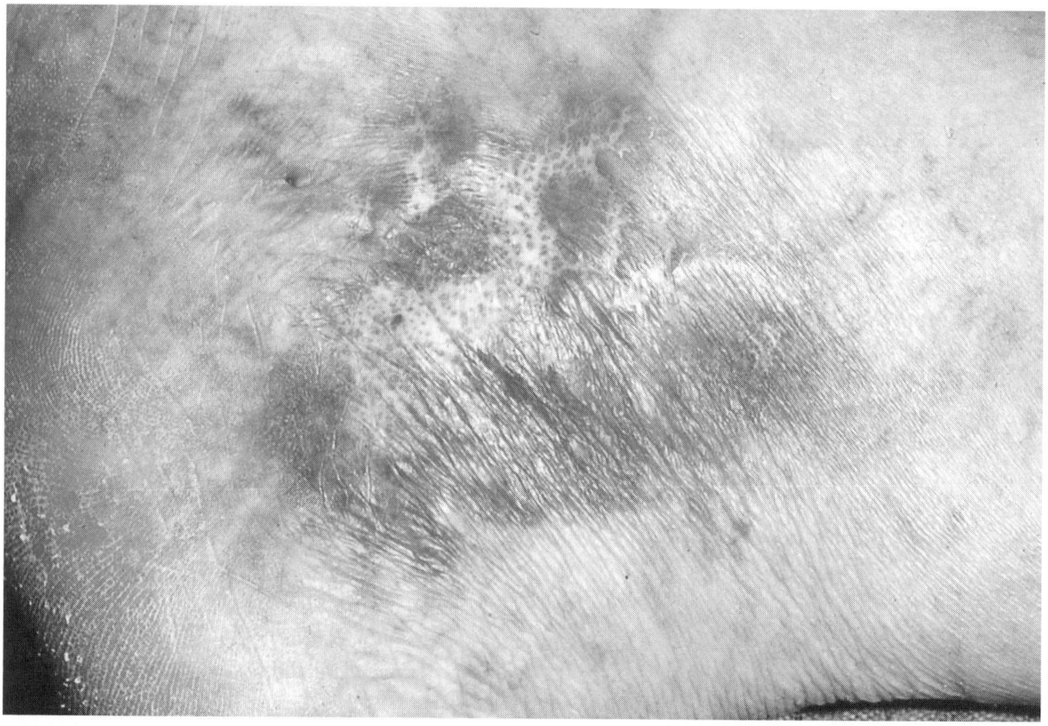

Fig. 25.5. Atrophie blanche in a leg with chronic venous disease (see colour plate section).

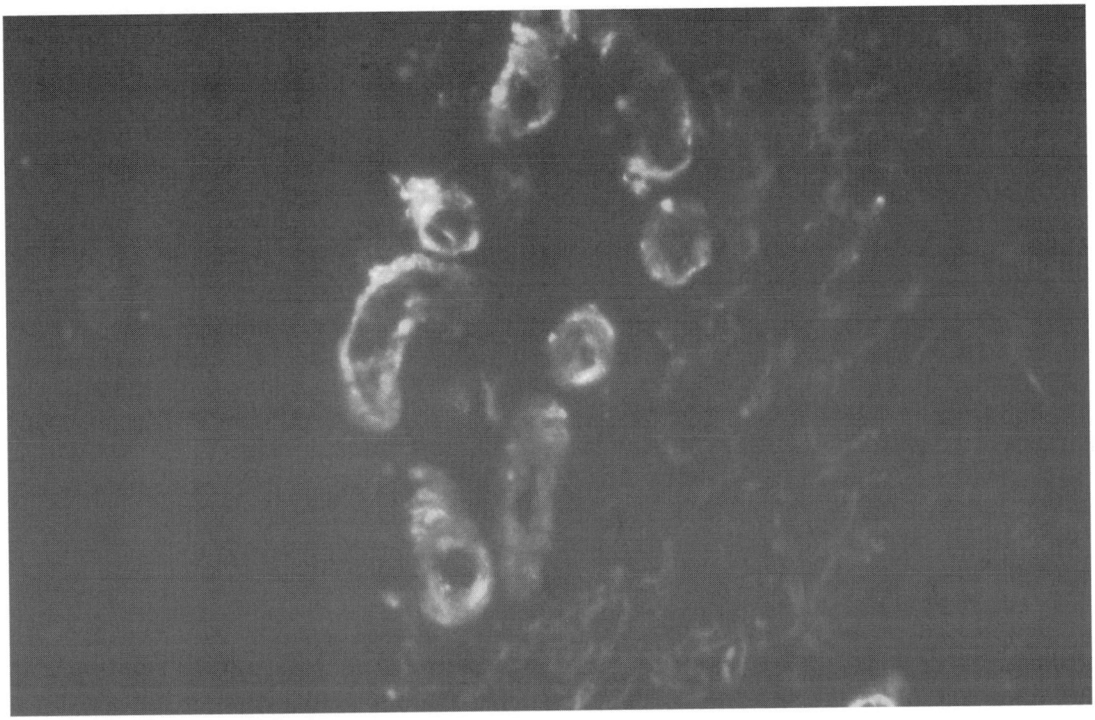

Fig. 25.6. Pericapillary deposit of protein – fibrinogen (see colour plate section).

inflammatory environment, with high levels of inflammatory cytokines, proteases and large numbers of immune cells [17; 18; 19]. The proteases that are elevated in venous ulcers compared with acute wounds include matrix metalloproteinase 2 and 9 (MMP2 and 9) (Figure 25.7) and collagenases (Figure 25.8). It is possible that this highly inflammatory environment may result in the destruction of factors that are important in the normal healing process. These factors may include growth factors, cell surface receptors, the matrix in the base of the wound and cellular adhesion molecules.

The increased inflammatory environment may also contribute to bacteria that colonize open wounds. The precise role that bacteria play in the impaired healing process has not been established, with no clear link being shown between the presence of bacteria and healing ability in venous ulcers [20].

The underlying causes of venous ulceration may affect both the ability to develop ulcers and the ability to heal ulcers, however, it is likely that additional factors will contribute to the impaired healing process once an ulcer has occurred. Further understanding of factors that impede the healing process may lead to better treatments to improve ulcer healing.

ASSESSMENT OF VENOUS FUNCTION

In patients with venous ulceration, the history and clinical signs on the leg will give a strong indication of the presence of venous disease. When surgical treatment is to be considered it is imperative to have a clear outline of the veins with reflux. If the deep veins are involved, the benefits of operating on surface or perforating veins are limited [21]. The current method that is used to assess for sites of incompetence is duplex scanning. Venography is used infrequently and usually only when there is uncertainty about the information from the duplex scan. Other methods of diagnosing venous disease such as plethysmography and hand held Doppler do not give a good indication of the sites of venous incompetence [22; 23]. When performing a duplex scan for chronic venous disease, the deep veins, superficial veins and the communicating veins should all be evaluated.

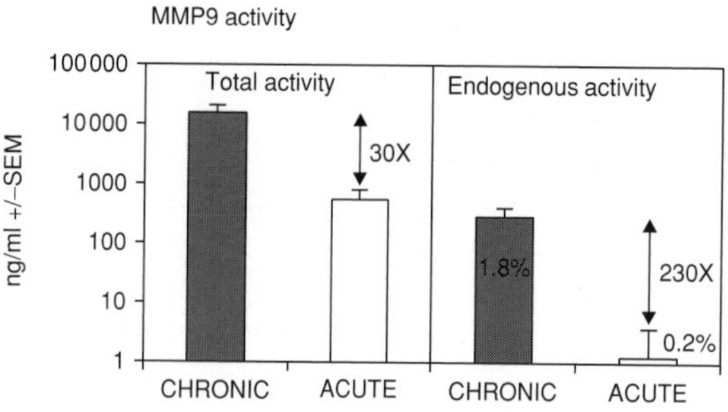

Fig. 25.7. Matrix metalloproteinase levels in wound fluid from acute and chronic wounds.

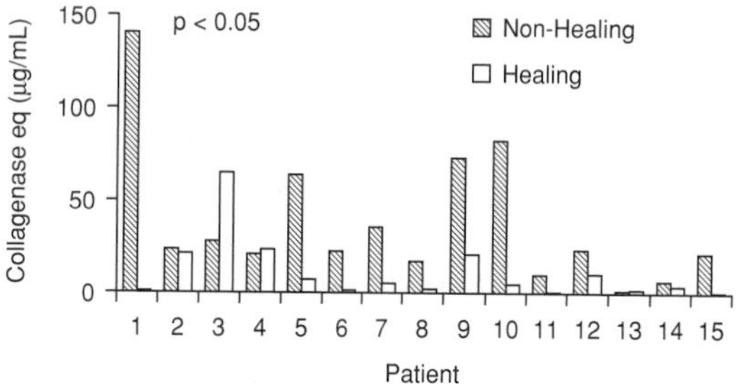

Fig. 25.8. Collagenase levels in wound fluid from chronic venous ulcers.

TREATMENT OF VENOUS ULCERATION

The objective of the treatment of venous ulceration is to improve the physiological abnormality of ambulatory venous hypertension. The two methods available are compression therapy applied to the leg, or direct treatment of the veins by surgery or other ablative techniques such as sclerotherapy. There is also ongoing study to identify topical and systemic therapies that will have a direct influence to improve the healing process in the ulcers. To date no such therapies have come into routine clinical practice.

Compression therapy

Compression applied to the leg improves venous return in the leg, primarily by reducing venous reflux into the leg and by reducing the leg volume [24]. Compression bandages have also been shown to significantly improve the time taken to heal venous ulcers [25]. This reduces oedema in the leg that is considered to impede the healing process. Compression is applied to the leg below the knee from the base of the toes to just below the knee. The level of compression that is recommended is to achieve a pressure of between 25 and 45 mm Hg at the ankle with a graduated reduction in pressure up the leg. The compression may be applied by either bandages or by compression stockings. In patients with an open ulcer, bandages are normally preferred because the exudate damages the stockings and shortens their life-span.

There are many different types of bandage systems that have been employed for venous ulcers. Most benefit has been shown to occur with systems that are multilayered [25]. To date no difference has been shown in the efficacy of inelastic (short stretch) or elastic (long stretch) bandages, as long as these are used as part of a multilayered system. The first layer consists of orthopaedic wool or similar padding as is placed beneath a plaster cast. This is to help protect the skin overlying bony prominences from excessive pressure. The next one or preferably two layers are the compression bandages that may be elastic or inelastic or a combination of the two. The top layer is one that helps prevent slippage of the bandage. This may be a bandage that adheres to itself or a tubular stockingette.

If a compression stocking is used this should be either class two (25–35 mm Hg at the ankle) or class three (35–45 mm Hg) and should aim to provide graduated compression. These come in a variety of sizes and should be fitted to the individual's leg. They come with and without zippers on one side that help with applying and removing the stocking. Patients with small or very large legs may need to have stockings custom made to fit their legs. Stockings can be difficult to both apply and remove, particularly in patients with arthritis or in frail patients. To assist with application there are frames onto which the stockings can be placed and into which the patient then places their foot. Stockings are often useful in younger patients who have active jobs and for whom wearing bulky bandages is difficult.

The dressing applied to the ulcer may be chosen from any of the vast number that are available. There is no one dressing that has a direct effect on improving the healing process [26]. Dressings are chosen according the needs of the patient and their wound. Different dressings may be chosen to absorb exudate, reduce pain, help liquefy slough, reduce bacterial contamination, reduce odour from the wound or protect the surrounding skin from maceration. The cost of the dressing also needs to be considered when making a selection. For patients who are using stockings a dressing that adheres to the skin is preferable as this aids with applying the stocking over it.

The dressings and compression may be left on the leg for up to one week and even longer in cooler climates. Commonly, however, the bandages and dressings may be changed anything from daily to weekly. The main determinants of the duration of application are the amount of exudate, the state of the wound and odour from the bandages.

Surgery

Surgery to the veins in the lower leg may include procedures on the superficial varicose veins, incompetent communicating veins or the deep veins in the leg. Surgery to the superficial veins includes surgery to the long and/or short saphenous vein by ligation and stripping, together with avulsion of varicosities [27; 28]. Incompetent communicating veins can be accurately located by duplex scanning, and may be approached directly by a small incision over the site and subfascial ligation. In order to avoid making incisions through areas of lipodermatosclerosis or ulceration, the perforators in the lower leg may be treated by subfascial endoscopic perforator surgery (SEPS) (Figure 25.9) [29]. The deep veins may be treated by direct repair of intact but incompetent valves. The repair may be directly by suture [30; 31], or may involve applying a cuff around the valve to reduce the diameter of the vein and to restore competence [32]. Veins that have had previous venous thrombosis and which have recanalized with destruction of the valve, can have a segment of vein containing competent valves taken from the arm and inserted to replace a segment of the femoral or popliteal vein [33].

The role of any of these operations in patients with venous ulcers remains uncertain and is supported only by anecdotal reports. The benefits of surgery to the deep veins for patients with open or healed venous ulcers remain unproven and should be confined to studies assessing their efficacy rather than be used in routine clinical practice. Surgery to the superficial veins or incompetent perforating veins may have an application in patients who do not have significant incompetence or evidence of post-thrombotic changes in the deep veins [27; 28]. A retrospective study demonstrated that in patients with healed ulcers, there was a higher incidence of recurrence of ulceration following superficial and perforator surgery if there was evidence of post-thrombotic changes in the deep veins [21]. While this has not been thoroughly evaluated to assess the effect on healing of venous ulcers, it is most likely that such patients would have less benefit from such surgery.

The need to treat incompetent communicating veins at the same time as treating superficial veins remains uncertain. Studies on patients with superficial venous incompetence and incompetent communicating veins, but without deep vein abnormalities, have indicated that in a majority of patients, the communicating veins cease to be incompetent after the superficial veins are ablated [34; 35]. Another study has indicated that, in the presence of deep vein reflux, ablation of superficial veins does not result in a return to competence in incompetent communicating veins [36].

Anecdotal reports have suggested that operating on the superficial and perforating veins does improve the healing of venous ulcers. The authors own anecdotal experience would support this observation, especially in patients who are not responding to optimal compression therapy and who have no or minimal reflux in the deep veins. In addition, in patients with very painful ulcers, this also seems to reduce their level of pain. It is still important to continue the compression after the surgery. A recent randomized controlled trial has, however, shown no improvement in venous ulcer healing when surgery is combined with compression bandaging compared with compression bandaging alone [37].

Surgery to correct venous obstruction has included vein bypass, transposition of a vein to bypass an obstruction [38] or balloon dilatation with stenting [39]. The efficacy of these procedures remains uncertain due to the infrequency with which they are performed and the consequent anecdotal nature of reports.

Prevention of venous ulcer recurrence

Once an ulcer has healed continued treatment should be implemented to help reduce the risk of ulcer recurrence. The simplest method is to use compression stockings [40]. These have been shown to significantly prolong the time before venous ulcers recur, however, they do not remove the risk completely. The stockings that are used are class three, however it is generally considered that class two stockings will have a similar benefit.

Surgery to the leg veins in patients with venous ulcers is most commonly used to help prevent ulcer

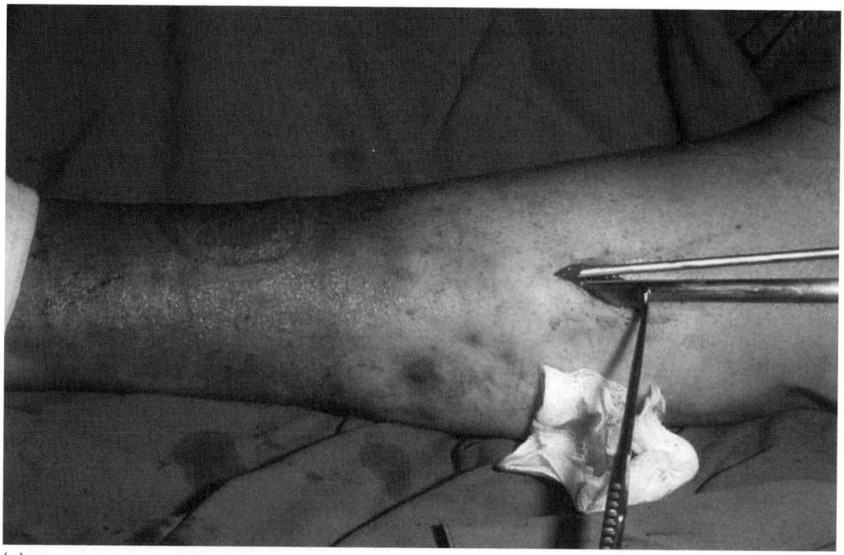

(a)

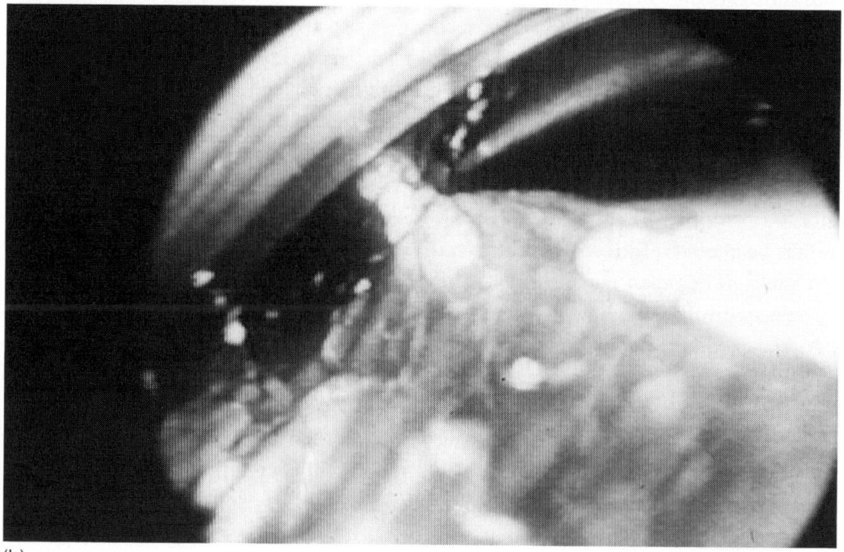

(b)

Fig. 25.9. Subfascial endoscopic perforator surgery – instruments in position and clip on a perforator (see colour plate section).

recurrence. This is usually performed after ulcers have healed, in order to not be operating with potential for contamination from an open ulcer. As indicated above the only form of surgery that is used in routine practice is surgery to the surface and/or perforating veins. The benefits of this surgery are greater in patients who have no evidence of post-thrombotic damage to the deep veins.

Sclerotherapy and other techniques to obliterate surface and perforating veins

Techniques other than surgery have been used to treat varicose veins and incompetent perforating veins. These include sclerotherapy [41], ultrasound guided sclerotherapy to incompetent perforating veins and saphenous veins [42], and laser or heat ablation of the long saphenous vein [43]. These techniques have not been specifically evaluated in the treatment of venous ulceration or the prevention of ulcer recurrence. It is likely that the benefit of these treatments would be commensurate with their efficacy in obliterating the appropriate veins compared with that achieved with the surgical techniques.

Other therapies

The use of other systemic or topical therapies is an area in which there is ongoing research. Many different therapies have been evaluated; however, to date no single therapy has been shown to be of sufficient benefit to be used in routine clinical practice. Therapies that have or are being assessed include aspirin, oxpentifylline, platelet lysate or releasate, a number of different recombinant growth factors, growth factors derived from bovine whey, protease inhibitors, topical antibacterial preparations or dressings, systemic or topical antibacterials and various vasoactive preparations. These have been selected for assessment based mainly on theoretical grounds, rather than detailed knowledge of the cellular and molecular abnormalities that result in venous ulcers forming and that impede their healing. There is a need to better understand these processes so that this knowledge can be used to help identify improved methods for treating venous ulcers.

REFERENCES

1. M. C. Stacey, Investigation and treatment of chronic venous ulcer disease. *Australian and New Zealand Journal of Surgery*, **71** (2001), 226–9.
2. J. J. Bergan, B. Eklof, R. L. Kistner *et al.*, Classification and grading of chronic venous disease in the lower limbs. A consensus statement. *Journal of Cardiovascular Surgery*, **38** (1997), 437–41.
3. S. R. Baker, M. C. Stacey, A. G. Jopp-McKay *et al.*, Epidemiology of chronic venous ulcers. *British Journal of Surgery*, **78** (1991), 864–7.
4. M. J. Callam, D. R. Harper, J. J. Dale & C. V. Ruckley, Chronic ulcer of the leg: clinical history. *British Medical Journal*, **294** (1987), 1389–91.
5. O. Nelzen, D. Bergqvist, A. Lindhagen & T. Halbook, Chronic leg ulcers: an underestimated problem in primary health care among elderly patients. *Journal of Epidemiology and Community Health*, **45** (1991), 184–7.
6. J. V. Cornwall, C. J. Dore & J. D. Lewis, Leg ulcers: epidemiology and aetiology. *British Journal of Surgery*, **73** (1986), 693–6.
7. N. L. Browse, K. G. Burnand & M. Lea-Thomas, *Diseases of the Veins*. (London: Edward Arnold, 1988).
8. D. Christopoulos, A. N. Nicolaides & A. Cook, Pathogenesis of venous ulceration in relation to the calf muscle pump function. *Surgery*, **106** (1989), 829–35.
9. M. Lea-Thomas, *Phlebography of the Lower Limb*. (Edinburgh: Churchill-Livingstone, 1982).
10. A. M. Van Rij, C. Solomon & R. Christie, Anatomic and physiologic characteristics of venous ulceration. *Journal of Vascular Surgery*, **20** (1994), 759–64.
11. K. G. Burnand, I. Whimster, A. Naidoo & N. L. Browse, Pericapillary fibrin in the ulcer bearing skin of the leg: the cause of lipodermatosclerosis and venous ulceration. *British Medical Journal*, **1** (1982), 478–81.
12. A. C. Brewer, Varicose ulceration, arteriovenous shunts. *British Medical Journal*, **2** (1950), 269–70.
13. N. L. Browse & K. G. Burnand, The cause of venous ulceration. *Lancet*, **2** (1982), 243–5.
14. P. Thomas, G. Nash & D. Dormandy, White cell accumulation in dependent leg of patients with venous hypertension: a possible mechanism for trophic changes in the skin. *British Medical Journal*, **296** (1988), 1693–5.
15. V. Falanga & W. Eaglstein, The trap 'hypothesis' of venous ulceration. *Lancet*, **341** (1993), 1006–7.
16. B. Bucalo, W. Eaglstein & V. Falanga, Inhibition of cell proliferation by chronic wound fluid. *Wound Repair and Regeneration*, **1** (1993), 181–6.
17. N. J. Trengove, H. Bielefeldt- Ohmann & M. C. Stacey, Mitogenic activity and cytokine levels in non-healing and healing chronic leg ulcers. *Wound Repair and Regeneration*, **8** (2000), 13–25.
18. N. J. Trengove, M. C. Stacey, S. MaCauley *et al.*, Analysis of the acute and chronic wound environments: the role of proteases and their inhibitors. *Wound Repair and Regeneration*, **7** (1999), 442–52.
19. M. C. Stacey, S. Lainez, T. Skender- Kalnenas & B. Morrison, Alterations in immune cells in human chronic leg ulcers. *Phlebology*, **1**(Suppl) (1995), 923–5.
20. N. J. Trengove, M. C. Stacey, D. F. McGechie, N. F. Stingemore & S. Mata, Qualitative bacteriology and leg ulcer healing. *Journal of Wound Care*, **5** (1996), 277–80.
21. K. Burnand, T. O'Donnell, M. Lea- Thomas & N. L. Browse, Relation between post-phlebitic changes in the deep veins and results of surgical treatment of venous ulcer. *Lancet*, **1** (1976), 936– 8.

22. M. C. Hoare & J. P. Royle, Doppler ultrasound detection of saphenofemoral and saphenopopliteal incompetence and operative venography to ensure precise saphenopopliteal ligation. *Australian and New Zealand Journal of Surgery*, **54** (1984), 49–52.
23. H. B. Abramowitz, L. A. Queral, W. R. Flinn *et al.*, The use of photoplethysmography in the assessment of venous insufficiency: a comparison to venous pressure measurement. *Surgery*, **86** (1979), 434–41.
24. D. Yang, Y. K. Vandongen & M. C. Stacey, The influence of minimal-stretch and elasticated bandages on calf muscle pump in patients with chronic venous disease. *Phlebology*, **14** (1999), 3–8.
25. A. Fletcher, N. Cullum & A. S. Sheldon, A systematic review of compression treatment for venous leg ulcers. *British Medical Journal*, **315** (1997), 576–80.
26. M. Stacey, V. Falanga, W. Marston *et al.*, Compression therapy in the treatment of venous leg ulcers: a recommended management pathway. *EWMA Journal*, **2** (2002), 9–13.
27. K. K. Sethia & S. G. Darke, Long saphenous incompetence as a cause of venous ulceration *British Journal of Surgery*, **71** (1984), 754–5.
28. M. C. Hoare, A. N. Nicolaieds, C. R. Miles *et al.*, The role of primary varicose venous in venous ulceration. *Surgery*, **92** (1982), 450–3.
29. M. Jugenheimer & T. Junginger, Endoscopic subfascial sectioning of incompetent perforating veins in treatment of primary varicosis. *World Journal of Surgery*, **16** (1992), 971–95.
30. R. L. Kistner, Surgical repair of the incompetent femoral vein valve. *Archives of Surgery*, **110** (1975), 1336–41.
31. S. Raju & R. Fredericks, Valve reconstruction procedures for non-obstructive venous insufficiency: rationale, technique and results in 107 procedures with two to eight year follow up. *Journal of Vascular Surgery*, **7** (1988), 301–9.
32. G. Jessup & R. L. Lane, Repair of incompetent venous valves: a new technique. *Journal of Vascular Surgery*, **8** (1988), 569–75.
33. T. P. Nash, Venous ulceration: factors influencing recurrence after standard surgical procedures. *Medical Journal of Australia*, **154** (1991), 48–50.
34. C. M. Sales, M. L. Bilof, K. A. Petrillo & N. L. Luka, Correction of lower extremity deep venous incompetence by ablation of superficial venous reflux. *Annals of Vascular Surgery*, **10** (1996), 186–9.
35. J. C. Walsh, J. J. Bergan, S. Beeman & T. P. Comer, Femoral venous reflux abolished by greater saphenous vein stripping. *Annals of Vascular Surgery*, **8** (1994), 566–70.
36. W. P. Stuart, D. J. Adam, P. L. Allan, C. V. Ruckley & A. W. Bradbury, Saphenous surgery does not correct perforator incompetence in the presence of deep venous reflux. *Journal of Vascular Surgery*, **28** (1998), 834–8.
37. M. Guest, J. J. Smith, G. Tripuraneni *et al.*, Randomised clinical trial of varicose vein surgery with compression versus compression alone for the treatment of venous ulceration. *Phlebology*, **19** (2003), 130–6.
38. E. A. Husni, Reconstruction of veins: the need for objectivity. *Journal of Cardiovascular Surgery*, **24** (1983), 525–8.
39. W. Blattler & I. K. Blattler, Relief of obstructive pelvic venous symptoms with endoluminal stenting. *Journal of Vascular Surgery*, **29** (1999), 484–8.
40. Y. K. Vandongen & M. C. Stacey, Graduated compression elastic stockings reduce lipodermatosclerosis and ulcer recurrence. *Phlebology*, **15** (2000), 33–7.
41. W. A. Fegan, The treatment of varicose veins during pregnancy. *Pacific Medicine and Surgery*, **72** (1964), 274–9.
42. A. Kanter & P. Thibault, Saphenofemoral incompetence treated by ultrasound guided sclerotherapy. *Dermatologic Surgery*, **22** (1996), 668–72.
43. N. Fassiadis, B. Kianifard, J. M. Holdstock & M. S. Whiteley, A novel endoluminal technique for varicose vein management: the VNUS closure. *Phlebology*, **16** (2002), 145–8.

26 • Pathophysiology and principles of management of the diabetic foot

MICHAEL STACEY AND ROBERT A. FITRIDGE

DEFINITION

The 'diabetic foot' is a collective term used to encompass the broad spectrum of problems that develop in the feet of patients with diabetes. These problems can affect patients with both type 1 and type 2 diabetes. Diabetes is implicated in approximately 50% of all lower limb amputations and most series have demonstrated a greater than 15 times increased risk of amputation in diabetics compared with the general population [1]. Approximately 15% of diabetics will develop foot ulceration during their lifetime. The 'diabetic foot' does not describe the specific problems encountered in an individual patient. The problems may encompass one or more of the following – neuropathy, contracture callus, ulceration, cellulitis, osteomyelitis, septic arthritis, ischaemic necrosis, or Charcot's deformity.

Neuropathy, contracture and peripheral vascular disease are all direct complications of diabetes. These themselves can produce significant symptoms and can present difficult clinical problems in their own right. Other complications of diabetes may indirectly contribute to the development of problems in the feet, including impaired eyesight and immune compromise leading to a susceptibility to infection (Table 26.1).

FACTORS THAT CONTRIBUTE TO THE DEVELOPMENT OF PROBLEMS IN THE FEET OF DIABETICS

In any individual diabetic patient who develops foot problems, one or more of the complications of diabetes that are listed in Table 26.1 may play a significant role.

Neuropathy

Approximately 30% of diabetics have clinically apparent peripheral neuropathy and up to 80% of diabetics with foot ulceration have detectable neuropathy [2]. The aetiology of diabetic neuropathy is multifactorial involving both metabolic and microvascular factors. Hyperglycaemia promotes oxidative stress resulting in the generation of reactive oxygen species which are neurotoxic. Increased oxidative stress may further impair nerve perfusion by increasing cyclo-oxygenase-2 (COX-2) activity [3]. Hyperglycaemia also results in binding of excess glucose to amino acids in tissue and circulating proteins. Early glycation end products (e.g. HbAIC) are reversible; however, further molecular modifications, commonly oxidation, ultimately result in advanced glycosylation end products (AGEs) being formed. Advanced glycosylation end products bind irreversibly to intravascular and intracellular proteins, and have multiple effects. Advanced glycosylation end products reduce endothelial barrier function and induce a pro-coagulant endothelium via binding to cell surface receptors. The receptor for AGEs (RAGE) functions as a signal transduction receptor on endothelial and smooth muscle cells, and neurons. Sustained expression of this receptor results in chronic cell activation and tissue damage [4]. It is also important to note that AGEs bind to low-density lipoprotein (LDL) resulting in disordered lipid metabolism and elevated levels of LDL [5]. Thus AGEs are likely to be implicated in the cardiovascular complications frequently associated with diabetes.

A proportion of intracellular glucose is metabolized to sorbitol via aldose reductase. Hyperglycaemia leads to intracellular accumulation of sorbitol causing depletion of intracellular myoinositol. Myoinositol is important in nerve cell functions including signal transduction [6]. Nerve ischaemia secondary to microvascular disease and depletion of nerve growth factors in diabetes have also been implicated in diabetic neuropathy [7].

It has been well-known for many years that the duration of diabetes and level of hyperglycemia are strong predictors of the likelihood of the development of neuropathy. However, the importance of tight glycaemic

Table 26.1. *Complications of diabetes that contribute to problems in the feet*

Neuropathy
Contracture
Vascular disease – large vessel
– microvascular
Impaired eyesight
Immune compromise

control in reducing the risk of progression of neuropathy has only recently been proven in the Diabetes Control and Complications Trial (DCCT) [8]. This study demonstrated a 60% reduction in the risk of developing neuropathy over the five year study period in the intensive therapy group unaffected at commencement of the study, compared with initially unaffected diabetics managed in the standard fashion.

Diabetic neuropathy generally develops in a glove and stocking distribution. It is frequently asymptomatic; however, if present symptoms can include numbness, paraesthesia, burning sensation or burning pain. Patients who have numbness will often not offer this symptom unless directly asked. It is therefore important that the clinician have a high index of suspicion and ensure that this is specifically asked in history taking. Testing for neuropathy in most diabetic patients who present with foot problems should ideally be performed using the Semmes-Weinstein monofilament test and vibration testing by 'on-off method' using a 128 Hz tuning fork. The monofilament test uses a nylon thread applied to non-callused areas of the foot with enough pressure to just bend the nylon (10 gm). Both of these simple non-invasive tests correlate well with nerve conduction studies and can be used by clinicians to diagnose diabetic peripheral neuropathy [9].

Neuropathy can lead to a number of problems for diabetics, the main one being reduced sensation in the feet which makes them more prone to local trauma. Injuries may be acute secondary to trauma from sharp or blunt objects, or may be more chronic in which the patient is unable to feel pressure on the feet and thereby make subconscious changes to their posture to prevent problems developing. This can then lead to the development of calluses which themselves can then directly damage the underlying tissues. Autonomic neuropathy can also affect the foot by reducing the production of sweat and sebaceous gland secretion, which results in drying of the skin and makes the skin prone to cracks and splitting.

Painful neuropathy is characterized by persistent burning discomfort, pins and needles or pain. At times this will be the reason for their referral to a vascular surgeon. It is important to distinguish neuropathic from an ischaemic cause of pain. This is usually straightforward due to the nature of the pain on history taking, the presence or absence of neuropathy on examination and the assessment of perfusion. Management of neuropathy includes an aggressive approach to glycaemic control. Patients with severe discomfort can be treated with medications such as carbamazepine, sodium valproate or amitriptyline. These or similar medications will often reduce the symptoms to a manageable level, but will not usually remove the discomfort completely (see Chapter 22). The dosage needs to be titrated according to the level of discomfort. This is purely for symptom control and does not affect the underlying neuropathy. As the neuropathy progresses, the discomfort may decrease and the medications can then be discarded.

Contracture

Contracture in the feet of diabetic patients is thought to occur as part of a motor neuropathy affecting the nerves supplying the intrinsic muscles of the foot. This results in the unopposed action of the anterior tibial compartment muscles which leads to clawing of the toes and subluxation of the metatarsal heads. These deformities make both the dorsal surface of the toe at the proximal interphalangeal joint and the pad of the apex of the toe, prone to trauma from shoes and during walking.

The trauma can result in the formation of calluses and ultimately ulceration which may lead to osteomyelitis. When deformities have developed, it is extremely important that the patient has a regular review by a podiatrist in order to adjust their footwear to try to prevent the development of complications. If they do develop ulceration this can be difficult to treat and at times may require amputation of a toe or toes. In patients who are having repeated problems progressing from one deformed toe to the next, there can be merit in amputating the remaining severely deformed toes to prevent repeated problems. In these patients, when a medially placed toe is removed, the next lateral toe is more exposed to increased pressure and trauma. (Thus the process of ulceration and infection may continue until all toes have been removed.)

Peripheral vascular disease

One of the major predisposing causes of arterial disease is diabetes mellitus. Diabetic patients develop accelerated atherosclerosis in all vascular beds but also seem predisposed to severe occlusive disease affecting the infragenicular arteries. The presence of small vessel or arteriolar disease in the lower limbs remains controversial but is probably important in a sub-group of diabetic patients.

Many diabetics give no history of claudication despite the presence of severe, chronic, distal arterial occlusive disease.

Assessment of foot perfusion in diabetics with foot ulcers is critical so that rational decision making can be made regarding the need for lower extremity revascularization. Clinical assessment can be unreliable due to the presence of autonomic neuropathy, resulting in a warm, pink foot with rapid capillary refill.

The ankle:brachial index (ABI) is widely used to assess the presence and extent of arterial occlusive disease. However, this test may be unreliable due to calcification of the media of calf arteries. Thus a low ABI (<0.5) will confirm severe ischaemia; however, an ABI >0.5 or an incompressible Doppler pressure in the absence of pulses will provide no useful diagnostic information.

In this situation perfusion studies should be performed. Toe pressures using a photoplethysmography probe, transcutaneous oxygen saturation or isotope perfusion studies can be used to assess foot perfusion and predict healing of ulcers or wounds following surgery. Vitti *et al.* [10] found that toe pressures of less than 40 mm Hg in diabetics were associated with no chance of healing and that a toe pressure of 68 mm Hg or more was highly predictive of healing. Other groups use a toe pressure of 30 mm Hg or a transcutaneous oxygen measurement ($tcPO_2$) of 35 mm Hg in association with clinical assessment as a cut off indicating the need for revascularization in diabetics [11]. Perfusion studies remain relatively imprecise but a useful adjunctive tool in the assessment of foot perfusion in the diabetic.

Duplex scanning and angiography demonstrate the anatomical distribution of arterial occlusive disease. However, they do not give an assessment of adequacy of perfusion and cannot be used to predict healing of foot lesions.

Peripheral vascular disease is not the dominant problem in most diabetic patients with foot problems. However, it is important to continually review the patient's vascular status as this may change with time and require intervention in the evolution of the individual patient's problems.

Impaired eyesight

Impaired eyesight is a common problem in diabetic patients due primarily to diabetic retinopathy but may also be secondary to other ocular diseases. The major impact of this is that patients may be unable to critically examine their feet on a regular basis. When poor eyesight is combined with impaired sensation in the feet, patients may be unaware that a significant problem is developing in their feet resulting in late presentation of ulceration, infection or even osteomyelitis. At times the only reason the patient is alerted to a foot problem is when they notice either a 'smell' or discharge from the foot.

It is important for the clinician to be aware of the status of the patient's eyesight, so that other strategies for regular foot inspection can be implemented to try to prevent late presentation of significant problems.

Immune impairment

Diabetic patients are known to have impaired white cell function and endothelial dysfunction which compromises their ability to counter infection. In addition, when an infection does develop diabetic control is compromised. The consequent elevation of blood sugars provides an ideal environment for bacterial growth and further impedes the ability to overcome infection. The impaired immune function may also influence the healing process reducing the ability to heal wounds.

SPECIFIC PROBLEMS IN THE FEET OF DIABETICS

Callus

Callus is a proliferative response in the skin secondary to continuously increased pressure. This may occur in many different areas of the foot depending on the

Table 26.2. *Pressure offloading techniques in the diabetic foot*

Bed rest/crutches
Ugg (sheepskin) boot
Post-operative boot
Orthotic inserts with customized shoes
Orthodiabetic walker
Airsplint
CROW (Charcot Restraint Orthotic Walker)
Total contact plaster

dynamics within the individual patient's foot. The most common areas are over the plantar aspect of the metatarsal heads, medial and lateral aspects of the first and fifth metatarsophalangeal joints, on the pads of the toes, on the dorsum of the interphalangeal joints, or on the heel. Calluses develop because of neuropathy and the inability to make minor, subconscious adjustments to the standing or walking position.

Calluses have the potential to damage the foot because they are rigid prominences that can themselves damage the underlying tissue. This damage first becomes clinically evident when there is bleeding into the callus from the underlying tissue. The bleeding is an indication that the callus has caused some degree of ulceration of the skin beneath, and signals the potential for greater problems. If there is bacterial invasion into the callus as can occur with splits or cracks in the callus, infection can then develop. This will often go unnoticed initially because of the neuropathy and because the callus keeps the infection contained within the foot. The infection therefore will spread into the surrounding tissues rather than discharging to the surface. This can result in the infection being quite advanced with cellulitis, or osteomyelitis present prior to clinical presentation.

Treatment of calluses is aimed at prevention of damage to the underlying tissue. The major method for doing this is 'conservative (sharp) debridement' of the callus to remove the hard 'nodule' that can damage the underlying tissue, but more importantly, adjusting the footwear to reduce pressure on the area where the callus is forming – 'pressure offloading'.

Frequently used pressure offloading techniques are summarized in Table 26.2.

Acute blisters and ulceration

Acute injury to the foot can occur at any time, particularly in a neuropathic foot. Apart from the obvious trauma from sharp or blunt objects in the shoe, the other major form of injury is from footwear itself. It is not uncommon to see blistering and acute ulceration occur when a diabetic patient has spent a number of hours walking in new or poorly fitting shoes. Once again the neuropathy prevents the individual from being aware of the problem until they stop walking.

The injuries that develop are usually blistering (that remains unbroken) or superficial ulceration. If there is an unbroken blister, this is often best left intact as it acts as a good biological dressing. Once a blister has broken there is a risk of infection and cellulitis. If there is any evidence that infection is present it is best to debride the blister and to dress it directly. Once again to encourage blisters or superficial ulcers to heal it is important to minimize pressure over the area.

Sepsis

Infection in a diabetic foot is a very significant problem because of the potential for considerable and rapidly progressive damage to occur within the foot. Diabetic foot sepsis is frequently polymicrobial with staphylococci, streptococci, enterococci, gram negative organisms and anaerobes frequently implicated. As mentioned previously, the patient may not be aware of foot sepsis in the early stages of the infection. Patients who have had several episodes of infection may become aware of the systemic signs of sepsis and be alerted to a problem in this way before they notice any foot abnormality. Such 'awareness' should be encouraged in patients who have significant neuropathy and poor eyesight.

Significant infection can lead to major systemic problems secondary to sepsis alone or because of the effect on the blood sugar levels. Blood sugar increases in the presence of infection and can at times lead to acute ketoacidosis. For some diabetic patients the diagnosis of diabetes is first made when they present with an infection in the foot and elevated blood sugar levels. These systemic effects require active treatment of the diabetes as well as the infection.

Infection in the foot may also cause tissue necrosis. When the patient has arterial disease this is more likely to occur. The arterial disease may warrant revascularization if underlying perfusion is inadequate. In some patients the disease may be microvascular and consequently infection can cause necrosis of tissue in the presence of palpable pedal pulses.

When cellulitis is present the source of infection should be sought and treated. If pus or wet gangrene is present, debridement and drainage should be undertaken. Frequently this may be associated with a callus or blister, which should then be debrided in order to assess the extent of the underlying injury and to effect drainage.

In diabetic foot sepsis, necrosis beneath the skin is often far more extensive than in the skin lesion itself, thus requiring extensive debridement in order to help to control the infection.

In any patient who has either cellulitis or ulceration in the foot, osteomyelitis and septic arthritis should be suspected and excluded. The possibility of this is greater if the infection or ulceration has been present for greater than two weeks. Clinical signs that are strongly suggestive and almost diagnostic of bone or joint involvement are excessive mobility in joints or toes, crepitus on moving a toe, contact with bone when an ulcer is probed and the presence of a serous 'sticky' discharge from an ulcer which may be synovial fluid. Bone involvement can be detected on x-ray if the infection has been present for some time. However, if there is no evidence on x-ray and the suspicion is strong, inflammatory markers (erythrocyte sedimentation rate (ESR) and C-reactive protein (CRP)) and further imaging, e.g. bone scan or magnetic resonance imaging (MRI), should be performed.

Treatment of the bone infection needs to be thorough and prolonged. Ideally confirmation of the responsible bacteria should be obtained by a swab from deep within the wound or if possible culture of a fragment of bone. The initial antibiotic therapy may need to be intravenous if there is major infection, however, this can be oral if there is not significant involvement of the surrounding soft tissues. As diabetic foot sepsis is frequently polymicrobial, broad coverage therapy should be commenced and modified as specific culture results become available. Depending on the clinical setting, intravenous treatment will generally be used for one to two weeks (frequently longer if significant bone involvement is found) and then can be converted to oral therapy. Oral treatment should continue for several months and cessation of antibiotics is determined by objective evidence that the infection has resolved. The most accurate way of determining this is demonstration that CRP and ESR have returned to normal. These should be performed at the initial diagnosis and repeated approximately once each month. In addition, one would expect healing of any ulceration or sinus and evidence of no further destruction of bone on x-ray.

Osteomyelitis is not itself an absolute indication for surgery to the foot. At times it is essential to debride devitalized tissue; however, after any excisional procedures the dynamics of the foot will change and new areas on the foot will be more susceptible to pressure. If osteomyelitis is not responding to antibiotics surgical debridement should be considered. In general if there is septic arthritis in an interphalangeal or metatarsophalangeal joint, this will not respond to antibiotics and surgical debridement should be considered early in the treatment. Septic arthritis is not always easy to diagnose. However, it is likely to be present if there is erosion of the bone that abuts a joint, if there is excessive mobility in a joint or if there is a discharge that resembles synovial fluid. In these circumstances amputation of a toe may be necessary, preserving the metatarsal head if this is not involved. If the involvement is just in a metatarsophalangeal joint the involved bone may be excised while still preserving the toe.

Ulceration

Moderate to severe peripheral neuropathy, is the most important predisposing cause of foot ulceration in diabetics. Sensory neuropathy allows injury or repetitive trauma to the foot resulting in ulceration or callus formation. The presence of callus further increases pressure on underlying tissues and if untreated will result in ulceration. Motor neuropathy causes atrophy of the intrinsic muscles of the foot, leading to biomechanical abnormalities which is also a strong aetiological factor in the development of ulceration.

The autonomic component of peripheral neuropathy causes decreased sweating, resulting in dry skin predisposed to cracking and hence ulceration.

Studies have demonstrated that elevated ambulatory plantar pressures are predictive of ulcer development [12]. However, abnormal foot pressures alone probably do not cause ulceration, rather the combination of high plantar pressures and neuropathy is a more potent predictor of predisposition to ulceration [13].

Further studies have demonstrated that both dynamic forefoot and rearfoot plantar pressures (increased when walking) are significantly elevated in moderate to severe neuropathy. Also the ratio between forefoot and rearfoot pressures is increased in severe neuropathy and this ratio is correlated with the development of ulceration [14].

Prevention and treatment of ulceration in the neuropathic foot is based on pressure relief/pressure offloading. Several types of pressure are important:

(1) Direct repetitive moderate pressure is the most important aetiological factor in the development of ulceration and delay in healing.
(2) Shear stress occurs parallel to the sole of the foot and occurs between the layers of the foot. This form of stress is particularly important after surgical debridement.

Offloading techniques are utilized by podiatrists and orthotists to decrease these forces on the neuropathic foot. Pressure relief is particularly important in allowing neuropathic ulceration to heal and prevent recurrence of ulceration.

The issues of pressure relief are considerably more important than the type of dressing applied to a foot wound.

Ischaemic necrosis

When the presenting problem is necrosis, it is important to determine whether there is contributory large vessel arterial disease and evidence of infection. As previously discussed, if the area of necrosis is infected and moist this should be debrided early. A major problem encountered in diabetic patients (and other individuals who are neuropathic or immobilized) is ischaemic necrosis of the heel which results from a combination of pressure and/or ischaemia. If perfusion is thought to be adequate and florid sepsis is not present, the necrotic areas may be left dry. Conservative management is frequently chosen if there is concern about the viability of the adjacent skin and subcutaneous tissues down to the calcaneus. If the necrosis is down to bone, the wound can at times heal and gradually the eschar will lift, whereas exposing the bone will mostly lead to major amputation. Clarification of the presence of osteomyelitis of the calcaneus can be undertaken by x-ray and if this shows no overt abnormality, a bone scan or MRI should be considered.

Charcot's arthropathy (diabetic neuropathic arthropathy)

Charcot's arthropathy refers to a progressive destruction of bone and soft tissues, most commonly occurring in the foot. Whilst diabetes is the most common cause of this condition, other causes of neuropathy can result in a Charcot joint. The condition may involve joint dislocations, pathological fractures and major bony deformities. The majority of individuals with Charcot's arthropathy have had poorly controlled diabetes for 15 to 20 years.

There are currently two theories proposed to explain the pathogenesis of this condition.

The 'neurotraumatic theory' suggests that this condition is due to unrecognized injury to the neuropathic foot. The individual is thus unaware of bony injury which can occur with walking as well as injury. This trauma results in bony destruction and damage to joints.

The 'neurovascular theory' suggests that the autonomic neuropathy results in a significant increase in blood flow to the foot resulting in osteopenia.

Currently, it is generally felt that Charcot's foot results from a combination of these two pathological processes.

Charcot's arthropathy may present acutely or in a more chronic phase of the disease.

Acute Charcot's foot presents with an acutely swollen, red, hot foot. Pain may or may not be present. Over 80% of cases involve the tarsometatarsal, naviculocuneiform, talonavicular and/or calcaneocuboid joints. Exclusion of osteomyelitis is of critical importance and this can be extremely difficult, particularly if ulceration is present.

Standard investigation of full blood count, x-ray, ESR and CRP should be performed routinely. If inflammatory markers are greatly raised, a high index of suspicion of osteomyelitis should be entertained. A bone scan will always be quite abnormal and if a high index of suspicion of osteomyelitis is held, a labelled white cell scan may be useful. Magnetic resonance imaging (or possibly spiral computed tomography (CT) scan) is probably the most useful diagnostic test for confirming or excluding osteomyelitis in acute Charcot's arthropathy. If ulceration is present, probing the ulcer down to joint or bone will be almost diagnostic of bony infection.

Management of acute Charcot's arthropathy requires immobilization of the foot, initially starting with bed rest if swelling is present. Total contact casting is the preferred technique once acute swelling has resolved and may be required for several months.

Chronic Charcot's arthropathy may present with ulceration or as an 'abnormal foot'. The principles of management in the chronic (or acute on chronic) situation are to exclude underlying bony infection (using the same approach as in the acute situation), assessment of neuropathy, assessment of diabetic control, and the use of pressure relief techniques to stabilize and prevent deterioration of the foot. Total contact casting, air splint or CROW may be used initially. Ultimately an orthotic shoe should be the long term aim of therapy [15].

PRINCIPLES OF TREATMENT

Classification

Management of the diabetic foot lesion requires a thorough assessment taking into account both the local and systemic issues discussed in this chapter. Classification of the foot pathology ought to be based on a widely accepted and reproducible system. A number of reliable grading systems are in clinical use, including the University of Texas Diabetic Wound Classification System which categorizes wounds on the basis of wound type (stage) and involvement of deep structures (grade).

Stage	A	clean
	B	infected, not ischaemic
	C	ischaemic, not infected
	D	ischaemic and infected
Grade	0	healed/pre- or post-ulcerative lesion
	1	superficial wound – not involving tendon capsule or bone
	2	wound penetrating to tendon or capsule
	3	wound penetrating to bone and joint

This classification can be used to clearly describe diabetic foot lesions, allow clinicians to discuss management of particular types of lesions and predict outcomes of ulcers [16].

Table 26.3. *Diabetics at highest risk of major amputation*

History of foot ulceration
Presence of – neuropathy
– peripheral vascular disease
Poor glycaemic control
Foot deformity

Preventive foot care

Ideally with a diabetic patient, preventing problems should be the main goal. Patients need to be well educated in problems of foot care and have regular contact with a podiatrist who has a good knowledge of diabetic foot problems. As new problems develop in a patient's foot the objective is not just to treat the specific problem, but rather to make adjustments that will help to prevent it from occurring again. Pressure offloading is vital in preventing ulceration. Whilst individuals with the highest risk of limb loss (Table 26.3) require frequent review by experienced podiatrists, this group are often least compliant, further increasing risk of complications.

Hyperbaric oxygen therapy (HBOT)

The role of HBOT in the non-healing diabetic foot lesion remains controversial, despite the theoretical benefits of enhanced neutrophil activity, increased tissue oxygenation, and improved angiogenesis and wound healing [17]. Hyperbaric oxygen therapy usually involves a five to six week course of daily treatments, and is thus expensive and time consuming. A recent small randomized controlled trial suggested significantly enhanced healing in ischaemic diabetic ulcers [18]. Further studies are required to clarify the indications for HBOT in this context.

Multidisciplinary treatment

Treating patients with diabetic foot problems clearly requires multidisciplinary treatment, preferably with

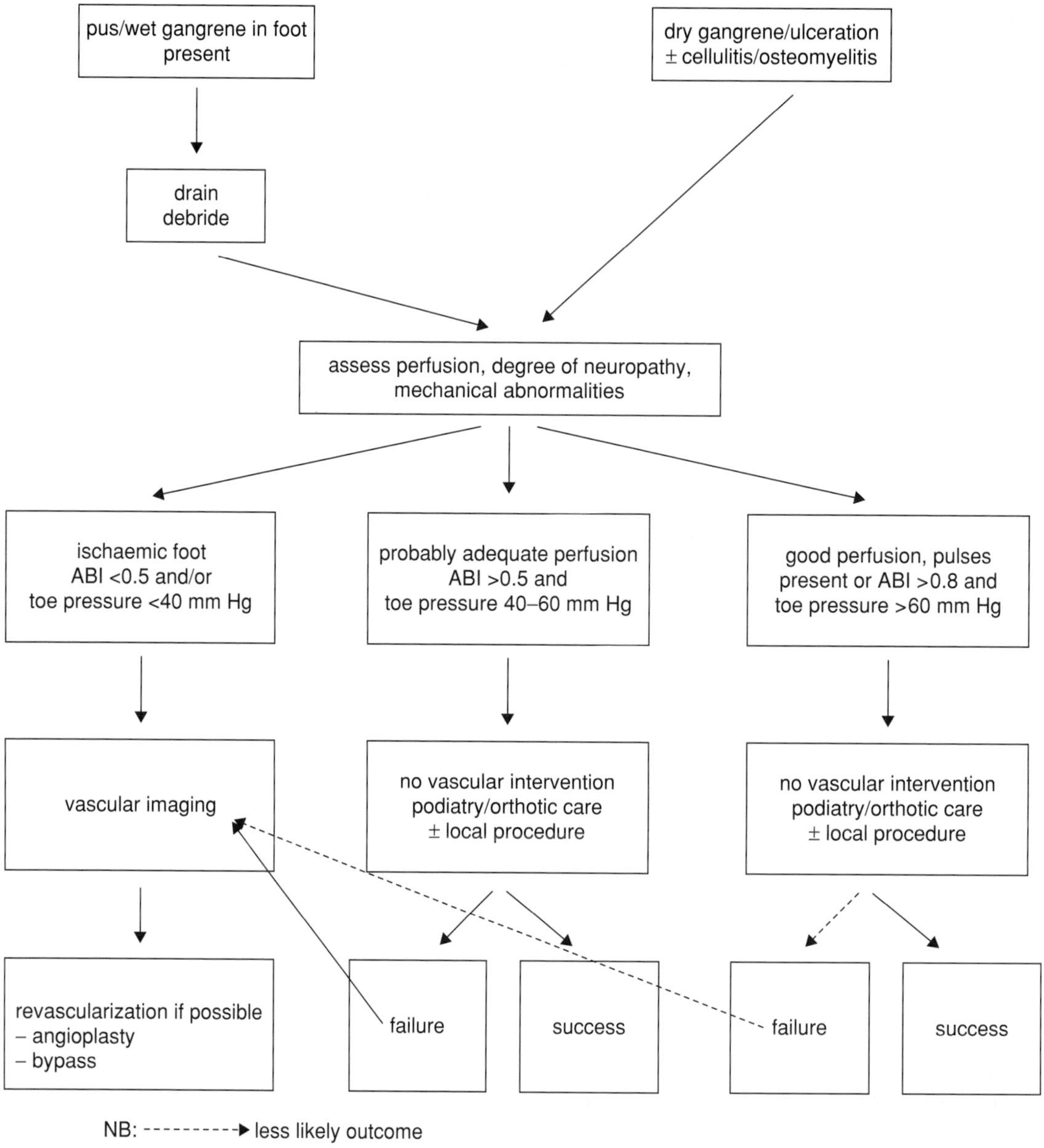

Fig. 26.1. Management algorithm for the diabetic foot lesion.

one contact professional who has extensive knowledge of the problem, who is able to recognize when new changes are appearing in the patient's foot and who can then enlist additional help from others when that is necessary. The team of professionals involved should include a diabetic physician, diabetes educator, vascular surgeon, podiatrist, orthotist and nurse.

A management algorithm for individuals with diabetic foot lesions is outlined above.

REFERENCES

1. C. M. Akbari & F. W. LoGerfo, Diabetes and peripheral vascular disease. *Journal of Vascular Surgery*, **30** (1999), 373–84.
2. G. M. Caputo, P. R. Cavanagh, J. S. Ulbrecht, G. W. Gibbons & A. W. Karchmer, Assessment and management of foot disease in patients with diabetes. *New England Journal of Medicine*, **331** (1994), 854–60.
3. R. Pop-Busui, V. Marinescu, C. van Huysen *et al.*, Dissection of metabolic, vascular and nerve conduction inter-relationships in experimental diabetic neuropathy by cyclo-oxygenase inhibition and acetyl-L-carnitine administration. *Diabetes*, **51** (2002), 2619–28.
4. A. M. Schmidt, S. D. Yan, J. L. Wautier & D. Stern, Activation of receptor for advanced glycation end products: a mechanism for chronic vascular dysfunction in diabetic vasculopathy and atherosclerosis. *Circulation Research*, **84** (1999), 489–97.
5. H. Vlassara, Protein glycation in the kidney: role in diabetes and aging. *Kidney International*, **49** (1996), 1795–804.
6. D. A. Greene, S. A. Lattimer & A. A. Sima, Sorbitol, phosphoinositides, and sodium-potassium ATPase in the pathogenesis of diabetic foot complications. *New England Journal of Medicine*, **316** (1987), 599–606.
7. P. C. Johnson, S. C. Doll & D. W. Cromey, Pathogenesis of diabetic neuropathy. *Annals of Neurology*, **19** (1986), 450–7.
8. The Diabetes Control and Complications Trial Research Group. The effect of intensive treatment of diabetes on the development and progression of long-term complications in insulin-dependent diabetes mellitus. *New England Journal of Medicine*, **329** (1993), 977–86.
9. D. Olaleye, B. A. Perkins & V. Bril, Evaluation of three screening tests and a risk assessment model for diagnosing peripheral neuropathy in the diabetic clinic. *Diabetes Research and Clinical Practice*, **54** (2001), 115–28.
10. M. J. Vitti, D. V. Robinson, M. Hauer-Jensen *et al.*, Wound healing in forefoot amputations: the predictive value of toe pressure. *Annals of Vascular Surgery*, **8** (1994), 99–106.
11. J. C. de Graaff, D. T. Ubbink, D. A. Legemate, G. P. Tijssen & M. J. M. Jacobs, Evaluation of toe pressure and transcutaneous oxygen measurements in management of chronic critical leg ischaemia: a diagnostic randomized clinical trial. *Journal of Vascular Surgery*, **38** (2003), 528–34.
12. A. Veves, H. J. Murray, M. J. Young & A. J. M. Bolton, The risk of foot ulceration in diabetic patients with high foot pressure: a prospective study. *Diabetologia*, **35** (1992), 660–3.
13. E. A. Masson, E. M. Hay, I. Stockley *et al.*, Abnormal foot pressure alone may not cause ulceration. *Diabetic Medicine*, **6** (1989), 426–8.
14. A. Coselli, H. Pham, J. M. Giurini, D. G. Armstrong & A. Veves, *Diabetic Care*, **25** (2002), 1066–71.
15. L. C. Schon, M. E. Easley & S. B. Weinfeld, Charcot neuroarthropathy of the foot and ankle. *Clinical Orthopaedics and Related Research*, **349** (1998), 116–31.
16. D. G. Armstrong, L. A. Lavery & L. B. Harkless, Validation of a diabetic wound classification system, the contribution of depth, infection and ischaemia to risk of amputation. *Diabetes Care*, **21** (1998), 855–9.
17. P. M. Tibbles & J. S. Edelsberg, Hyperbaric-oxygen therapy. *New England Journal of Medicine*, **334** (1996), 1642–8.
18. A. Abidia, G. Laden, G. Kuhan *et al.*, The role of hyperbaric oxygen therapy in ischaemic diabetic lower extremity ulcers: a double-blind randomized controlled trial. *European Journal of Vascular and Endovascular Surgery*, **25** (2003), 513–18.

27 • Lymphoedema: principles, genetics and pathophysiology

TAHIR ALI AND KEVIN BURNAND

INTRODUCTION

A reduction in the lymphatic drainage of tissues leads to excessive accumulation of interstitial fluid in the interstitial space. Lymphoedema most frequently affects the lower limbs, but can also cause swelling of the external genitalia, arms and face. (Figure 27.1). Lymphoedema may be unilateral or bilateral, symmetrical or asymmetrical in appearance. Lymphoedema is classified as primary when the cause is unknown or secondary if there is a clearly defined cause.

Primary lymphoedema is rare with an incidence of 1 in 6000 and is three times more common in women compared with men [1]. It is associated with a defective function of the lymphatic vessels or lymph nodes, leading to the inability to conduct lymph back to the circulation.

Secondary lymphoedema is more common. Filarial infiltration of lymphatic vessels leading to inflammatory fibrosis of the draining lymph nodes interferes with lymph flow [2; 3; 4]. This is the commonest cause of secondary lymphoedema worldwide and is especially common in Africa, the Far East and parts of South America. In Europe and North America, secondary lymphoedema is most often associated with malignancy and its treatment with surgery or radiotherapy. For example, lymphoedema of the upper limb following treatment of carcinoma of the breast [5]. The complications of lymphoedema include recurrent cellulitis, lymphangitis, and rarely skin ulceration and lymphangiosarcomatous change [6; 7].

CLASSIFICATION OF LYMPHOEDEMA

Primary lymphoedema was originally classified by Kinmonth on the basis of its lymphangiographic appearances into distal aplasia, distal hypoplasia with or without proximal hypoplasia, obstruction of the lymphatic pathways, numerical hyperplasia or megalymphatics [8; 9].

It was also classified by the age of its onset into the following categories [9]:

- Congenital: lymphoedema present at birth.
- Praecox: lymphoedema which occurs after birth and before 35 years of age.
- Tarda: lymphoedema which occurs after the age of 35.

More recently, Browse and Stewart proposed a new classification based upon the known physiology, and the potential abnormalities of the collection and passage of lymph from the interstitial space to the blood system. They suggested that there were three groups of patients with primary lymphoedema in whom the functional abnormality and its cause were known [10]:

- Large vessel abnormalities such as congenital aplasia, or incompetence of the thoracic duct or cysterna chyli.
- Congenital lymphatic valvular incompetence or congenital aplasia of the collecting ducts.
- Fibrosis in the lymph nodes [11; 12].

Patients with acquired lymphoedema were classified as having:

- Intraluminal or intramural lymphangio-obstructive oedema which was divided into distal, proximal and combined types. The lymphatic vessels could be obliterated in the distal limb or obliterated in the proximal limb (with possible distal dilatation of lymphatics). A combination of both proximal and distal obliteration was also recognized.
- Intra lymph gland (hilar) fibrosis. The lymph nodes had to be found to have hilar fibrosis on histology which blocks the lymph-conducting pathways, possibly causing lymphatic valvular incompetence.

Recent advances in the understanding of the genetics of lymphoedema have led to a modification of this classification. The word 'congenital' has been replaced with the more specific 'genetic' and the term

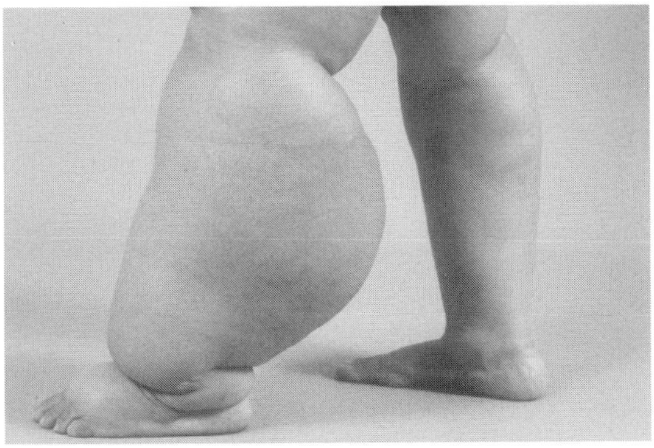

(a)

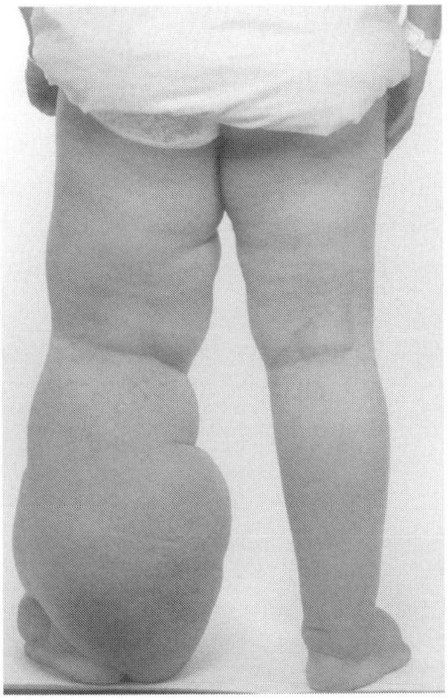

(b)

Fig. 27.1. (a) Unilateral left lower limb lymphoedema with pedal involvement (lateral view). (b) Unilateral left lower limb lymphoedema (posterior view).

'lymphangio-obstructive' has been altered to 'lymphangio-obliterative' to more accurately indicate the underlying pathology [13].

The current classification of lymphatic abnormalities in use at St. Thomas' hospital, requires both anatomical and chronological information for a functional appreciation of the lymphatic channels. This is outlined below:

(1) Genetically determined abnormalities
- Aplasia, malformation and valvular incompetence of the central lymphatic ducts, namely the cisterna chyli and thoracic duct.
- Aplasia, hypoplasia or dilatation and valvular incompetence of the collecting ducts in the subcutaneous tissues of the limb and trunk. This group therefore includes the familial conditions such as Milroy's, Meige's and lymphoedema-distichiasis syndromes. This group also includes the sporadic congenital lymphoedemas associated with recognized congenital abnormalities (Table 27.1).

(2) Acquired abnormalities
- Lymphangio-obliterative lymphoedema
  - (a) Distal
  - (b) Proximal
  - (c) Combined
- Intra lymph gland (hilar) fibrosis. Representing the lymphangio-obliterative process in the lymph conducting parts of the lymph gland.

(3) Kinmonth's numerical hyperplasia.

Table 27.1. *Clinical syndromes associated with primary lymphoedema*

Distichiasis (familial)
Klippel-Trenaunay
Mixed lymphatic and vascular deformities
Maffuci's syndrome
Lymphangiomatosis
Neurofibromatosis
Proteus syndrome
Turner's syndrome
Noonan's syndrome
Amniotic bands
Yellow nail syndrome

The pathological process in numerical hyperplasia does not fit into the above classification and is therefore listed separately. Here, the lymphangiographical abnormality is of increased numbers of normally sized lymphatic channels associated with excessive numbers of small lymph glands.

THE GENETICS OF LYMPHOEDEMA AND LYMPHANGIOGENESIS

Milroy's disease

Milroy first described a syndrome of hereditary lymphoedema seen at birth in 1892 [16]. The family

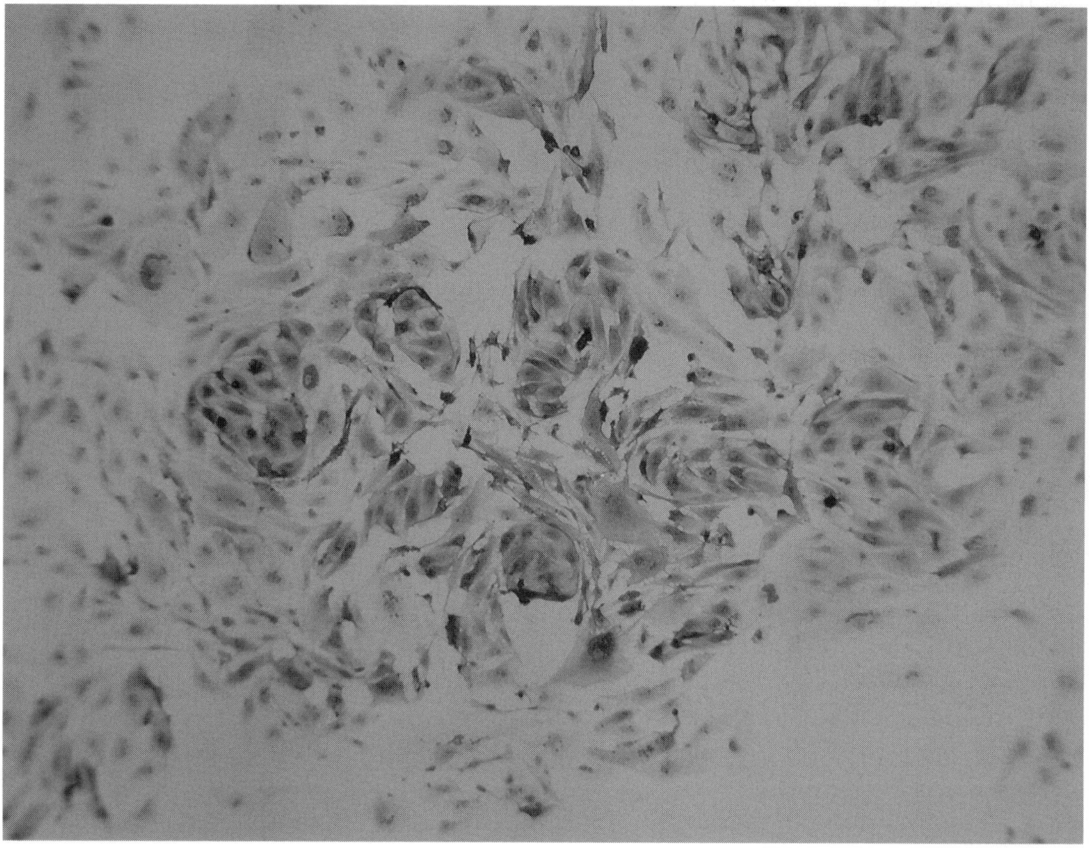

Fig. 27.2. Human dermal tissue stained with specific marker anti-LYVE-1 (see colour plate section).

genology of the affected clergyman was followed across six generations and 22 out of 97 descendants were thought to have limb swelling indicative of lymphoedema.

Linkage studies in families with primary congenital lymphoedema have mapped the diseased allele to chromosome 5q35.3 [17]. This region codes for vascular endothelial growth factor receptor-3 (VEGFR-3), a tyrosine kinase receptor for vascular endothelial growth factor-C (VEGF-C) [18]. Vascular endothelial growth factor was originally thought to increase vascular permeability but is now known to be the most powerful factor responsible for the growth of new blood vessels (angiogenesis). Lymphatic endothelium selectively expresses VEGFR-3 [19], while vascular endothelium expresses a different receptor (VEGFR-2) [20].

Vascular endothelial growth factor-C stimulates lymphangiogenesis and is one of two ligands that binds to VEGFR-3 [21] (the other ligand being VEGF-D). The ability to specifically target lymphatic endothelium has allowed the visualization of channels in mouse and human lymphatics with specific markers such as anti-LYVE-1 [22]. (Figure 27.2). Transfection of adenoviral VEGF-C into the skin of mice causes massive dermal lymphangiogenesis [23; 24; 25]. Transgenic expression of VEGF-C and VEGF-D in mice (the ligands to the above receptor), also increases lymphatic endothelial cell proliferation and causes lymphatic channel hyperplasia with normal lymph drainage.

Transgenic mice that over express VEGFR-3 have selective proliferation of lymphatic endothelial cells and hyperplasia of the lymphatic vasculature [26]. Targeted deletion of VEGFR-3 in mice causes defective vasculogenesis and embryonic death, and therefore cannot be used as a model of human lymphoedema [27]. Transgenic mice that over express VEGFR-3

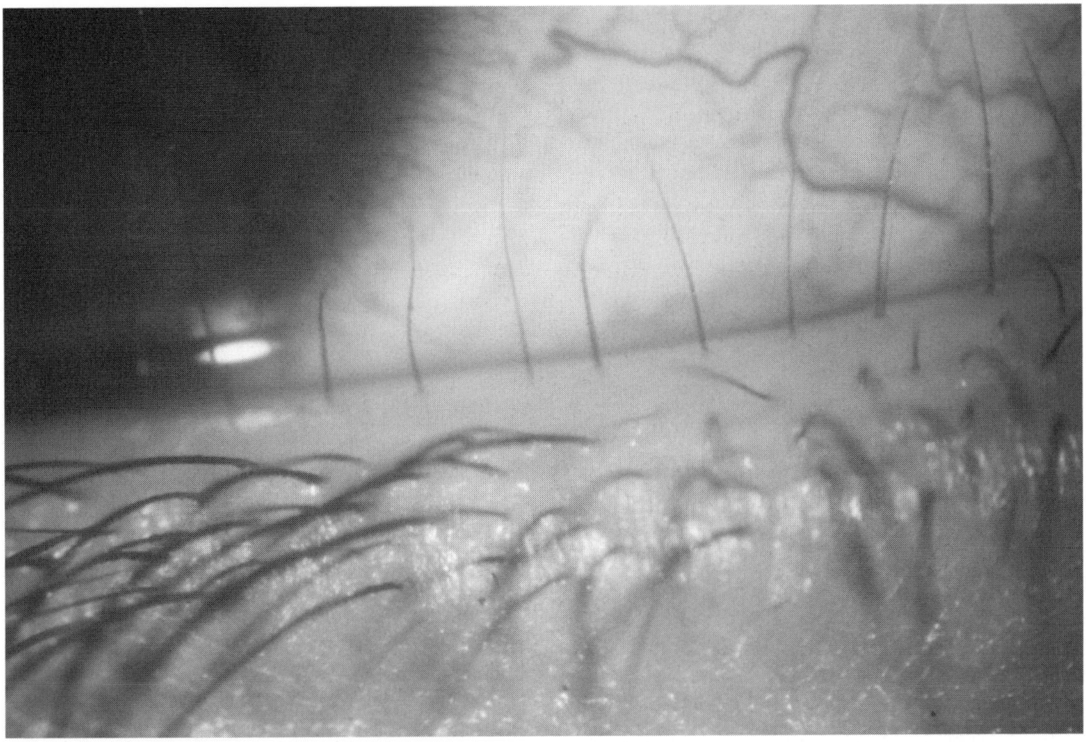

Fig. 27.3. Distichiasis with accessory eyelashes along the inferior posterior border of the lid margin in the position of the Meibomian glands (see colour plate section).

immunoglobulin, a soluble blocking epitope to VEGFR-3, do, however, survive into adulthood if a keratinocyte promotor is used to deliver the genetic mutation selectively to the dermis. These animals have no evidence of any deleterious effects on angiogenesis. Regression of formed dermal lymphatics occurs when this transgene is expressed in the embryo. Lymphatic endothelial apoptosis and involution is seen in the new born mice. Phenotypically these mice have absent cutaneous lymphatics, and have dermal and subcutaneous thickening associated with limb oedema due to the inhibition of VEGFR-3 [28]. These studies show that VEGFR-3 has an essential role in lymphangiogenesis [29].

Lymphoedema-distichiasis

In this syndrome peripubertal onset lymphoedema is associated with an extra row of eyelashes along the posterior border of the lid margin (distichiasis). There is often an associated ptosis and the condition has been classified as the lymphoedema-distichiasis syndrome [30] (Figure 27.3). The distichiasis often causes corneal irritation, conjunctivitis and photophobia. The condition is often associated with other congenital abnormalities which include congenital heart defects, cleft lip or palate, Pierre Robin syndrome (micrognathia, cleft soft palate, macroglossia), venous abnormalities and spinal extradural cysts [31].

The variable penetrance and autosomal dominant expression of the syndrome is similar to that seen in Milroy's disease [32]. The lymphoedema phenotype is, however, more prevalent in males and occurs at an earlier age of onset. In half the cases it is associated with the early onset of varicose veins [33]. The specific genetic abnormality in this syndrome has been located to chromosome 16q24.3 [34]. The gene has been identified as the forkhead transcription factor, FOXC2. The mutational analysis of 14 families with lymphoedema-distichiasis syndrome has provided support that alteration of the FOXC2 gene produces haploinsufficiency [35].

Targeted deletion or 'knock-out' of the FOXC2 gene in mice results in occular, cranio-facial, cardiovascular and vertebral anomalies in keeping with the associated congenital abnormalities witnessed in humans. Homozygous null animals die embryologically or shortly after birth. The use of oil contrast lymphography in heterozygote FOXC2+/− mice demonstrated that almost all had numerical lymphatic hyperplasia [36; 37]. Some 8% of the heterozygote mice had demonstrable hind limb swelling and a further 8% had demonstrable periorbital oedema.

Meige's disease

In 1898, Henri Meige described the most common variety of primary lymphoedema (38; 39). Meige's disease is a familial lymphoedema developing at or soon after puberty in which no other congenital abnormality is identified. The lymphoedema is often symmetrical and rarely extends above the knee. It occurs three times more commonly in females than males and has a genetic predisposition in about one-third of cases. Lymphography demonstrates peripheral lymphatic hypoplasia with more proximal lymphatic channels remaining patent (Kinmonth's hypoplasia) [40].This may represent peripheral lymphatic occlusion rather than true congenital hyopoplasia, as suggested by Browse and Stewart [10]. The genetic abnormality in this syndrome has not been found. It may be difficult to determine because of genetic heterogeneity within this group of patients.

Hypotrichosis-lymphoedema-telangiectasia

Three families with hypotrichosis, lymphoedema and telangiectasia have recently been reported [41]. All affected subjects presented with progressive alopecia, with loss of eyebrows and eyelashes, associated with pubertal onset lymphoedema. Two of the families had children with severe lymphatic agenesis presenting with fatal non-immune hydrops fetalis, and surviving offspring demonstrating the lymphoedema phenotype. Vascular endothelial growth factor receptor-3 and FOXC2 were excluded as causative genes for the disease by microsatellite marker analysis. A homozygous and heterozygous mutation in the gene encoding for the transcription factor SOX18 was identified as the cause. Consanguinity was identified in two families, which was characterized by a heterozygote and a homozygote mutation in the SOX18 protein. An error in the coding sequence led to a substitution of alanine with proline at position 104 in the SOX18 protein in one family. The second family had a homozygous substitution of trytophan with arginine at position 95 and in the third family, a heteozygous premature stop codon instead of cysteine residue at position 240.

Incontinentia pigmenti

Incontinentia pigmenti is a rare X-linked dominant genetic disorder. Male offspring with this condition die antenatally of sepsis. The immunological and infectious features observed in affected subjects result from impaired NF-κ B signalling and impaired cellular humoral response [42]. Mutations of the NF-κ B essential modulator gene (NEMO) results in undetectable NEMO protein and absent NF-κ B activation. This transcription factor, NF-κ B, regulates the expression of numerous genes controlling the immune and inflammatory responses, cell adhesion, and apoptosis [43; 44]. Those affected also develop ectodermal dysplasia with osteopetrosis and lymphoedema (OL-EDA-ID) [45].

Other clinical syndromes associated with primary lymphoedema (Table 27.2)

Noonan's syndrome

This autosomal dominant condition is associated with congenital heart defects such as dysplastic pulmonary stenosis and cardiomyopathy [46]. Those affected can also have ptosis, a short stature, webbed neck with a low hair line, facial abnormalities [47], intra-uterine cystic hygromas [48], hyperkeratosis and mental retardation [49]. They also commonly develop lymphoedema of the lower limbs, which is usually present from birth but presentation may vary from prenatal period to adulthood [50]. The Noonan's syndrome gene has been mapped to chromosome 12q, using linkage analysis in Dutch families [51; 52]. Missense mutations in PTPN11, the gene encoding the non-receptor-type protein tyrosine phosphatase SHP-2 (src homology region 2-domain phosphatase-2), has been identified as the cause of Noonan's syndrome [53].

Table 27.2. *Mendelian disorders with primary effects on lymphatics*

Yellow nail syndrome	*FOXC2* mutation(14)
Noonan's syndrome	12q24.1, *PTPN11* gene
Lymphoedema-distichiasis	16q24.3, *FOXC2* gene
Meige's syndrome	Not known
Incontinentia pigmenti	NEMO mutation
Hennekam Lymphagiectasia-lymphoedema	Not known
Turner's syndrome	Xp11.4 (15)
Milroy's disease	5q 34–5q 35, *VEGFR-3* gene

Cholestasis-lymphoedema syndrome

The syndrome of hereditary neonatal cholestasis and severe lymphoedema from birth was originally described in South Western Norwegian kindred in 1968 [54]. It has an autosomal recessive mode of inheritance. The genetic abnormality is located on chromosome 15q [54; 55; 56]. This locus has been mapped to a 6.6.cM interval on chromosome 15 [57]. More recently a separate second locus has been found which suggests that there is genetic heterogeneity in this syndrome [58].

LYMPHANGIOGENESIS

Venous endothelial cells originating in the region of the embryonic cardinal veins have been shown to direct lymphangiogenesis, possibly through polarization of endothelial cells [59; 60]. *Prox-1*, a homeobox gene, which determines cell differentiation, appears to control lymphatic development before birth. *Prox-1* knock-out mice have no viable progeny and demonstrate an absence of lymphatic vessels in homozygous littermates [61; 62].

Neuropilin-2 is another receptor, which has been identified and targeted, in knock-out studies. The neuropilin-2 knock-out mouse phenotypically has hypoplasia of endothelial lymphatic cells and reduced numbers of small lymphatic channels, but with normal development of arterial and venous vasculature. The larger lymphatic channels such as the thoracic duct and jugular lymph sacs are preserved. This suggests that selective lymphangiogenic failure may be classified into the absence of larger central lymphatic channels which are derived from the cardinal vein under the influence of *Prox-1* gene and an absence of smaller peripheral lymphatics (which may branch from these larger lymphatic trunks), perhaps dependent on the neuropilin-2 gene. [63; 64].

Angiopoietin-1 and -2 (Ang-1 and Ang-2) are members of the VEGF family that are known to orchestrate blood vessel and lymphatic growth by stimulating specific endothelial VEGF receptors (Tie 2) [65]. Angiopoietin-2 can both stimulate and antagonize the Tie 2 receptor, leading to angiogenic vessel sprouting and regression [66]. Angiopoietin-2 is thus capable of remodelling angiogenesis depending upon the circumstances [66; 67]. Angiopoietin-2 is not a prerequisite for blood vessel development unlike VEGF and Ang-1. Studies in *Ang-2* knock-out mice have demonstrated that these mice develop subcutaneous oedema and chylous ascites before dying. The lymphatics of these mice display a disorganized appearance, which may account for the abnormal permeability of these vessels. The circumferential smooth muscle coat of the major lymphatic is also poorly developed and disorganized. Central lacteals in the intestine are also often absent or underdeveloped, and the dermal lymphatics disorganized, disorientated and irregularly spaced. Replacing the *Ang-2* gene with *Ang-1*, reversed the lymphatic phenotype in the *Ang-2* deficient mice [68]. *Tie 2* knock-out animals have also confirmed the importance of Tie 2 signalling in angiogenesis [69]. The binding of Ang-2 to the Tie 2 receptor is therefore an important signal not only for angiogenic remodelling but also for lymphatic organization.

PATHOPHYSIOLOGY OF LYMPH FORMATION

The lymphatic system consists of the lymphatic collecting vessels, lymphoid cells and lymphoid tissue, such as lymph nodes, spleen, intestine, bone marrow and thymus gland.

Interstitial fluid is present in all regions of the body except the eye and central nervous system, where cerebrospinal fluid is circulated and absorbed through specialized cells lining the ventricles and intracranial venous sinuses. Lymphatics return the protein rich interstitial fluid formed in the rest of the body to the venous system in the neck through the thoracic and accessory thoracic ducts [70]. Dye injected in the inter-digit web space of the lower limb appears in the blood

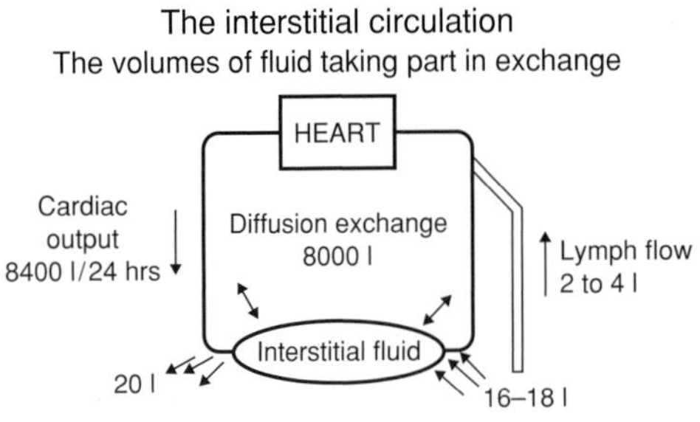

	FILTRATE	ABSORBATE	LYMPH
Fluid	20 l	16–18 l	2–4 l
Protein	80–200 g	0–5 g	75–195 g

After Landis and Pappenheimer

Fig. 27.4. Extravascular circulation of fluid and plasma protein in a 65 kg human.

within two minutes. This rapid circulation is aided by intrinsic contractility of the smooth muscle surrounding lymphatic vessels [71]. Contraction is seen in the lymphatics regardless of their distension or innervation. The rate of lymphatic return can be increased by factors that influence the rhythm and amplitude of spontaneous contractions [72].

Four litres of lymph is returned each day to the circulation. This fluid contains plasma proteins (mainly albumin which is principally derived from hepatic fenestrated capillaries), hydrophillic solutes, glucose, urea and hyaluronan [73] (Figure 27.4).

The volume of the lymph filtrate is governed principally by the capillary blood pressure, hydraulic permeability, capillary wall surface area and the opposing hydrostatic pressure of the surrounding pericapillary interstitial space [74; 75]. As flow along a lymph vessel decreases with decreasing lumen size and compliance, the interstitial filtrate is also reduced and the net interstitial colloid pressure therefore rises. The difference in colloid pressure between luminal and abluminal surfaces would approach equilibrium if flow approached zero. This would result in no net absorption of filtrate. The production of filtrate and thereby afferent lymph fluid is dependent upon the hydrostatic capillary pressure and the maintenance of a difference between the plasma and interstitial colloid pressure. This maximizes filtrate absorption in low flow areas, especially the postcapillary venule.

Tissues with numerous capillaries, which are fenestrated and discontinuous, such as the hepatic sinusoids, intestinal mucosal vessels and renal vessels, generate more filtrate when compared with skin, fat or connective tissue where the capillary density is less [76]. The pore size of these latter tissues is less. The gap junctions between endothelial cells are covered by a glycocalyx layer of fibrous molecules which acts as a semipermeable membrane and reduces the gap junction from 20 nm to 4 nm, thereby reducing plasma protein leakage into the interstitium [77].

In tissues with fenestrated capillaries interstitial colloid pressure is prevented from rising by water 'flushing' the interstitial space. This reduces protein accumulation on the abluminal surface of the vessel and minimizes the interstitial colloid pressure [78]. Dilution of interstitial colloid pressure allows continuous absorption of fluid into the venular capillaries. [79]. This increases the colloid pressure difference across the endothelial membrane and results in less lymph production [80].

FACTORS INFLUENCING OEDEMA FORMATION

Inflammation

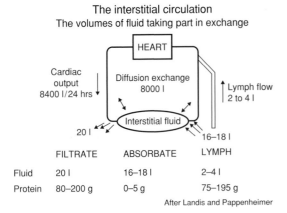

Inflammation increases endothelial hydraulic permeability by increasing the diameter of the intercellular clefts. This is as a consequence of the release of vasoactive peptides such as bradykinin, serotonin, interleukin-1 and -10, tumour necrosis factor, vascular epidermal growth factor, histamines and bacterial lipopolysaccharides. All these act to increase blood flow and vessel permeability [81]. The associated hyperaemia increases protein transport across the lymphatic endothelium [82]. In the presence of poorly functioning lymphatics, interstitial fluid becomes stagnant and can become infected. *Streptococcus pyogenes* is the most common pathogen. Patients often present with recurrent episodes of cellulitis. Each episode of infection predisposes the patient to fibrosis and further lymphatic damage. The acute inflammation not only induces hyperaemia and increased hydrostatic pressure but also increases protein rich interstitial fluid accumulation as a consequence of increased vascular permeability. This abolishes the plasma-interstitial pressure difference and increases the amount of interstitial fluid [83]. Inflammation also causes the release of endothelial derived nitrous oxide and oxygen free radicals which act as vasodilators, and inhibit the spontaneous tonic and phasic contractions of the smooth muscle of the lymphatic vessel wall further reducing lymphatic flow [84].

Hypoproteinaemia

Any reduction in plasma colloid pressure reduces lymph formation [85]. Cirrhotic liver failure, severe malnutrition, protein losing enteropathy and nephrotic syndrome reduce the albumin concentration in the intravascular compartment, and in some instances initiate neuro-humoral responses to maintain an effective circulating plasma volume [86]. This is mediated by the renin-angiotensin-aldosterone pathway, atrial natriuretic peptides (Henry-Gauer reflex) [87] and prostacyclins [88]. The glomerular filtration rate is reduced as the result of renal arteriolar vasoconstriction which leads to increased sodium and water reabsorption in the loop of Henle. Antidiuretic hormone increases the permeability of the collecting tubules to water and acts to increase the intravascular volume.

Increased capillary and venous pressure

Distension of the right atrium caused by high venous pressures leads to the release of natriuretic peptides. Natriuretic peptides inhibit the effect of antidiuretic hormone on the collecting ducts and cause a diuresis thereby reducing venous filling. This leads to a reduction in venous hydrostatic pressure. Veno-dilation further reduces the atrial stretch and optimizes contractility as predicted by the Frank-Starling curve. This leads to a reduction of hydrostatic pressure in the post-capillary venules and encourages fluid absorption from the interstitium. In chronic oedematous states, end organ resistance to these peptides increases interstitial fluid accumulation through reduced sodium excretion and increased venous hydrostatic pressure [89].

The gravitational loading which affects the lower limbs increases the pooling of blood in the venules and increases the hydrostatic pressure. The pressure exerted on the capillaries of the foot and ankle below the level of the heart is approximately 95 mm Hg. This causes fluid to accumulate in the interstitial space [90]. This tendency towards oedema is resisted by the increased dermal lymphatic density [91]. This delicate balance is overcome in pathological conditions which raise microvascular pressure, such as right heart failure, deep vein thrombosis, iatrogenic excessive fluid resuscitation and portal hypertension [92; 93].

Exercise prevents the accumulation of lymphatic fluid by the action of the axial musculature on lymph propulsion in competent lymphatic vessels [94]. The action of the calf muscle pump reduces capillary pressure at the ankle on ambulation to 30 mm Hg. Obstruction of the deep veins from a previous thrombosis or valvular damage causes excessive accumulation of interstitial fluid, because the calf pump does not work efficiently and the venous pressure remains persistently high during exercise.

Interstitial fluid compartment

The pressure in the interstitial space is negligible in comparison to the hydrostatic pressure present within the capillaries. In the subcutaneous fat the interstitial pressure is estimated at −2 mm Hg [95; 96]. This allows the movement of the capillary filtrate through the interstitial matrix towards the lymphatic plexus.

Small molecules are transported through the afferent lymphatics at 10 microns per second with microlymphatic vessels having a diameter of 60 microns [97]. Macromolecules such as albumin take longer to traverse the interstitial space because they are impeded by the large glycoaminoglycan polymer chain structures on the abluminal surface of the capillary endothelium [98]. Preferential channels may be present in the interstitium which allow some large molecules to rapidly traverse the interstitium and enter the afferent lymphatic channels [99]. Although the apparent reduction in transit time of the large molecules may simply be related to the greater distribution of the smaller molecules.

Filling of lymphatic capillaries

Endothelial cells of lymphatic capillaries are placed obliquely to one another with adjacent cells overlapping. This may allow the junctions between cells to act as flap valves, being opened up when the intraluminal pressure is exceeded by the interstitial pressure and closed when the converse occurs.

Lymph formation and propulsion

Blind ended lymphatic channels join together in the skin and subpapillary dermal plexus, around arterioles and venules. The lymphatic plexuses so formed unite to form larger collecting vessels [10]. The initial lymphatic channels are permeable to small solutes which enter through the endothelial gap junctions and pinocytic vesicles [100; 101]. The basal lamina of the lymphatics are held open by tethering radial filaments which prevent rises in interstitial pressure collapsing the lumen of the vessels [102]. As interstitial pressure exceeds intraluminal pressure, fluid enters the lymphatic vessel. As there is no smooth muscle layer in these terminal lymphatics passive movement and arteriolar contraction may encourage filling [103; 104]. The rising intraluminal pressure then causes the overlapping endothelial cells to close preventing lymph from refluxing into the interstitium.

A small hydraulic gradient may be the force responsible for encouraging the interstitial fluid to enter the lymphatics through the intercellular gaps in the lymphatic capillaries. The favourable pressure gradient that must exist if this flow is to be encouraged may be the result of lymphatic recoil, after cessation of compression, sucking fluid into the lumen. Lymph flow is coupled to capillary filtration if tissue oedema is to be prevented in normal individuals. Changes in the interstitial volume may pull open the intercellular junctions and encourage interstitial fluid to enter the lymphatics.

The lymphatics contain many bicuspid valves which prevent bi-directional flow, encouraging drainage to regional lymph nodes aided by the intrinsic contractility of the vessels [105]. The strength of this contraction is dependent upon the lymphatic wall stretch [106]. The rhythmical oscillation in pressure, which can be measured within the interstitium and lymphatics, is related to the respiratory rate and surrounding arterial pulsation [107; 108; 109; 110]. This is thought to aid lymph flow [111]. Skeletal muscle contraction may also increase lymph flow [112]. Over-filling of lymphatic vessels leads to a decrease in their contractile strength. Calcium antagonists have also been shown to reduce both lymph propulsion and frequency of spontaneous contraction [113]. Alpha-1 blockade of adrenergic receptors similarly reduces lymphatic pressure [114; 115].

The identification of action potentials across endothelial cell membranes and the modulation of this electrochemical gradient across lymphatic vessels has confirmed the presence of sino-atrial type pacemaker cells in lymphatic smooth muscle [113; 116].

The formation and propulsion of lymphatic fluid is seen to be a complex process and a better understanding of the mechanisms may provide new therapeutic approaches for the treatment of lymphoedema.

PATHOLOGY

Lymphatic channels

Initial lymphatic channels, in the upper one-third of the dermis, consist solely of endothelial cells without smooth muscle cells or anchoring filaments. These channels easily distend when interstial fluid enters them through the endothelial gap junctions. These initial lymphatics drain into pre-collecting lymphatic channels through a series of one-way valves. The basal lamina in these pre-collecting channels is incomplete allowing peripheral tethering filaments to bind to the abluminal surface of the endothelial cells through defects in the basal lamina. This prevents the lumen becoming occluded when the interstitial pressure rises.

Lymph fluid drains from the pre-collecting lymphatics into collecting lymphatics which lie in the upper or middle part of the dermis. These channels acquire a smooth muscle layer and continuous basal lamina. Fluid is directed from these collecting channels into larger subcuticular lymphatics which pass up to drain into the local lymph nodes. Efferent lymph fluid drains from the lymph nodes into central lymph trunks before eventually entering the thoracic duct. The thoracic duct has distinct layers of intima, media and adventitia.

The lymphatic endothelium in patients with chronic lymphoedema has an increased number of pinocytic vesicles in the cytoplasm and other various tubulo-reticular inclusion bodies. There is a reduction in the number of tethering filaments to the endothelial cell membrane, resulting in widened gap junctions. This may encourage lymph to reflux back into the interstitial space.

The endothelial lined intraluminal valves are thickened and the cells which cover the free edge of the valves develop abnormal filamentous changes [117; 118; 119; 120; 121; 122]. Luminal dilatation and valvular incompetence further increases lymphatic reflux. The perilymphatic space becomes chronically thickened with a granulofilamentous material containing degenerate elastic fibres and collagen [121; 122]. This ground substance is mixed with inflammatory cells and extravasated red cells. The mixed cellular infiltrate of polymorphonuclear leucocytes, lymphocytes, histiocytes and macrophages leads to the enzymatic release of collagenases and elastases [123]. These cells may target and deform the lysine and hydroxylysine components of dermal collagen fibres degrading the normal perilymphatic spiral arrangement of elastic fibres. This leads in turn to abundant amorphous hyalin-like deposits and a reduction in elastic fibres in the ground substance. A perivascular cuff of inflammatory cells is also seen around the small venules and arterioles.

Epidermal and dermal appearances in lymphoedema

Release of cytokines causes thickening of the dermal prickle cell layer. This cell-mediated proliferation of keratinocytes and the accumulation of protein-rich interstitial oedema leads to an acanthotic appearance of the dermis. Inflammatory cells migrate from the papillary dermal layers into the epidermal cell layer. Microfilament deposition in the dermo-epidermal junction leads to a thickened epidermal basal lamina. The keratinocytes become vacuolated indicating intracellular oedema and they develop pseudopodial projections. Hyperplasia and hypertrophy of the dermal vascular endothelial and epidermal cells, with a reduction in the intercellular desmosomes and tonofilaments, is responsible for the abnormal papillomatosis which develops in the skin of many patients with chronic lymphoedema.

Lymph nodes in lymphoedema

Lymph nodes filter lymph as it passes toward the thoracic or accessory cervical ducts. Intrinsic lymph node damage from surgical resection or radiotherapy results in secondary lymphoedema. The concept that nodal disease might be a cause of lymphoedema seems plausible. Excessive nodal fibrosis has been postulated by Kinmonth [12], Wolfe [124] and Fyfe, to be an important factor in the development of lymphoedema in some patients. These patients were thought to develop proximal lymphatic obstruction which eventually led to the afferent lymphatics dying back. The aetiology of the fibrosis within the lymph node has not been satisfactorily elucidated.

SUMMARY

The importance of genetic abnormalities in the development of different types of primary lymphoedema is now being elucidated. As the genetic abnormalities are discovered it will become clear which factors are responsible for lymphatic development and distribution. The pathophysiological changes which accompany lymphoedema and normal lymph function are also being investigated, and greater knowledge of the basic mechanisms may lead to better treatments.

REFERENCES

1. R. F. Dale, The inheritance of primary lymphoedema. *Journal of Medical Genetics*, **22**(4) (1985), 274–8.
2. N. C. Fyfe & E. W. Price, The effects of silica on lymph nodes and vessels – a possible mechanism in the pathogenesis of non-filarial endemic elephantiasis. *Transactions of the Royal Society of Tropical Medicine and Hygiene*, **79**(5) (1985), 645–51.
3. E. W. Price & W. J. Henderson, Silica and silicates in femoral lymph nodes of barefooted people in Ethiopia with special reference to elephantiasis of the lower legs. *Transactions of the Royal Society of Tropical Medicine and Hygiene*, **73**(6) (1979), 640–7.
4. E. W. Price, The relationship between endemic elephantiasis of the lower legs and the local soils and climate. *Tropical and Geographical Medicine*, **26**(3) (1974), 225–30.
5. A. L. Hoe, D. Iven, G. T. Royle & I. Taylor, Incidence of arm swelling following axillary clearance for breast cancer. *British Journal of Surgery*, **79**(3) (1992), 261–2.
6. F. W. Stewart & N. Treves, Classics in oncology: lymphangiosarcoma in postmastectomy lymphedema: a report of six cases in elephantiasis chirurgica. CA: *Cancer Journal for Clinicians*, **31**(5) (1981), 284–99.
7. H. Gajraj, S. G. Barker, K. G. Burnand & N. L. Browse, Lymphangiosarcoma complicating chronic primary lymphoedema. *British Journal of Surgery*, **74**(12) (1987), 1180.
8. J. B. Kinmonth, [Classification of primitive lymphedemas with special references to thoracic duct obstructions]. *Chirurgie*, **100**(3) (1974), 231–6.
9. J. B. Kinmonth, Primary lymphoedema of the lower limb. *Proceedings of the Royal Society of Medicine*, **58**(12) (1965), 1021–3.
10. N. L. Browse & G. Stewart, Lymphoedema: pathophysiology and classification. *Journal of Cardiovascular Surgery (Torino)*, **26**(2) (1985), 91–106.

11. J. H. Wolfe & J. B. Kinmonth, The prognosis of primary lymphedema of the lower limbs. *Archives of Surgery*, **116**(9) (1981), 1157–60.
12. J. B. Kinmonth & J. H. Wolfe, Fibrosis in the lymph nodes in primary lymphoedema. Histological and clinical studies in 74 patients with lower-limb oedema. *Annals of the Royal College of Surgeons of England*, **62**(5) (1980), 344–54.
13. N. L. Browse, K. Burnand & P. Mortimer, *Diseases of the Lymphatics*. 1. (London: Arnold, 2003).
14. R. Bell, G. Brice, A. H. Child *et al.*, Analysis of lymphoedema-distichiasis families for FOXC2 mutations reveals small insertions and deletions throughout the gene. *Human Genetics* **108**(6) (2001), 546–51.
15. C. A. Boucher, C. A. Sargent, T. Ogata & N. A. Affara, Breakpoint analysis of Turner patients with partial Xp deletions: implications for the lymphoedema gene location. *Journal of Medical Genetics*, **38**(9) (2001), 591–8.
16. M. A. Kanter, The lymphatic system: an historical perspective. *Plastic and Reconstructive Surgery*, **79**(1) (1987), 131–9.
17. A. L. Evans, G. Brice, V. Sotirova *et al.*, Mapping of primary congenital lymphedema to the 5q35.3 region. *American Journal of Human Genetics*, **64**(2) (1999), 547–55.
18. R. E. Ferrell, K. L. Levinson, J. H. Esman, Hereditary lymphedema: evidence for linkage and genetic heterogeneity. *Human Molecular Genetics*, **7**(13) (1998), 2073–8.
19. K. Hamada, Y. Oike, N. Takakura *et al.*, VEGF-C signaling pathways through VEGFR-2 and VEGFR-3 in vasculoangiogenesis and hematopoiesis. *Blood*, **96**(12) (2000), 3793–800.
20. A. Kaipainen, J. Korhonen, T. Mustonen *et al.*, Expression of the fms-like tyrosine kinase 4 gene becomes restricted to lymphatic endothelium during development. *Proceedings of the National Academy of Sciences of the USA*, **92**(8) (1995), 3566–70.
21. M. G. Achen, M. Jeltsch, E. Kukke *et al.*, Vascular endothelial growth factor D (VEGF-D) is a ligand for the tyrosine kinases VEGF receptor 2 (Flk1) and VEGF receptor 3 (Flt4). *Proceedings of the National Academy of Sciences of the USA*, **95**(2) (1998), 548–53.
22. S. Banerji, J. Ni, S. X. Wang *et al.*, LYVE-1, a new homologue of the CD44 glycoprotein, is a lymph-specific receptor for hyaluronan. *Journal of Cell Biology*, **144**(4) (1999), 789–801.
23. B. Enholm, T. Karpanen, M. Jeltsch *et al.*, Adenoviral expression of vascular endothelial growth factor-C induces lymphangiogenesis in the skin. *Circulation Research*, **88**(6) (2001), 623–9.
24. M. J. Karkkainen, A. Saaristo, L. Jussila *et al.*, A model for gene therapy of human hereditary lymphedema. *Proceedings of the National Academy of Sciences of the USA*, **98**(22) (2001), 12677–82.
25. A. Saaristo, T. Veikkola, B. Enholm *et al.*, Adenoviral VEGF-C overexpression induces blood vessel enlargement, tortuosity, and leakiness but no sprouting angiogenesis in the skin or mucous membranes. *FASEB Journal*, **16**(9) (2002), 1041–9.
26. M. Jeltsch, A. Kaipainen, V. Joukov *et al.*, Hyperplasia of lymphatic vessels in VEGF-C transgenic mice. *Science*, **276**(5317) (1997), 1423–5.
27. D. J. Dumont, L. Jussila, J. Taipale *et al.*, Cardiovascular failure in mouse embryos deficient in VEGF receptor-3. *Science*, **282**(5390) (1998), 946–9.
28. T. Makinen, L. Jussila, T. Veikkola *et al.*, Inhibition of lymphangiogenesis with resulting lymphedema in transgenic mice expressing soluble VEGF receptor-3. *Nature Medicine*, **7**(2) (2001), 199–205.
29. T. Veikkola, L. Jussila, T. Makinen *et al.*, Signalling via vascular endothelial growth factor receptor-3 is sufficient for lymphangiogenesis in transgenic mice. *EMBO Journal*, **20**(6) (2001), 1223–31.
30. J. Mangion, N. Rahman, S. Mansour *et al.*, A gene for lymphedema-distichiasis maps to 16q24.3. *American Journal of Human Genetics*, **65**(2) (1999), 427–32.
31. Z. Pap, T. Biro, L. Szabo & Z. Papp, Syndrome of lymphoedema and distichiasis. *Human Genetics*, **53**(3) (1980), 309–10.
32. J. L. Rosbotham, G. W. Brice, A. H. Child *et al.*, Distichiasis-lymphoedema: clinical features, venous function and lymphoscintigraphy. *British Journal of Dermatology*, **142**(1) (2000), 148–52.
33. G. Brice, S. Mansour, R. Bell *et al.*, Analysis of the phenotypic abnormalities in lymphoedema-distichiasis syndrome in 74 patients with FOXC2 mutations or linkage to 16q24. *Journal of Medical Genetics*, **39**(7) (2002), 478–83.
34. J. Mangion, N. Rahman, S. Mansour *et al.*, A gene for lymphedema-distichiasis maps to 16q24.3. *American Journal of Human Genetics*, **65**(2) (1999), 427–32.

35. R. Bell, G. Brice, A. H. Child *et al.*, Analysis of lymphoedema-distichiasis families for FOXC2 mutations reveals small insertions and deletions throughout the gene. *Human Genetics*, **108**(6) (2001), 546–51.
36. B. M. Kriederman, T. L. Myloyde, M. H. Witte *et al.*, FOXC2 haploinsufficient mice are a model for human autosomal dominant lymphedema-distichiasis syndrome. *Human Molecular Genetics*, **12**(10) (2003), 1179–85.
37. J. Fang, S. L. Dagenais, R. P. Erickson *et al.*, Mutations in FOXC2 (MFH-1), a forkhead family transcription factor, are responsible for the hereditary lymphedema-distichiasis syndrome. *American Journal of Human Genetics*, **67**(6) (2000), 1382–8.
38. R. F. Dale, The inheritance of primary lymphoedema. *Journal of Medical Genetics*, **22**(4) (1985), 274–8.
39. H. Meige, Dystrophie oedemateuse hereditaire. *Presse Medicale*, **6** (1898), 341–3.
40. J. B. Kinmonth, Primary lymphoedema of the lower limb. *Proceedings of the Royal Society of Medicine*, **58**(12) (1965), 1021–3.
41. A. Irrthum, K. Devriendt, D. Chitayat *et al.*, Mutations in the transcription factor gene SOX18 underlie recessive and dominant forms of hypotrichosis-lymphedema-telangiectasia. *American Journal of Human Genetics*, **72**(6) (2003), 1470–8.
42. S. Aradhya & D. L. Nelson, NF-kappaB signaling and human disease. *Current Opinion in Genetics and Development*, **11**(3) (2001), 300–6.
43. A. Smahi, G. Courtois, S. H. Rabia *et al.*, The NF-kappaB signalling pathway in human diseases: from incontinentia pigmenti to ectodermal dysplasias and immune-deficiency syndromes. *Human Molecular Genetics*, **11**(20) (2002), 2371–5.
44. I. Garcia-Cao, M. J. Lafuente & L. M. Criado, Genetic inactivation of Par4 results in hyperactivation of NF-kappaB and impairment of JNK and p38. *EMBO Reports*, **4**(3) (2003), 307–12.
45. R. Doffinger, A. Smahi, C. Bessia *et al.*, X-linked anhidrotic ectodermal dysplasia with immunodeficiency is caused by impaired NF-kappaB signaling. *Nature Genetics*, **27**(3) (2001), 277–85.
46. M. Chery, C. Philippe, A. M. Worms & S. Gilgenkrantz, The Noonan syndrome. The Nancy experience revisited. *Genetics Counseling*, **4**(2) (1993), 113–18.
47. G. Neri, M. Zollino & J. F. Reynolds, The Noonan-CFC controversy. *American Journal of Medical Genetics*, **39**(3) (1991), 367–70.
48. M. J. Edwards & J. M. Graham, Jr., Posterior nuchal cystic hygroma. *Clinical Perinatology*, **17**(3) (1990), 611–40.
49. D. R. Witt, H. E. Hoyme, J. Zonana *et al.*, Lymphedema in Noonan syndrome: clues to pathogenesis and prenatal diagnosis and review of the literature. *American Journal of Medical Genetics*, **27**(4) (1987), 841–56.
50. P. Lanning, S. Simila, I. Suramo & T. Paavilainen, Lymphatic abnormalities in Noonan's syndrome. *Pediatric Radiology*, **7**(2) (1978), 106–9.
51. C. R. Jamieson, I. van der Burgt, A. F. Brady *et al.*, Mapping a gene for Noonan syndrome to the long arm of chromosome 12. *Nature Genetics*, **8**(4) (1994), 357–60.
52. A. F. Brady, C. R. Jamieson, I. van dB *et al.*, Further delineation of the critical region for Noonan syndrome on the long arm of chromosome 12. *European Journal of Human Genetics*, **5**(5) (1997), 336–7.
53. M. Tartaglia, K. Kalidas, A. Shaw *et al.*, PTPN11 mutations in Noonan syndrome: molecular spectrum, genotype-phenotype correlation, and phenotypic heterogeneity. *American Journal of Human Genetics*, **70**(6) (2002), 1555–63.
54. O. Aagenaes, H. Sigstad & R. Bjorn-Hansen, Lymphoedema in hereditary recurrent cholestasis from birth. *Archives of Disease in Childhood*, **45**(243) (1970), 690–5.
55. M. Fruhwirth, A. R. Janecke, T. Muller *et al.*, Evidence for genetic heterogeneity in lymphedema-cholestasis syndrome. *Journal of Pediatrics*, **142**(4) (2003), 441–7.
56. A. Heiberg, [Aagenaes syndrome – lymphedema and intrahepatic cholestasis.] *Tidsskrift for den Norske Laegeforening*, **121**(14) (2001), 1718–19.
57. L. N. Bull, E. Roche, E. J. Song *et al.*, Mapping of the locus for cholestasis-lymphedema syndrome (Aagenaes syndrome) to a 6.6-cM interval on chromosome 15q. *American Journal of Human Genetics*, **67**(4) (2000), 994–9.
58. M. Fruhwirth, A. R. Janecke, T. Muller *et al.*, Evidence for genetic heterogeneity in lymphedema-cholestasis syndrome. *Journal of Pediatrics*, **142**(4) (2003), 441–7.
59. J. T. Wigle & G. Oliver, Prox1 function is required for the development of the murine lymphatic system. *Cell*, **98**(6) (1999), 769–78.

60. F. R. Sabin, On the origin of the lymphatic system from the veins and the development of the lymph hearts and thoracic duct in the pig. *American Journal of Anatomy*, **1** (1902), 367–91.
61. J. T. Wigle, N. Harvey, M. Detmar *et al.*, An essential role for Prox1 in the induction of the lymphatic endothelial cell phenotype. *EMBO Journal*, **21**(7) (2002), 1505–13.
62. Y. K. Hong, N. Harvey, Y. H. Noh *et al.*, Prox1 is a master control gene in the program specifying lymphatic endothelial cell fate. *Developmental Dynamics*, **225**(3) (2002), 351–7.
63. L. Yuan, D. Moyon, L. Pardanaud *et al.*, Abnormal lymphatic vessel development in neuropilin 2 mutant mice. *Development*, **129**(20) (2002), 4797–806.
64. M. J. Karkkainen & K. Alitalo, Lymphatic endothelial regulation, lymphoedema, and lymph node metastasis. *Seminars in Cell and Developmental Biology*, **13**(1) (2002), 9–18.
65. T. Veikkola & K. Alitalo, Dual role of Ang2 in postnatal angiogenesis and lymphangiogenesis. *Developmental Cell*, 3(3) (2002), 302–4.
66. J. Holash, P. C. Maisonpierre, D. Compton *et al.*, Vessel cooption, regression, and growth in tumors mediated by angiopoietins and VEGF. *Science*, **284**(5422) (1999), 1994–8.
67. A. Stratmann, W. Risau & K. H. Plate, Cell type-specific expression of angiopoietin-1 and angiopoietin-2 suggests a role in glioblastoma angiogenesis. *American Journal of Pathology*, **153**(5) (1998), 1459–66.
68. N. W. Gale, G. Thurston, S. F. Hackett *et al.*, Angiopoietin-2 is required for postnatal angiogenesis and lymphatic patterning, and only the latter role is rescued by Angiopoietin-1. *Developmental Cell*, 3(3) (2002), 411–23.
69. T. N. Sato, Y. Tozawa, U. Deutsch *et al.*, Distinct roles of the receptor tyrosine kinases Tie-1 and Tie-2 in blood vessel formation. *Nature*, **376**(6535) (1995), 70–4.
70. L. E. Davis, A. R. Hohimer & R. A. Brace, Changes in left thoracic duct lymph flow during progressive anemia in the ovine fetus. *American Journal of Obstetrics and Gynecology*, **174**(5) (1996), 1469–76.
71. M. Aas, A. Skretting, A. Engeset, R. Westgaard & G. Nicolaysen, Lymphatic drainage from subcutaneous tissue in the foot and leg in the sitting human. *Acta Physiologica Scandinavica*, **125**(3) (1985), 505–11.
72. J. N. Benoit & D. C. Zawieja, Effects of f-Met-Leu-Phe-induced inflammation on intestinal lymph flow and lymphatic pump behavior. *American Journal of Physiology*, **262**(2) (Pt 1) (1992), G199–202.
73. H. Zoltzer & A. Castenholz, [The composition of lymph]. *Zeitschrift fur Lymphologie*, **9**(1) (1985), 3–13.
74. H. J. Zdolsek, B. Lisander, A. W. Jones & F. Sjoberg, Albumin supplementation during the first week after a burn does not mobilise tissue oedema in humans. *Intensive Care Medicine*, **27**(5) (2001), 844–52.
75. P. Kjellgren, A. Gupta & F. Sjoberg, Volume replacement during cardiac surgery-influence on microcirculation. *Acta Anaesthesiologica Scandinavica*, **39**(5) (1995), 709–10.
76. M. Taherzadeh, A. K. Das & J. B. Warren, Nifedipine increases microvascular permeability via a direct local effect on postcapillary venules. *American Journal of Physiology*, **275**(4) (Pt 2) (1998), H1388–94.
77. A. Castenholz, Functional microanatomy of initial lymphatics with special consideration of the extracellular matrix. *Lymphology*, **31**(3) (1998), 101–18.
78. J. R. Levick, Fluid exchange across endothelium. *International Journal of Microcirculation: Clinical and Experimental*, **17**(5) (1997), 241–7.
79. M. Aas, A. Skretting, A. Engeset, R. Westgaard & G. Nicolaysen, Lymphatic drainage from subcutaneous tissue in the foot and leg in the sitting human. *Acta Physiologica Scandinavica*, **125**(3) (1985), 505–11.
80. X. Hu, R. H. Adamson, B. Liu, F. E. Curry & S. Weinbaum, Starling forces that oppose filtration after tissue oncotic pressure is increased. *American Journal of Heart and Circulatory Physiology*, **279**(4) (2000), H1724–36.
81. J. N. Benoit & D. C. Zawieja, Effects of f-Met-Leu-Phe-induced inflammation on intestinal lymph flow and lymphatic pump behavior. *American Journal of Physiology*, **262**(2) (Pt 1) (1992), G199–202.
82. C. C. O' Morchoe, W. R. Jones, III, H. M. Jarosz, P. J. O'Morchoe & L. M. Fox, Temperature dependence of protein transport across lymphatic endothelium *in vitro*. *Journal of Cell Biology*, **98**(2) (1984), 629–40.
83. A. Szuba & S. G. Rockson, Lymphedema: classification, diagnosis and therapy. *Vascular Medicine*, **3**(2) (1998), 145–56.

84. A. A. Gashev & D. C. Zawieja, Physiology of human lymphatic contractility: a historical perspective. *Lymphology*, **34**(3) (2001), 124–34.
85. K. Aukland & R. K. Reed, Interstitial-lymphatic mechanisms in the control of extracellular fluid volume. *Physiology Reviews*, **73**(1) (1993), 1–78.
86. A. M. Chonko, W. H. Bay, J. H. Stein & T. F. Ferris, The role of renin and aldosterone in the salt retention of edema. *American Journal of Medicine*, **63**(6) (1977), 881–9.
87. N. Perico & G. Remuzzi, Edema of the nephrotic syndrome: the role of the atrial peptide system. *American Journal of Kidney Diseases*, **22**(3) (1993), 355–66.
88. N. Perico, A. Benigni, M. Gabanelli *et al.*, Atrial natriuretic peptide and prostacyclin synergistically mediate hyperfiltration and hyperperfusion of diabetic rats. *Diabetes*, **41**(4) (1992), 533–8.
89. I. S. Anand, R. Ferrari, G. S. Kalra *et al.*, Edema of cardiac origin. Studies of body water and sodium, renal function, hemodynamic indexes, and plasma hormones in untreated congestive cardiac failure. *Circulation*, **80**(2) (1989), 299–305.
90. V. Aarli, R. K. Reed & K. Aukland, Effect of longstanding venous stasis and hypoproteinaemia on lymph flow in the rat tail. *Acta Physiologica Scandinavica*, **142**(1) (1991), 1–9.
91. A. W. Stanton, H. S. Patel, J. R. Levick & P. S. Mortimer, Increased dermal lymphatic density in the human leg compared with the forearm. *Microvascular Research*, **57**(3) (1999), 320–8.
92. J. R. Levick & C. C. Michel, The effects of position and skin temperature on the capillary pressures in the fingers and toes. *Journal of Physiology*, **274** (1978), 97–109.
93. A. Bollinger, G. Isenring & U. K. Franzeck, Lymphatic microangiopathy: a complication of severe chronic venous incompetence (CVI). *Lymphology*, **15**(2) (1982), 60–5.
94. E. Havas, T. Parviainen, J. Vuorela, J. Toivanen *et al.*, Lymph flow dynamics in exercising human skeletal muscle as detected by scintography. *Journal of Physiology*, **504**(1) (1997), 233–9.
95. H. Noddeland, A. R. Hargens, R. K. Reed & K. Aukland, Interstitial colloid osmotic and hydrostatic pressures in subcutaneous tissue of human thorax. *Microvascular Research*, **24**(1) (1982), 104–13.
96. H. O. Fadnes, R. K. Reed & K. Aukland, Interstitial fluid pressure in rats measured with a modified wick technique. *Microvascular Research*, **14**(1) (1977), 27–36.
97. M. Fischer, U. K. Franzeck, I. Herrig *et al.*, Flow velocity of single lymphatic capillaries in human skin. *American Journal of Physiology*, **270**(1) (Pt 2) (1996), H358–63.
98. P. D. Watson, D. R. Bell & E. M. Renkin, Early kinetics of large molecule transport between plasma and lymph in dogs. *American Journal of Physiology*, **239**(4) (1980), H525–31.
99. A. Castenholz, G. Hauck & U. Rettberg, Light and electron microscopy of the structural organization of the tissue-lymphatic fluid drainage system in the mesentery: an experimental study. *Lymphology*, **24**(2) (1991), 82–92.
100. L. V. Leak, Lymphatic endothelial-interstitial interface. *Lymphology*, **20**(4) (1987), 196–204.
101. L. V. Leak, The structure of lymphatic capillaries in lymph formation. *Federation Proceedings*, **35**(8) (1976), 1863–71.
102. A. Bollinger, Microlymphatics of human skin. *International Journal of Microcirculation: Clinical and Experimental*, **12**(1) (1993), 1–15.
103. D. A. Berk, M. A. Swartz, A. J. Leu & R. K. Jain, Transport in lymphatic capillaries. II. Microscopic velocity measurement with fluorescence photobleaching. *American Journal of Physiology*, **270**(1) (Pt 2) (1996), H330–7.
104. M. A. Swartz, D. A. Berk & R. K. Jain, Transport in lymphatic capillaries. I. Macroscopic measurements using residence time distribution theory. *American Journal of Physiology*, **270**(1) (Pt 2) (1996), H324–9.
105. K. H. Albertine, L. M. Fox C. C. O'Morchoe, The morphology of canine lymphatic valves. *Anatomical Record*, **202**(4) (1982), 453–61.
106. A. R. Hargens & B. W. Zweifach, Contractile stimuli in collecting lymph vessels. *American Journal of Physiology*, **233**(1) (1977), H57–65.
107. J. G. McGeown, Splanchnic nerve stimulation increases the lymphocyte output in mesenteric efferent lymph. *Pflugers Arch*, **422**(6) (1993), 558–63.
108. J. G. McGeown, N. G. McHale & K. D. Thornbury, The effect of electrical stimulation of the sympathetic chain on peripheral lymph flow in the anaesthetized sheep. *Journal of Physiology*, **393** (1987), 123–33.

109. J. G. McGeown, N. G. McHale, I. C. Roddie & K. Thornbury, Peripheral lymphatic responses to outflow pressure in anaesthetized sheep. *Journal of Physiology*, **383** (1987), 527–36.
110. J. G. McGeown, N. G. McHale & K. D. Thornbury, The role of external compression and movement in lymph propulsion in the sheep hind limb. *Journal of Physiology*, **387** (1987), 83–93.
111. T. C. Skalak, G. W. Schmid-Schonbein & B. W. Zweifach, New morphological evidence for a mechanism of lymph formation in skeletal muscle. *Microvascular Research*, **28**(1) (1984), 95–112.
112. E. Ikomi, B. W. Zweifach & G. W. Schmid-Schonbein, Fluid pressures in the rabbit popliteal afferent lymphatics during passive tissue motion. *Lymphology*, **30**(1) (1997), 13–23.
113. K. D. McCloskey, H. M. Toland, M. A. Hollywood, K. D. Thornbury & N. G. McHale, Hyperpolarisation-activated inward current in isolated sheep mesenteric lymphatic smooth muscle. *Journal of Physiology*, **521**(1) (1999), 201–11.
114. D. E. Dobbins & A. J. Premen, Receptor mechanisms of bradykinin-mediated activation of prenodal lymphatic smooth muscle. *Regulatory Peptides*, **74**(1) (1998), 47–51.
115. D. E. Dobbins, Catecholamine-mediated lymphatic constriction: involvement of both alpha 1- and alpha 2-adrenoreceptors. *American Journal of Physiology*, **263**(2) (Pt 2) (1992), H473–8.
116. H. M. Toland, K. D. McCloskey, K. D. Thornbury, N. G. McHale & M. A. Hollywood, Ca(2+)-activated Cl(−) current in sheep lymphatic smooth muscle. *American Journal of Physiology – Cell Physiology*, **279**(5) (2000), C1327–35.
117. G. Azzali, M. Vitale & M. L. Arcari, Ultrastructure of absorbing peripheral lymphatic vessel (ALPA) in guinea pig Peyer's patches. *Microvascular Research*, **64**(2) (2002), 289–301.
118. J. Trzewik, S. K. Mallipattu, G. M. Artmann, F. A. Delano & G. W. Schmid-Schonbein, Evidence for a second valve system in lymphatics: endothelial microvalves. *FASEB Journal*, **15**(10) (2001), 1711–17.
119. J. Zhang, H. Li & R. Xiu, The role of the microlymphatic valve in the propagation of spontaneous rhythmical lymphatic motion in rat. *Clinical Hemorheology and Microcirculation*, **23**(2–4) (2000), 349–53.
120. S. Bannykh, A. Mironov, Jr., G. Bannykh & A. Mironov, The morphology of valves and valve-like structures in the canine and feline thoracic duct. *Anatomy and Embryology*, **192**(3) (1995), 265–74.
121. B. V. Vtiurin, V. G. Istratov & T. V. Savchenko, [Electron microscopic and mass spectrometric studies of lymphedema pathogenesis aspects]. *Vestnik Rossiikoi Akademii Meditsinskikh Nauk*, (7) (1999), 45–9.
122. M. Foldi, [Lymphological aspects of the pathophysiological basis of edema formation]. *Acta Medica Austriaca*, **3**(4) (1976), 105–12.
123. H. Galkowska & W. L. Olszewski, Cellular composition of lymph in experimental lymphedema. *Lymphology*, **19**(4) (1986), 139–45.
124. J. H. Wolfe, R. Rutt & J. B. Kinmonth, Lymphatic obstruction and lymph node changes – a study of the rabbit popliteal node. *Lymphology*, **16**(1) (1983), 19–26.

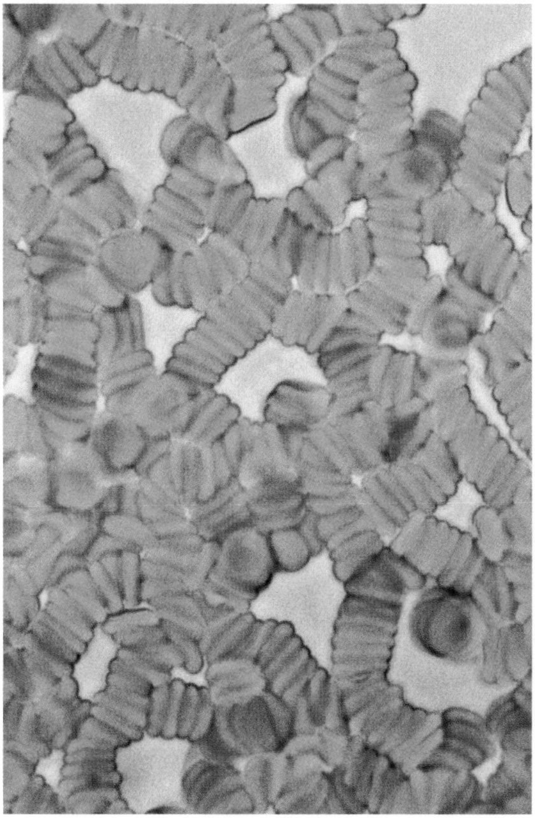

Fig. 3.5. Rouleaux blood cell network.

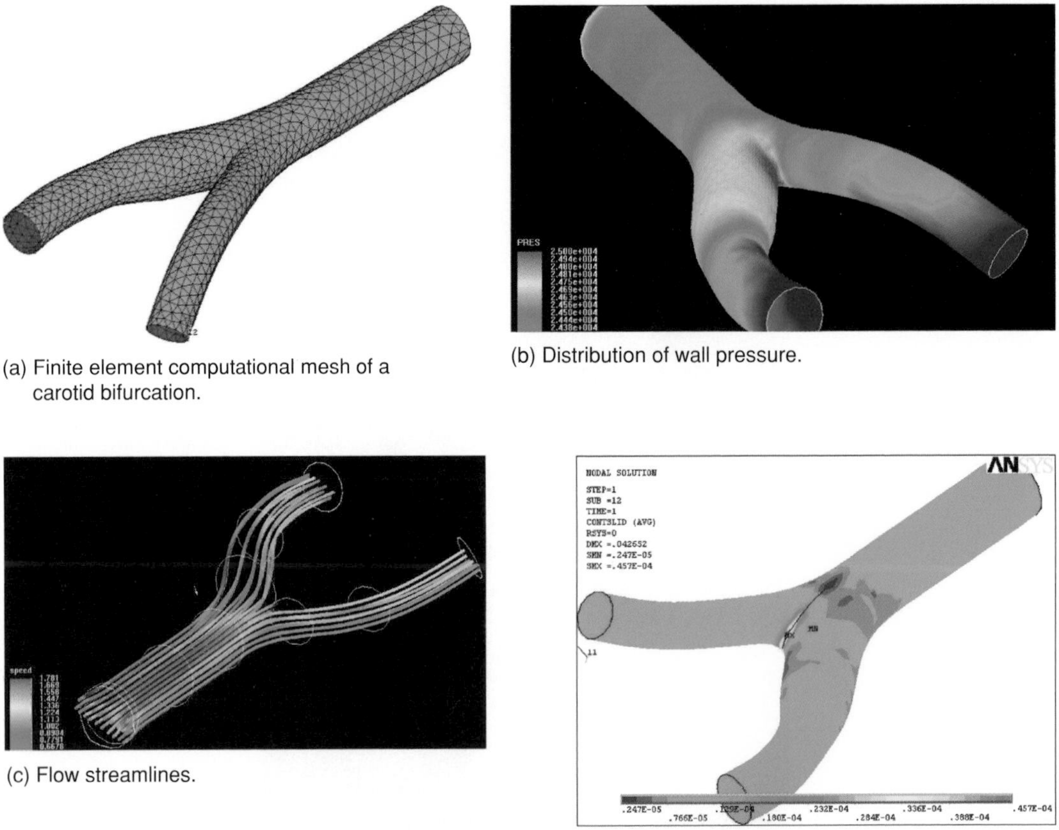

(a) Finite element computational mesh of a carotid bifurcation.

(b) Distribution of wall pressure.

(c) Flow streamlines.

(d) Inter-layer sliding distance.

Fig. 3.12. Finite element stress/strain and computational fluid dynamic model of a carotid bifurcation.

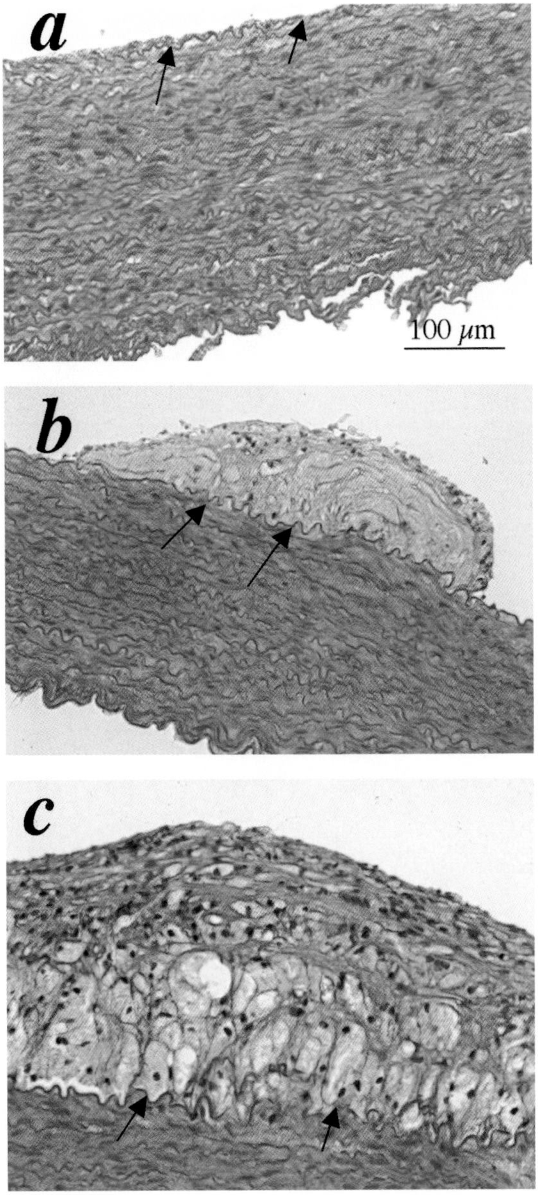

Fig. 7.1. Sections of the vessel wall. Rabbits were fed with: (a) a standard chow-diet; or (b) a cholesterol-enriched diet (0.2%) for three weeks; or (c) for 16 weeks. Their aortas were harvested, and sections prepared and stained with haematoxilin and eosin. Arrows indicate the internal elastic lamina, the border between the intima and media of the arterial wall.

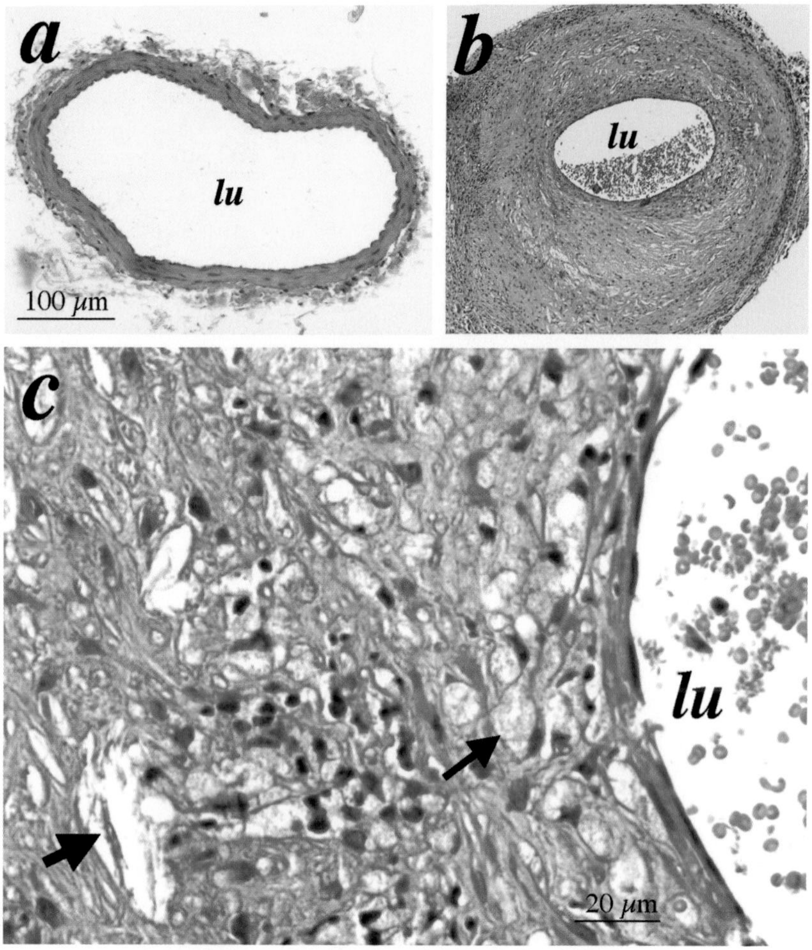

Fig. 7.3. Haematoxilin and eosin-stained sections of mouse vein grafts. Under anaesthesia, vena cava veins were removed and isografted into (a) carotid arteries of (b) apoE-/- mice. Animals were sacrificed eight weeks after surgery. The grafted tissue fragments were fixed in 4% phosphate phosphate-buffered (pH 7.2) formaldehyde, embedded in paraffin, sectioned and stained with haematoxilin-eosin. Panel (c) is a photograph of a vein graft section with higher magnification. Smaller arrow indicates a foam cell, whilst a larger one indicates a cholesterol crystal structure. The lumen of the vessel is inicated by *lu*.

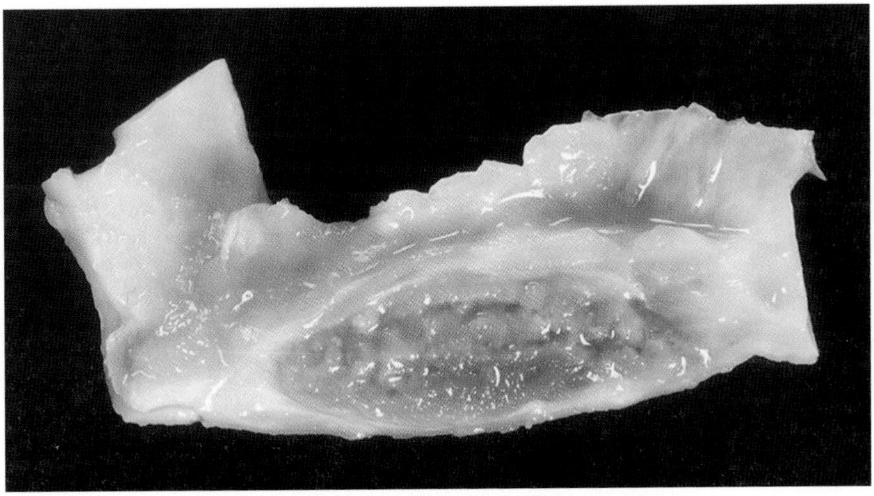

Fig. 8.3. Longitudinal section of carotid plaque demonstrating a large volume lipid core.

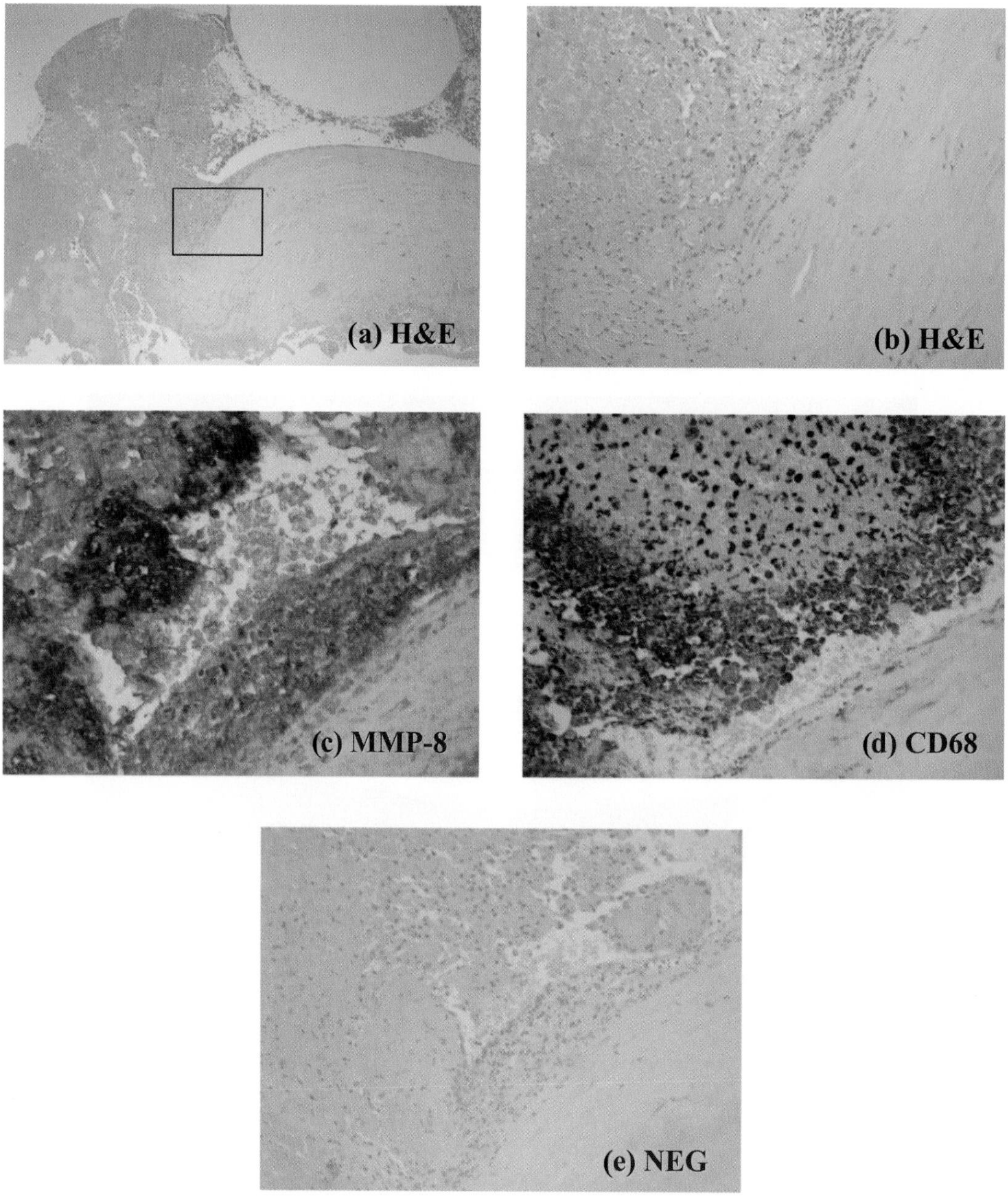

Fig. 8.7. Histological sections taken from the shoulder region of a symptomatic carotid plaque. Some sections show disruption of the friable plaque. (a) Low power haematoxilin and eosin (H&E) section with boxed area delineating high power view shown in (b–e). (b) High power H&E section demonstrating a cellular infiltrate. (c) Strong reactivity for MMP-8 in cells. (d) Positive staining for CD68. (d) Negative immunochemistry control.

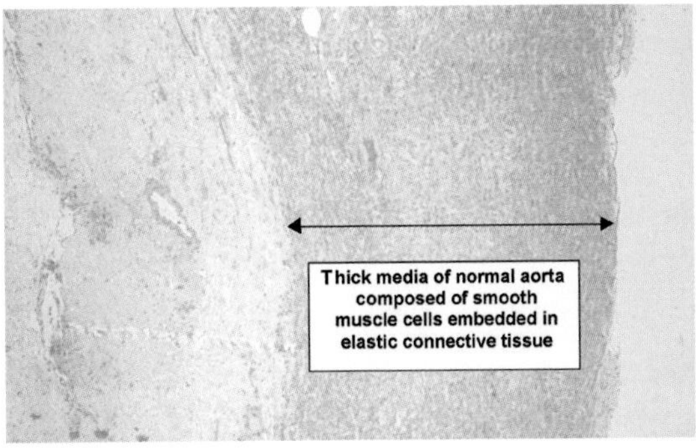

Fig. 15.2. The thick normal aortic media. Haematoxilin and eosin stained section of abdominal aorta showing the thick media.

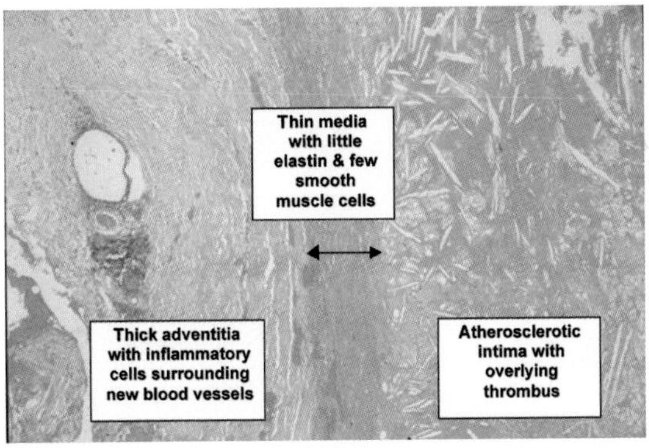

Fig. 15.3. The thin media in an abdominal aortic aneurysm. The section has been stained with haematoxilin and eosin.

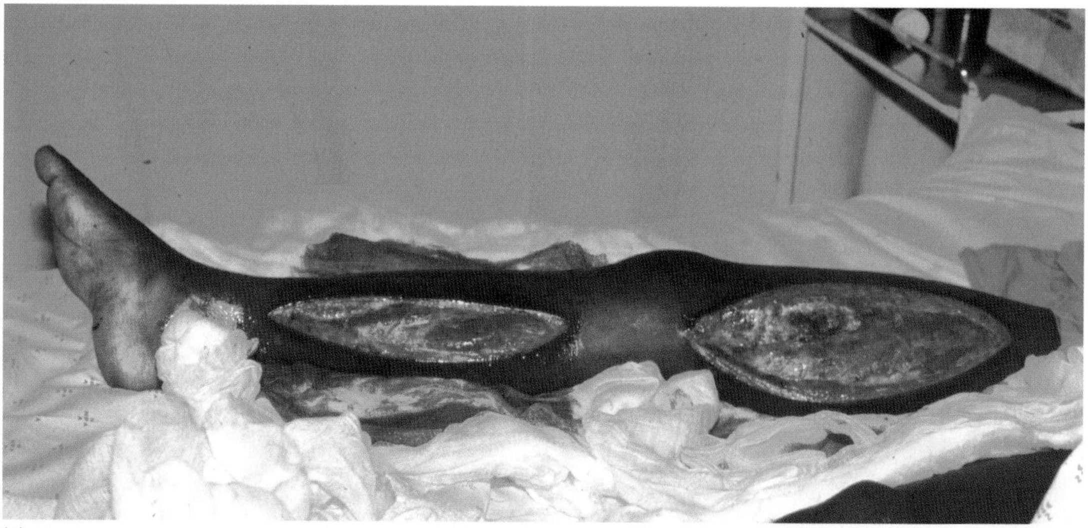

(a)

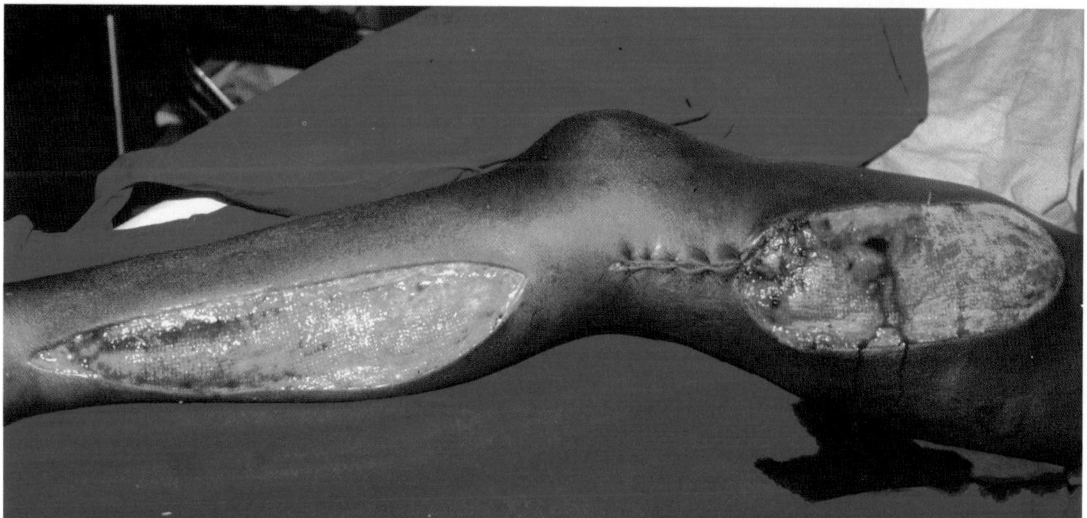

(b)

Fig. 19.6. (a) Medial thigh and calf fasciotomies following lower limb ischaemia after traumatic vascular injury, and (b) the same wounds after five days showing healthy granulation tissue.

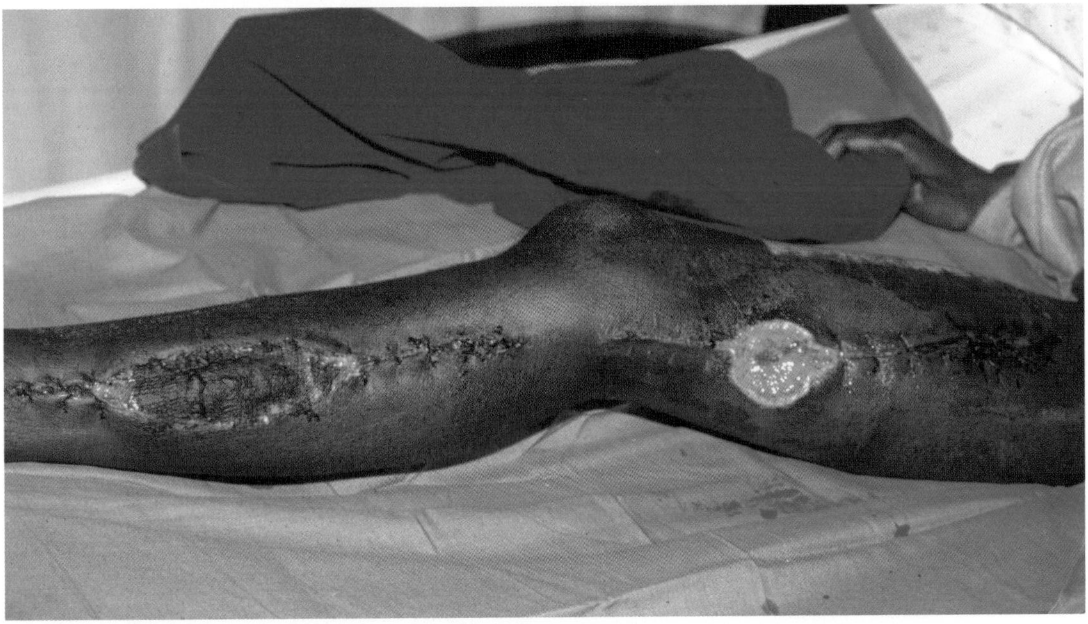

Fig. 19.8. Split skin grafting to calf fasciotomy two weeks post-injury (same patient as figure 19.6). The thigh fasciotomy has been treated by delayed closure leaving a small defect to heal by secondary intention.

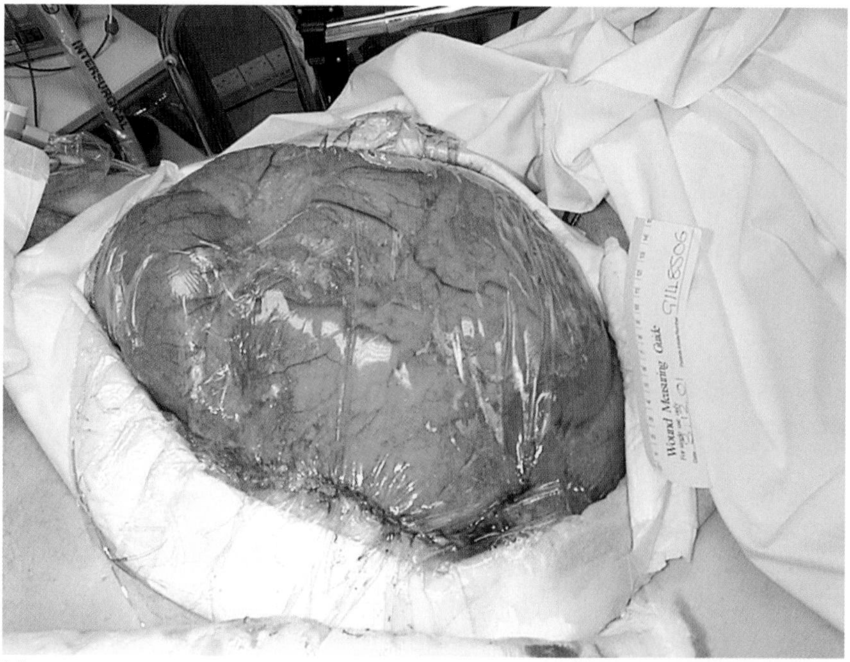

(a)

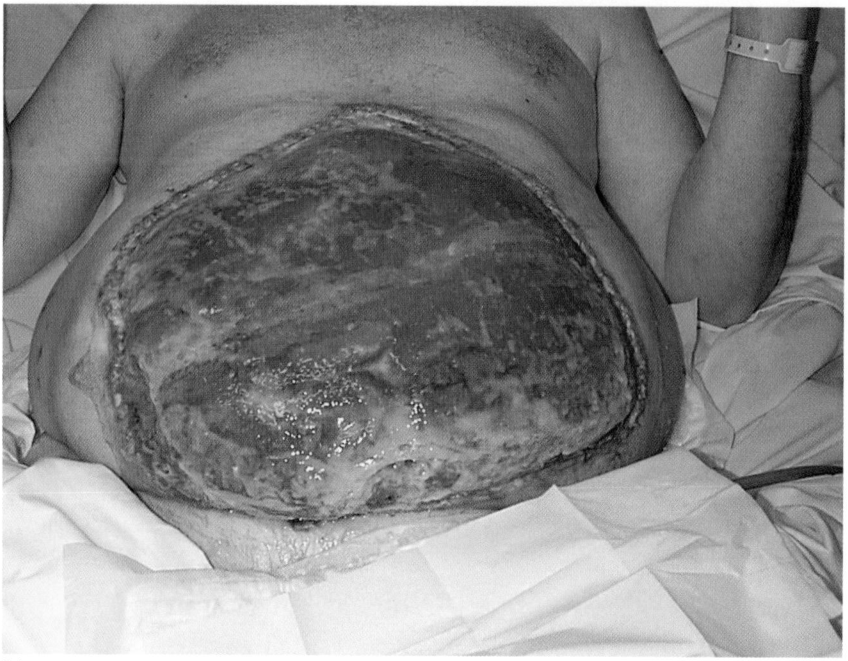

(b)

Fig. 19.9. (a) Immediate containment of abdominal contents using a plastic bowel bag after decompressive laparostomy following a ruptured abdominal aortic aneurysm repair; and (b) the same wound after four weeks, the viscera having granulated over.

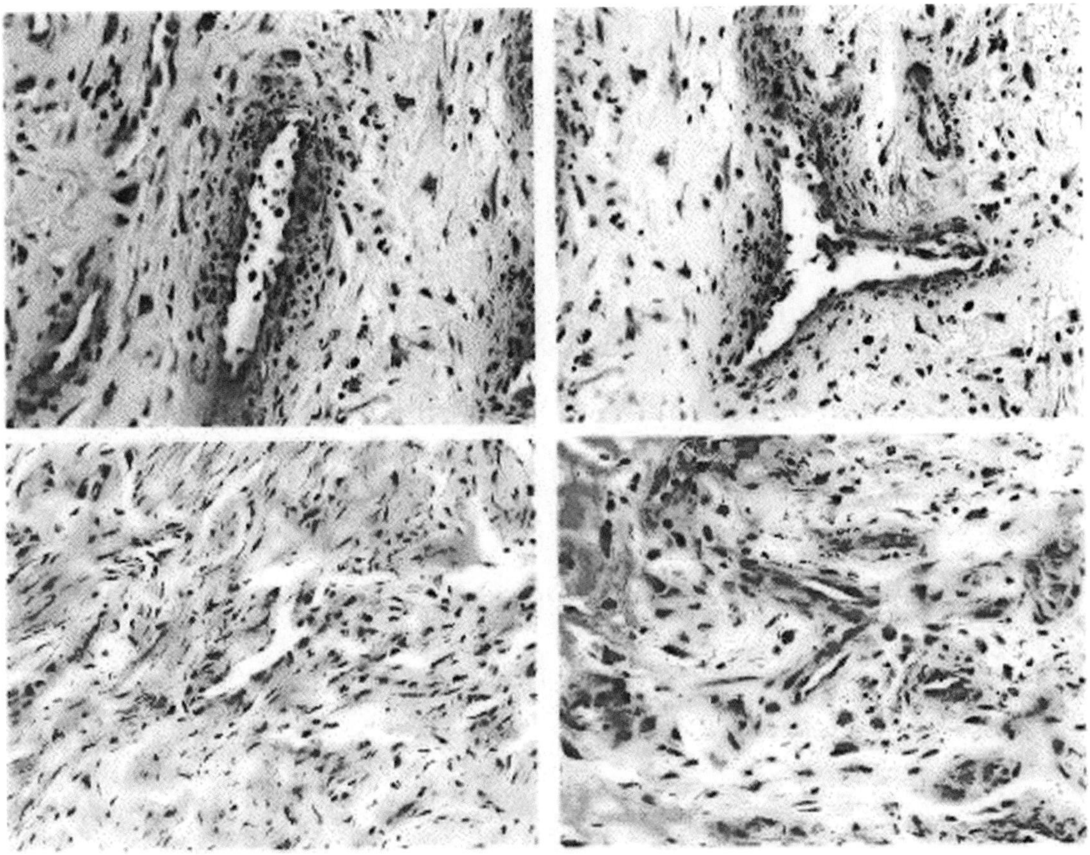

Fig. 23.9. Oral doxycycline reduced inflammation in chronic pressure ulcer. Top panels show pressure before oral doxycycline treatment (100 mg bid, seven days). Note the large numbers of inflammatory cells (neutrophil) around inflamed vessels and reduced matrix (faint pink staining). Bottom panels show biopsies from the same patient following doxycycline treatment. Note reduced inflammation and increased matrix (intense pink staining).

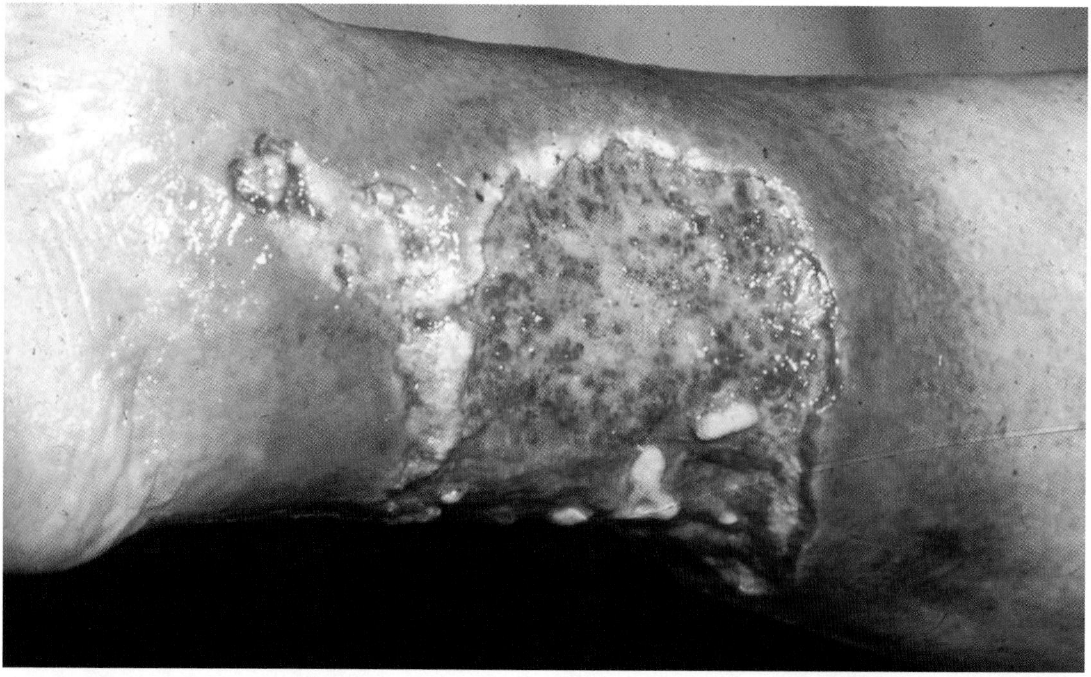

Fig. 25.4. Lipodermatosclerosis and ulceration in a leg with chronic venous diease.

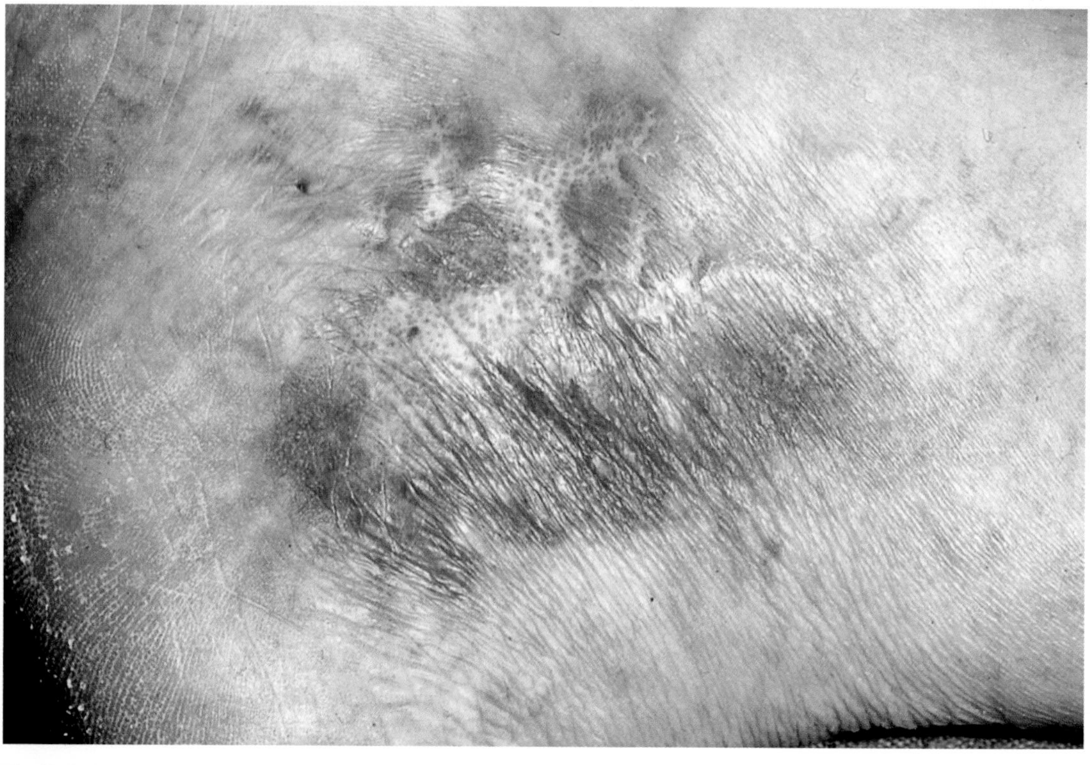

Fig. 25.5. Atrophie blanche in a leg with chronic venous disease.

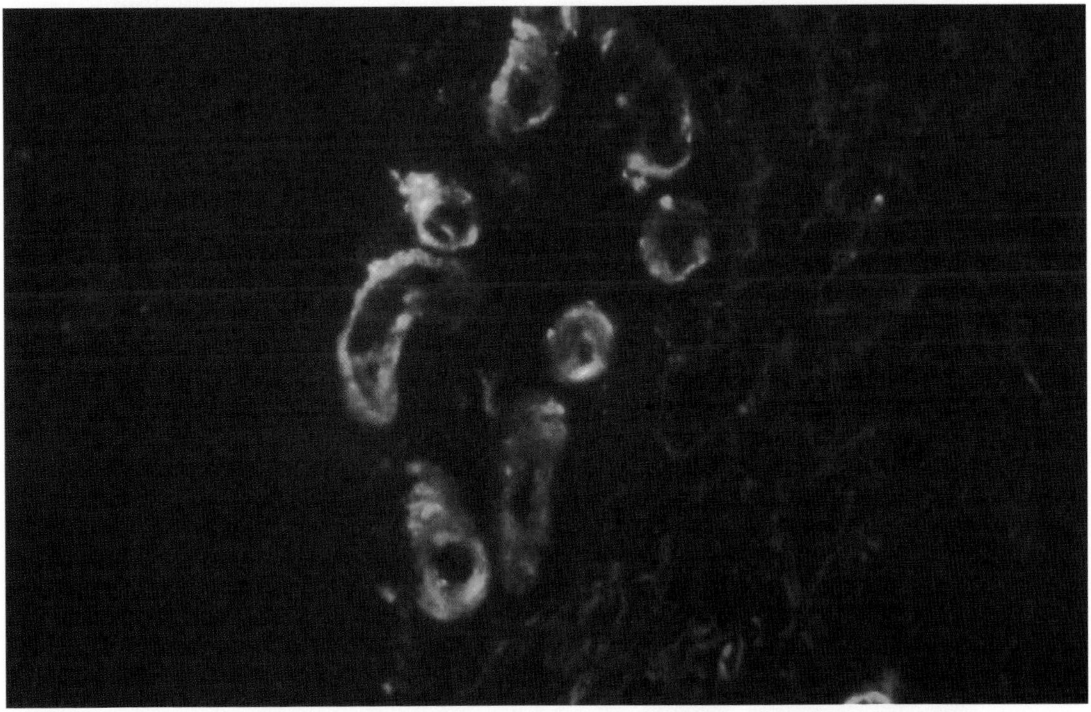

Fig. 25.6. Pericapillary deposit of protein – fibrinogen.

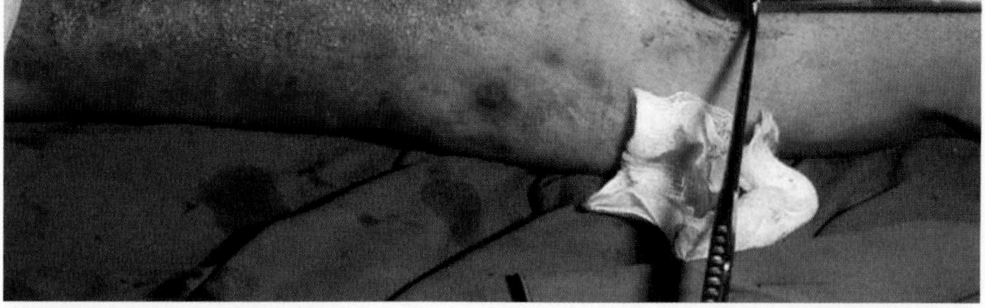
(a)

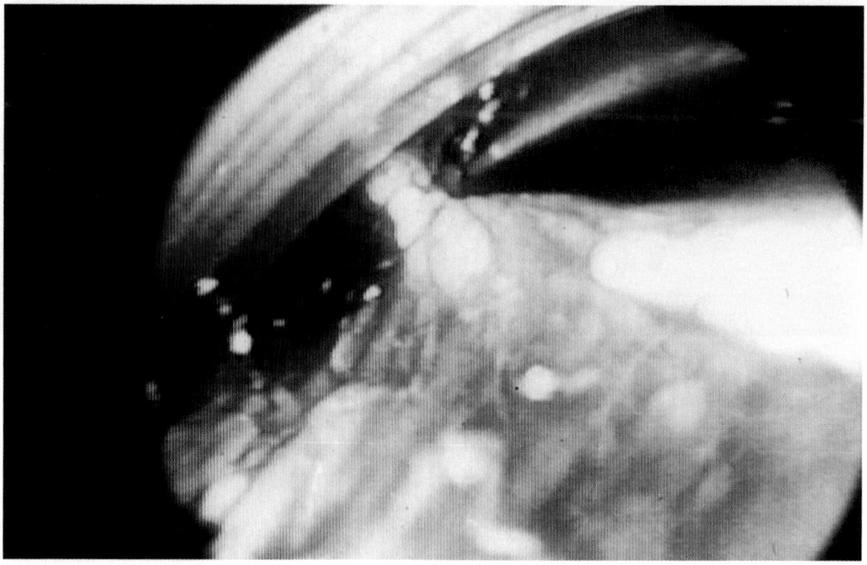
(b)

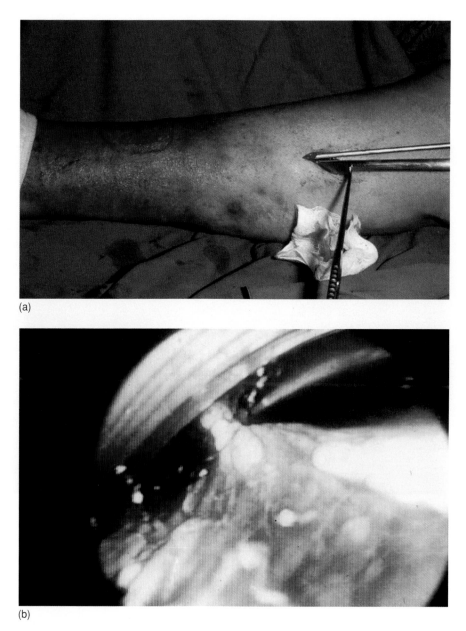

Fig. 25.9. Subfascial endoscopic perforator surgery – instruments in position and clip on a perforator.

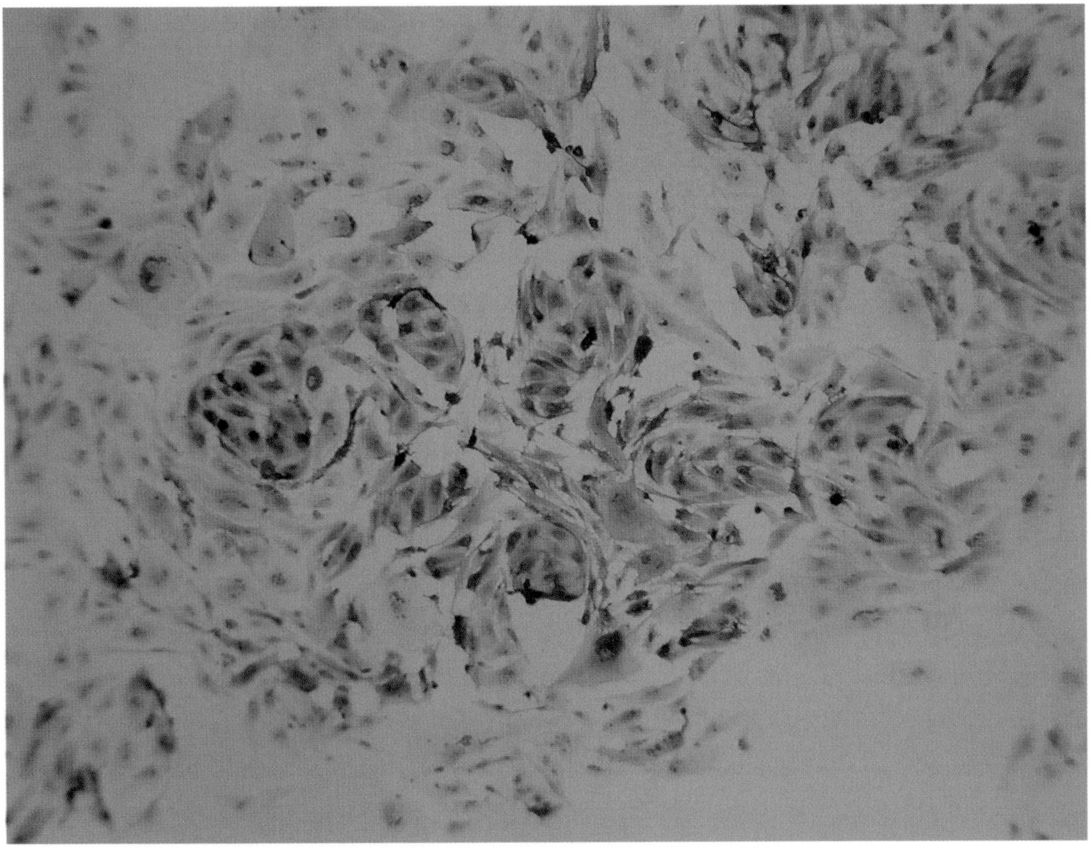

Fig. 27.2. Human dermal tissue stained with specific marker anti-LYVE-1.

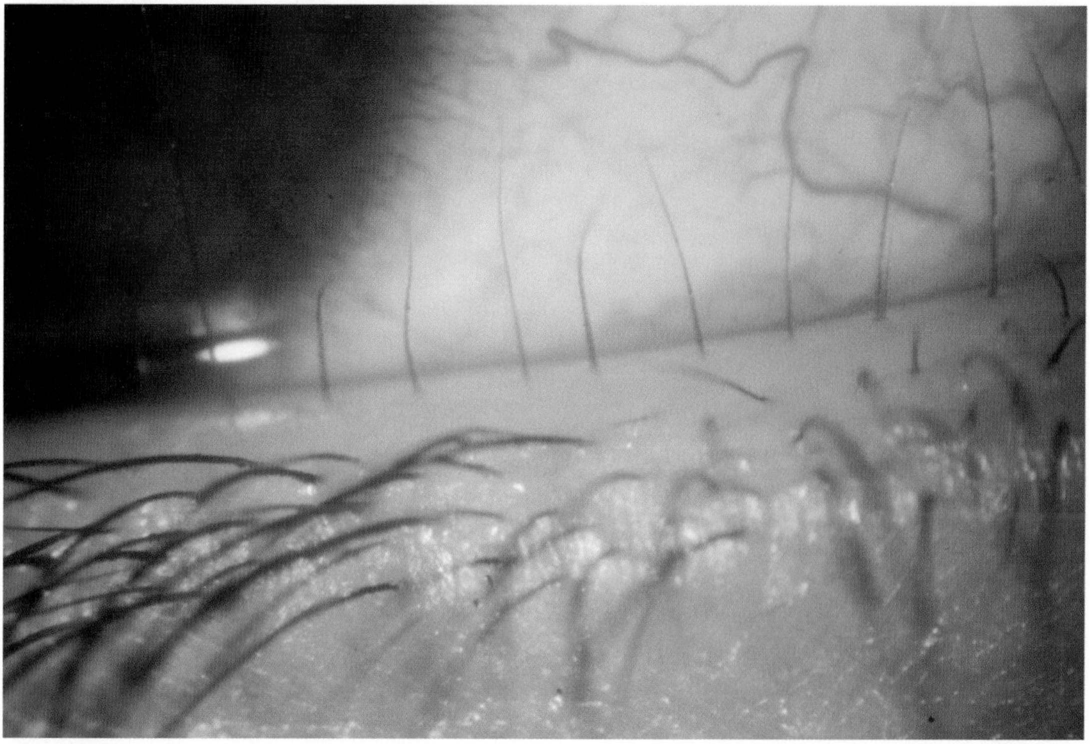

Fig. 27.3. Distichiasis with accessory eyelashes along the inferior posterior border of the lid margin in the position of the Meibomian glands.

28 • Graft materials past and future

GEORGE HAMILTON

INTRODUCTION

The search for better materials with which to replace diseased blood vessels has been a constant theme in the development of vascular surgery. Of several prosthetic materials two have dominated, dacron (polyethylene terephthalate) and expanded PTFE (polytetrafluoroethylene) or ePTFE. Both have proved to be durable but have a record of poor performance in small diameter arterial bypass grafts (<8 mm).

The internal mammary and radial arteries are used in coronary artery bypass surgery. The radial artery is used in lower limb bypass grafting. These all have excellent and durable results [1; 2]. The long saphenous vein remains the most common source of lower limb grafts, while other veins are more difficult to harvest and are not as adequate in length, calibre or wall integrity [3]. Veins have been shown to have superior patency rates in many individual studies, but a recent Cochrane Review suggested that the evidence for this is not as strong as commonly perceived [4].

The development of prosthetic grafts has been driven by the absence of autogenous conduits in up to 30% of patients, and by the desire for convenient and reliable 'off the shelf' small diameter grafts. The design of prosthetic grafts has focused primarily on strong and impervious conduits.

THE PATHOPHYSIOLOGY OF GRAFT HEALING

The mechanisms of graft healing are of central importance in understanding the successes and failures of current bypass grafts. The tissue response to implantation of a prosthetic graft is complex with many variable factors involved such as the material used, its construction, its porosity and its length. Further important factors relate to the interaction between the graft and the host artery at the anastomotic areas. Until recently graft design focused on simple conduits for blood flow which were strong (resistant to pressure), biologically inert (resistant to biodegradation) and non-porous. Each of the major graft failure causes, luminal thrombogenicity, compliance mismatch and anastomotic intimal hyperplasia, have the potential to be modulated if their aetiology could be better understood.

The peri-anastomotic area

Intimal or neointimal hyperplasia is a characteristic healing reaction to prosthetic vascular reconstruction [5]. In prosthetic grafting the injury typically involves the direct trauma of implantation and subsequent exposure of the anastomotic areas to haemodynamic stress (compliance mismatch, turbulent flow and altered shear stress). This results in injury which is transmural with endothelial removal, and variable disruption of the internal elastic lamina and medial smooth muscle cells [6]. This process is discussed in detail in Chapter 12.

The endothelial cell plays a pivotal role in graft failure, via its mechanoreceptors which are sensitive to changes in flow and shear stress. High shear stress, as found in laminar flow, promotes endothelial cell survival and quiescence, and secretion of nitric oxide (NO). Low or changing shear stress direction (turbulent flow), promotes endothelial proliferation and apoptosis, shape change, and reduced secretion of NO. A process of flow change towards high shear stress and endothelialization by regrowth in the injured area, may alter the balance between stimulatory and inhibitory factors, and ameliorate intimal hyperplasia. Conversely, lack of endothelial cover, major haemodynamic disturbance, turbulent flow with areas of stagnation and low shear stress, may stimulate intimal hyperplasia and graft failure.

Healing of prosthetic grafts

Healing of prosthetic grafts takes place by two main mechanisms, capillary in-growth through the graft wall and growth of endothelial cells along the luminal surface of the graft from each anastomosis [7]. Studies of prosthetic graft healing in various animal models typically used short lengths of graft (10 cm or less), which readily developed a full lining of endothelial cells. In man, however, endothelialization is restricted to the first centimetre or two of the anastomotic regions with no evidence of healing beyond this region. This observation has led to the conviction that man is different from other species in the inability to endothelialize a graft.

The effect of graft porosity on graft healing

There is quite a body of animal-based experimental evidence that prosthetic grafts can show a degree of endothelialization related to the porosity of the graft and the graft type.

ePTFE

The threshold for endothelialization appears to lie between an internodal distance of 30 μm and 45 μm. Low porosity ePTFE grafts (<30 μm) showed no spontaneous endothelialization. Within two weeks of implantation the surface of these grafts is covered with fibrin and platelet thrombus, typically 15 μm thick, which over following months increases to 80–300 μm. This pannus persists for years and remains actively thrombogenic. The ingrowth of connective tissue is limited to the outer graft wall in low porosity grafts.

High porosity ePTFE grafts (>45 μm internodal distance) behave quite differently in animal models. The first layering on the luminal surface is similar to that of low porosity ePTFE grafts, but spontaneous endothelialization of the lumen has been described. These changes occur one to two weeks after implantation, with patches of endothelial cells and capillary orifices being found approximately 100–500 μm apart.

These cells then achieve confluence [8]. The endothelial cells lie over a layer of arterial smooth muscle cells probably derived from pericytes. This complex develops into a stable neointima evenly distributed along the surface of the graft. This extensive endothelialization can only arise from cells reaching the luminal surface by transmural ingrowth [9].

Dacron

Immediately after implantation, a thin pannus of fibrin and platelets is deposited on the surface of low porosity woven dacron grafts. This thrombus becomes compacted over time and in man stabilizes after one year [10]. Endothelialization does not happen in animals or humans, although small islands of endothelial cells have been reported after many years of implantation in explanted woven dacron grafts in man [11; 12]. Underneath this layer of thrombus, the very narrow graft interstices are filled with fibrin. Typically a foreign body giant cell reaction will be present, and a variable spread of some capillaries and fibroblasts into interstitial spaces may develop, but this never breaks through the compacted fibrin of the inner lining [13].

High porosity dacron grafts are knitted. The initial pannus is the same as that found in woven dacron but will develop to a thickness of 100–120 μm increasing to 500 μm by six months. In animal experiments, this inner lining becomes replaced with a confluent layer of smooth muscle cells resting directly on the graft surface, covered by endothelium. These come from anastomotic ingrowth but in longer grafts endothelialization in the midgraft region fails to occur despite partial ingrowth of capillary fibroblasts from the adventitia.

The healing process at the anastomosis

Endothelialization from the host artery occurs more aggressively in animals as compared with man. In all of these studies the short graft lengths utilized makes it likely that anastomotic ingrowth was the sole avenue for endothelialization [9].

The speed of trans-anastomotic endothelialization differs between species, but more importantly, trans-anastomotic endothelialization is seven to eight times more pronounced in any animal compared with man [9]. Two factors are foremost among the possible explanations, the first is the exclusive clinical use of low or zero porosity grafts (see earlier). The second is that clinical revascularization is often performed in elderly patients with severe medical co-morbidity. Endothelial cells from such patients grow poorly in tissue culture.

Graft permeability

Permeability is the property of material that allows passage of substances through the interstices. Classically it is measured by the volume of water traversing a given area and pressure. Porosity refers to the spaces or pores that exist within the graft material which, depending on the material, may not traverse its entire thickness but end blindly. Furthermore, graft wall characteristics may be affected in different ways at different levels of the graft wall after exposure to the pressure changes of the cardiac cycle.

Zilla has suggested that to facilitate transmural healing and endothelialization, graft spaces should be wide enough to allow ingrowth of a capillary tuft, with accompanying fibroblasts or pericytes requiring minimum pore diameters of 60–80 μm [9; 14]. Currently available grafts, even those described as having high porosity, fail in this regard.

PHYSICAL PROPERTIES OF PROSTHETIC MATERIALS

Arterial wall pulsatility has long been recognized as an essential component of normal blood flow. This important property is due to a combination of elastic and viscous components inherent in the structure of the artery. This visco-elasticity is measured as compliance, defined as the ratio of change in diameter over change in blood pressure (percentage/mm Hg $\times 10^{-2}$).

Arterial compliance is complex, having both longitudinal and circumferential components. Compliance mismatch has been implicated as an important factor in the performance of vascular grafts since 1976 [15]. This mismatch should be considered to have two major components, tubular and anastomotic.

Tubular compliance mismatch

Mismatch of tubular compliance is present when there is a significant difference in elasticity between the prosthetic graft and native artery. A compliant vessel acts as an elastic reservoir absorbing energy during systole that is released during diastole. A rigid conduit will consequently diminish this secondary pulsatile energy and reduce distal perfusion. At the interface between a compliant artery and a non-compliant graft, changes in impedance (defined as the resistance to pulsatile flow) will diminish pulsatile energy by as much as 60% [16]. Furthermore, optimal organ perfusion depends on pulsatile blood flow, and a change from pulsatile to static increases peripheral resistance by 10% [17]. Finally, at the graft to artery interface wave reflection of pulsatile energy occurs, that can lead to increased velocity gradients and turbulence. As a result of these increased vibratory movements and mechanical stresses, endothelial damage occurs.

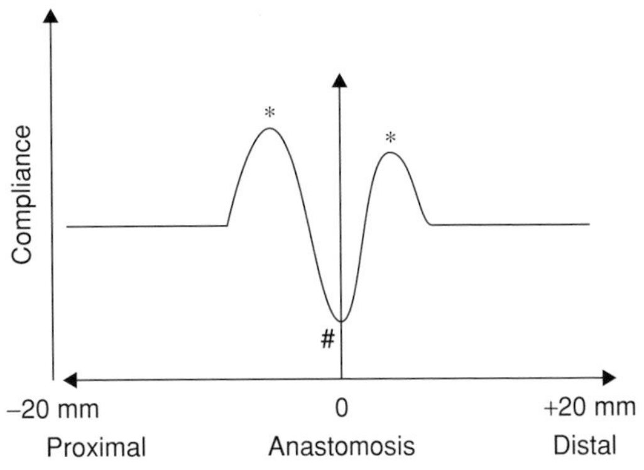

Fig. 28.1. The peri-anastomotic hyper compliant zones (PHZs). Compliance at the anastomosis is lower due to the suture (#), while compliance is increased compared with the vessel wall several millimetres from the anastomosis (*). This effect further aggravates compliance mismatch in bypass grafting.

Anastomotic compliance mismatch

A sutured anastomosis generates a decrease in diameter and drop in compliance caused by the lack of elasticity of the suture material. Interrupted sutures give a more compliant anastomosis, whilst a continuous technique results in a ring of non-compliant suture material. Within a few millimetres on either side of the suture line, there is a paradoxical increase of compliance which is known as the para-anastomotic hyper compliant zone (PHZ) [18] (Figure 28.1). Intimal hyperplasia develops typically in these areas of hyper compliance.

The compliance hypothesis of graft failure

Compliance mismatch will lead to a region of excessive mechanical stress that can give rise to subtle arterial wall injuries and initiate intimal hyperplasia. Cyclical stretching is known to have a positive influence on proliferation of vascular smooth muscle cells and production of extracellular matrix. This increased cyclical stretch at the PHZ will therefore cause proliferation of smooth muscle cells. Changes in compliance are also known to affect flow and shear stress. Where there is turbulent flow, there will be areas of low shear stress that will promote endothelial proliferation, apoptosis and reduced production of NO.

The clinical evidence for the compliance mismatch hypothesis is largely speculative, but analysis of the clinical performance of grafts of differing compliance reveals

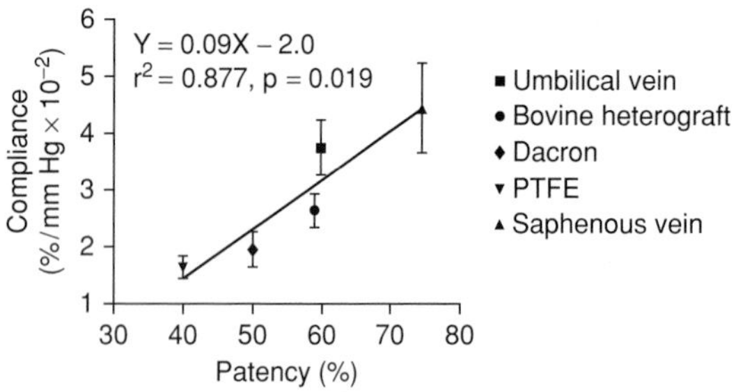

Fig. 28.2. Correlation between typical compliance and two year patency of several graft materials in clinical use.

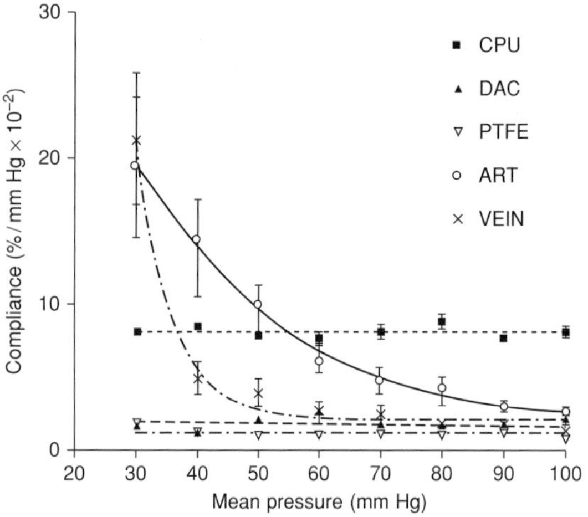

Fig. 28.3. Compliance/Pressure curve for compliant polyurethane (CPU), dacron (DAC), ePTFE (PTFE), human femoral artery (ART) and saphenous vein (VEIN). None of the prosthetic materials possess the visco-elastic properties of artery and vein which give higher compliance at lower pressures. CPU maintains higher compliance at all pressures compared with dacron or ePTFE.

a positive correlation between compliance and patency rates (Figure 28.2). The most commonly used prosthetic grafts, namely PTFE and dacron are profoundly rigid over the physiological pressure range. A feature of the visco-elastic nature of human artery is compliance which diminishes with increasing pressure but which increases exponentially as the mean pressure falls below 80 mm Hg (Figure 28.3). The ideal prosthetic graft would share this property but to date no such material has been developed.

SYNTHETIC GRAFTS

The history of prosthetic grafts began in 1952 with a serendipitous finding by Voorhees. A silk thread lying loose in the ventricle of a dog, was found to have a glistening smooth covering which had not attracted any thrombus formation [19]. This finding led to successful placement of vinyon N tubes into the abdominal aorta of dogs and subsequent human implantation in 1954 [20]. An explosion of interest followed with synthetic grafts being made from various textiles, but their major problem was loss of tensile strength. Two materials proved to be resistant (dacron and PTFE) and have dominated graft development to this day.

Dacron grafts

Dacron is a thread-like material, made into grafts by either weaving, knitting or braiding. The basic dacron yarn is multi-filament, which in preparation can be textured with spiral or coil spring formulation to vary the softness and elasticity of the cloth.

Woven dacron

Woven dacron fabrics are comprised of threads interlaced in simple over and under patterns, with two of sets of yarns, the warp and the weft, interlaced at right angles to each other (Figure 28.4). The warp refers to lengthways fibres and weft to fibres in circumferential orientation. Woven dacron grafts are rigid with no stretch in either the longitudinal or circumferential direction. The cut ends of this graft fray and to minimize this are tightly constructed. As a result these grafts are very strong with high burst strength and very low permeability. This results in minimal bleeding at the time of implantation, and little long term dilatation or kinking. The disadvantages include poor handling characteristics, an enduring tendency to fraying and very low compliance [21].

Knitted dacron

Knitted grafts have yarns that are inter-looped around each other as opposed to interlaced. These can be orientated in either a predominantly longitudinal or warp knitted manner, or predominantly circumferential or weft knitted manner. The longitudinal or warp knitted grafts are more stable and for this reason most grafts are manufactured using this method (Figure 28.5). The

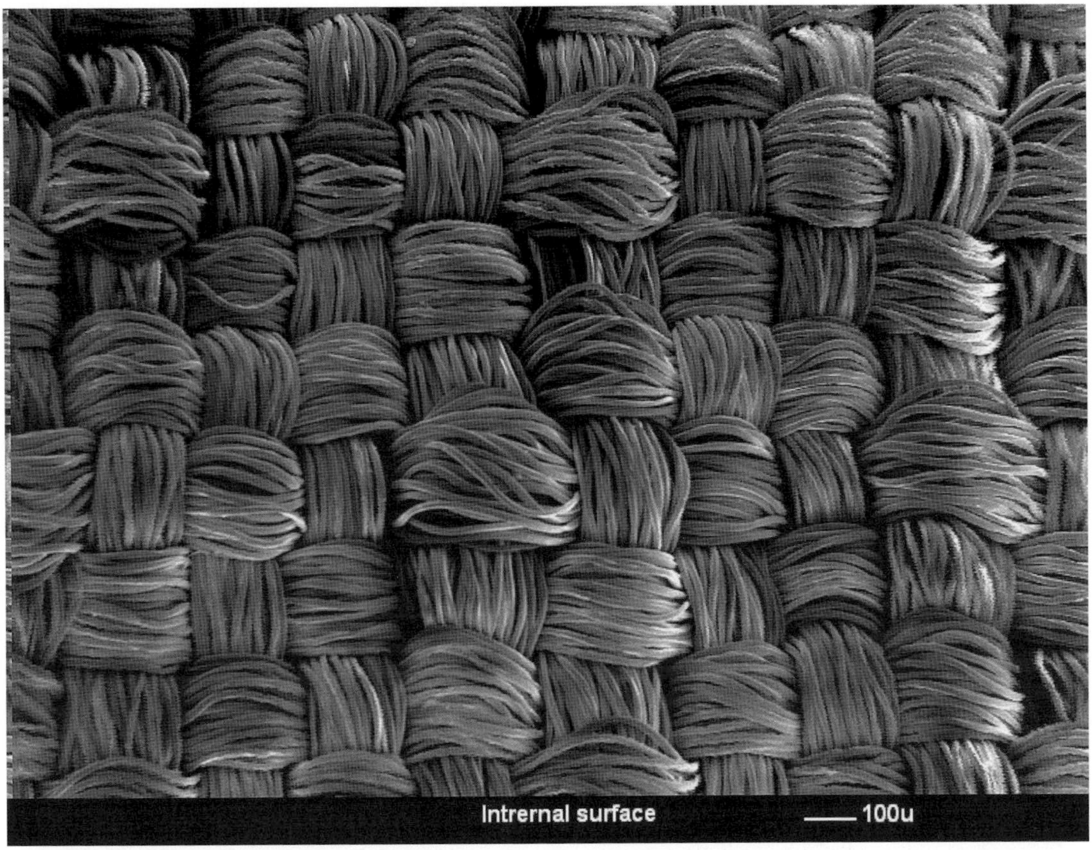

Fig. 28.4. Scanning electron micrograph of a woven dacron graft. Note the tight interlacing of the yarn and minimal potential for porosity.

space between the yarns can be varied according to the size of the needles, thus allowing variable porosity. A further advantage of inter-looping is increased elasticity.

Knitted grafts have better healing and tissue ingrowth, and are more attractive to the surgeon because of flexibility and ease of suturing. The disadvantage is the need for pre-coating and the subtle but greater propensity to dilatation with time. Pre-clotting of knitted grafts has been eliminated as a consequence of impregnation with biodegradable substances such as bovine collagen, albumen and gelatin. These are all absorbed within a few weeks allowing tissue healing to take place. Original concerns regarding allergic reactions have been allayed by their excellent clinical performance. A further advantage is the increased ability of these grafts to absorb antibiotics when risk of infection is high.

Any graft fabric can have its outer or inner surface made softer by adding additional yarns extending upwards and at right angles to the fabric surface [22]. All commercially provided velour grafts, however, have been with knitted designs. Outer wall velour gives better tissue incorporation, while inner wall velour allows development of a stable neointima. Despite these theoretical advantages no benefit has been shown from any velour grafts [23].

PTFE grafts

Expanded PTFE grafts are made by extrusion of the PTFE polymer initially developed in 1969 by W. L. Gore. The first clinical use as an arterial graft was in 1976 [24]. Extrusion of the heated and stretched polymer through a dye produces a microporous material with solid nodes interconnected by fine fibrils (Figure 28.6).

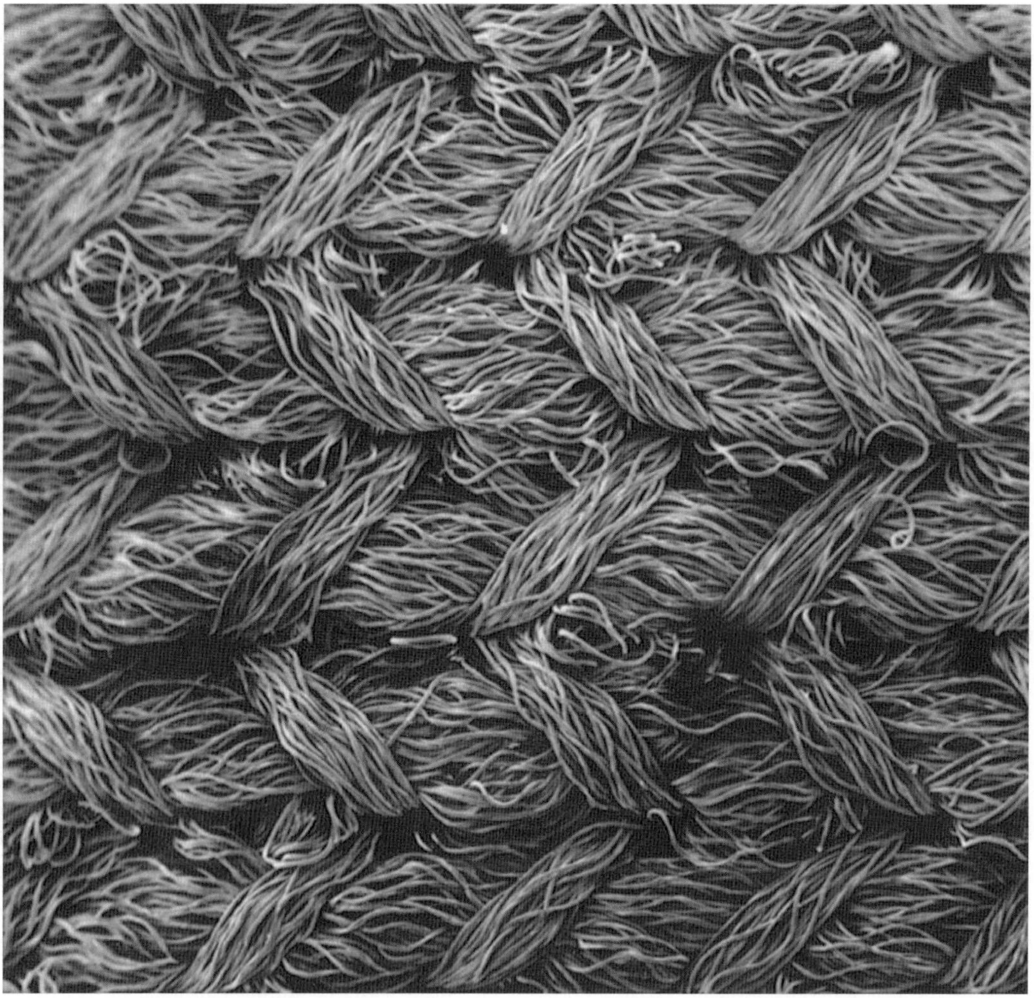

Fig. 28.5. Scanning electron micrograph of a knitted dacron graft. Note loose interlocking yarn configuration.

Porosity varies with fibril length but grafts currently available have pore sizes of 30 μm.

Polytetrafluoroethylene is inert with a marked electronegative charge that renders the graft hydrophobic. The unique node and fibril structure means that the polymer occupies about 20% of the total volume with air spaces forming the remaining 80%. The spaces between the individual fibrils are significantly smaller than those between the fibres of a dacron graft. Thus while the porosity of an ePTFE graft is high, its permeability is low. This feature together with its hydrophobic nature provides a graft that has minimal leakage when exposed to blood flow. Furthermore, because of a tendency to aneurysmal change, contemporary grafts have a thin outer reinforcing wrap of ePTFE to increase wall strength and abolish permeability. This allows their use without pre-clotting [25].

The ePTFE graft has been modified in various ways. Thin walled ePTFE grafts have improved handling characteristics but still have an outer wrap to provide strength. Stretch ePTFE grafts have improved longitudinal rather than circumferential elasticity, with improved handling characteristics. External support, either rings or spirals, is thought to be beneficial in extra-anatomic (axillo-femoral or femoro-femoral) or below knee grafts. However, the only randomized comparison

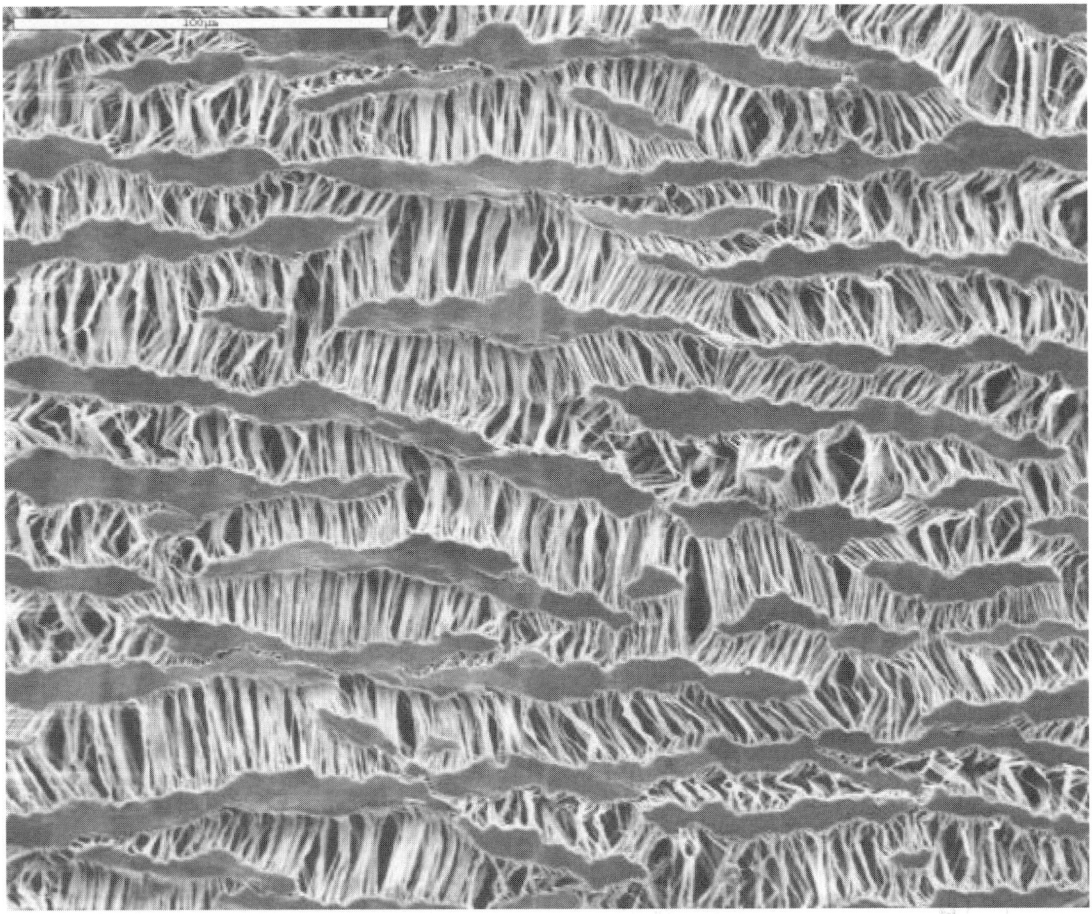

Fig. 28.6. Scanning electron micrograph of the inner surface of an ePTFE graft. Note the characteristic node-fibril structure.

between ringed and non-ringed grafts demonstrated no benefit [26].

Anticoagulation has been reported to increase long term patency although this treatment option is often not applicable to elderly patients [27]. A further valuable adjunct to improve below knee PTFE graft patency is an interposition vein cuff or patch at the distal anastomosis [28]. This appears to improve haemodynamic parameters at the distal anastomosis through minimized compliance mismatch and improved blood flow [29].

Several reports indicate potential benefit with ePTFE aortic grafts, including reduced bleeding and a lower risk of infection. The only prospective randomized comparison of ePTFE and dacron aortic grafts, however, failed to show any benefit between the two graft types [30]. The predilection of ePTFE in lower limb bypass grafting has recently been challenged in a randomized trial which showed no difference between ePTFE and gelatin sealed dacron [31; 32].

Polyurethane grafts

Polyurethanes are segmented polymers initially formulated in the early 1960s to provide elasticity in garment materials (lycra). The most important component of polyurethanes is the urethane group present in repeating sequences on the main chain of the polymer that forms the hard segment providing strength. The second important component is the soft segment which is derived from a macromonomer ranging from several hundred to over a thousand Daltons molecular weight. These hard and soft components have a degree of incompatibility, which allows microphase separation to occur

Table 28.1. *Results of clinical grafting using conventional polyurethanes prone to biodegradation*

Reference and Year	Indication	Number of grafts	Patency
39 (1989)	Vascular access	15	73% at 6 months
37 (1992)	Fem-pop bypass	15	47% at 6 months
40 (1993)	Fem-pop bypass	57	59% at 6 months
42 (1995)	Vascular access	39	53% at 12 months
38 (1996)	Vascular access	145	45% at 12 months

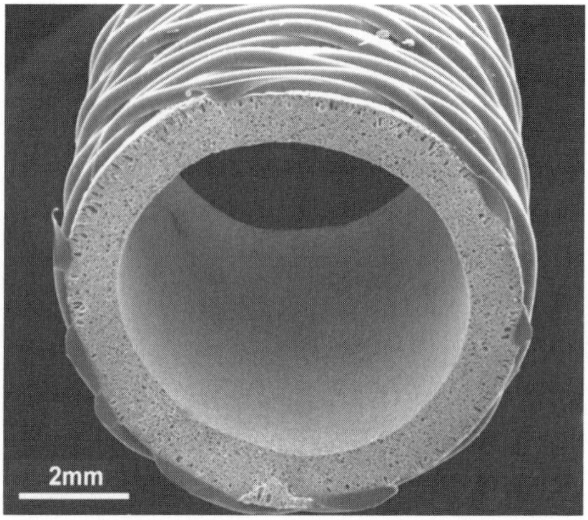

Fig. 28.7. Compliant polyurethane graft with external support. The sponge-like structure of the wall allows pulsatile elastic recoil even with external support and after perigraft tissue incorporation has taken place.

within the wall. It is this that gives their superior visco-elastic and compliant nature.

Polyurethanes also possess excellent blood and tissue compatibility, and are in extensive use in access catheters and linings of various prosthetic devices. Clinical experience of conventional polyurethane grafts has confirmed their superior thrombo-resistance, rapid ingrowth of living tissue and reduced anastomotic hyperplasia [33; 34; 35; 36].

Polyurethane vascular access grafts for haemodialysis have several advantages, including easy cannulation, rapid compression haemostasis and early use after implantation. Disadvantages with polyurethane grafts include poor patency rates when compared with PTFE and most problematically hydrolytic degradation leading to aneurysm formation. It is this complication that has limited their clinical use despite the advantages of good compliance [37; 39; 40; 42] (Table 28.1).

Newer developments of polyurethane vascular grafts
Conventional polyurethanes are biodegradable with the site of degradation being the soft segment of the polymer, particularly at the ester and ether groups in poly(ester)urethane and poly(ether)urethane. Polyester is subject to rapid degradation by hydrolysis and polyether by oxidative degradation [44; 45]. Recent interest has focused on replacing these susceptible groups with other moieties, in particular polycarbonate which is more hydrolytically and oxidatively stable. Two polycarbonate polyurethanes are currently available for clinical use, Corvita (Corvita Inc.) and Expedial (Le Maitre, Figure 28.7). A renal access graft composed of polyether polyurethane, the Vectra graft (Bard Inc.), was licensed by the Food and Drug Administration (FDA) in 2000 for use in renal access and coronary artery bypass grafting [46; 47; 48].

One bio-resistant compliant polyurethane graft has undergone pilot clinical studies both for dialysis access and in lower limb bypass grafting. In over 100 implantations with a follow-up of up to 18 months, no aneurysmal change or significant dilatation of the graft has been found. The graft therefore appears to be resistant to biodegradation.

Biological vascular grafts
Biografts, vascular grafts made from biological sources (i.e. not from autologous tissue), have been used over many years. Allografts in current use include umbilical and saphenous vein. Xenografts have a long history of disappointing results and there is no xenograft currently in clinical use.

The major problems with biografts are biodegradation and immunogenicity, which can be counteracted by chemical treatment and cryopreservation. The first clinical use of an allograft was in 1948 in the treatment of aortic coarctation [50]. Arterial allografts harvested from cadavers were first used in the 1960s to perform lower limb bypass, but these were prone to significant degeneration, aneurysm formation and wall calcification [51].

Improved cryo-preservation with solutions to prevent intracellular ice crystals on thawing allowed the development of tissue banks to provide a ready source of allografts. Clinical use of cryopreserved allografts in the 1960s showed good short term function and the attractive possibility that cryo-preservation might reduce immunogenicity [52]. Further clinical experience, however, revealed disappointing one year patency rates of less than 50% [53].

Sparks in 1973 reported the use of a mandril that was implanted subcutaneously in the lower limb. After eight weeks the mandril was removed and the remaining fibrous conduit incorporated about a polyester mesh was used as a bypass graft [54]. Unfortunately these grafts were prone to aneurysmal degeneration and were abandoned in the 1970s.

Xenografts were introduced in the 1970s, most commonly the bovine carotid artery. Various chemicals including glutaraldehyde were used to cross-link collagen to provide stability and reduced immunogenicity. Clinical success rates of these xenografts were poor with biodegradation after six months due to progressive breakdown of the collagen cross-linkages. Newer formulations may be more effective.

Dardik and Dardik [55] developed human umbilical cord vein as a bypass graft. This graft was stabilized using glutaraldehyde and supported by an external dacron mesh. The initial popularity of this graft waned because of aneurysmal degeneration after six to 12 months. Deficiencies in the manufacturing process were corrected in the late 1980s with apparent significant resolution of this problem. The graft, however, never regained popularity despite very impressive results reported by Dardik *et al.* in a very large series of 1275 cases [56].

PROSTHETIC GRAFT MODIFICATIONS

Modifications to reduce graft infection (see Chapter 29)

Graft infection is a devastating complication, particularly if with methicillin resistant *Staphylococcus aureus* (MRSA). Several different strategies have been employed to reduce the risk of infection. The simplest approach is soaking grafts coated with albumin, collagen or gelatin with antibiotics, in particular rifampicin [57]. *In vitro* studies show that antibacterial levels of rifampicin will remain present for 48 to 72 hours, with reduced risk of graft infection to bacterial challenge [58]. The clinical experience of rifampicin bonded dacron grafts has been investigated in two randomized controlled trials. Both trials demonstrated no long term benefit in terms of reduced graft infection, although early wound infection rates were significantly reduced [59; 60].

A further approach to reducing infection is the binding of triclosan (irgason) to grafts. This is an antimicrobial with broad-spectrum activity, which in experimental studies appears to bind effectively to dacron grafts for four weeks [61]. Silver bonded grafts have been shown experimentally to reduce the risk of infection and are currently available for clinical use [62] (InterVascular, France). However, *in vivo* comparison in a dog model between rifampicin/gelatin sealed and silver/collagen coated dacron grafts, revealed significantly greater resistance to infection for rifampicin bonding [63]. The haematogenous route used for microbial administration may have biased this result.

Modifications to improve patency

Grafts have also been modified in an attempt to provide a less thrombogenic luminal surface. Carbon has been used because of its lack of reactivity with flowing blood, and experimental studies have suggested improved primary and secondary patency rates [64]. Prospective randomized comparison of carbon impregnated PTFE grafts for infrainguinal bypass with standard PTFE found no significant difference at two years, but with a trend for improved patency in the carbon graft [65].

A prospective randomized comparison of a heparin bonded dacron graft (InterVascular, France) with PTFE in femoropopliteal bypass confirmed significantly improved patency rates of 70% and 50% at one year, and 56% and 42% at three years, respectively [66]. A further commercially available graft is Fluoropassiv (Terumo-Vascutek), a dacron graft coated with a fluoropolymer which has been shown in experimental studies to cause less tissue reaction and to have reduced thrombogenicity [67]. There are no clinical data available to confirm any beneficial effect of this graft.

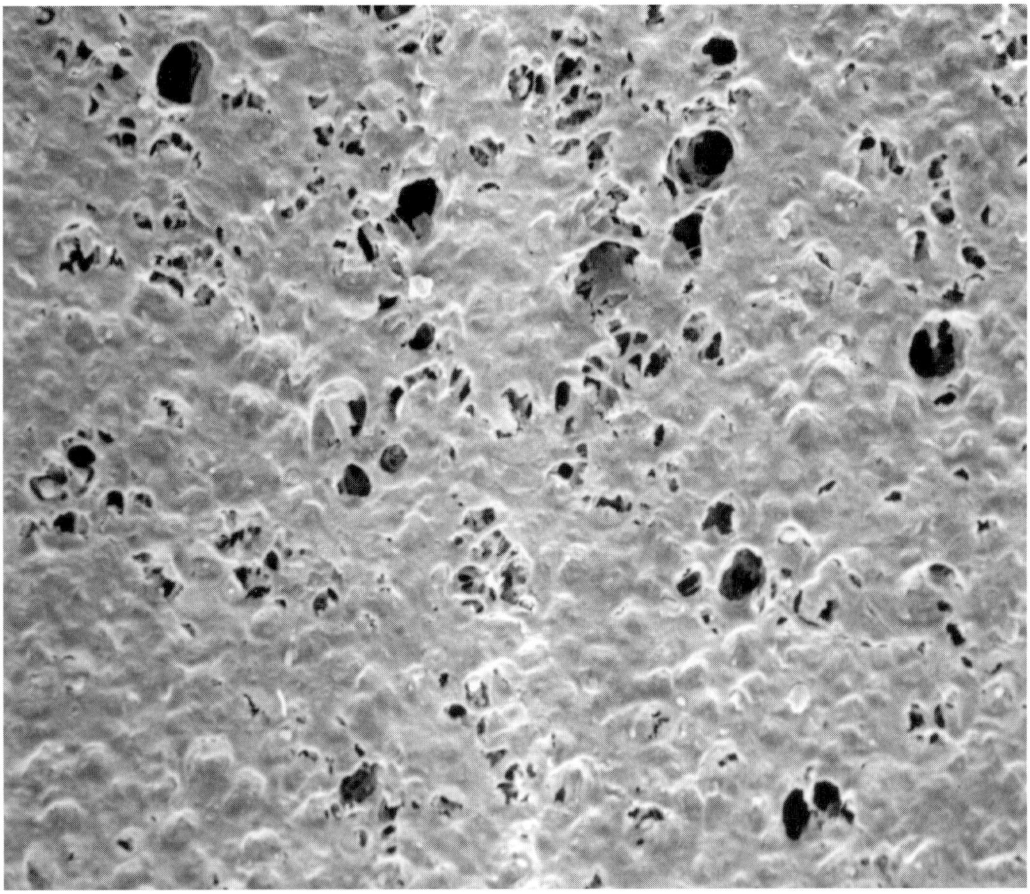

Fig. 28.8. Significantly improved endothelial cell attachment onto myolink coated with fibronectin derivative FEPP1.

ENDOTHELIAL CELL SEEDING

One of the major differences between prosthetic vascular grafts and autologous conduits is the lack of an endothelial monolayer on the prosthetic graft surface. The concept of endothelial cell seeding was introduced to address this problem. Endothelial cell seeding involves the attachment of autologous endothelial cells to the luminal graft surface, in an attempt to line the graft with a confluent endothelial monolayer (Figure 28.8).

Endothelial cells can be harvested from three main sources – vein, subcutaneous fat and omentum [68]. Further potentially promising sources are from bone marrow, circulating blood and mesenchymal stem cells.

Endothelial cell seeding may be achieved by two methods; single-stage and two-stage [69; 70]. Two-stage seeding involves harvesting a modest quantity of endothelial cells typically from a peripheral vein and culturing sufficient numbers of cells to completely line the graft with a confluent endothelial monolayer. This process takes a considerable time as amplifying the endothelial cells in culture may take six to eight weeks between endothelial harvest and graft implantation.

Single-stage seeding requires sourcing larger numbers of endothelial cells to allow immediate seeding of the graft at implantation. With this method seeding is not expected to be fully confluent but rather is achieved over the early post-implantation period by endothelial cell replication. The major disadvantage of single-stage seeding is a lack of sources of sufficient cells to allow immediate seeding.

There is good animal evidence to support the benefit of endothelial cell seeding of bypass grafts. Endothelial seeded grafts have better patency rates, are less thrombogenic, will tolerate low flow states and have been shown to have normal endothelial cell activity [14; 72; 73; 74; 75; 76; 77]. In addition, seeded grafts have been shown to resist bacteraemic infection in animal models.

Deutsch *et al.* reported the largest study in man using two-stage seeding with endothelial cells harvested from cephalic or jugular veins [77]. Expanded PTFE grafts were pre-coated with fibrin glue and then seeded with the patient's own cultured endothelial cells. Patency was 65% at nine years [79]. This group's experience now is of 213 patients with patency for below knee reconstructions of 68% at five and seven years. Endothelial cell seeding has been successful in coronary artery bypass with a recent trial using two-stage seeding of ePTFE reporting a 90.5% patency rate at 28 months [79].

These early clinical results are very promising but two-stage cell seeding is cumbersome, and not easily applicable [80; 81].

Single-stage seeding is feasible. The entire process should take a maximum of two hours and be performed in the operating room. Much improved endothelial cell retention for single-stage seeding of prosthetic grafts has been achieved by covalent bonding of substances such as RGD. Retention rates of 80% are obtained after only one hour of seeding, compared with 35%–40% cell retention seen with ePTFE [82; 83]. This combination of a compliant graft with a non-thrombogenic surface achieved by single-stage seeding has shown much experimental promise and will shortly be assessed in clinical studies.

VASCULAR TISSUE ENGINEERING

Broadly speaking there are three major research approaches to creating the ideal graft. The first is the addition of vascular cells to synthetic polymers of which seeding existing graft materials forms the most basic example (Figure 28.9). The second approach is the development of bioresorbable or biodegradable grafts made of polymers that will be absorbed at varying speeds and degrees with eventual replacement by host tissue. The third approach is that of growing new grafts in tissue culture made from endothelial cells, vascular smooth muscle cells, collagen and matrix.

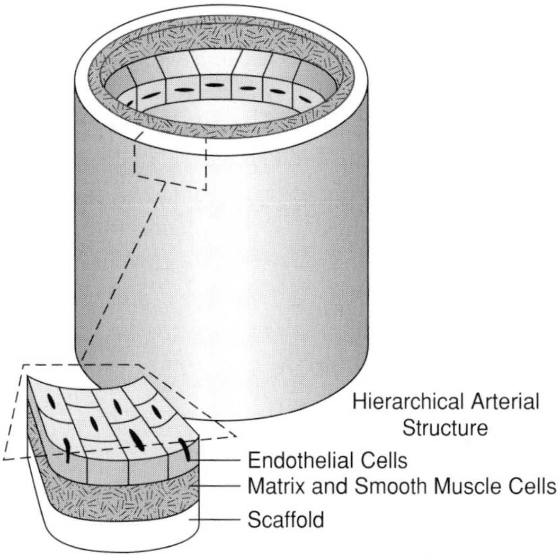

Fig. 28.9. Vascular graft composed of autologous endothelial cells, a neomedia of vascular smooth muscle cells and matrix, and a scaffold to provide structural strength. The scaffold can be bioresorbable or permanent.

Non-degradable polymer and cell seeding

Deutsch and colleagues in Vienna showed that explants of endothelial cell seeded PTFE grafts developed a neo-media between the prosthesis and the endothelium [84; 85]. Cells in the neomedia contained actin filaments and a true internal elastic membrane had developed to separate them from the endothelial layer. The original inoculums of endothelial cells obtained from the cephalic or jugular vein had probably been contaminated with vascular smooth muscle cells or pericytes. There has been much debate in the past as to whether endothelial cells for seeding should be pure or whether it would be beneficial to include vascular smooth muscle cells or pericytes. This finding of a neomedia with a well developed internal elastic membrane providing an inner structure very similar to that of a normal artery is exciting and lends support to the argument that co-culturing of cells of vascular origin would be beneficial.

The reintroduction of high porosity prosthetic grafts (i.e. pores >90 μm) merits further study. Impermeability at the time of implantation using established impregnation methodology avoids the risk of haemorrhage. Once the sealant is absorbed, capillary tuft ingrowth with development of a media and intima may result.

Bioresorbable and biodegradable polymers

The concept of degradable or absorbable graft materials, providing initial vessel integrity but eventually replaced by the host's own tissues, has been under development for some time [86; 87]. While biodegradable polymer fragments linger at the site of implantation stimulating a significant inflammatory reaction, bioresorbable polymers are completely absorbed avoiding chronic inflammatory reactions.

Polyglycolic and polylactic acid are the two bioresorbable polymers which have been most fully investigated [86; 88].

Greisler's group in Chicago initially made grafts from woven polyglycolic acid for a rabbit model [87; 89]. Four weeks after implantation a confluent layer of endothelial cells with a medial layer of myofibroblasts surrounded by dense collagen fibres was revealed. There was macrophage infiltration and phagocytosis present during reabsorbtion of the polyglycolic acid. By three months after implantation no polyglycolic acid could be found. Some 10% of these grafts became aneurysmal due to graft reabsorbtion before the adequate ingrowth of host tissue. Grafts made of polydioxanone (PDS) were more slowly reabsorbed. Polydioxanone was present for up to six months, at which time the grafts developed full endothelialization over a neomedia. These grafts were able to withstand very high static bursting pressures (600–2000 mm Hg) [90]. Alternative compositions for bioresorbable grafts have demonstrated encouraging results [91; 92], but no bioresorbable small diameter graft has yet been produced for human implantation.

Combined bioresorbable and tissue engineered grafts

Later work focused on the concept of a graft composed of autologous vascular cells with a bioresorbable scaffold [93; 94; 95; 96]. The majority of research in this area has focused on the development of the optimum polymer for the graft scaffold, the ideal attachment substrate and mechanical properties of the cells used to populate the graft [97, 98; 99; 100; 101; 102; 103; 104; 105; 106; 107; 108].

Tissue-engineered autologous grafts

Blood vessels made purely from biological materials and vascular cells have the major potential advantage of a vaso-active biological conduit, which can both heal and remodel according to the changing environment. The first totally autologous tissue engineered graft was made by Weinberg and Bell in 1986 from bovine endothelial cells, smooth muscle cells and fibroblasts co-cultured with collagen [109]. L'Heureux's group in Quebec reported a similarly constructed graft made from cultured human vascular cells but with the same structural weakness [110]. In Japan Hiraj and Matsuda developed a similar graft from canine vascular cells and collagen, which proved resistant to physiological pressures with only a dacron backbone [111]. In 1998 the Quebec group reported the first successful totally biological graft made from cultured human umbilical vein cells which withstood physiological pressures [112]. Their method used sheets of smooth muscle cells cultured with ascorbic acid. These were wrapped around a tubular support and allowed to mature into a media, with an outer sheet of cultured fibroblasts to provide an adventitia. Once the tubular support was removed a confluent layer of endothelial cells was seeded onto the luminal surface. The resulting graft had good functional characteristics; smooth muscle cells were shown to produce extracellular matrix and desmin, and the endothelial cells produced prostacyclin, expressed von Willebrand factor and inhibited platelet adhesion.

Structural integrity in fully tissue engineered grafts depends on a suitably mature extracellular matrix in the media with resistance to physiological pressure provided principally by cross-linked collagen. The addition of a period of pulsatile culture following an initial static culture of smooth muscle cells and collagen reliably produces grafts which are strong and resistant to supra-physiological burst pressures [113; 114].

All work in this field has been based on young cells. The successful translation of these promising developments to clinical application requires proof that adult or senile vascular cells will behave similarly. Such cells will have to come from each individual vascular patient until such time as pluri-potential, non-immunogenic cells can be sourced. It has recently been shown that such grafts can be produced using smooth muscle cells harvested from the saphenous vein of elderly vascular patients undergoing coronary artery bypass [115]. Despite the considerable advances over this last decade, many questions regarding optimal culture methods and long term stability of these grafts remain to be answered, before autologous tissue engineered human vascular grafts can be introduced to clinical application.

THE FUTURE

Over the next five years improved prosthetic grafts may become available with the introduction of biodurable and compliant polyurethane grafts. Indeed such grafts are already available for vascular access in renal dialysis patients. Lumen modulation by anticoagulant molecules, cell ligands and growth factors will further enhance performance, thus adding thrombo-resistance to compliance. Attachment technology will allow standard grafts such as dacron and PTFE to be similarly modified, although these can never be sufficiently compliant to abolish compliance mismatch.

Endothelial cell seeding of standard ePTFE grafts brings improved patency and resistance to infection. Advances in cell harvesting techniques, improved cell adhesion to the graft lumen and the growing evidence that a neomedia is probably as important as a neo-intima, will lead to efficient and practical cell seeding of small diameter grafts. Seeding protocols are already under pilot clinical study and promise to be widely clinically applicable within the next five years. Cell seeding, or durable antibiotic or antibacterial bonding will reduce graft infection in all sizes of prosthetic grafts.

New compliant graft materials will be developed using novel spinning technologies to incorporate collagen and elastin polymers resistant to degradation. Hybrid grafts composed of strong and porous non-degradable scaffolds, and autologous neomedia and neointima are on the horizon. The technology for totally bioresorbable grafts is already with us but assessment of the safety of this approach is needed before clinical use can be contemplated. Similarly the development of totally autologous tissue engineered grafts is in its infancy but progressing rapidly with the potential for clinical application within the next five to ten years.

New graft development to match as closely as possible the mechanical characteristics and functions of normal human arteries will remain a major priority for vascular and cardiovascular surgeons for at least the next decade.

ACKNOWLEDGEMENTS

Dr Alex Seifalian, Reader in Biophysics and Tissue Engineering, University Department of Surgery, Royal Free Hospital for help with the figures and manuscript.

Jennifer Carlyle, Vascutek-Terumo, Scotland for the scanning electron micrographs of dacron and PTFE.

REFERENCES

1. V. J. Teodorescu, J. K. Chun, N. J. Morrisey *et al.*, Radial artery flow-through graft: a new conduit for limb salvage. *Journal of Vascular Surgery*, **37**(4) (2003), 816–20.
2. G. S. Treiman, P. F. Lawrence & W. B. Rockwell, Autogenous arterial bypass grafts: durable patency and limb salvage in patients with inframalleolar occlusive disease and end-stage renal disease. *Journal of Vascular Surgery*, **32**(1) (2000), 13–22.
3. P. L. Faries, S. Arora, F. B. Pomposelli, Jr. *et al.*, The use of arm vein in lower-extremity revascularization: results of 520 procedures performed in eight years. *Journal of Vascular Surgery*, **31** (2000), 50–9.
4. N. Mamode & R. N. Scott, Graft type for femoro-popliteal bypass surgery. *Cochrane Database Systematic Reviews*, (2) (2000), CD001487.
5. L. W. Kraiss & A. W. Clowes, Response of the arterial wall to injury and intimal hyperplasia. In *The Basic Science of Vascular Disease*, ed. A. N. Sidaway, B. E. Sumpio and R. G. De Palma. (Armonk, NY: Futura Publishing Company Inc., 1997), pp. 289–317.
6. V. Lindner & A. Reidy, Expression of basic fibroblast growth factor and its receptor by smooth muscle cells and endothelium in injured rat arteries: an en face study. *Circulation Research*, **73** (1993), 589–95
7. Q. Shi, M. H. Wu, N. Hayashida *et al.*, Proof of fall out endothelialization of impervious dacron grafts in the aorta and inferior vena cava of the dog. *Journal of Vascular Surgery*, **20** (1994), 546–56.
8. A. W. Clowes, R. K. Zacharias & T. R. Kirkman, Early endothelial coverage of synthetic arterial grafts: porosity revisited. *American Journal of Surgery*, **153** (1987), 501–4.
9. L. Davids, T. Dower & P. Zilla, The lack of healing in conventional vascular grafts. In *Tissue Engineering of Prosthetic Vascular Grafts*, ed. P. Zilla and H. P. Greisler. (R. G. Lands Co Ltd, 1999), pp. 4–44.
10. M. S. Pepper, D. Belin, L. Montesano, L. Orchi & J. D. Vassalli, Transforming growth factor-b1 modulates basic fibroblast growth factor-induced proteolytic and

angiogenic properties of endothelial cells *in vitro*. *Journal of Cell Biology*, **111** (1990), 743–55.
11. M. H. Wu, Q. Shi, A. R. Wecheak *et al.*, Definitive proof of endothelialisation of a dacron arterial prosthesis in a human being. *Journal of Vascular Surgery*, **21** (1995), 862–7.
12. Q. Shi, M. Hong, Y. Onuki *et al.*, Endothelium on the flow surface of human aortic dacron vascular grafts. *Journal of Vascular Surgery*, **25** (1997), 736–42.
13. K. Berger, L. R. Sauvage, A. M. Rao & S. J. Wood, Healing of arterial prostheses in man: its incompleteness. *Annals of Surgery*, **175** (1972), 118–27.
14. M. B. Herring, S. Baughman, G. Glover *et al.*, Endothelial seeding of dacron and polytetrafluoroethylene grafts: the cellular events of healing. *Surgery*, **96** (1984), 745–54.
15. R. N. Baird & W. M. Abbott, Pulsatile blood flow in arterial grafts. *Lancet*, **30** (1976), 948–9.
16. D. E. Strandness & D. S. Summer, *Hemodynamics for the Surgeon*. (New York: Grune and Stratton Inc Pub, 1975).
17. F. Giron, W. S. Bertwell, H. S. Soroff & R. A. Deterling, Hemodynamic effects of pulsatile and non-pulsatile flow. *Archives of Surgery*, **93** (1966), 802–10.
18. J. E. Hasson, J. M. Megerman & W. M. Abbott, Increased compliance near vascular anastomosis. *Journal of Vascular Surgery*, **2** (1985), 419–23.
19. A. B. Voorhees, Jr., A. L. Jaretzke, III & H. Blakemore, The use of tubes constructed from vinyon N cloth in bridging arterial defects. *Annals of Surgery*, **135** (1952), 332.
20. A. H. Blakemore & A. B. Voorhees, Jr., The use of tubes constructed from vinyon N cloth and bridging arterial defects: experimental and clinical. *Annals of Surgery*, **140** (1954), 324.
21. G. J. Stewart, K. H. Y. Essan Chang & F. A. Reichle, Scanning and transmission electron microscope study of the luminal coating on dacron prostheses in the canine thoracic aorta. *Journal of Laboratory and Clinical Medicine*, **85** (1975), 208–6.
22. L. R. Sauvage, K. Verger, S. G. Wood, Y. Nakagawa & P. B. Mansfield, An external velour surface for porous arterial prostheses. *Surgery*, **70** (1971), 940–53.
23. M. Goldman, C. N. McCollum, R. G. Hawker, Z. Drolcz & G. Slaney, Dacron arterial grafts; the influence of porosity, velour and maturity on thrombogenecity. *Surgery*, **92** (1982), 947–52.
24. C. D. Campbell, D. H. Brooks, N. W. Webster & H. T. Bahnson, The use of expanded microporous polytetrafluoroethylene for limb salvage: a preliminary report. *Surgery*, **79** (1976), 485–91.
25. C. D. Campbell, D. H. Brooks, N. W. Webster *et al.*, Aneurysm formation in expanded polytetrafluoroethylene prostheses. *Surgery*, **79** (1976), 491–3.
26. S. K. Gupta, F. J. Veith, H. P. Kram & K. R. Wengerter, Prospective randomised comparison of ringed and non-ringed polytetrafluoroethylene femoropopliteal bypass grafts: a preliminary report. *Journal of Vascular Surgery*, **13** (1991), 162–72.
27. L. W. Kraiss & K. Johansen, Pharmacologic intervention to prevent graft failure. *Surgical Clinics of North America*, **75** (1995), 761–72.
28. P. A. Stonebridge, R. J. Prescott & C. V. Ruckley, Ramdomised trial comparing infrainguinal polytetrafluorothylene bypass grafting with and without vein interposition cuff at the distal anastomosis. The Joint Vascular Research Group. *Journal of Vascular Surgery*, **26** (1997), 543–50.
29. M. R. Tyrrell, J. F. Chester, M. N. Vipond *et al.*, Experimental evidence to support the use of interposition vein collars/patches in distal PTFE anastomoses. *European Journal of Vascular Surgery*, **4** (1990), 95–101.
30. P. Polterauer, M. Parger, T. H. Holzenbian *et al.*, Dacron versus polytetrafluoroethylene for Y-aortic bifurcation grafts: a six year prospective randomised trial. *Surgery*, (1992), 111–626.
31. B. I. Robinson, J. P. Fletcher, P. Tomlinson *et al.*, A prospective multi-centre comparison of expanded polytetrafluoroethylene and gelatin-sealed knitted dacron grafts for femoropopliteal bypass. *Cardiovascular Surgery*, **7** (1999), 214–18.
32. W. M. Abbott, R. M. Green, T. Matsumoto *et al.*, Prosthetic above knee femoropopliteal bypass grafting: results of a multi-centre randomised prospective trial. *Journal of Vascular Surgery*, **25** (1997), 19–28.
33. G. J. Wilson, D. C. MacGregor, P. Klement *et al.*, The composite corethane/dacron vascular prosthesis. Canine *in vivo* evaluation of four mm diameter grafts with one year follow up. *ASAIO Transactions*, **37** (1991), M475–6.
34. M. G. Jeschke, V. Hermanutz, S. E. Wolf & G. B. Kovekar, Polyurethane vascular prosthesis decreases neointimal inflammation compared with expanded

polytetrafluoroethylene. *Journal of Vascular Surgery* **29** (1999), 168–76.

35. D. J. Lyman, F. J. Fazzio, H. Voorhees *et al.*, Compliance as a factor effecting the patency of a co-polyurethane vascular graft. *Journal of Biomedical Materials Research*, **12** (1978), 337–45.
36. L. De Cossart, T. V. How & D. Annis, A two year study of the performance of a small diameter polyurethane (biomer) arterial prosthesis. *Journal of Cardiovascular Surgery (Torino)*, **30** (1989), 388–94.
37. P. G. Bull, H. Denck, R. Guidoin & H. Gruber, Preliminary clinical experience with polyurethane vascular prostheses in femoropopliteal reconstruction. *European Journal of Vascular Surgery*, **6** (1992), 217–24.
38. R. D. Allen, E. Yuill, B. J. Nankivell & D. M. Francis, Australian multi-centre evaluation of a new polyurethane vascular access graft. *Australian and New Zealand Journal of Surgery*, **66** (1996), 738–42.
39. K. Ota, T. Kawai, S. Teraoka & Y. L. Nakagawa, Clinical application of a self sealing poly (ether) urethane graft applicable to blood access for haemodialysis. *Artificial Organs*, **13** (1989), 498–503.
40. J. P. Dereume, A. van Romphey, G. Vincent & E. Engelmann, Femoropopliteal bypass with a compliant composite polyurethane/dacron graft: short term results of a multi-centre trial. *Cardiovascular Surgery*, **1** (1993), 499–503.
41. Y. Nakagawa, K. Ota, Y. Sato *et al.*, Complications in blood access for haemodialysis. *Artificial Organs*, **18** (1994), 283–8.
42. Y. Nakagawa, K. Ota, Y. Sato, S. Teraoka & T. Agisi, Clinical trial of a new polyurethane vascular graft for haemodialysis compared with expanded polytetrafluoroethylene grafts. *Artificial Organs*, **19** (1995), 1227–32.
43. T. E. Brothers, J. C. Stanley, W. E. Burkel & L. M. Graham, Small calibre polyurethane and polytetrafluoroethylene grafts: a comparative study in a canine aortoiliac model. *Journal of Biomedical Materials Research*, **24** (1990), 761–71.
44. J. M. Anderson, Inflammatory response to implants. *ASAIO Transactions*, **34** (1988), 101–7.
45. Y. B. Aldenhoff, F. H. DerVeen, J. TerWoorst *et al.*, Performance of a polyurethane vascular prosthesis carrying a dipyridamole (Persantin R) coating on its luminal surface. *Journal of Biomedical Materials Research*, **54** (2001), 224–33.
46. A. Aberhart, Z. Zhang, R. Guidon *et al.*, A new generation of polyurethane vascular prostheses: *rara avis* or *ignis fatuus*? *Journal of Biomedical Materials Research*, **48** (1999), 546–58.
47. H. J. Salacinski, N. R. Tai, R. J. Carson *et al.*, *In vitro* stability of a novel compliant poly (carbonate-urea) urethane to oxidative and hydrolytic stress. *Journal of Biomedical Materials Research*, **59** (2002), 207–18.
48. N. R. Tai, H. Salacinski, A. M. Seifalian & G. Hamilton, An *in vitro* assessment of the resistance of compliant polyurethane vascular grafts to degradative oxidative and hydrolytic stress. *Cardiovascular Pathology*, **9**(4) (2000), 219.
49. N. R. Tai, A. Giudiceandrea, H. J. Salacinski, A. Seifalian & G. Hamilton, *In vivo* femoropopliteal arterial wall compliance in subjects with and without lower limb vascular disease. *Journal of Vascular Surgery*, **30**(5) (1999), 936–45.
50. R. E. Gross, E. S. Huwitt, A. H. Bill Jr. *et al.*, Preliminary observations on the use of human arterial grafts and the treatment of certain cardiovascular defects. *New England Journal of Medicine*, **239** (1948), 578–9.
51. J. W. Meade, R. R. Linton, R. C. Darling & C. V. Menendez, Arterial homografts. A long term clinical follow up. *Archives of Surgery*, **93** (1966), 392–9.
52. D. A. Tsee & V. R. Zerpino, Clinical experience with preserved human allografts for vascular reconstruction. *Surgery*, **72** (1972), 260–7.
53. K. Wengerter & H. Dardik, Biological vascular grafts. *Seminars in Vascular Surgery*, **12** (1999), 46–51.
54. C. H. Sparks, Silicone mandril method for growing reinforced autogenous femoral popliteal artery grafts *in situ*. *Annals of Surgery*, **177** (1973), 293–300.
55. I. Dardik & H. Dardik, Vascular heterograft; human umbilical cord vein as an aortic substitute in baboon. A preliminary report. *Journal of Medical Primatology*, **2** (1973), 269–301.
56. H. Dardik, K. Wengerter, F. Quin *et al.*, Comparative decades of experience with glutaraldehyde-tanned human umbilical cord vein graft for lower limb revascularisation: an analysis of 1,275 cases. *Journal of Vascular Surgery*, **35** (2002), 624–71.
57. G. Torsello & W. Sandmann, Use of antibiotic-bonded grafts and vascular graft infection. *European Journal of Vascular and Endovascular Surgery*, **14** (1997), 84.
58. K. LaChapelle, A. M. Graham & J. R. Symes, Antibacterial activity, antibiotic retention and infection

resistance of a rifampicin impregnated gelatine-sealed dacron graft. *Journal of Vascular Surgery*, **19** (1994), 675–82.

59. M. D. Abbato, T. Curti & A. Freyvic, Prophylaxis of graft infection with rifampicin bonded gel-seal graft: two year follow up of a prospective clinical trial. Italian Investigative Group. *Cardiovascular Surgery*, **4** (1996), 200–4.
60. J. J. Earnshaw, B. Whitman & B. P. Heather Two year results of a randomised trial of rifampicin-bonded extra-anatomic dacron grafts. *British Journal of Surgery*, **87** (2000), 758–9.
61. T. Hernandez Richter, H. M. Schardey, F. Lohlein *et al.*, Binding kinetics of triclosan (irgasan) to alloplastic vascular grafts: an *in vitro* study. *Annals of Vascular Surgery*, **14** (2000), 370–5.
62. B. Illingworth, K. Tweden, R. F. Schroeder & J. D. Cameron, *In vivo* efficacy of silver coated (silzore) infection resistant polyester fabric against biofilm producing bacteria, *Staphylococcus epidermidis*. *Journal of Heart Valve Disease*, **7** (1998), 524–30.
63. O. A. Goeau-Brissonniere, D. Fabre, V. Leflon-Guibout *et al.*, Comparison of the resistance to infection of rifampicin-bonded gelatin-sealed and silver/collagen coated polyester prostheses. *Journal of Vascular Surgery*, **36** (2002), 916.
64. H. Tsuchida, B. L. Cameron, C. S. Marcus & S. E. Wilson, Modified polytetrafluoroethylene: indium 111-labelled platelet deposition on carbon-lined and high porosity polytetrafluoroethylene grafts. *Journal of Vascular Surgery*, **16** (1992), 643–50.
65. F. Bacourt, Prospective randomised study of carbon-impregnated polytetrafluoroethylene grafts for below-knee popliteal and distal bypass: results at two years. The Association Universitaire de Recherche Chirurgie. *Annals of Vascular Surgery*, **6** (1997), 596–603.
66. C. Devine & C. N. McCollum, Prosthetic femoral-popliteal bypass: PTFE or heparin bonded dacron? *British Journal of Surgery*, **87** (2000), 491.
67. R. Y. Rhee, P. Gloviczki, A. Cambria & V. M. Miller, Experimental evaluation of bleeding complications, thrombogenicity and neointimal characteristics of prosthetic patch materials used for carotid angioplasty. *Cardiovascular Surgery*, **4** (1996), 746–52.
68. A. Tiwari, H. J. Salacinski & G. Hamilton, Tissue engineering of vascular bypass grafts: role of endothelial cell extraction. *European Journal of Vascular and Endovascular Surgery*, **21** (2001), 193–201.
69. P. Zilla, R. Fasol, M. Deutsch *et al.*, Endothelial cell seeeding of polytetrafluoroethylene vascular grafts in humans: a preliminary report. *Journal of Vascular Surgery*, **6** (1987), 535–41.
70. B. E. Jarrell, S. K. Williams, G. Stokes *et al.*, Use of freshly isolated capillary endothelial cells with the immediate establishment of a mono-layer on a vascular graft at surgery. *Surgery*, **100** (1986), 392–9.
71. J. S. Budd, K. Allen, J. Hartley *et al.*, Prostacyclin production from seeded prosthetic vascular grafts. *British Journal of Surgery*, **79** (1982), 1151–15.
72. L. K. Biriniyi, E. C. Douville, S. A. Lewis, H. S. Bjornson & R. F. Kempczinski, Increased resistance to bacteremic graft infection after endothelial cell seeding. *Journal of Vascular Surgery*, **5** (1987), 193–7.
73. M. B. Herring, A. Gardiner & J. L. Glover, A single-stage technique for seeding vascular grafts with autogenous endothelial cells. *Surgery*, **84** (1978), 498.
74. M. B. Herring, A. Gardiner & J. L. Glover, Seeding human arterial prostheses with mechanically derived endothelium; the detrimental effect of smoking. *Journal of Vascular Surgery*, **2** (1984), 279.
75. M. B. Herring, S. Baugham & J. L. Glover, Endothelium develops on seeded arterial prosthesis. A brief clinical report. *Journal of Vascular Surgery*, **2** (1985), 727.
76. P. Ortenwall, H. Wadenvik & B. Risberg, Reduced platelet deposition on seeded versus unseeded segments of expanded polytetrafluoroethylene grafts: clinical observations after six month follow up. *Journal of Vascular Surgery*, **10** (1989), 374–80.
77. M. Deutsch, J. Meinhart, T. Fischlein, P. Preiss & P. Zilla, Clinical autologous *in vitro* endothelialisation of infrainguinal ePTFE grafts in one hundred patients: a nine year experience. *Surgery*, **126** (1999), 847–55.
78. J. G. Meinhart, M. Deutsch, T. Fischlein *et al.*, Clinical autolologus in vitro endothelialisation of 153 infrainguinal ePTFE grafts. *Annals of Thoracic Surgery*, **71** (2001), S327–31.
79. H. R. Laube, J. Duwe, W. Rutsch & W. Konetz, Clinical experience with autolologous endothelial cell seeded polytetrafluoroethylene coronary artery bypass grafts. *Journal of Thoracic and Cardiovascular Surgery*, **120** (2000), 134–41.
80. H. J. Salacinski, M. R. Tai, G. Punshon *et al.*, Optimal endothelialisation of a new compliant

poly(carbonate-urea)urethane vascular graft with the effect of physiological shear stress. *European Journal of Vascular and Endovascular Surgery*, **20** (2000), 342–52.
81. H. J. Salacinski, G. Punshon, B. Krijgsman, G. Hamilton & A. M. Seifalian, A hybrid compliant vascular graft seeded with microvascular endothelial cells extracted from human omentum. *Artificial Organs*, **25** (2001), 974–82.
82. B. Krijgsman, A. M. Seifalian, H. J. Salacinski *et al.*, An assessment of covalent grafting of RGD peptides to the surface of a compliant poly(carbonate-urea)urethane vascular conduit versus conventional biological coatings: its role in enhancing cellular retention. *Tissue Engineering*, **8** (2002), 673–80.
83. A. Tiwari, A. Kidane, H. Salacinski *et al.*, Improving endothelial cell retention of the single stage seeding of prosthetic grafts: use of polymer sequences of arginine-glycine-aspartate. *European Journal of Vascular and Endovascular Surgery*, **25** (2003), 325–9.
84. M. Deutsch, J. Meinhart & P. Zilla, *In vitro* endothelialization elicits tissue re-modelling emulating native artery structures. In *Tissue Engineering of Prosthetic Vascular Grafts*, ed. P. Zilla and H. P. Greisler. (Georgetown, Texas: R. G. Landes Co., 1999), pp. 179–87.
85. P. Zilla, Neo-media formation in explanted endothelial seeded ePTFE grafts in lower limb bypass in man. (personal communication, 2003).
86. S. Bowald, C. Busch & I. Eriksson, Arterial regeneration following polyglactin 910 suture mesh grafting. *Surgery*, **86** (1979), 722–9.
87. H. P. Greisler, Arterial regeneration over absorbable prostheses. *Archives of Surgery*, **177** (1982), 1425–31.
88. A. J. Putnam & D. J. Mooney, Tissue engineering using synthetic extra cellular matrices. *Nature Medicine*, **2** (1996), 824–6.
89. H. P. Greisler, D. U. Kim, J. B. Price & A. B. Voorhees, Arterial regenerative activity after prosthetic implantation. *Archives of of Surgery*, **120** (1985), 315–23.
90. H. P. Greisler, J. Ellinger, T. H. Schwarcz *et al.*, Arterial regeneration over polydioxanone prostheses in a rabbit. *Archives of Surgery*, **122** (1987), 715–21.
91. H. P. Greisler, E. D. Endean, J. G. Klosak *et al.*, Polyglactin 910/polydioxanone bicomponent totally resorbable vascular prostheses. *Journal of Vascular Surgery*, **7** (1988), 697–705.
92. H. P. Greisler, C. W. Tattersall, J. J. Klosak, Partially bioresorbable vascular grafts in dogs. *Surgery*, **110** (1991), 645–55.
93. J. P. Vacanti & R. Langer, Tissue engineering: the design and fabrication of living replacement devices for surgical reconstruction and transplantation. *Lancet*, **354** (1999), 32–34T.
94. X. Yue, B. van der Lei, J. M. Schakenradd *et al.*, Smooth muscle cell seeding in biodegradable grafts in rats: a new method to enhance the process of arterial wall regeneration. *Surgery*, **103** (1998), 206–12.
95. T. Shinoka, D. Schum-Tim, P. X. Ma *et al.*, Creation of viable pulmonary artery autografts through tissue engineering. *Journal of Thoracic and Cardiovascular Surgery*, **115** (1998), 536–46.
96. D. Shum-Tim, U. Stock, J. Hrkach *et al.*, Tissue engineering of autologous aorta using a new biodegradable polymer. *Annals of Thoracic Surgery*, **69** (1999), 298–305.
97. J. Gao, L. Niklason & R. Langer, Surface hydrolysis of poly(glycolic) acid meshes increases the seeding density of vascular smooth muscle cells. *Journal of Biomedical Materials Research*, **42** (1998), 417–24.
98. S. P. Massia & J. A. Hubbell, Vascular endothelial cell adhesion and spreading promoted by the peptide REDV of the IIICS region of plasma fibronectin is mediated by integrin alpha 4 beta 1. *Journal of Biological Chemistry*, **267** (1992), 14019–26.
99. L. E. Niklason, J. Gao, W. M. Abbott *et al.*, Functional arteries grown *in vitro*. *Science*, **284** (1999), 489–93.
100. L. E. Niklason, W. M. Abbott, J. Gao *et al.*, Morphologic and mechanical characteristics of engineered bovine arteries. *Journal of Vascular Surgery*, **33** (2001), 628–38.
101. U. A. Stuck, D. Wiederschain, S. M. Kilroy *et al.*, Dynamics of ECM production and turnover in tissue engineered cardiovascular structures. *Journal of Cellular Biochemistry*, **81** (2001), 220–8.
102. A. Rademacher, M. Paulitschke, R. Meyer & R. Hetzer, Endothelialisation of PTFE vascular grafts under flow induces significant cell changes. *International Journal of Artificial Organs*, **4** (2001), 235–42.
103. R. Buttemeyer, J. W. Mall, M. Paulitschke, A. Radermacher & Phillipp. In a pig model ePTFE grafts will sustain for 6 weeks a confluent endothelial cell layer formed *in vitro* under shear stress conditions. *European Journal of Vascular and Endovascular Surgery*, **26** (2003), 156–60.

104. D. W. Urry & A. Pattanaik, Elastic protein-based materials in tissue reconstruction. *Annals of the New York Academy of Sciences*, **831** (1997), 32–46.
105. A. Nicol, D. C. Gowda & D. W. Ullay, Cell adhesion and growth on synthetic elastomeric matrixes containing Arg-Gly-Asp-Ser-3. *Journal of Biomedical Materials Research*, **26** (1992), 393–413.
106. G. J. Wilson, H. Yeger, P. Klement, J. M. Lee & D. W. Courtman, Acellular matrix allograft small caliber vascular prostheses. ASAIO *Transactions*, **36** (1990), M340–3.
107. A. Bader, G. Steinhoff, K. Stroble Engineering of human vascular aortic tissue based on xenogeneic starter matrix. *Transplantation*, **70** (2000), 7–14.
108. O. E. Teebken, A. M. Pichlmaier & A. Haverich, Cell seeded decellularised allogeneic matrix grafts and biodegradable polydioxanone-prostheses compared with arterial autografts in porcine model. *European Journal of Vascular and Endovascular Surgery*, **22** (2001), 139–45.
109. C. B. Weinberg & E. Bell, A blood vessel model constructed from collagen and cultured vascular cells. *Science*, **231** (1986), 397–400.
110. N. L-Heureux, L. Germain, R. Labbe & F. A. Auger, *In vitro* construction of a human blood vessel from cultured vascular cells: a morphologic study. *Journal of Vascular Surgery*, **17** (1993), 499–509.
111. J. Hiraj & T. Matsuda, Venous reconstruction using hybrid vascular tissue composed of vascular cells and collagen-tissue regeneration process. *Cell Transplant*, **5** (1996), 93–105.
112. N. L'Heureux, S. Paquet, R. Labbe, L. Germain & F. A. Auger, A completely biological tissue-engineered human blood vessel. *FASEB Journal*, **12** (1998), 47–56.
113. S. Goldner, A. M. Seifalian, M. S. Baguneid *et al.*, Effect of preconditioning living vascular graft matrices. *Cardiovascular Pathology*, 9(4), (2000), 224.
114. M. S. Baguenid, A. Seifalian, G. Hamilton & Walker, Unpublished data on tissue engineered arterial graft in long term porcine aortic implantation model. Royal Free Hospital and Manchester Royal Infirmary.
115. M. C. J. Button, B. J. Fuller & G. Hamilton, The enzymatic extraction of adult human venous smooth muscle cells and their incorporation into a wholly biological tissue engineered arterial bypass conduit. *British Journal of Surgery*, **90** (2003), 622.

29 • Graft infections

MAURO VICARETTI AND JOHN FLETCHER

The introduction of prosthetic grafts has revolutionized the management of vascular disease, but graft infection although uncommon is still a dreaded complication, with significant morbidity and mortality. Mortality occurs in approximately one-third of all graft infections [1], with mortality highest when an aortic prosthesis is involved [2; 3]. As many as 75% of survivors of an infected aortic prosthesis require amputation of a limb [3], with the incidence of amputation highest when the infection involves more distal prosthetic grafts [4]. The incidence of graft infections is difficult to quantify as infection may manifest many years after implantation [1]. Nevertheless, the reported incidence is in the order of 5%. This varies according to the site of operation, being higher following use of a groin incision, an emergency or a redo procedure.

NATURAL HISTORY OF PROSTHETIC VASCULAR GRAFT INFECTIONS

Early prosthetic vascular graft infections occurring in the first four months following placement are relatively uncommon (1%) and are usually caused by the more virulent micro-organisms, such as *Staphylococcus aureus*, *Escherichia coli*, *Pseudomonas*, *Klebsiella*, *Proteus* and *Enterobacter* [1]. Late prosthetic vascular graft infections are the result of two possible mechanisms. Firstly, by haematogenous seeding from a septic focus elsewhere [5] or by becoming infected with enteric contents following a graft-enteric erosion [6]. In both situations the usual causative organisms are those with high virulence, and clinical manifestations are signs and symptoms of sepsis. The second mode of presentation is insidious, caused by the less virulent coagulase negative staphylococci such as *Staphylococcus epidermidis*. Contamination is likely to occur at the time of implantation [1].

MECHANISMS OF GRAFT CONTAMINATION AT OPERATION

Prosthetic grafts most commonly become infected at the time of implantation, either by contamination from the surgical team or by colonized micro-organisms on the patient. It has been demonstrated that the majority of patients undergoing arterial revascularization are colonized with coagulase negative staphylococci [7]. Colonization of patients with nosocomial bacteria is enhanced when the pre-operative hospitalization is lengthy [8].

The incidence of infection following emergency aneurysmorrhapy has been reported to be increased to 7.5% [9]. The evidence for other potential mechanisms, such as division of lymph nodes [10; 11; 12], infected transudated fluid during aortic surgery [13; 14; 15] and infected laminated thrombus [4; 14; 16; 17] is conflicting.

PATHOGENESIS OF GRAFT INFECTIONS

The exact aetiology of vascular graft infections is not completely understood and is likely to be multifactorial. According to Bandyk and Esses [18] the risk of vascular graft infection as demonstrated by animal models can be predicted by the formula:

$$\text{Risk of biomaterial infection} = \frac{\text{Dose of bacterial contamination} \times \text{virulence}}{\text{Host resistance}}$$

The dose of bacterial contamination is dependent on the infecting micro-organism. Experimentation in a canine aortic model has demonstrated that the infective threshold for bacteria to cause graft infection in over 50% of grafts was 10^7, 10^9 and 10^2 for *S. aureus*, *S. epidermidis* and *P. aeruginosa*, respectively [19]. Virulence of micro-organisms is often associated with the production of secreted toxins and enzymes. There is a resultant decline in structural integrity of the vessel wall [18], and the release of toxins and enzymes to control the perigraft environment and cause graft infection [19; 20]. Many bacterial strains, including *S. aureus, S. epidermidis* and *P. aeruginosa* are known to produce extracellular polymer substances (slime), forming a capsule incorporating the bacteria. This is referred to as a biofilm, and protects the micro-organism against host defences and antibiotic therapy [21]. It also allows greater adherence of the micro-organism to the biomaterial [22; 23].

BACTERIOLOGY OF VASCULAR GRAFT INFECTIONS

Gram positive, gram negative, anaerobic and fungal micro-organisms all have the potential to infect a vascular prostheses, but in general the majority of infections are the result of a small number of micro-organisms. Staphylococci are the most prevalent organism associated with prosthetic graft infection [2; 24; 25; 26]. Of the staphylococci, *S. aureus* is generally regarded as the most common causative bacteria [2; 25; 27; 28], particularly methicillin resistant *Staphylococcus aureus* (MRSA) [26]. *Staphylococcus epidermidis* has been recognized as the leading cause of vascular graft infection, particularly chronic and late onset infections [17; 28; 29; 30; 31].

The gram negative organisms, *E. coli, Pseudomonas, Klebsiella, Enterobacter* and *Proteus,* although relatively uncommon causative organisms for graft infections, are of particular interest and concern because of their high virulence and their tendency to destroy the vessel wall [18; 32; 33].

Candidia, Mycobacteria and *Aspergillus* infections are uncommon but pose a significant risk to patients who are immunocompromised [2]. Although uncommon they are all expected to increase in frequency because of their increasing resistance to standard prophylactic antibiotics [34].

There is an association between the type of infecting organism, type of vascular complication and arteries that are involved in the anastomosis to the prosthetic graft. Bandyk and Bergamini [2], in a collective survey of 1258 patients who had a vascular graft infection, found that the majority of aortoenteric fistulas were the result of either streptococci or *E. coli.* Also if the anastomosis involved the femoral artery, thoracic aorta, or the subclavian, carotid or innominate arteries, *S. epidermidis* or *S aureus* were the most likely causative organisms. *E. coli,* enterococci and *Enterobacter* were the more likely organisms to be involved in aortoiliac anastomoses.

INVESTIGATIONS FOR DETECTION OF PROSTHETIC GRAFT INFECTIONS

The diagnosis of vascular prosthetic infection can be difficult as the presentation may be subtle, especially if it is a late onset infection, the prosthesis is intra-abdominal and the micro-organism is one of low virulence. The diagnosis is aided by multiple available microbiological and imaging testing but in general is directed more at proving the absence of infection rather its presence.

History and physical examination

The clinical clues suggesting graft infection, especially those placed superficially, include: an inflammatory perigraft mass; overlying cellulitus; presence of exposed prosthetic graft; a sinus tract with persistent purulent drainage and/or bleeding; and/or a palpable anastomotic pseudoaneurysm, graft thrombosis and distal septic embolization [2; 3; 4; 35; 36]. The presence of intra-abdominal prosthetic graft infection may be nonspecific, such as fever of unknown origin, septicaemia or abdominal pain [3]. Upper or lower gastrointestinal haemorrhage either of an acute or chronic nature may indicate a graft-enteric fistula [17; 36; 37].

Laboratory investigations

Routine laboratory studies such as white cell count, differential erythrocyte sedimentation rate and blood cultures are obtained. However, the results may be nonspecific and even normal if the organism is *S. epidermidis* [2]. Wherever possible pus, exudates, tissue specimens, blood and wound cultures should be analysed microbiologically to aid in micro-organism identification, and to allow the commencement of appropriate and specific chemotherapy [38]. To aid in the diagnosis of *S. epidermidis* all solid material should be mechanically or ultrasonically disrupted [39; 40; 41; 42].

Diagnostic imaging

Various diagnostic modalities (computerized tomography, ultrasonography, magnetic resonance imaging, leucocyte or immunoglobulin labelled scanning, angiography) may assist the vascular surgeon in determining the presence and extent of prosthetic graft infection. These modalities are also helpful in planning definitive surgery. In general the features suggestive of graft infection include perigraft fluid and/or gas, graft disruption, absence of graft incorporation and pseudoaneurysm formation. The presence of periprosthetic gas more than six weeks following graft implantation is an abnormal finding and should alert the physician to the possibility of a graft infection [43].

MANAGEMENT OF PROSTHETIC GRAFT INFECTIONS

Prevention

Preventive measures, such as the routine use of skin preparations [44], the use of a depilatory agent [45], and limiting the length of pre-operative hospitalization [8], operating time and intensive care stay, all contribute to the reduction in wound infection and more importantly the chance of developing resistant multiple nosocomial infections [44]. Antimicrobial prophylaxis has been shown to reduce wound infections in vascular surgery [46]. Ideally it should be given as close to the time of incision, and repeated in the event of haemorrhage and lengthy operations every four hours.

As a preventive measure host resistance may be enhanced by the antimicrobial impregnation of grafts. A number of novel combinations of grafts and antibiotic with or without various forms of treatment have been trialled at both the *in vitro* and *in vivo* levels [47; 48; 49; 50; 51; 52; 53; 54; 55; 56; 57; 58; 59; 60; 61] (Table 29.1).

Table 29.1. *Enhancement of host resistance: antimicrobial impregnation of grafts*

Antibiotics used in experimental models	Vehicles, agents
Silver allontoin-heparin [47]	Silver [47; 48; 49; 51]
Norflaxacin [48]	Triododecylmethylammonium chloride (cationic surfactant) [48; 50]
Penicillin [50]; oxacillin [49; 52; 56; 57]	
Amikacin [61]	Benzalkonium chloride [50; 52]
Cephazolin [50], cefoxitin [53], ciprofloxacin [51; 59; 60], oflaxacin [56]	Luminal coated glucosaminoglycan-keratin fibrin glue (cryoprecipitate, bovine thrombin, aminocaproic acid) [53; 54]
Tobramycin [54; 55]	N-butyl-2 cyanoacrylate [55]
Gentamicin [58]	PTFE threads [56]

Rifampicin, a known anti-staphylococcal agent, particularly methicillin resistant [62], is a hydrophobic semi-synthetic substance with a high affinity for gelatin [63]. It inhibits DNA dependent RNA polymerase activity in bacterial cells without affecting mammalian cells [64] and has been passively incorporated into gelatin sealed dacron grafts as a mode of staphylococcal protection at the time of implantation. It has been shown to be resistant to experimental bacterial contamination [65; 66; 67; 68] with *in vivo* bioactivity to 22 days [69], and *in vitro* bioactivity to four days [70; 71; 72]. It is these qualities plus its excellent tissue and intracellular penetration [62] that make rifampicin an ideal antibiotic to be bonded to prosthetic grafts in order to prevent subsequent graft infection.

An *in vitro* study [73] examined the effect of soaking four clinically available prosthetic grafts (polytetrafluoroethylene (PTFE^{TM}), gelsoft^{TM}, thoratec^{TM} and fluoropassiv^{TM}) in known concentrations of rifampicin against staphylococcal (MRSA and methicillin resistant *S. epidermidis* (MRSE)) infection. Graft segments were soaked in rifampicin concentrations of 1.2, 10 or 30 mg/ml and placed on a bacterial lawn of either MRSA or MRSE. In all the graft types, with increasing rifampicin concentration there was a significant increase in the average zone of inhibition and the total antibacterial activity of the rifampicin soaked graft (Figures 29.1, 29.2, 29.3, 29.4, 29.5, 29.6). No significant differences were apparent between the staphylococcal species when adjusting for graft type and rifampicin concentration. The dacron grafts were

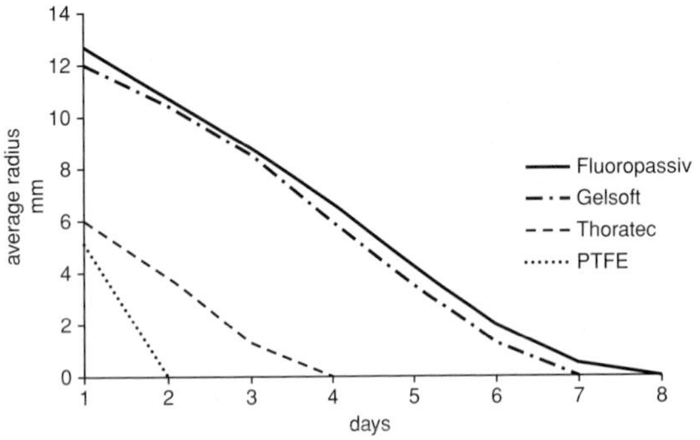

Fig. 29.1. MRSA + 1.2 mg/ml rifampicin.

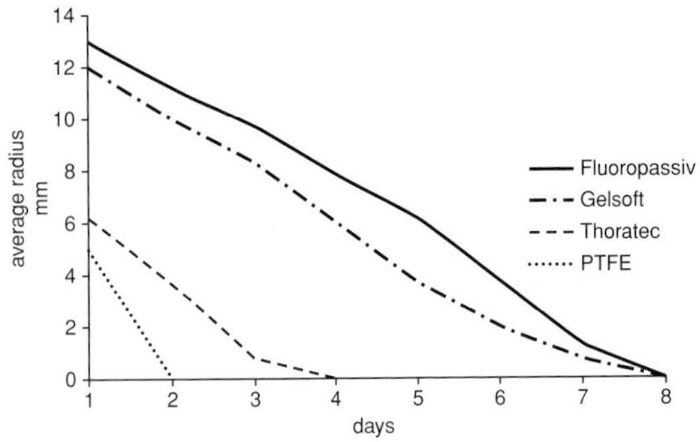

Fig. 29.2. MRSE + 1.2 mg/ml rifampicin.

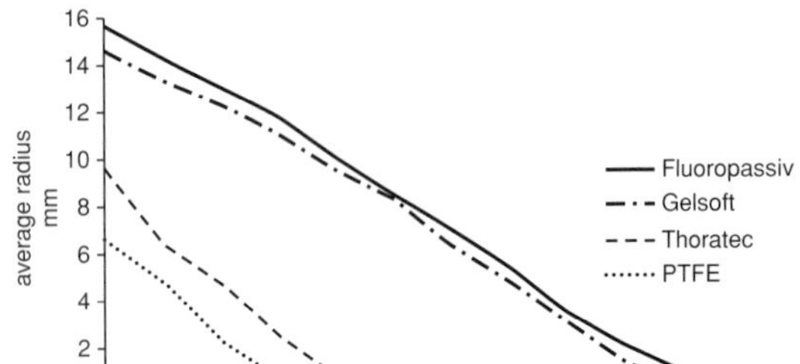

Fig. 29.3. MRSA+ 10 mg/ml rifampicin.

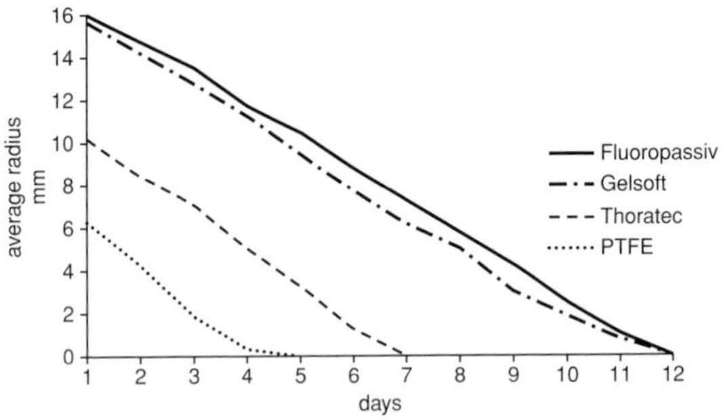

Fig. 29.4. MRSE + 10 mg/ml rifampicin.

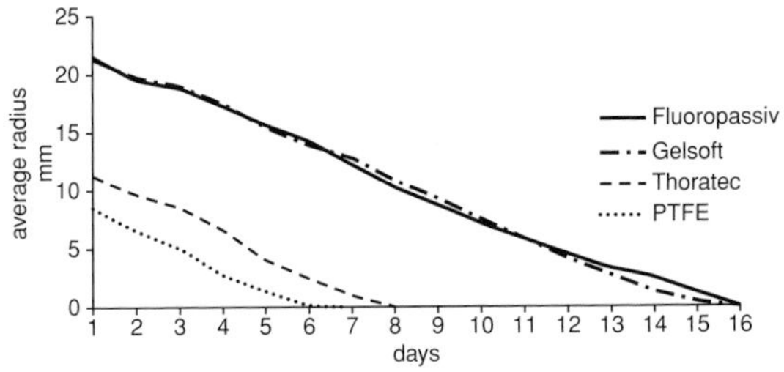

Fig. 29.5. MRSA + 30 mg/ml rifampicin.

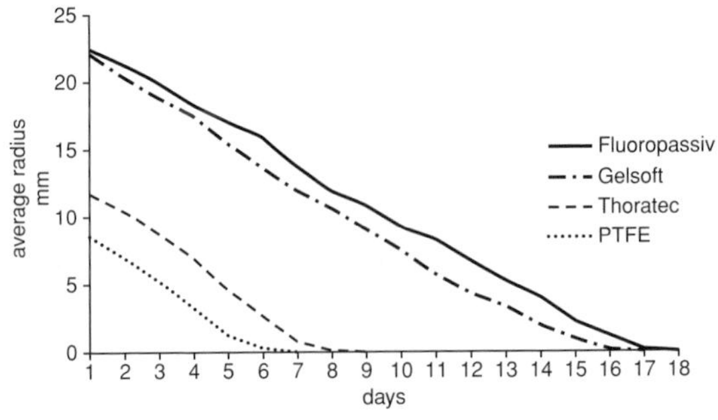

Fig. 29.6. MRSE + 30 mg/ml rifampicin.

significantly better compared with the other grafts at all studied rifampicin concentrations.

An established sheep model [74] was used, in which a segment of carotid artery was replaced with a rifampicin soaked gelsoft graft. The rifampicin (1.2 mg/ml or 10 mg/ml) soaked graft was directly inoculated with 10^8 colony forming units of either MRSA or methicillin resistant *Staphylococcus epidermidis* (MRSE). It was demonstrated that the rifampicin soaked graft offered significant prophylaxis [75; 76; 77].

For the MRSE arm, in the 10 mg/ml rifampicin group there was a significant reduction in graft infection when compared to both the control group ($p < 0.05$) and the 1.2 mg/ml group ($p < 0.05$) [77]. Similarly, for the MRSA group, in the 10mg/ml treatment group there was a significant reduction in the total number of possible cultures when compared to the control group ($p < 0.05$) and the 1.2 mg/ml group ($p < 0.05$) [77].

ESTABLISHED INFECTION

Antibiotic therapy

Once the diagnosis or suspicion of prosthetic vascular graft infection is made then broad spectrum antimicrobial therapy is initiated and subsequently converted to organism specific antibiotics [3]. The length of antibiotic therapy following excision of the infected graft is unclear but Bandyk and Bergamini [2] advocate parenteral antibiotics for two weeks and oral for six months.

Operative

The 'gold standard' although technically challenging is the removal of all infected tissue and extra-anatomic revascularization [78]. A number of more conservative approaches have been advocated depending on the site of infection and the micro-organism involved. The most conservative of treatments is aggressive local wound care with graft preservation. This is providing the graft and anastomoses are intact, and the patient has no systemic features of sepsis [79]. Calligaro *et al.* [33], in a report of a series of patients who had graft preservation, concluded that with the exception of *Pseudomonas*, vascular graft infections could be managed with debridement, antibiotic therapy and wound closure. The skeletonized prosthetic graft can be covered using viable regional rotational flaps [80]. Others have proposed graft excision and replacement with cadaveric arterial allografts [81], venous autografts [82], cryopreserved saphenous vein homografts [83], autogenous arteries, and/or veins [84] or prosthesis [85]. The major drawback with in situ reconstruction is sepsis [86].

Schmitt *et al.* [22], in an *in vitro* model, compared the bacterial adherence of four strains of bacteria (*S. aureus*, 'mucin' and 'non-mucin' producing *S. epidermidis*, and *E. coli*) with ePTFE, woven dacron and velour knitted dacron. They found that bacterial adherence was greatest to velour knitted dacron and least with ePTFE. In addition, Schmitt *et al.* [87] found that 'mucin' producing *S. epidermidis* adhered to dacron in 10- to 100-fold greater numbers compared to ePTFE. Bandyk and Bergamini [2] have postulated that the differential adherence of staphylococci relates to capsular adhesins.

Using the established sheep model [74] studies have been performed to determine if the replacement of a staphylococcal infected vascular graft with a graft impregnated with rifampicin would be considered appropriate surgical management in preventing early recurrent infection. Gelsoft grafts without any antibiotic treatment were infected with overwhelming concentrations of either MRSA or MRSE. The grafts were removed at three weeks and replaced with either control (no rifampicin) grafts or grafts soaked in either 1.2 mg/ml or 10 mg/ml of rifampicin. The replacement grafts were removed three weeks following placement.

For MRSA [88] there were no statistically significant differences between the groups for any of the macroscopic or microbiological parameters recorded.

For MRSE [88] there were no statistical differences between the concentrations for macroscopic findings. There were, however, statistically significant reductions in the number of total infected specimens in the 10 mg/ml when compared to both the control ($p < 0.001$) and the 1.2 mg/ml ($p < 0.005$) [88]. Conclusions from the studies [88] were that the established MRSE bacterial biofilm graft infections model can be treated by the *in situ* replacement of the infected prosthesis with a 10 mg/ml rifampicin impregnated gelsoft graft. However, such management for MRSA established infections cannot be recommended from the results obtained in this particular animal model.

To date a number of groups [89; 90] have successfully managed prosthetic graft infections with rifampicin impregnated grafts, with zero mortality, no requirement for limb amputation and to date no recurrence of infection.

The future management of vascular graft infections will be reliant on a better understanding of the interaction between the micro-organism, prosthesis and immune system. This will allow a more directed approach towards prevention and treatment. A possibility could be more powerful antibiotics either administered parenterally or incorporated into the prosthesis, acting as a local delivery system for prolonged periods of time. The role of the biofilm in the pathogenesis of graft infection needs further understanding from both a molecular and immune level.

REFERENCES

1. M. R. Back & S. R. Klein, Infections and antibiotics in vascular surgery. In *Vascular Surgery: Basic Science and Clinical Correlations*, ed. R. A. White and L. H. Hollier.

(Philadelphia: J. B. Lippincott Company, 1994), pp. 613–24.

2. D. F. Bandyk & T. M. Bergamini, Infection in prosthetic vascular grafts. In *Vascular Surgery,* 4th edn, ed. R. B. Rutherford. (Philadelphia: W. B. Saunders Company, 1995), pp. 588–604.
3. W. S. Moore & D. H. Deaton, Infection in prosthetic vascular grafts. In *Vascular Surgery: A Comprehensive Review,* 4th edn, ed. W. S. Moore. (Philadelphia: W. B. Saunders, 1993), pp. 694–706.
4. J. A. Buckels & S. E. Wilson, Prevention and management of prosthetic graft infection. In *Vascular Surgery: Principles and Practice,* 2nd edn, ed. F. J. Veith, H. R. W. Hobson, R. A. Williams and S. E. Wilson. (New York: McGraw-Hill Inc, 1994), pp. 1081–9.
5. W. S. Moore & C. W. Cole, Infection in prosthetic vascular grafts. In *Vascular Surgery: A Comprehensive Review,* 3rd edn, ed. W. S. Moore. (Philadelphia: W. B. Saunders, 1991), pp. 598–609.
6. G. R. Seabrook, Pathobiology of graft infections. *Seminars in Vascular Surgery*, 3 (1990), 81–8.
7. M. F. Levy, D. D. Schmitt, C. E. Edmiston *et al.*, Sequential analysis of staphylococcal colonization of body surface cultures on patients undergoing vascular surgery. *Journal of Clinical Microbiology*, **28** (1990), 664–9.
8. M. O. Perry, Infection in vascular surgery. In *Principles and Management of Surgical Infections*, ed. J. M. Davis and G. T. Shires. (Philadelphia: J. B. Lippincott, 1991), pp . 371–82.
9. G. Jamieson, J. DeWeese & C. Rob, Infected arterial grafts. *Annals of Surgery*, **181** (1975), 850–2.
10. T. J. Bunt, Synthetic vascular graft infections. II. Graft-enteric erosions and graft-enteric fistulas. *Surgery*, **94** (1983b), 1–9.
11. J. Bouhoutsos, D. Chavatzas, P. Martin & T. Morris, Infected synthetic arterial grafts. *British Journal of Surgery*, **61** (1974), 108–11.
12. J. R. Rubin, J. M. Malone & J. Goldstone, The role of the lymphatic system in acute arterial prosthetic graft infections. *Journal of Vascular Surgery*, **2** (1985), 92–7.
13. H. E. Russell, R. W. Barnes & W. A. Baker, Sterility of intestinal transudate during aortic reconstructive procedures. *Archives of Surgery*, **110** (1975), 402–4.
14. C. B. Ernst, H. C. Campbell, M. E. Daugherty, C. R. Sachatello & W. O. Griffin, Incidence and significance of intraoperative bacterial cultures during abdominal aortic aneurysmectomy. *Annals of Surgery*, **85** (1977), 626–33.
15. K. Scobie, N. McPhail, G. Barber & R. Elder, Bacteriologic monitoring in abdominal aortic surgery. *Canadian Journal of Surgery*, **22** (1979), 368–71.
16. C. Brandimarte, C. Santini, M. Venditti *et al.*, Clinical significance of intra-operative cultures of aneurysm walls and contents in elective abdominal aortic aneurysmectomy. *European Journal of Epidemiology*, **5** (1989), 521–5.
17. T. O'Brien & J. Collin, Prosthetic vascular graft infection. *British Journal of Surgery*, **79** (1992), 1262–7.
18. D. F. Bandyk & G. E. Esses, Prosthetic graft infection. *Surgical Clinics of North America*, **74** (1994), 571–90.
19. J. V. White, C. C. Nessel & K. Whang, Differential effect of type of bacteria on peripheral graft infections. In *Management of Infected Arterial Grafts*, ed. K. D. Calligaro and F. J. Veith. (St Louis: Quality Medical Publishing Incorporated, 1994), pp. 25–42.
20. J. O. Cohen, *Staphylococcus*. In *Medical Microbiology*, 3rd edn, ed. S. Baron. (New York: Churchill Livingstone, 1991), pp. 203–214.
21. G. K. Richards & R. F. Gagnon, An assay of *Staphylococcus epidermidis* biofilm responses to therapeutic agents. *International Journal of Artificial Organs*, 16 (1993), 777–87.
22. D. D. Schmitt, D. F. Bandyk, A. J. Pequet & J. B. Towne, Bacterial adherence to vascular prostheses. A determinant of graft infectivity. *Journal of Vascular Surgery*, **3** (1986b), 732–40.
23. M. A. Malangoni, D. H. Livingston & M. S. Peyton, The effect of protein binding on the adherence of staphylococci to prosthetic vascular grafts. *Journal of Surgical Research*, **54** (1993), 168–72.
24. J. E. Lorentzen, O. M. Nielson, H. Arendrup *et al.*, Vascular graft infection: an analysis of sixty-two infections in 2411 consecutively implanted synthetic vascular grafts. *Surgery*, **98** (1985), 81–6.
25. J. F. Golan, Vascular graft infection. *Infectious Disease Clinics of North America*, **3** (1989), 247–58.
26. J. P. Fletcher, M. Dryden & T. C. Sorrell, Infection of vascular prosthesis. *Australian and New Zealand Journal of Surgery*, **61** (1991), 432–5.
27. T. J. Bunt, Synthetic vascular graft infections. I. Graft infections. *Surgery*, **93** (1983a), 733–46.
28. D. F. Bandyk, Vascular graft infection. In *Complications in Vascular Surgery,* 2nd edn, ed. V. M. Bernhard and J. B. Towne. (Orlando: Grune and Stratton, 1985), pp. 471–85.

29. D. F. Bandyk, G. A. Berni, B. L. Thiele & J. B. Towne, Aortofemoral graft infection due to *Staphylococcus epidermidis*. *Archives of Surgery*, **119** (1984), 102–8.
30. D. F. Bandyk, Vascular graft infections: epidemiology, microbiology, pathogenesis and prevention. In *Complications in Vascular Surgery*, 2nd edn, ed. V. M. Bernhard and J. B. Towne. (St Louis: Quality Medical Publishing, 1991), pp. 223–34.
31. K. D. Calligaro, C. J. Westcott, R. M. Buckley, R. P. Savarese & D. A. DeLaurentis, Infrainguinal anastomotic arterial graft infections treated by selective graft preservation. *Annals of Surgery*, **216** (1992a), 74–9.
32. K. J. Geary, A. M. Tomkiewicz, H. N. Harrison *et al.*, Differential effects of a gram-negative and a gram-positive infection on autogenous and prosthetic grafts. *Journal of Vascular Surgery*, **11** (1990), 339–47.
33. K. D. Calligaro, F. J. Veith, M. L. Schwartz, R. P. Savarese & D. A. DeLaurentis, Are gram-negative bacteria a contraindication to selective preservation of infected vascular grafts. *Journal of Vascular Surgery*, **16** (1992c), 337–46.
34. G. S. Treiman, Bacteriology of aortic graft infections. In *Surgery of the Aorta and its Branches*, ed. B. L. Gewartz and L. B. Schwartz. (Philadelphia: W. B. Saunders Company, 2000), pp. 375–83.
35. J. Goldstone & W. S. Moore, Infection in vascular prosthesis. Clinical manifestations and surgical management. *American Journal of Surgery*, **128** (1974), 225–33.
36. S. P. Murray & J. Goldstone, Diagnostic advances. In *Management of Infected Arterial Grafts*, ed. K. D. Calligaro & F. J. Veith. (St Louis: Quality Medical Publishing Incorporated, 1994), pp. 43–53.
37. J. Goldstone & C. Cunningham, Diagnosis, treatment, and prevention of aorto-enteric fistulas. *Acta Chirrugia Scandinavia Supplement*, **555** (1990), 165–72.
38. D. H. M. Gröschel & B. A. Strain, Arterial graft infections from a microbiologist's view: In *Management of Infected Arterial Grafts*, ed. K. D. Calligaro and F. J. Veith. (St Louis: Quality Medical Publishing Incorporated, 1994), pp. 3–15.
39. E. D. Tollefson, D. F. Bandyk, H. W. Kaebnick, G. R. Seabrook & J. B. Towne, Surface biofilm disruption. Enhanced recovery of microorganisms from vascular prosthesis. *Archives of Surgery*, **122** (1987), 38–43.
40. T. M. Bergamini, D. F. Bandyk, D. Govostis, H. W. Kaebnick & J. B. Towne, Infection of vascular prostheses caused by bacterial biofilms. *Journal of Vascular Surgery*, **7** (1988), 21–30.
41. T. M. Bergamini, D. F. Bandyk, D. Govostis, R. Vetsch & J. B. Towne, Identification of *Staphylococcus epidermidis* vascular graft infections. A comparison of culture techniques. *Journal of Vascular Surgery*, **9** (1989), 665–70.
42. M. Wengrovitz, S. Spangler & L. F. Martin, Sonication provides maximal recovery of Staphylococcus epidermidis from slime-coated vascular prosthetics. *American Surgery*, **57** (1991), 161–4.
43. P. G. Qvarfordt, L. M. Reilly, A. S. Mark *et al.*, Computerized tomographic assessment of graft incorporation after aortic reconstruction. *American Journal of Surgery*, **150** (1985), 227–31.
44. P. J. Cruse & R. Foord, A five year prospective study of 23 649 surgical wounds. *Archives of Surgery*, **107** (1973), 206–10.
45. R. Seropian & B. M. Reynolds, Wound infections after preoperative depilatory versus razor preparation. *American Journal of Surgery*, **121** (1971), 251–4.
46. D. F. Bandyk, T. M. Bergamini, E. V. Kinney, G. R. Seabrook & J. B. Towne, *In situ* replacement of vascular prosthesis infected by bacterial biofilms. *Journal of Vascular Surgery*, **13** (1991), 575–83.
47. R. E. Clark & H. W. Margraf, Antibacterial vascular grafts with improved thromboresistance. *Archives of Surgery*, **109** (1974), 159–62.
48. P. M. Shah, S. Modak, C. L. Fox *et al.*, PTFE graft treated with silver norfloxacin (AgNF): drug retention and resistance to bacterial challenge. *Journal of Surgical Research*, **42** (1987), 298–303.
49. A. I. Benvenisty, G. Tannenbaum, T. N. Ahlborn *et al.*, Control of prosthetic bacterial infection: evaluation of an easily incorporated, tightly bound, silver antibiotic PTFE graft. *Journal of Surgical Research*, **44** (1988), 1–7.
50. R. A. Harvey & R. S. Greco, The noncovalent bonding of antibiotics to a polytetrafluoroethylene benzalkonium graft. *Annals of Surgery*, **194** (1981), 642–7.
51. E. V. Kinney, D. F. Bandyk, G. A. Seabrook, H. M. Kelly & J. B. Towne, Antibiotic-bonded PTFE vascular grafts: the effect of silver antibiotic on bioactivity following implantation. *Journal of Surgical Research*, **50** (1991), 430–5.
52. L. X. Webb, R. T. Myers, A. R. Cordell *et al.*, Inhibition of bacterial adhesion by antibacterial surface pretreatment of vascular prostheses. *Journal of Vascular Surgery*, **4** (1986), 16–21.

53. K. R. Sobinsky & D. P. Flanigan, Antibiotic binding to polytetrafluoroethylene via glucosaminoglycan-keratin luminal coating. *Surgery*, **100** (1986), 629–33.
54. A. L. Ney, P. H. Kelly, D. T. Tsukayama & M. P. Bubrick, Fibrin glue antibiotic suspension in the prevention of prosthetic graft infection. *Journal of Trauma*, **30** (1990), 1000–6.
55. J. S. Shenk, A. L. Ney, D. T. Tsukayama, M. E. Olson & M. P. Bubrick, Tobramycin adhesive in preventing and treating PTFE vascular graft infections. *Journal of Surgical Research*, **47** (1989), 487–92.
56. K. Okahara, J. Kambayashi, T. Shibuya *et al.*, An infection resistant PTFE vascular graft; spiral coiling of the graft with ofloxacin-bonded PTFE thread. *European Journal of Vascular and Endovascular Surgery*, **9** (1995), 408–14.
57. W. B. Shue, S. C. Worosilo, A. P. Donetz *et al.*, Prevention of vascular prosthetic infection with an antibiotic-bonded dacron graft. *Journal of Vascular Surgery*, **8** (1988), 600–5.
58. A. Haverich, S. Hirt, M. Karck, F. Siclari & H. Wahlig, Prevention of graft infection by bonding of gentamicin to dacron prostheses. *Journal of Vascular Surgery*, **15** (1992), 187–93.
59. M. D. Phaneuf, C. K. Ozaki, M. J. Bide *et al.*, Application of the quinolone antibiotic ciprofloxacin to dacron utilizing textile dyeing technology. *Journal of Biomedical Materials Research*, **27** (1993), 233–7.
60. C. K. Ozaki, M. D. Phaneuf, M. J. Bide *et al.*, *In vivo* testing of an infection-resistant vascular graft material. *Journal of Surgical Research*, **55** (1993), 543–47.
61. W. S. Moore, M. Chvapil, G. Seiffert & K. Keown, Development of an infection-resistant vascular prosthesis. *Archives of Surgery*, **116** (1981), 1403–7.
62. J. Turnbridge & M. L. Grayson, Optimum treatment of staphylococcal infections. *Drugs*, **45** (1993), 353–66.
63. T. R. Ashton, J. D. Cunningham, D. Patan & R. Maini, Antibiotic loading of vascular grafts. *Proceedings of the 16th Annual Meeting of the Society for Biomaterials*, **13** (1990), 235.
64. B. Farr & G. L. Mandell, Rifampicin. *Medical Clinics of North America*, **66** (1982), 157–68.
65. T. W. Powell, S. J. Burnham & G. Johnson, Jr., A passive system using rifampicin to create an infection resistant vascular prosthesis. *Surgery*, **94** (1983), 765–9.
66. E. G. MacDougal, S. J. Burnham & G. Johnson, Jr., Rifampicin protection against experimental graft sepsis. *Journal of Vascular Surgery*, **4** (1986), 5–7.
67. J. R. Avramovic & J. P. Fletcher, Rifampicin impregnation of a protein sealed dacron graft: an infection resistant vascular graft. *Australia and New Zealand Journal of Surgery*, **61** (1991), 436–40.
68. A. Chervu, W. S. Moore, H. A. Gelabert, M. Colburn & M. Chvapil, Prevention of graft infection by use of prosthesis bonded with a rifampicin/collagen release system. *Journal of Vascular Surgery*, **14** (1991), 521–5.
69. A. Chervu, W. S. Moore, M. Chvapil & T. Henderson, Efficacy and duration of anti-staphylococcal activity comparing three antibiotics bonded to dacron vascular grafts with a collagen release system. *Journal of Vascular Surgery*, **13** (1991), 897–901.
70. O. Goeau-Brissonniere, C. Leport, F. Bacourt *et al.*, Prevention of vascular graft infection by rifampicin bonding to a gelatin sealed dacron graft. *Annals of Vascular Surgery*, **5** (1991), 408–12.
71. K. Lachapelle, A. M. Graham & J. F. Symes, Antibacterial activity, antibiotic retention, and infection resistance of a rifampicin-impregnated gelatin-sealed dacron graft. *Journal of Vascular Surgery*, **19** (1994), 675–82.
72. V. Gahtan, G. E. Esses, D. F. Bandyk *et al.*, Anti-staphylococcal activity of rifampicin-bonded gelatin-impregnated dacron grafts. *Journal of Surgical Research*, **58** (1995), 105–10.
73. M. Vicaretti, W. J. Hawthorne, P. Y. Ao & J. P. Fletcher, *In vitro* study determining the optimal vascular material and dose of rifampicin impregnation to prevent graft infection. *Annual Scientific Meeting of the Royal Australasian College of General Surgeons*. (Sydney, 1998).
74. J. P. Fletcher, M. Dryden, B. Munro, J. H. Xu & M. D. Hehir, Establishment of a vascular graft infection model in the sheep carotid artery. *Australian and New Zealand Journal of Surgery*, **60** (1990), 801–3.
75. F. Sardelic, P. Y. Ao, D. A. Taylor & J. P. Fletcher, Prophylaxis against *Staphylococcus epidermidis* vascular graft infection with rifampicin-soaked, gelatin-sealed dacron. *Cardiovascular Surgery*, **4**, (1996), 389–92.
76. J. P. Fletcher, J. R. Avramovic, J. Kenny F. Sardelic, Increased resistance to staphylococcal graft infection by rifampicin impregnation of gelatin sealed dacron. In *Modern Vascular Surgery*. Vol. 6, ed. J. B. Chang. (New York: Springer Verlag, 1994), pp. 483–7.
77. M. Vicaretti, W. J. Hawthorne, P. Y. Ao & J. P. Fletcher, An increased concentration of rifampicin bonded to gelatin-sealed dacron reduces the incidence of

subsequent graft infections following a staphylococcal challenge. *Cardiovascular Surgery*, **6** (1998), 268–73.

78. G. R. Curl & J. J. Ricotta, Total prosthetic graft excision and extra-anatomic bypass. In *Management of Infected Arterial Grafts*, ed. K. D. Calligaro and F. J. Veith. (St Louis: Quality Medical Publishing Incorporated, 1994), pp. 82–94.
79. K. D. Calligaro, F. J. Veith, M. L. Schwartz *et al.*, Management of infected lower extremity autologous vein grafts by selective graft preservation. *American Journal of Surgery*, **164** (1992b), 291–4.
80. W. D. Turnispeed & D. G. Dibbell, Sr., Rotational muscle flaps in localized infections. In *Management of Infected Arterial Grafts*, K. D. Calligaro and F. J. Veith. (St Louis: Quality Medical Publishing Incorporated, 1994), pp. 142–59.
81. E. Kieffer, A. Bahnini, F. Koskas *et al.*, *In situ* allograft replacement of infected infrarenal aortic prosthetic grafts: results in forty three patients. *Journal of Vascular Surgery*, **17** (1993), 349–56.
82. G. P. Clagett, B. L. Bowers, M. A. Lopez-Viago *et al.*, Creation of a neo-aortoiliac system from lower extremity deep and superficial veins. *Annals of Surgery*, **218** (1993), 239–49.
83. R. M. Fujitani, H. S. Bassinouny, B. L. Gewertz, S. Glagoz & C. K. Zarins, Cryopreserved saphenous vein allogenic homografts: an alternative conduit in lower extremity arterial reconstruction in infected fields. *Journal of Vascular Surgery*, **15** (1992), 519–26.
84. J. M. Seeger, J. R. Wheeler, R. T. Gregory, S. O. Snyder & R. G. Gayle, Autogenous graft replacement of infected prosthetic grafts in the femoral position. *Surgery*, **93** (1983), 39–45.
85. J. B. Towne, G. R. Seabrook, D. Bandyk, J. A. Freischlag & C. E. Edmiston, *In situ*-replacement of arterial prosthesis infected by bacterial biofilms: long-term follow-up. *Journal of Vascular Surgery*, **19** (1994), 226–35.
86. J. A. Robinson & K. Johansen, Aortic sepsis: is there a role for *in situ* graft reconstruction? *Journal of Vascular Surgery*, **13** (1991), 677–84.
87. D. D. Schmitt, D. F. Bandyk, A. J. Pequet, M. A. Malangoni & J. B. Towne, Mucin production by *Staphylococcus epidermidis*. *Archives of Surgery*, **121** (1986), 89–95.
88. M. Vicaretti, W. J. Hawthorne, P. Y. Ao & J. P. Fletcher, Does *in situ* replacement of an infected vascular graft with a rifampicin soaked gelatin sealed dacron graft reduce the incidence of subsequent infection? *International Angiology*, **19** (2000), 158–65.
89. G. Torsello, W. Sandmann, A. Gehrt & R. M. Jungblut, *In situ* replacement of infected vascular prosthesis with rifampicin-soaked vascular grafts: early results. *Journal of Vascular Surgery*, **17** (1993), 768–73.
90. A. R. Naylor, S. Clark, N. J. London *et al.*, Treatment of major aortic graft infection: preliminary experience with total graft excision and *in situ* replacement with a rifampicin bonded prosthesis. *European Journal of Vascular and Endovascular Surgery*, **9** (1995), 252–6.

Index